RSSDI
Diabetes Update
2018

Celebrating 50 Years
Passion, Quality and Innovation in Healthcare Publishing

RSSDI Diabetes Update 2018

Editor-in-Chief

Rajeev Chawla MD FDiab FRSSDI FACP (USA) FRCP UK (Edin) FACE (USA)
Senior Consultant Diabetologist and Director
North Delhi Diabetes Center
New Delhi, India

Associate Editor

Shalini Jaggi Dip Diab (UK) Dip Endo (UK) FRSSDI FRCP (Glas, Edin)
Consultant and Head
Department of Diabetology
Dr Mohans' Diabetes Specialities Center
New Delhi, India

JAYPEE BROTHERS MEDICAL PUBLISHERS
The Health Sciences Publisher
New Delhi | London | Panama

Jaypee Brothers Medical Publishers (P) Ltd

Headquarters

Jaypee Brothers Medical Publishers (P) Ltd
4838/24, Ansari Road, Daryaganj
New Delhi 110 002, India
Phone: +91-11-43574357
Fax: +91-11-43574314
Email: jaypee@jaypeebrothers.com

Overseas Offices

J.P. Medical Ltd
83 Victoria Street, London
SW1H 0HW (UK)
Phone: +44 20 3170 8910
Fax: +44 (0)20 3008 6180
Email: info@jpmedpub.com

Jaypee-Highlights Medical Publishers Inc
City of Knowledge, Bld. 235, 2nd Floor, Clayton
Panama City, Panama
Phone: +1 507-301-0496
Fax: +1 507-301-0499
Email: cservice@jphmedical.com

Jaypee Brothers Medical Publishers (P) Ltd
17/1-B Babar Road, Block-B, Shaymali
Mohammadpur, Dhaka-1207
Bangladesh
Mobile: +08801912003485
Email: jaypeedhaka@gmail.com

Jaypee Brothers Medical Publishers (P) Ltd
Bhotahity, Kathmandu, Nepal
Phone: +977-9741283608
Email: kathmandu@jaypeebrothers.com

Website: www.jaypeebrothers.com
Website: www.jaypeedigital.com

Inquiries for bulk sales may be solicited at: jaypee@jaypeebrothers.com

RSSDI Diabetes Update–2018 **/ Rajeev Chawla, Shalini Jaggi**

First Edition: **2019**

ISBN: 978-93-5270-618-1

Printed at Rajkamal Electric Press, Kundli, Haryana.

Contributors

EDITOR-IN-CHIEF

Rajeev Chawla MD FDiab FRSSDI FACP (USA) FRCP UK (Edin) FACE (USA)
Senior Consultant Diabetologist and Director
North Delhi Diabetes Center
New Delhi, India

ASSOCIATE EDITOR

Shalini Jaggi Dip Diab (UK) Dip Endo (UK) FRSSDI FRCP (Glas, Edin)
Consultant and Head
Department of Diabetology
Dr Mohans' Diabetes Specialities Center
New Delhi, India

CONTRIBUTING AUTHORS

A Muruganathan MBBS MD
Governor American College of Physicians
India Chapter
Department of General Medicine
AG Hospital
Tirupur, Tamil Nadu, India

Aastha Chawla MD (DVL)
Resident
Department of Skin, VD and Leprosy
Sardar Patel Medical College
Bikaner, Rajasthan, India

Abhijit Das MD (Pathology)
Assistant Professor
Department of Pathology
Janakpuri Super Speciality Hospital
Delhi, India

Alan Jones PhD FRCP FRCPath
Consultant Chemical Pathologist
Department of Clinical Biochemistry
University Hospitals Birmingham NHS
Foundation Trust
West Midlands, England, United Kingdom

Alok Jain MD DM
Director and Head
Nephrology and
Kidney Transplant
CK Birla Hospital
Rukmani Birla Hospital
Jaipur, Rajasthan, India

Amandeep Singh MD Medicine
Senior Resident
Department of Medicine
All India Institute of Medical Sciences
New Delhi, India

Anand Moses MD FRCP (Glas)
Emeritus Professor
Tamil Nadu Dr MGR Medical University
Chennai
Formerly Director and Professor
Institute of Diabetology
Madras Medical College and
Rajiv Gandhi Government General
Hospital
Chennai, Tamil Nadu, India

Anil Kumar Virmani MD DRM FICP
FIACM FACP
Consultant Physician
Viru's Diabetic Center
Jamshedpur, Jharkhand, India

Anil S Bhoraskar MD
Chair
South East Asia
International
Diabetes Federation
Diabetologist
Department of Diabetology
Raheja Hospital
Asian Heart Institute
Asian Cancer Institute
Mumbai, Maharashtra, India

Anuj Maheshwari MD FICP FIACM
FACP FACE FRCP (London)
Professor and Head
Department of General Medicine
Babu Banarasi Das University
Lucknow, Uttar Pradesh, India

Anupama Kaul MD DM
Professor
Department of Nephrology
Sanjay Gandhi Postgraduate Institute of Medical Sciences
Lucknow, Uttar Pradesh, India

Anupam Prakash MBBS MD PGCC PDCDM FICP MNAMS
Professor
Department of Medicine
Lady Hardinge Medical College
New Delhi, India

Arpan Dev Bhattacharya MBBS MD (Internal Medicine) DM Endocrinology MRCP
Consultant Endocrinologist
Manipal Hospital
Bengaluru, Karnataka, India

Arvind Gupta MD FACE FICP
Director and Consultant Physician
Internal Medicine and Diabetes
Jaipur Diabetes Research Center
Jaipur, Rajasthan, India

Ashish Reddy MD
Senior Resident
Department of Endocrinology
Ramaiah Medical College
Bengaluru, Karnataka, India

Ashish Sharma MD
Professor and Head
Department of Renal TransplantSurgery
Postgraduate Institute of Medical Education and Research
Chandigarh, Punjab, India

Ashok K Taneja MD DIP CARD FRCP (UK) FACP (USA) FICP FIAE FDI FAPSC (Taiwan)
Medical Director
Taneja Heart–Diabetes Center
Gurugram, Haryana, India

Ashu Rastogi MBBS MD DM
Assistant Professor
Department of Endocrinology and Metabolism
Postgraduate Institute of Medical Education and Research
Chandigarh, Punjab, India

Ashutosh Chaturvedi MD (Medicine)
Consultant Physician
Maxwell Hospital and Jain Chest Care Center
Jaipur, Rajasthan, India

Ashwin Pillai MBBS DNB
Fellow
Department of Medicine
Ruby Hall Clinic
Pune, Maharashtra, India

Banshi Saboo MD MSc (Endo - UK) PhD
Chairman, Chief Diabetologist
Dia Care - Diabetes and Hormone Clinic
Ahmedabad, Gujarat, India

Benny V Negalur MD FICP
Ex Associate Professor
Department of Medicine
Dr Negalur's Diabetes Specialities Center
Mumbai, Maharashtra, India

Chandrasekhar Valupadas MD General Medicine
Professor
Kakatiya Medical College
Mahatma Gandhi Memorial Hospital
Warangal, Telangana, India

CL Nawal MD Internal Medicine FICP FACP (USA) FRSSDI
Professor and Head
Department of Medicine
Sawai Man Singh Medical College and Hospital
Jaipur, Rajasthan, India

Debaleena Mukherjee MBBS
Postgraduate Trainee 3rd year
Junior Resident
Institute of Post Graduate Medical Education and Research
Seth Sukhlal Karnani Memorial Hospital
Kolkata, West Bengal, India

Deep Dutta MD DM DNB MRCP FACE
Assistant Professor
Department of Endocrinology
Post Graduate Medical Education and Research and Ram Manohar Lohia Hospital
New Delhi, India

Deependra Vikram Singh MD Ophthalmology (AIIMS)
Senior Registrar
Retina (AIIMS)
Senior Research Associate (Retina) AIIMS
Medical Director
Retina Services
Eye-Q Superspecialty Eye Hospitals
Gurugram, Haryana, India

Dharini Krishnan Doctorate in Foods Nutrition and Dietetics
Director
DV Living Science Enterprises Pvt. Ltd.
Chennai, Tamil Nadu, India

Dheeraj Kapoor MD DM
Head
Department of Endocrinology
Artemis Hospital
Gurugram, Haryana, India

Diksha Shirodkar MBBS MD Pediatrics
Fellow in Pediatric Endocrinology
Manipal Hospital
Bengaluru, Karnataka, India

Dinesh Chandra Sharma DM
Director Endocrinology
Department of Endocrinology
Institute of Endocrinology and Diabetes
Sarajan Hospital
Udaipur, Rajasthan, India

Gaikwad Mahesh MBBS
Junior Resident
Department of Medicine
Pandit Bhagwat Dayal Sharma Post Graduate Institute of Medical Sciences
Rohtak, Haryana, India

Geena Susan George MBBS MD
Senior Resident
Department of Endocrinology
Government Medical College
Thiruvananthapuram, Kerala, India

Girish Mathur MD FRCP (Glasgow) FICP FACP (USA) FIACM
Senior Consultant Internal Medicine
Vice Dean
Indian College of Physicians
Past Vice President API
Kota, Rajasthan, India

Hamid Ashraf MD (Medicine) DM (Endocrinology)
Assistant Professor
Department of Endocrinology
Rajiv Gandhi Center For Diabetes and Endocrinology
Jawaharlal Nehru Medical College
Aligarh Muslim University
Aligarh, Uttar Pradesh, India

Hardeva Ram Nehara MD (Medicine) DM (Endocrinology)
Senior Resident
Department of Endocrinology
Sawai Man Singh Medical College
Jaipur, Rajasthan, India

Harpreet Pasricha MBBS MD
Consultant, Department of Medicine
Pasricha Hospital
Gurugram, Haryana, India

Harpreet Singh MD (General Medicine)
Senior Professor and Incharge of Rheumatology
Department of Medicine
Pandit Bhagwat Dayal Sharma Post Graduate Institute of Medical Sciences
Rohtak, Haryana, India

Hemraj B Chandalia MD FACP
Director
Endocrinology, Diabetes, Metabolism
Jaslok Hospital and Research Center
Director
Diabetes, Endocrine Nutrition Management and Research Center
Mumbai, Maharashtra, India

Jamal Ahmad MD (Med) DM (Endo) PhD (Med) FCCP FRCP (UK) DSc (Endocrinology)
Former Professor of Endocrinology
Chairman, Department of Medicine and Dean Faculty of Medicine
Ex-Director
Rajiv Gandhi Center for Diabetes and Endocrinology
Aligarh Muslim University
Aligarh
Diabetes and Endocrinology
Super Speciality Center
Aligarh, Uttar Pradesh, India

Jayanta Kumar Panda MBBS (Hons) MD (Internal Medicine) FICP FACP FRSSDI
Professor and Head
Department of Medicine
Saheed Laxman Nayak Medical College
Koraput, Odisha, India

Jaydeep Khalpada Masters in Medical Technology
Medical Technologist

Jothydev Kesavadev MD FRCP (London, Glasg, Edin) FACP FACE (USA) FRSSDI
Chairman and Managing Director
Jothydev's Diabetes Research Centers
Trivandrum, Attingal and Kochi, Kerala, India

Jotideb Mukhopadhyay MBBS MD
Professor
Institute of Post Graduate Medical Education and Research
Seth Sukhlal Karnani Memorial Hospital
Kolkata, West Bengal, India

Jugal Kishor Sharma MD FICP FACE FRCP (Glasgow and Edinburgh) FACP FRSSDI FDI FGSI FIACM FIMSA FISH
Medical Director and Senior Consultant
Central Delhi Diabetes Center
New Delhi, India

K Kiranmala MD
Ex-PG Resident
Department of Medicine
University College of Medical Sciences
New Delhi, India

Kamlakar Tripathi MBBS MD DM MNAMS FRCP
Retired Professor of Medicine and Ex Head
Department of Medicine
Institute of Medical Sciences
Banaras Hindu University
Varanasi, Uttar Pradesh, India

Kavita S Gupta MSc CDE
Dietician
Department of Dietetics
Sunil's Diabetes Care N' Research Center Pvt. Ltd.
Nagpur, Maharashtra, India

Kingshuk Bhattacharjee M. Pharm MBA PhD Scholar
Research Scholar
Department of Medical Sciences
JJT University
Jhabarmal, Rajasthan, India

Lalit Kumar Meher MD (Medicine)
Dean cum Principal
Bhima Bhoi Medical College and Hospital
Balangir, Odisha, India

Leena Singh MBBS DCP
Managing Director
Diabetes and Heart Research Center
Dhanbad, Jharkhand, India

Leepica Dahiya Kapoor BSc MSc (Food and Nutrition) UGC (NET) PhD
School of Bio Sciences and Technology
Vellore Institute of Technology
Vellore, Tamil Nadu, India

M Gowri Sankar MBBS MD
Asistant Professor
Department of General Medicine
Government Medical College and ESI Hospital
Coimbatore, Tamil Nadu, India

Madhur Rai MBBS MD Physiology
Senior Tutor, Post Graduate
Department of Physiology
Mahatma Gandhi Mission Institute of Health Sciences
Navi Mumbai, Maharashtra, India

Mahesh Rath MBBS MD
PG Tutor
Hitech Medical College and Hospital
Bhubaneswar, Odisha, India

Mala Dharmalingam MD DM (AIIMS)
Professor and Head
Department of Endocrinology
Ramaiah Medical College
Bengaluru, Karnataka, India

Mangesh Harihar Tiwaskar MBBS MD FRCP (London/Ireland/Glasgow) FACP FICP FGSI
Consultant Physician and Diabetologist
Shilpa Medical Center
Mumbai, Maharashtra, India

Manisha SahayMD DNB MAMS
Professor and Head
Department of Nephrology
Osmania Medical College and
General Hospital
Hyderabad, Telangana, India

Man Mohan MehndirattaMD DNB DM (Neurology) FAAN FANA FAMS FRCP FICP FIAN FIACM
Director Professor
Department of Neurology
Govind Ballabh Pant Institute of
Postgraduate Medical Education and
Research (Delhi University)
Director
Janakpuri Super Speciality Hospital
New Delhi, India

Manoj ChadhaMD (Med) DM (Endo)
Consultant Endocrinologist
Department of Endocrinology
P.D. Hinduja Hospital
Mumbai, Maharashtra, India

Manoj SalujaMD (Medicine)
Professor
Department of Medicine
Government Medical College
Kota, Rajasthan, India

Manoj YadavMD (Medicine)
Senior Resident
Department of Medicine
Pandit Bhagwat Dayal Sharma Post
Graduate Institute of Medical Sciences
Rohtak, Haryana, India

Manoranjan BeheraMD FICP
Associate Professor
Department of Medicine,
SBB Medical College
Cuttack, Odisha, India

Manshi KashyapMD
Senior Resident
Department of Medicine
Lady Hardinge Medical College
New Delhi, India

Mayur AgrawalMD
Senior Resident
Department of Endocrinology
Sanjay Gandhi Postgraduate Institute of
Medical Sciences
Lucknow, Uttar Pradesh, India

Meena ChhabraMD Medicine GMC (Bhopal) Diploma in Diabetes from Middlesex University
Senior Consultant Medicine and Diabetes
Specialist at Dr Meena Chhabra's
Diabetes Clinic
Visiting Consultant
Department of Medicine
Sir Ganga Ram Hospital
New Delhi, India

Minal MohitMBBS MD (Internal Medicine) FDE FPAE FACP (US) FICN (UK) FIACM FDI
Consultant and Head
Department of Endocrinology
Manipal Hospital
Jaipur, Rajasthan, India

Mithun BhartiaMBBS MRCGP (UK) MRCP (UK) FECSM
Consultant Endocrinologist
Apollo Hospitals, Guwahati
Director
Dr Bhartia's Diabetes and
Thyroid Clinic
Guwahati, Assam, India

Mudit KhuranaMD
Senior Resident
Department of Nephrology
Sanjay Gandhi Postgraduate Institute of
Medical Sciences
Lucknow, Uttar Pradesh, India

NagarajMD
Professsor
Department of Medicine
P.E.S. Institute of Medical Sciences and
Research
Kuppam, Andhra Pradesh, India

Naval K VikramMD
Professor
Department of Medicine
Metabolic Research Group
All India Institute of Medical
Sciences
New Delhi, India

Navneet AgrawalMD PhD FCCP FIACM
Consultant Diabetologist
Diabetes, Obesity and
Thyroid Center
Gwalior, Madhya Pradesh, India

Neeta DeshpandeMD FRCP (Edin) PG Endo (London) ASBP Cert Obesity (USA)
Consultant Diabetologist and Bariatric
Physician
Belgaum Diabetes Center
Professor and Head
Department of Medicine
Maratha Mandal Dental College
Associate Professor
Department of Medicine
USM-KLE International Medical
Programme
Belgaum, Karnataka, India

Nihal Jacob ThomasMBBS MD MNAMS DNB (Endo) FRACP (Endo) FRCP (Edin) FRCP (Glas) FRCP (London) PhD (Copenhagen)
Professor and Head, Unit-1
Department of Endocrinology, Diabetes
and Metabolism
Christian Medical College
Vellore, Tamil Nadu, India

Nikhil NasikkarDNB (Internal Medicine)
Assistant Professor
Department of Medicine
KJ Somaiya Medical College and
Hospital
Mumbai, Maharashtra, India

Nitin KapoorMBBS MD (Medicine) DM (Endo) ABBM (USA) Post doc Fellowship (Endo)
Associate Professor
Department of Endocrinology
Diabetes and Metabolism
Christian Medical College
Vellore, Tamil Nadu, India

NK SinghMD FICP
Director
Diabetes and Heart Research Center
Dhanbad, Jharkhand, India
Chairman
Research Society for the Study of
Diabetes in India
Jharkhand, India

NK SoniMD FRCP FACP FICP FIACM
Head
Department of Medicine
Yashoda Super Speciality Hospital
Ghaziabad, Uttar Pradesh, India

OP Sharma MD (Medicine), FICN FICP FIAMS FCGP FGSI FACM FIMSA FRCP (Eden)
Senior Consultant
Department of Geriatric Medicine
Indraprastha Apollo Hospitals
New Delhi, India

P Jabbar MD DNB (Med) DM (Endo) DNB (Endo)
Additional Director and Professor
Department of Endocrinology
Indian Institute of Diabetes
Trivandrum, Kerala, India

Prakash Keswani MD DM DNB MNAMS
Senior Professor
Department of Medicine
Sawai Man Singh Medical College
Jaipur, Rajasthan, India

Prasanna Kumar Kanakatte MD DM (Endo)
Director and Consultant Endocrinologist
Center for Diabetes and Endocrine Care
Bengaluru, Karnataka, India

Rajeev Gupta MD PhD
Chairman and Head
Preventive Cardiology and Internal Medicine
Eternal Heart Care Center and Research Institute
Jaipur, Rajasthan, India

Rajesh Datt Mehta MD(DVL)
Senior Professor and Head
Department of Skin, VD and Leprosy
Sardar Patel Medical College
Bikaner, Rajasthan, India

Rajesh K Marya MBBS MD (Medicine) FIAMS
Fellow Diabetes India
Post Graduate Diploma Diabetes
Middlesex University, UK
Consultant Physician and Diabetologist
Marya Clinic- Center for Diabetes and Lifestyle Diseases
New Delhi, India

Rajesh Rajput MD DM (Endocrinology) FRCP (Edin) FACE (USA) FICP FIACM FISH FIMSA
Senior Professor and Head
Department of Endocrinology
Post Graduate Institute of Medical Sciences
Rohtak, Haryana, India

Rajesh Upadhyay MRCP FRCP FACP FICP FIAMS
Director and Head
Department of Gastroenterology and Hepatology, Max Super Speciality Hospital
New Delhi, India

Raj Kumar Lalwani MBBS MD (Med) GDDC-Diploma Diabetes (Australia) FIMSA FDI
Senior Consultant Diabetologist
PG Medical Center and National Heart Institute
New Delhi, India

Rakesh Sahay MD DNB DM (Endo) FICP FACE
Professor and Head, Endocrinology
Osmania Medical College and Hospital
Hyderabad, Telangana, India

Ranjana Bhatt MBBS DNB Medicine
Registrar
Department of Endocrinology
Artemis Hospital
Gurugram, Haryana, India

Ranjit Mohan Anjana MD PhD
Diabetologist and
Joint Managing Director
Madras Diabetes Research Foundation
Chennai, Tamil Nadu, India

Ranjit Unnikrishnan MD FRCP (Lond, Glasg and Edin) FACP FICP
Vice-Chairman
Dr Mohan's Diabetes Specialities Center
Chennai, Tamil Nadu, India

Rashmi Rajput MD
Senior Resident, Department of Medicine
Lady Hardinge Medical College
New Delhi, India

Richa Manaswita MBBS DCH DNB (Obstetrics and Gynecology)
Research Fellow
Diabetes and Heart Research Center
Dhanbad, Jharkhand, India

Richard Charles Strange PhD FRCPath
Professor, Department of Clinical Biochemistry
Institute for Science and Technology in Medicine, Keele University
Staffordshire, England,United Kingdom

Richik Tripathi BDS MDS
Assistant Professor
Department of Oral and Maxillofacial Surgery
Deparment of Dentistry
Institute of Medical Sciences
Banaras Hindu University
Varanasi, Uttar Pradesh, India

Rishabh Kapoor MBBS
Senior Resident
Department of Medicine
Care Well Heart and Super Speciality Hospital
Amritsar, Punjab, India

Rohit Kapoor FACC (USA) FACP(USA) ECNU FCSI FISC FICP FDI FRSSDI
Medical Director and Head of Department
Department of Medicine and Endocrinology
Care Well Heart and Super Speciality Hospital
Amritsar, Punjab, India

RP Agrawal MD (Medicine)
Principal and Controller
Senior Professor
Department of Medicine
Sardar Patel Medical College
Bikaner, Rajasthan, India

Rujul Jain MD
Senior Resident
Department of Endocrinology and Metabolism
Institute of Medical Sciences
Varanasi, Uttar Pradesh, India

S Charles Bronson MBBS D Diab (MMC)
Diabetologist
Institute of Diabetology
Stanley Medical College and Government Stanley Hospital,
Chennai, Tamil Nadu, India

Sambit Das MD (Medicine) DM (Endocrinology, PGIMER Chandigarh) PGD Endocrinology (New South Wales University)
Associate Professor
Department of Endocrinology
Hitech Medical College and Hospital,
Bhubaneswar, Odisha
Senior Consultant Endocrinologist
ACODE and Apollo Sugar Clinics
Bhubaneswar, Odisha, India

Sandeep K Mathur MD DM FACE
Senior Professor and Head
Deparment of Endocrinology
Sawai Man Singh Medical College
Jaipur, Rajasthan, India

Sandeep Rai MBBS DNB (Medicine) MNAMS PGDHS (Diabetology) FRCP (UK)
Professor and Unit Head
Post Graduate Department of Medicine and Diabetology
Mahatma Gandhi Mission Institute of Health Sciences
Navi Mumbai, Maharashtra, India

Sanhita Walawalkar MBBS MD
Consultant
Panikar's Speciality Care Centers
Mumbai, Maharashtra, India

Sanjay Agarwal MD FACE
Director, Aegle Clinic-Diabetes Care
Head, Deparment of Medicine
Ruby Hall Clinic, Pune
Senior Consultant in Diabetes and Medicine
Jehangir Hospital
Pune, Maharashtra, India

Sanjay K Bhadada DM
Professor
Department of Endocrinology
Postgraduate Institute of Medical Education and Research
Chandigarh, Punjab, India

Sanjay Kalra MD DM
Consultant
Department of Endocrinology
Bharti Hospital
Karnal, Haryana, India

Sanjay Reddy ACMD
Consultant Diabetologist
Center for Diabetes and Endocrine Care
Bengaluru, Fortis Hospitals
Vice President
Primer Academy of Medical Sciences
Bengaluru, Karnataka, India

Sanjiv Shah MD
Consultant
Apollo Sugar Clinic
Mumbai, Maharashtra, India

Santosh Yadav PhD (Medicine)
Research Head
Department of Cardiology
Institute of Medical Sciences
Banaras Hindu University
Varanasi, Uttar Pradesh, India

Satinath Mukhopadhyay MD DM FRCP
Professor
Department of Endocrinology and Metabolism
Institute of Post Graduate Medical Education and Research
Kolkata, West Bengal, India

Saumik Datta MBBS DTCD MD (Gen. Medicine) DM (Endocrinology) FICP
Associate Professor
Department of General Medicine
Calcutta National Medical College and Hospital
Kolkata, West Bengal, India

Shahla Shafique MD (Biochemistry)
Senior Resident
Department of Biochemistry
Janakpuri Super Speciality Hospital
Delhi, India

Shaila Shamanur Bhattacharyya MBBS MD (Pediatrics) DM Endocrinology MRCP
Consultant Pediatric Endocrinologist
Manipal Hospital
Bengaluru, Karnataka, India

Shilpa S Joshi MSc RD
Consultant
Department of Nutrition
Mumbai Diet and Health Center
Mumbai, Maharashtra, India

Shivam Kapoor MBBS
Senior Resident
Medicine Department
Care Well Heart and Super Speciality Hospital
Amritsar, Punjab, India

Shrikant Sharma MD
Associate Professor
Department of Medicine
Sawai Man Singh Medical College
Jaipur, Rajasthan, India

Siddhant Trehan
Senior Medical Officer
Department of Pediatric Cardiology
Artemis Hospital
Gurugram, Haryana, India

SK Sharma MD (Medicine) DM (Endocrinology)
Department of Endocrinology
Galaxy Speciality Center
Jaipur, Rajasthan, India

SK Singh MD DM
Professor and Head
Department of Endocrinology and Metabolism, Institute of Medical Sciences
Varanasi, Uttar Pradesh, India

Smina TP MSc PhD
Scientist cum Medical Writer
MV Hospital for Diabetes and
Prof M Viswanathan Diabetes Research Center
Royapuram, Chennai, Tamil Nadu, India

Sneha Kothari MD (Med) DNB (Endo)
Consultant Endocrinologist
Department of Endocrinology
Global Hospital
Mumbai, Maharashtra, India

Soumitra Ghosh MD (Cal) FRCP (Edin) FACE (USA) FACP (USA) DTCD MSc Diabetes (UK) PG Dip Diabetes (UK) FICP
Professor and Head
Department of Medicine
Head, Obesity and Lifestyle Diseases Division, Institute of Post Graduate Medical Education and Research
Kolkata, West Bengal, India

Subhash B Yadav MD DNB (Endocrinology)
Professor, Department of Endocrinology
Sanjay Gandhi Postgraduate Institute of Medical Sciences
Lucknow, Uttar Pradesh, India

Subhash Kumar Wangnoo MD DM
Senior Consultant, Endocrinologist and Diabetologist
Apollo Centre for Obesity, Diabetes and Endocrinology
Indraprastha Apollo Hospital
New Delhi, India

Sudarshan Ramachandran PhD FRCPath
Professor of Metabolic Medicine
Department of Clinical Biochemistry
University Hospitals Birmingham NHS Foundation Trust
West Midlands, England, United Kingdom
Department of Clinical Biochemistry
University Hospitals of North Midlands / Faculty of Health Sciences, Staffordshire University
Staffordshire, England, United Kingdom

Sudha Vidyasagar MD
Professor
Department of Medicine
Kasturba Medical College
Manipal, Karnataka, India

Sujeet Jha MRCP
Director
Department of Endocrinology, Diabetes and Metabolism
Max Healthcare Institute Ltd.
New Delhi, India

Sujoy Ghosh DM (Endocrinology)
Associate Professor
Department of Endocrinology
Institute of Post Graduate Medical Education and Research and Seth Sukhlal Karnani Memorial Hospital
Kolkata, West Bengal, India

Sundeep Ruder MBChb (Wits) FCP (SA) FSEM (SA)
Clinical Endocrinologist
Life Fourways Hospital
Johannesburg
Honorary Consultant
Charlotte Maxeke Johannesburg Academic Hospital
Associate Lecturer
University of the Witwatersrand
Executive Committee Member
Society of Endocrinology, Metabolism and Diabetes of South Africa (SEMDSA)
South Africa

Sunil Kumar Kota MD (Medicine) DNB (Endocrinology)
Chief Consultant Diabetologist and Endocrinologist
Diabetes and Endocare Clinic
Berhampur, Odisha, India

Sunil Surajprasad Gupta MD FRCP(Glasgow) FRCP(Edinburgh) FACP FICP FIAMS FIACM FRSSDI
Managing Director
Department of Diabetology
Sunil's Diabetes Care n' Research Center Pvt. Ltd.
Nagpur, Maharashtra, India

SV Madhu MD DM (Endocrinology)
Professor and Head
Department of Medicine
Head
Center for Diabetes
Endocrinology, and Metaboloism
University College of Medical Sciences
Guru Teg Bahadur Hospital
New Delhi, India

Swati Waghdhare MD
Associate Consultant
Department of Endocrinology
Diabetes and Metabolism
Max Healthcare Institute Ltd.
New Delhi, India

Swati Tayal Goray MBBS MD (AIIMS)
Clinical Associate
Apollo Centre for Obesity, Diabetes and Endocrinology
Indraprastha Apollo Hospital
New Delhi, India

Trupti Amaresh Kulkarni PG Dip in Dietetics CDE
Dietician and Diabetes Educator
Apollo Sugar Clinics Ltd.
Mumbai, Maharashtra, India

Urman Dhruv MD (Internal Medicine) LLB
Consulting Physician
Director
Department of Internal Medicine and Diabetes
HCG Hospitals
Mithakhali, Ahmedabad, Gujarat, India

V Sanjay Moses MD
Diabetologist
Moses Diabetes and Medical Center
Chennai, Tamil Nadu, India

V Seshiah MD FRCP DSc DSc DSc (Hony)
Consultant
Dr V Balaji Diabetes Care Centre and Dr V Seshiah Diabetes Research Institute
Chennai, Tamil Nadu, India

Vaibhav Agnihotri MBBS DCH DNB (Ped)
Research Fellow
Diabetes and Heart Research Center
Dhanbad, Jharkhand, India

VB Jindal MD FICP FIAMS FIACM
Head
Department of Medicine
Sant Joseph Hospital, Nand Gram
Ghaziabad, Uttar Pradesh, India

Vijay G Negalur MD FICP
Honourable Assistant Professor
Department of Medicine
Dr Negalur's Diabetes Specialities Center
Mumbai, Maharashtra, India

Vijay Panikar MD FCPS DNB
Consultant
Department of Endocrinology and Diabetes
Lilavati Hospital
Mumbai, India

Vijay Viswanathan MD PhD FRCP (London and Glasgow)
Head and Chief Diabetologist
MV Hospital for Diabetes and Prof M Viswanathan Diabetes Research Center
Royapuram, Chennai, Tamil Nadu, India

Vikrant Bapuji Tari MD PG Dip Diab (UK) Fellowship in Diabetology [DRC (WHO) Chennai]
Consultant, Apollo Sugar Clinics Ltd.
Mumbai, Maharashtra, India

Vinod Mittal MD (Medicine) FRSSDI FIAMS FCAM FCCP FGSI FICP FDI FACP(USA)
Senior Consultant Diabetologist and Head
Center for Diabetes and Metabolic Diseases
Delhi Heart and Lung Institute
Director
Delhi Diabetes Care Center
New Delhi, India

Preface

"The worth of a book is to be measured by what you can carry away from it." This famous quote by James Bryce, British academic and historian very aptly describes the purpose behind our efforts to present the 2018 edition of the RSSDI Update Book to you with great pleasure and pride. Our knowledge today pertaining to all the aspects of diabetes, right from its basics to its types, etiopathogenesis, diagnosis and management as well as complications has increased by leaps and bounds with advancements in scientific research and technology. This update has been designed to give the readers a complete overview of all these aspects of diabetes, including its complications as well as comorbidities by means of chapters, well-illustrated with numerous figures and tables based on the scientific discussions at the RSSDI 2018 Annual Conference. The text has been segregated into–sections with related subtopics in each section to make it well organised and reader friendly.

This update comprises a wide range of topics extending from the basic anatomy and physiology of the islet, the alterations in cell biology and functioning, aetiology and pathogenesis to types of diabetes, its epidemiology, screening, diagnosis and management– diet, lifestyle, pharmacotherapy, latest RCTs and studies and their translation into evidence based clinical medicine. Latest advancements in the clinical management of diabetes, reversal of diabetes, special situations, technological advancements, other related comorbidities, acute as well as chronic complications and futuristic issues- this update covers them all!

Every effort has been made to match the standard and benchmarks set by the previous RSSDI Update books. Simple language and presentation enables this update to serve as a handy reference guide to not only diabetes physicians and endocrinologists, but also primary care practitioners, post graduate students and internists.

I am thankful to all the speakers and faculty of the RSSDI 2018 Annual Conference who so kindly transformed their scientific presentations into chapters at our request. Compiling everything in one book has been a herculean task managed by a well-coordinated team effort, sifting through the manuscripts, editing and finalising them to their current form to bring out all the scientific discussions at the conference into this compact yet comprehensive book. My gratitude and thanks to all contributors and my editing and publishing team who raced against time to successfully bring out this update well in time to reach your hands. Happy Reading

Rajeev Chawla

Contents

Section 1: Etiopathogenesis of Diabetes Mellitus

Section 2: Management of Diabetes Mellitus—Nutrition, Lifestyle and Education

Section 3: Management of Type 1 Diabetes Mellitus

Section 4: Management of Type 2 Diabetes Mellitus

Section 8: Diabetes Care in Special Populations

Section 11: Recent Advances in Diabetes Care

Section 12: Diabetes and Infections

PLATE 1

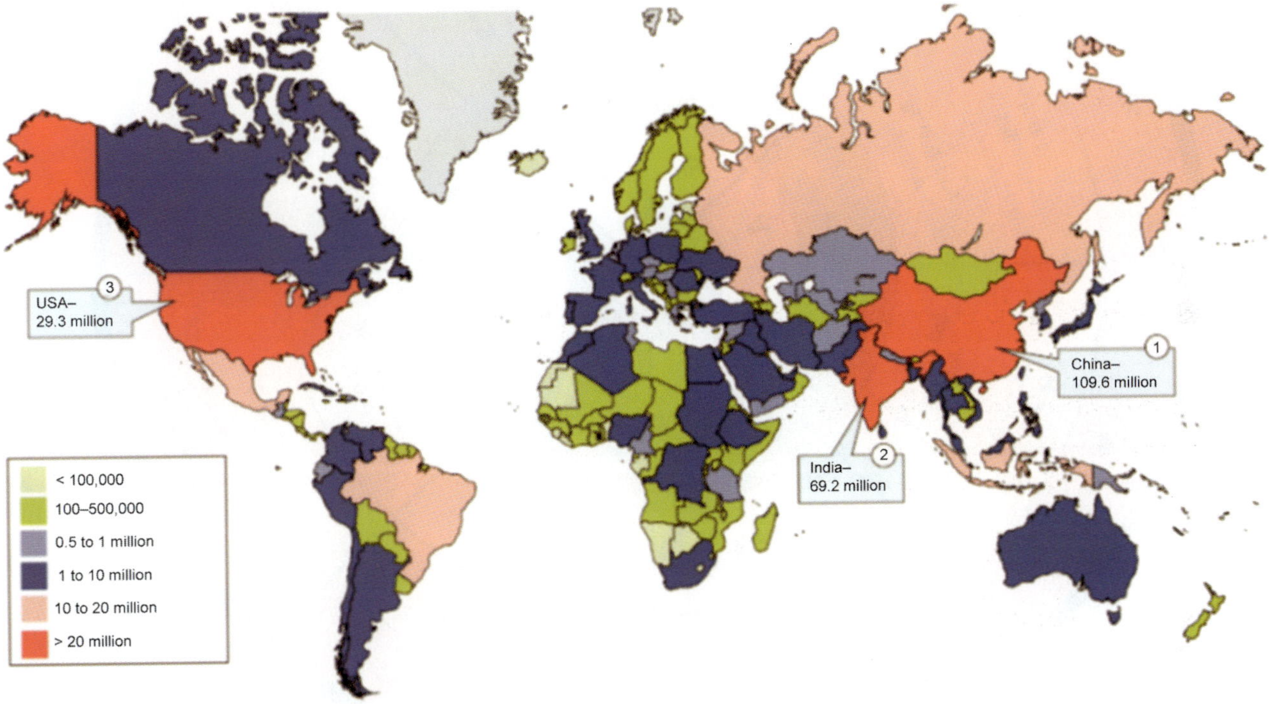

Figure 1 Estimated total number of adults (20–79 years) living with diabetes mellitus. ***(Chapter 31)***

PLATE 2

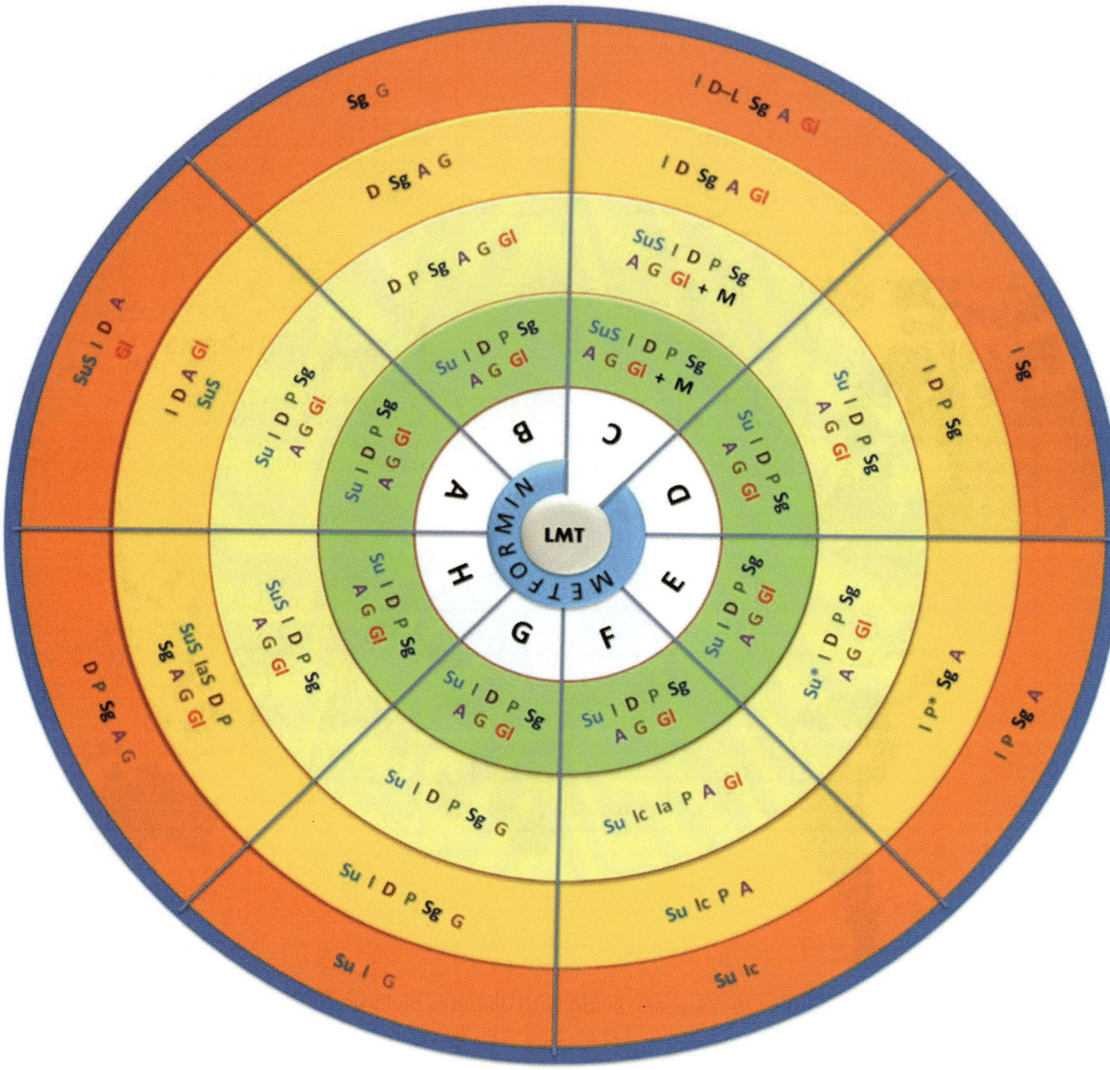

Su – Sulfonylurea
Su* – Preferably glimiperide or gliclazide
SuS – Short-acting sulfonylureas
I – Insulin
Ic – Conventional insulins
Ia – Insulin analogs
IaS – Short-acting insulin analogs
D – DPP-4 inhibitors
D-L – Linagliptin
P – Pioglitazone
P* – Pioglitazone if EF >40%
Sg – SGLT2 inhibitors
A – Alphaglucosidase inhibitors
G – GLP analogs
Gl – Glinides

From innermost to outermost: A: Age = Advancing Age; B: BMI = Increasing BMI; C: CKD = Advancing CKD; D: Duration of diabetes = Increasing duration; E: Established CVD = Low CVD risk to Established CVD risk; F: Finance = Adequate-to-limited; G: Glycemic status = Worsening glycemic control; H: Hypoglycemia = Hypoglycemia concern.

Lesser options available

Wider options available

(BMI: body mass index; CKD: chronic kidney disease; CVD: cardiovascular disease; DPP-4: dipeptidyl peptidase-4; EF: ejection fraction; GLP: glucagon-like peptide; SGLT2: sodium-glucose cotransporter 2.)

Figure 1 RSSDI diabetes therapeutic wheel. ***(Chapter 34)***

PLATE 3

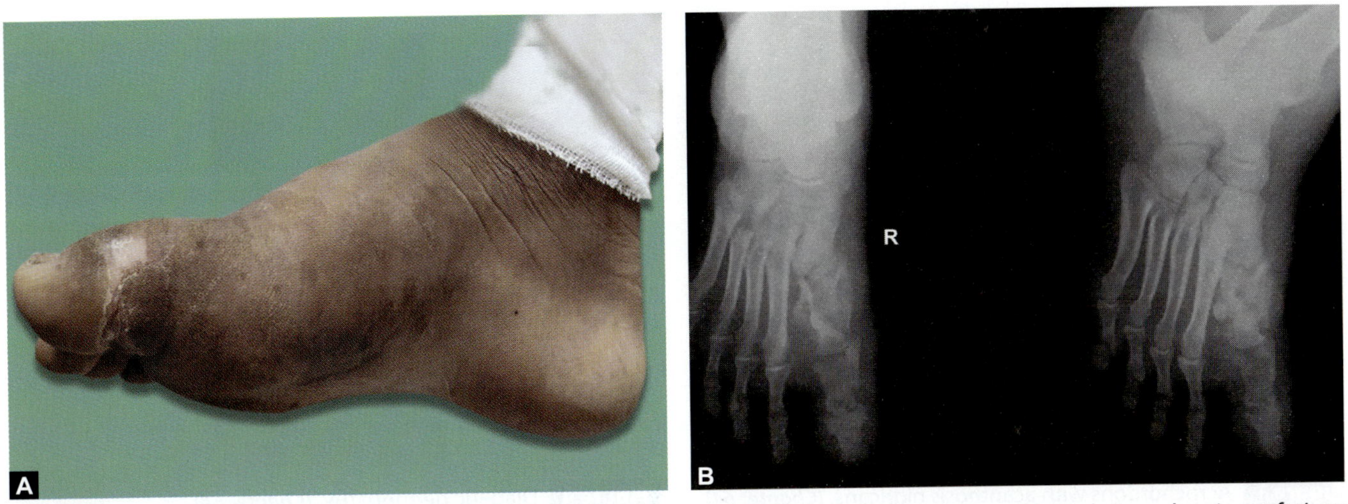

Figure 2 (A) Swelling and midfoot deformity in Charcot foot; (B) X-ray right foot anteroposterior and lateral views showing soft tissue swelling and destruction of bones. ***(Chapter 48)***

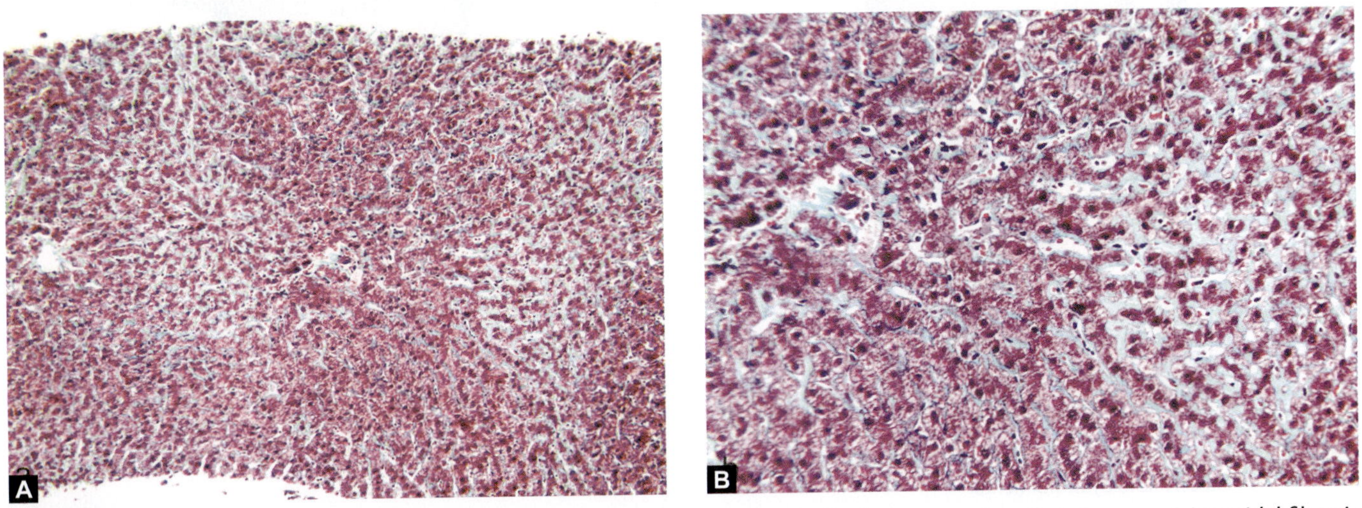

Figure 2 Diabetic hepatosclerosis: Masson's trichrome staining. The upper half is low power view that shows perisinusoidal fibrosis and lack of steatosis. The lower half is a higher power showing dense collagen deposition in the perisinusoidal spaces of the involved regions.[16] ***(Chapter 50)***

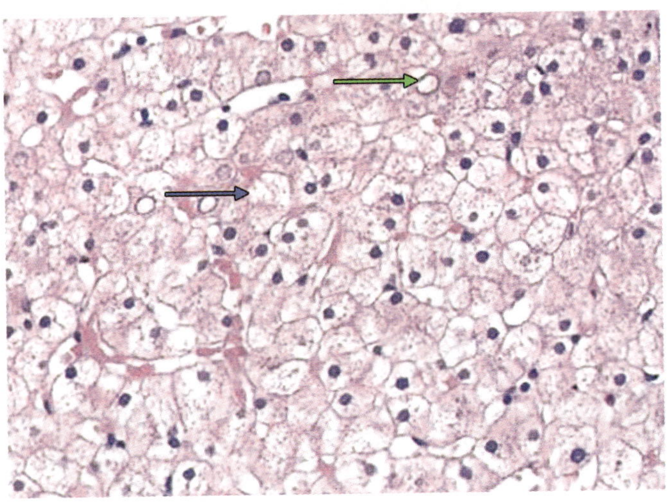

Figure 3 Glycogenic hepatopathy: Liver biopsy section. Hematoxylin and Eosin staining shows enlarged hepatocytes with cytoplasmic pallor. Reddish pink areas of glycogen accumulation (blue arrow) and prominent glycogenated nucleoli (green arrow) are seen.[17] ***(Chapter 50)***

PLATE 4

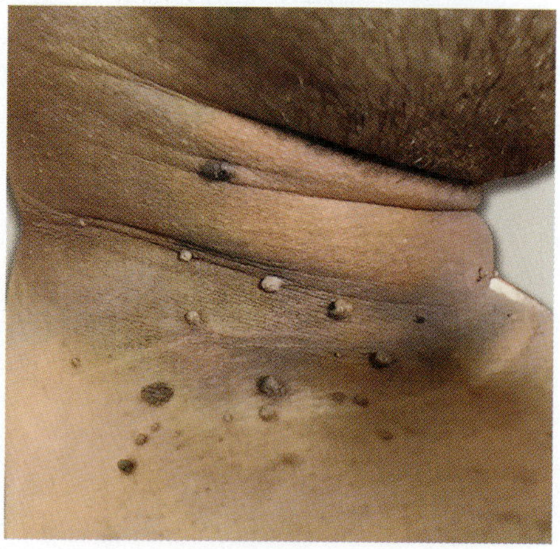

Figure 1 Acrochordons with acanthosis nigricans. ***(Chapter 64)***
Source: Photo by Dr RD Mehta.

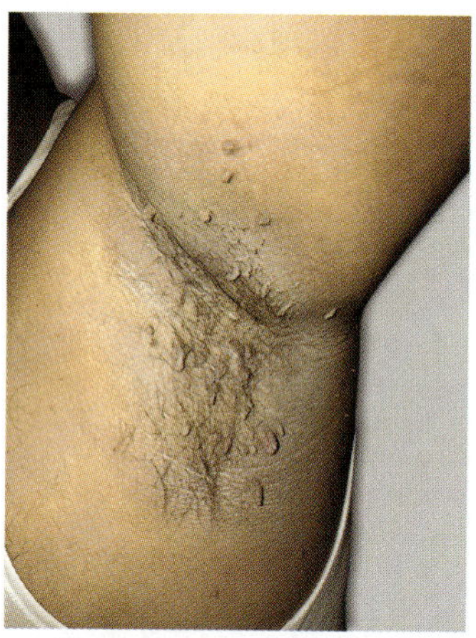

Figure 2 Acrochordons in the axillary fold. ***(Chapter 64)***
Source: Photo by Dr RD Mehta.

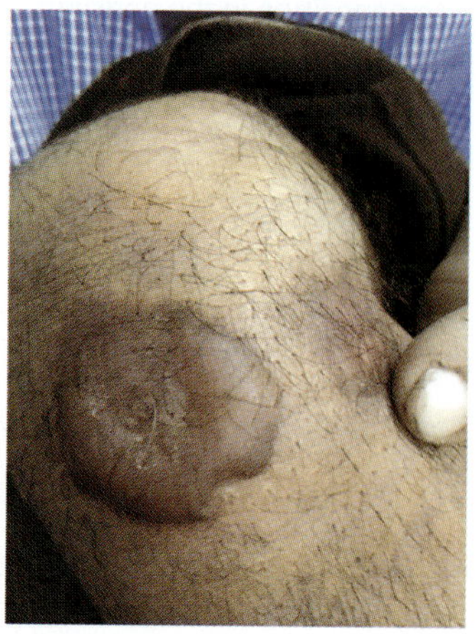

Figure 3 Bullosis diabeticorum over the extensor surface of the knee. ***(Chapter 64)***
Source: Photo by Dr RD Mehta.

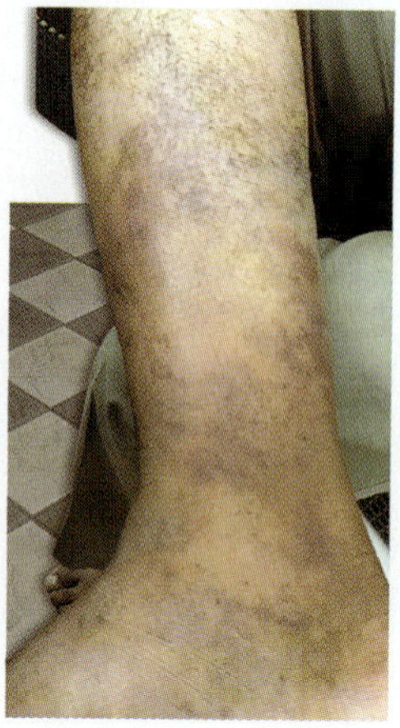

Figure 4 Diabetic dermopathy. ***(Chapter 64)***
Source: Photo by Dr Aastha Chawla.

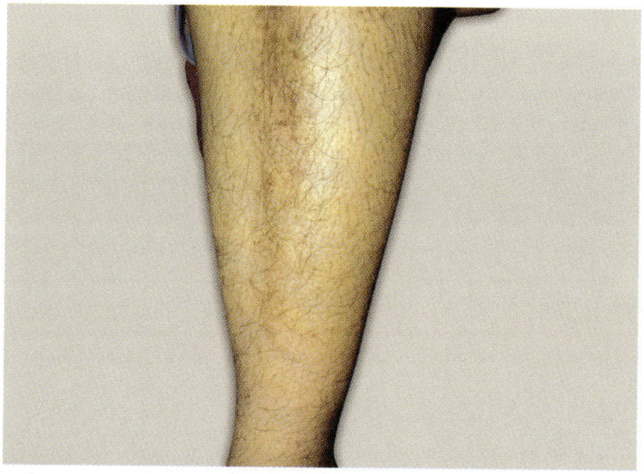

Figure 5 Evoluting necrobiosis lipoidica diabeticorum over the shin. ***(Chapter 64)***
Source: Photo by Dr RD Mehta.

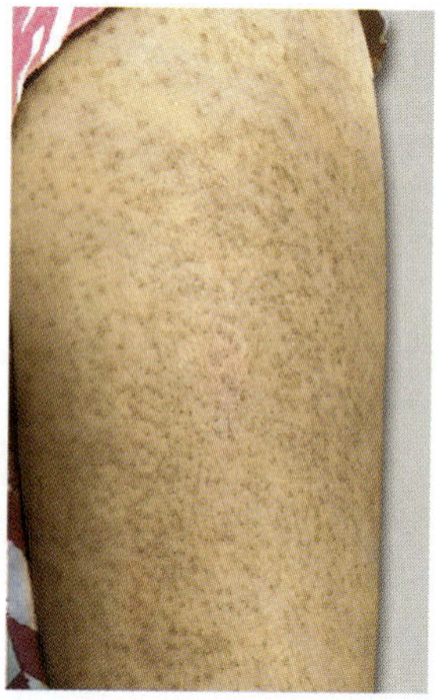

Figure 6 Follicular keratosis over the extensor surface of the arm. ***(Chapter 64)***
Source: Photo by Dr Aastha Chawla.

PLATE 5

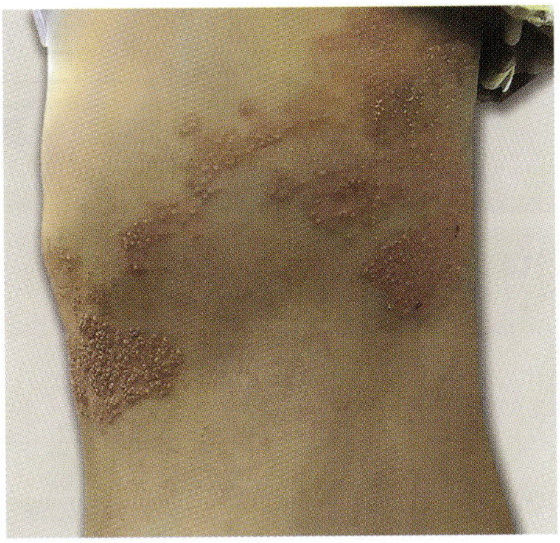

Figure 7 Herpes zoster along the thoracic dermatome. ***(Chapter 64)***
Source: Photo by Dr Aastha Chawla.

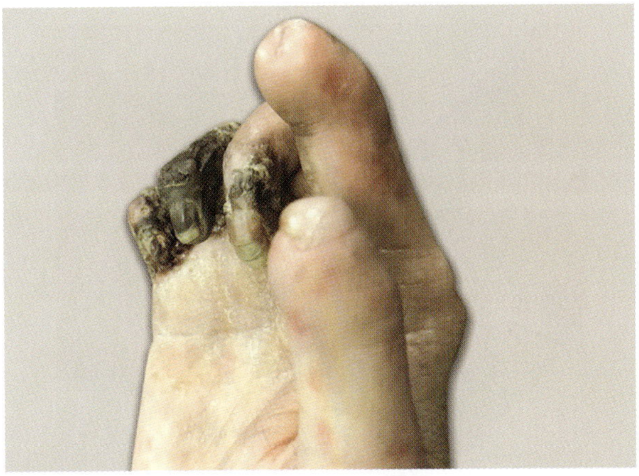

Figure 10 Gangrenous changes of the fingers. ***(Chapter 64)***
Source: Photo by Dr RD Mehta.

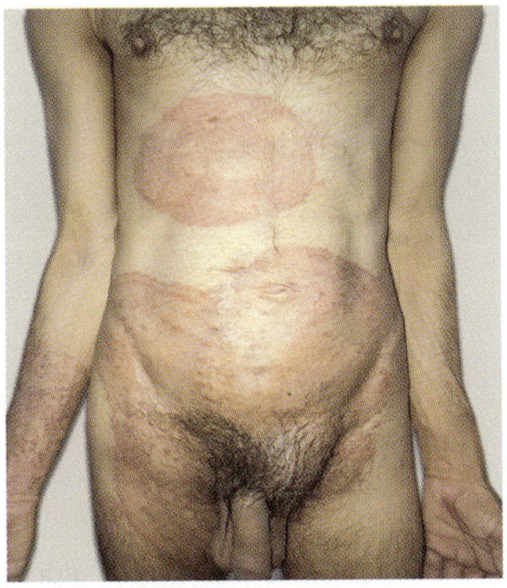

Figure 8 Extensive tinea. ***(Chapter 64)***
Source: Photo by Dr RD Mehta.

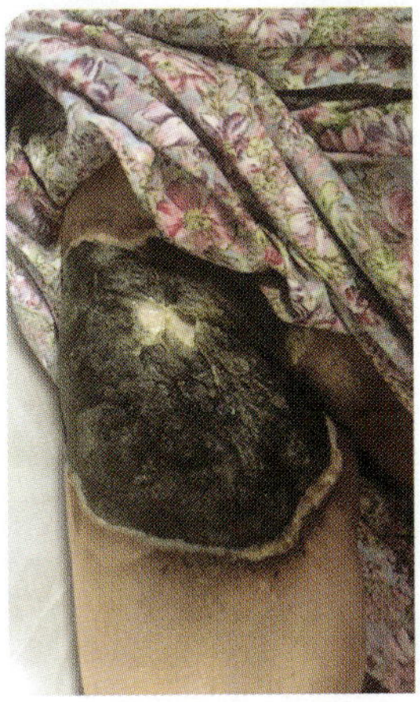

Figure 11 Ecthyma gangrenosum. ***(Chapter 64)***
Source: Photo by Dr Aastha Chawla.

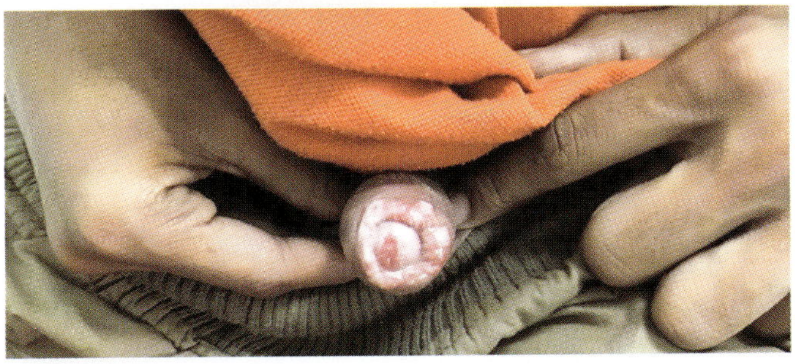

Figure 9 Candidal balanoposthitis. ***(Chapter 64)***
Source: Photo by Dr RD Mehta.

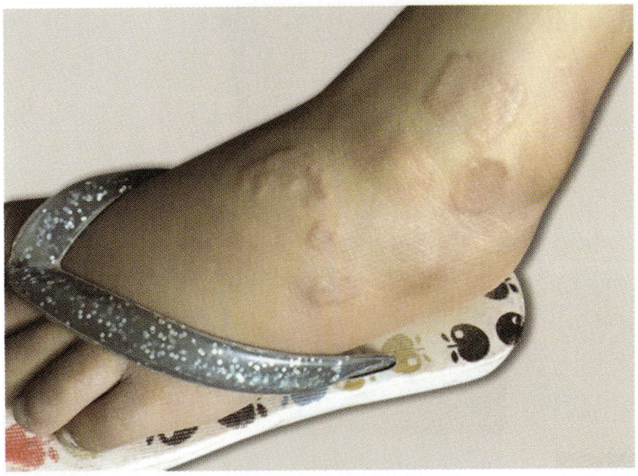

Figure 12 Granuloma annulare. ***(Chapter 64)***
Source: Photo by Dr Aastha Chawla.

PLATE 6

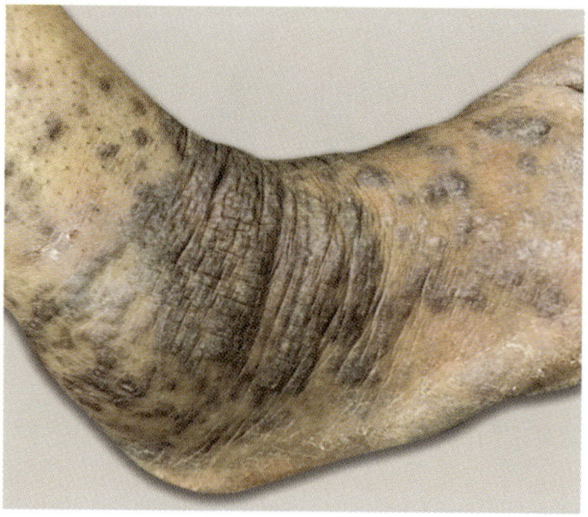

Figure 13 Lichen planus over foot. ***(Chapter 64)***
Source: Photo by Dr RD Mehta.

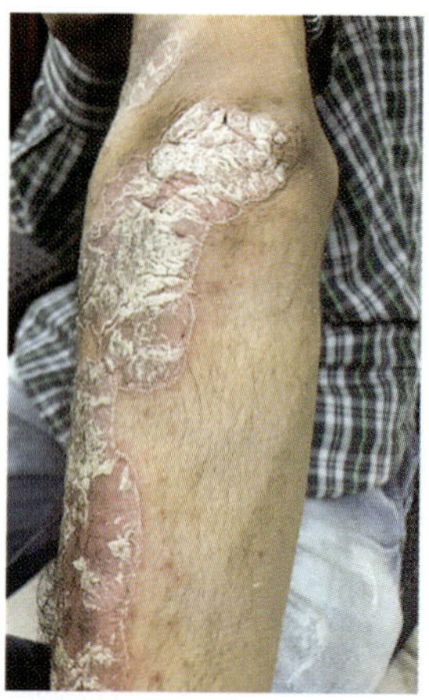

Figure 14 Psoriasis vulgaris. ***(Chapter 64)***
Source: Photo by Dr RD Mehta.

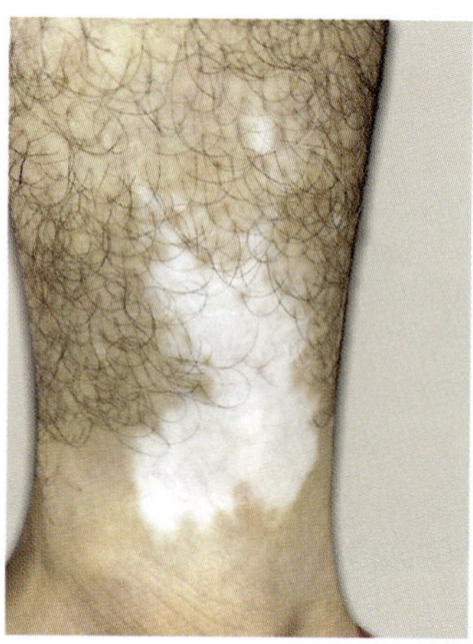

Figure 15 Localized vitiligo. ***(Chapter 64)***
Source: Photo by Dr Aastha Chawla.

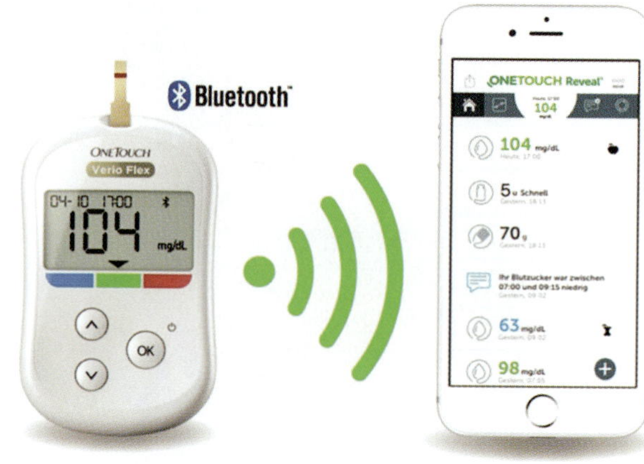

Figure 1 OneTouch Verio Flex™ Meter and the OneTouch Reveal™ app. ***(Chapter 77)***

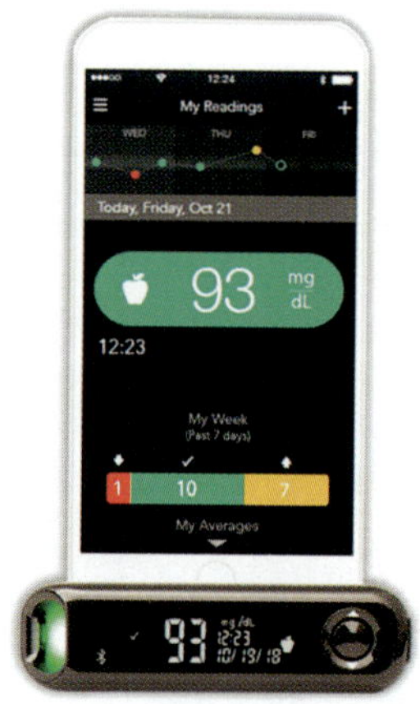

Figure 2 CONTOUR® NEXT ONE blood glucose monitoring system. ***(Chapter 77)***

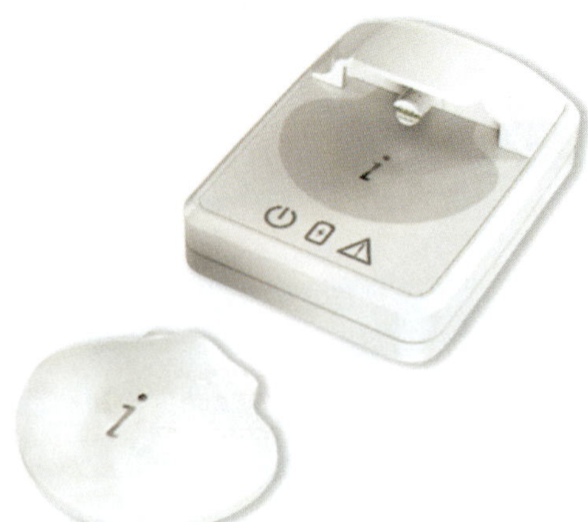

Figure 3 iPro®2 professional continuous glucose monitoring system. ***(Chapter 77)***

PLATE 7

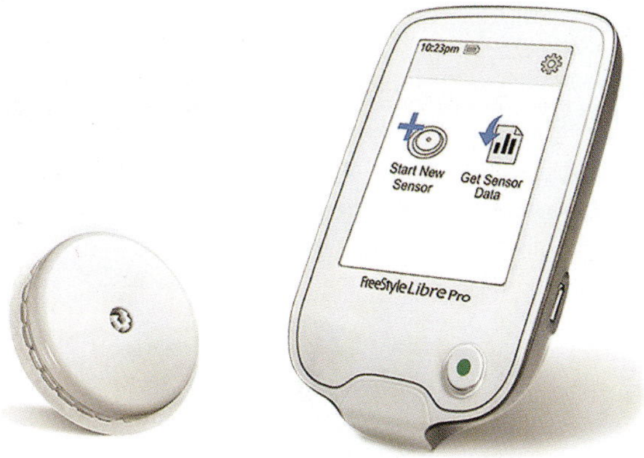

Figure 4 FreeStyle Libre™ Pro continuous glucose monitoring system. ***(Chapter 77)***

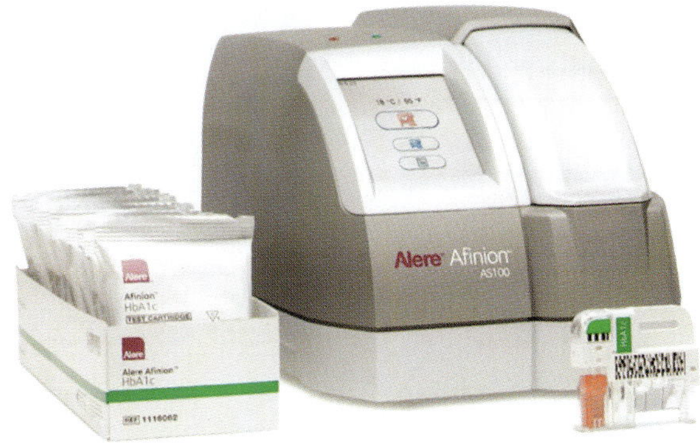

Figure 7 Point-of-Care HbA1c testing device alere Afinion™ HbA1c Dx. ***(Chapter 77)***

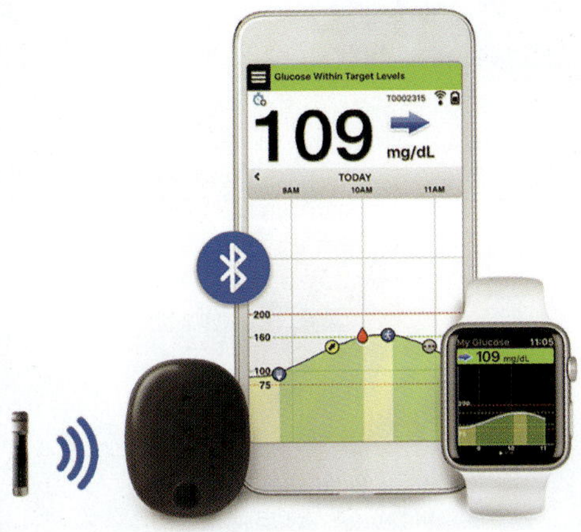

Figure 5 Eversense® 90-day implantable continuous glucose monitoring system. ***(Chapter 77)***

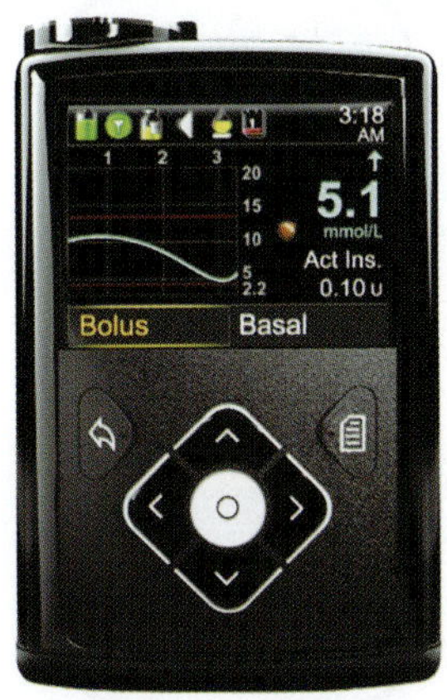

Figure 8 MiniMed™ 640G Insulin Pump. ***(Chapter 77)***

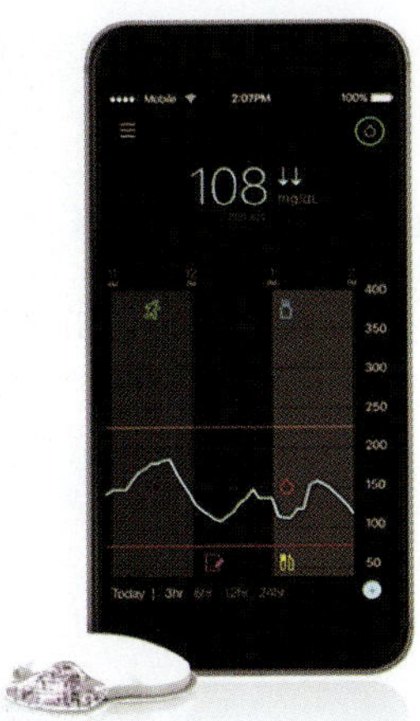

Figure 6 Guardian™ Connect continuous glucose monitoring system. ***(Chapter 77)***

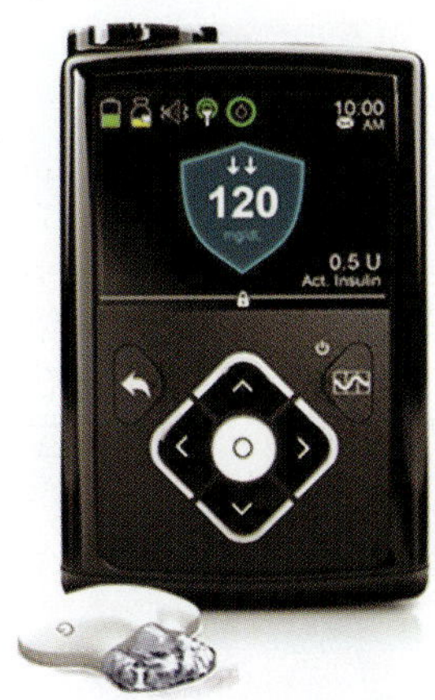

Figure 9 MiniMed™ 670G hybrid closed-loop insulin pump. ***(Chapter 77)***

PLATE 8

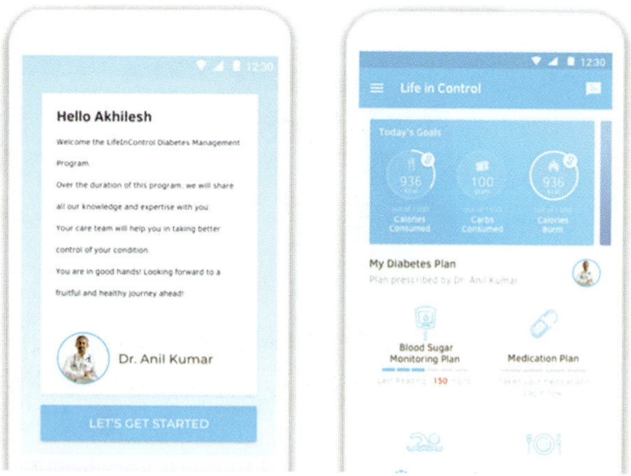

Figure 10 Life in Control™ Diabetes Coach. ***(Chapter 77)***

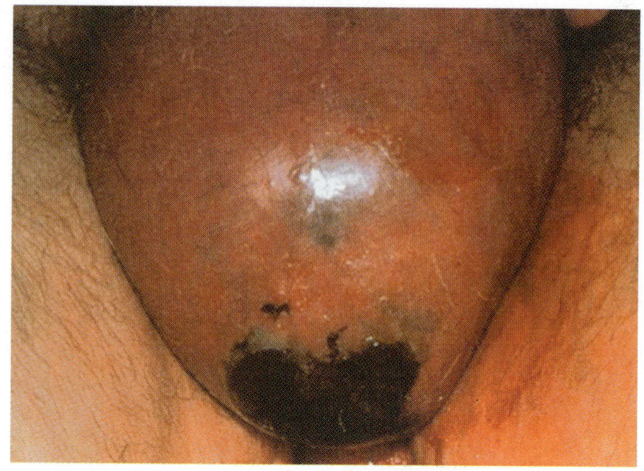

Figure 5 Fournier's gangrene. ***(Chapter 87)***

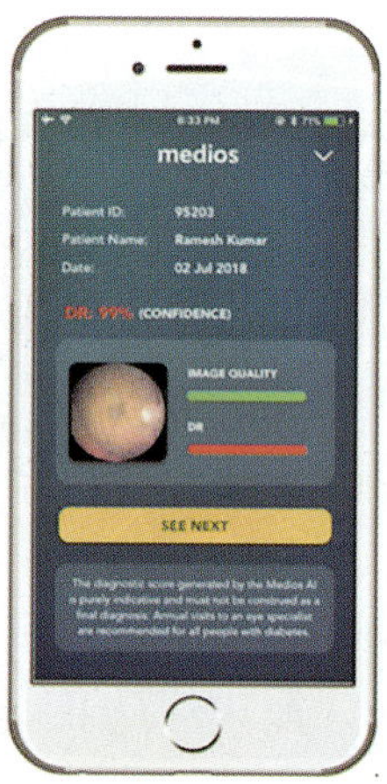

Figure 11 Medios Technologies AI assistant to detect diabetic retinopathy. ***(Chapter 77)***

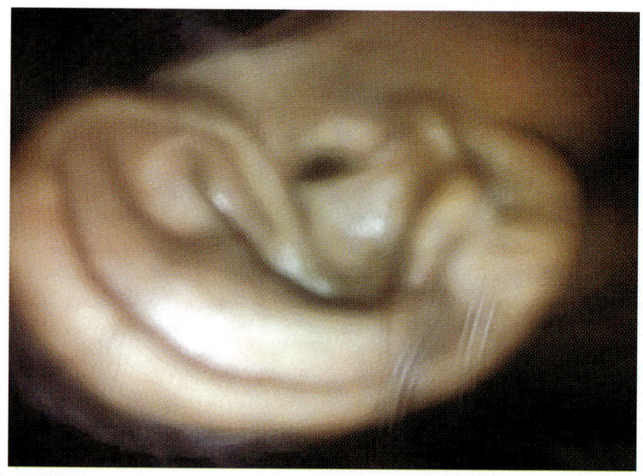

Figure 6 Malignant otitis externa. ***(Chapter 87)***

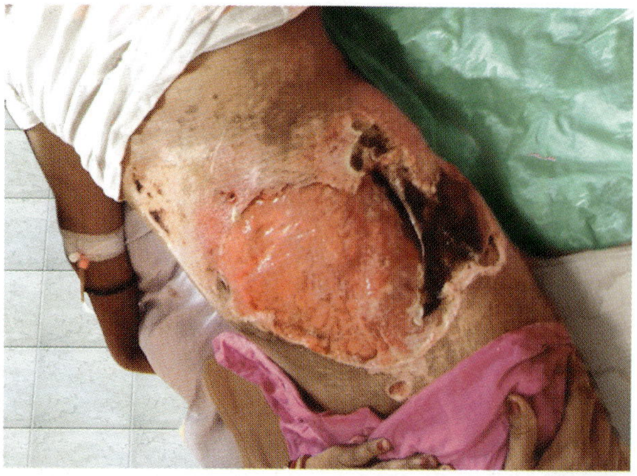

Figure 4 Necrotizing fasciitis of abdomen and chest wall. ***(Chapter 87)***

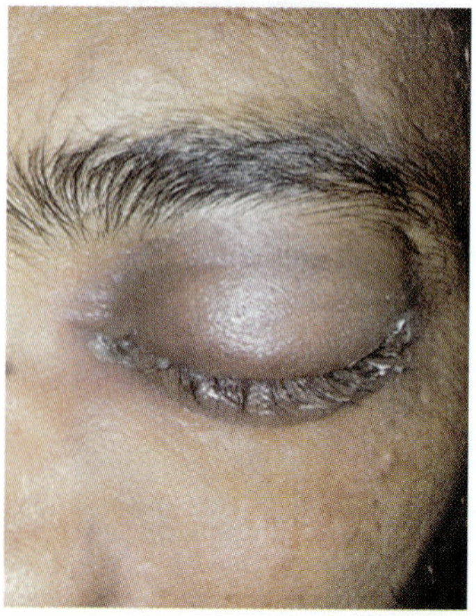

Figure 7 Rhino-orbital-cerebral-mucormycosis showing proptosis and drooping of left eyelid. ***(Chapter 87)***

Chapter 1

Conceptual Advances in Innate Immunity and Diabetes Mellitus

Sandeep K Mathur, Hardeva Ram Nehara

INTRODUCTION

Prevalence of diabetes mellitus (DM) is about 8.8%, with more than 425 million people affected as of 2017, and expected to increase to approximately 629 million people by 2045. India, have the second largest number of diabetes cases (73 million in 2018) and over half of people currently living with diabetes are estimated to be undiagnosed.[1] Chronic inflammation is an important proposed mechanism for the development of both DM and its vascular complication.[2]

Insults caused by majority of microorganisms can be sensed and eliminated within minutes or hours, by the innate immune system, by identification of pathogen-associated molecular patterns (PAMPs) by pattern recognition receptors (PRRs).[3] The innate immune system can also recognize endogenous danger signals through the sensing of danger-associated molecular patterns (DAMPs).[4] DAMPs are by-products of damaged or dying cells, and are small molecules [adenosine triphosphate (ATP) and deoxyribonucleic acid (DNA)], particles (uric acid crystals and exogenous noxious factors), and environmental factors such as ultraviolet radiation. Both local and systemic inflammation and upregulation of proinflammatory cytokines are implicated in the etiopathogenesis of type 1 diabetes mellitus (T1DM) and type 2 diabetes mellitus (T2DM).[5]

INNATE IMMUNITY

Innate immunity is defined as the immune responses that are present since birth. The innate immune system protects the host during the initial period of immune response that is between exposure to microbe and first adaptive responses. The innate immune system senses microorganisms by PRRs, which are specific to molecular components of microorganisms.[6,7]

Components of Innate Immunity

Components of the innate immune system include both host components and resident microbiomes.

Host Components[8,9]

- *Physical barriers*: The skin, epithelial surfaces, mucous membrane, mucus, and vascular endothelial cells
- Enzymes presents in epithelial and phagocytic cells (e.g. lysozyme)
- *Inflammation-related serum proteins*: Complement system, C-reactive protein (CRP), lectins (carbohydrate-binding proteins), and ficolins
- *Antimicrobial peptides (AMPs)*: Cathelicidins, defensins, etc. on the cell surfaces and within phagocyte granules
- Cell receptors that recognize microorganisms and produce a defensive response like, toll-like receptors (TLRs), NOD (nucleotide-binding oligomerization domain)-like receptors (NLRs)
- Inflammatory cells that release cytokines and other inflammatory mediators like, macrophages, mast cells, natural killer (NK) cells, and innate lymphoid cells
- *Phagocytic cells*: Neutrophils, monocytes, macrophages.

The Microbiomes

The human microbiomes includes bacteria, fungi and viruses that live within and on the human body, and are component of the innate immune system, as they affects mechanisms of host defence.[10] The body's microbial composition directly effects the maturation of the immune response and its continued effectiveness, protects against pathogen overgrowth, and modulates the balance between inflammation and immune homeostasis.[11]

Toll-like Receptors

The innate immune system includes various PRRs, like membrane-bound TLRs and C-type lectin receptors, which detect PAMPs and DAMPs in the extracellular space and endosomal compartment. TLRs are type 1 membrane glycoproteins that have a characteristic cytoplasmic Toll/interleukin (IL)-1 receptor (TIR) domain and a leucine-rich repeat domain.[12] Activation of TLR causes subsequent activation of other signaling molecules, such as nuclear factor-κB (NF-κB), mitogen-activated protein kinases (MAPKs), and interferon regulatory factor (IRF), which causes subsequent production and release of various cytokines and chemokines.[13]

Nucleotide-binding Oligomerization Domain-like Receptors

Nucleotide-binding oligomerization domain-like receptors are another intracellular sensing PRRs, present in the cytosol and are essential for recognition of invading pathogens and subsequent innate immune response.[14] NLRs initiate signaling complexes, like NOD signalosomes (a protein complex which causes regulation of protein degradation by ubiquitination) and inflammasomes (a multiprotein molecular scaffold complex).[15] NOD1 and NOD2 are NLRs in the NOD signalosome, which upon activation causes homo-oligomerization and recruitment of signaling molecules that causes NF-κB-dependent and AP1-dependent production of proinflammatory cytokines. Some inflammasomes causes activation of caspase-1 and convert premature forms of IL-1β, IL-18, and IL-33 to mature forms, and secrete these cytokines into the extracellular space.[16]

TYPE 1 DIABETES MELLITUS

Various studies have established role of the T-cell-mediated adaptive immune response in etiopathogenesis of T1DM. Understanding of various signaling pathways involved in innate immunity, which is implicated in promoting the autoreactive T-cell response that can leads to T1DM, have been improved after the discovery of TLRs.[17]

Role of TLR 2 and TLR4 in T1DM

Toll-like receptor 2 and TLR4 are the main receptors for the DAMP on pancreatic β-cells and can trigger an inflammatory response responsible for causation of DM in nonobese diabetic mice.[18] Activation of TLR2 and TLR4 with lipopolysaccharide (LPS) and peptidoglycans leads failure of transplanted islet grafts with infiltration of mononuclear cell. Transplantation of islets from TLR2–/– and TLR4–/– mice into wild type mice decreased the proinflammatory cytokines production and improved islet cell survival. These findings proposed role of TLR2 and TLR4 signaling in sustained inflammation in pancreatic islets.[19]

Role of NLR in T1DM

Activation of TLRs causes activation of NF-κB, which leads to enhanced transcription of pro-IL-1β. Pro-IL-1β is subsequently processed and cleaved to IL-1β by the NLRP3 inflammasome. TLRs and IL-1β are unregulated in T1DM and IL-1β trigger apoptosis of pancreatic β-cells.[20] Two multicenter randomized controlled trials were conducted to see the effects of IL-1 antagonist on pancreatic β-cells.[21]Canakinumab (anti-IL-1β antibody) and anakinra (IL-1 receptor antagonist) were found safe but not as effective as immunomodulatory drugs in preservation of pancreatic β-cells. *Nlrp1b* was found as a strong candidate gene for T1DM susceptibility in both nonobese diabetic mice and nonobese diabetes resistant (NOR) mice that were insulitis resistant and diabetes free despite being genetically similar to nonobese diabetic mice at a number of chromosomal regions. *Nlrp1b* is a part of the NLR gene family, which facilitates the assembly of the inflammasome, helps in the recruitment of caspase-1, and also release of IL-β.[22] Research about the role of inflammasome in the development of T1DM is limited and more investigations are required to answer the question that whether targeting inflammasomes will exert beneficial effects in development of T1DM.

TYPE 2 DIABETES MELLITUS

Type 2 diabetes mellitus with obesity is now considered a chronic inflammatory disease. Subclinical and chronic inflammation in obesity and the metabolic syndrome can results in insulin resistance and T2DM.[23] Excess of nutrient intake results in low-grade inflammatory state in adipose tissue, skeletal muscle, liver, gastrointestinal tract, and pancreas, and activation of the innate immune response mediated by TLRs and NLRs, leads to insulin resistance.[24] Adipose tissue is a most important site of inflammation and is host to various inflammatory cells, such as neutrophils, basophils, M1 and M2 macrophages, Th1, Th2, and regulatory T-cells (TREG cells), cluster of differentiation (CD8+) T-cells, and B-cells, and is also an important source of various chemokines, cytokines, and adipokines that mediate inflammatory responses in obesity and T2DM.[25]

Role of Toll-like Receptors

Mice lacking TLR2 are protected from diet-induced adiposity, hypercholesterolemia insulin resistance, hepatic steatosis, and macrophage infiltration, and levels of inflammatory cytokines are less compared to wild-type mice.[26] Absence of TLR2 was associated with attenuated local inflammatory cytokine expression and enhanced insulin action in the liver.[27] TLR2 is also implicated in the inflammatory response in high-fat diet (HFD)-induced obesity in rodents and in human gene expression studies.[28]

Obesity-associated Inflammation

Sustained obesity-associated inflammation is due to three apparently distinct mechanisms, and includes TLR4 activation, changes in the gut microbiota, and endoplasmic reticulum stress.

Toll-Like Receptor 4

Reduced defense barriers in the intestine, increased leakage of LPS and fatty acids, and changes in the gut microbiota causes activation of TLR4 pathways and subsequent inflammation.[29] Lack of TLR4 in mice fed on a HFD are protected from obesity, insulin resistance, and chronic inflammation in liver, adipose tissues, skeletal muscle, and vasculature.[30] Deletion of TLR4 in hematopoietic cells causes improvement in insulin resistance in liver and adipose tissue[31] and deletion of TLR4 in hepatocytes improved glucose tolerance, increased insulin sensitivity, and improved hepatic steatosis in mice.[32] The agonists for TLR2 and TLR4, like LPSs and saturated free fatty acids, are implicated in the signaling cascades via NF-κB nuclear translocation and subsequent proinflammatory cytokine production in adipose, liver, muscle, and pancreatic β-cells in animal models of insulin resistance and obesity.[33] The inflammatory pathway mediated by IL-6 and tumor necrosis factor (TNF) is mainly induced by the activation of TLR2 and TLR4, as seen in adipose tissue samples obtained from adolescents with the metabolic syndrome.[34]

Endogenous ligand for TLR4 is not known, as free fatty acids do not directly bind to TLR4. Fetuin-A has been proposed as an endogenous ligand for TLR4 and knockdown mice with HFD-induced insulin resistance have downregulation of TLR4-mediated inflammatory signaling cascades in adipose tissue.[35] S100A8 and S100A9 are members of S100 calgranulin family and are endogenous DAMPs. These DAMPs can lead to TLR4 and NLRP3 inflammasome mediated IL-1β production in adipose tissue, macrophages, and neutrophils and induce insulin resistance in both mice and humans.[36]

Gut Microbiota

Research regarding the link between the pathophysiology of metabolic diseases and the gut microbiota, are proposed from various evidences that the composition of the gut microbiota is different in healthy individuals, obese, and patients with T2DM. TLR2 knockout mice bred and maintained under germ-free conditions have no diet-induced insulin resistance.[37] While, due to changes in the gut microbiota, under nongerm-free conditions these mice are associated with insulin resistance and obesity.[38]

These finding suggested that TLR2 has an important role in maintaining healthy gut microbiota and protection from obesity and insulin resistance. Similarly, TLR4 knockout mice fed with HFD are associated with decreased intestinal permeability, increased plasma endotoxin, and proinflammatory cytokine levels.[39] Apart from these, bacterial flagellin-recognizing TLR5 knockout mice have hyperphasia and metabolic syndrome, which was transmissible to wild type mice by gut microbiota transplantation.[40] These data concludes that upregulation of TLRs leads to enhanced the inflammatory response and development of insulin resistance and obesity. The interaction between the microbiota and TLRs can result in whole-body chronic inflammation and subsequent insulin resistance and its consequences.[41]

Endoplasmic Reticulum Stress

There is crosstalk between TLRs and endoplasmic reticulum stress. As assessed by monitoring markers of endoplasmic reticulum stress, TLR4 knockout mice fed a HFD were protected from endoplasmic reticulum stress in comparison to wild-type mice.[42] Mice fed a HFD or administered a prolonged low dose of LPSs to induce TLR4 before cold adaptation, had reduced heat release, core body temperature, and increased endoplasmic reticulum stress in comparison to mice that had received a low-fat diet or had not received LPSs.[43] Endoplasmic reticulum stress also activate the NLRP3 inflammasome leading to apoptosis of pancreatic β-cells. Endoplasmic reticulum stress via the activation of NF-κB and the NLRP3 inflammasome leads to increased production of IL-1β.[44]

INSULIN RESISTANCE

Obesity, metabolic syndrome, and T2DM are interrelated metabolic diseases associated with chronic low-grade inflammation, in which chronic inflammation leads to alteration in metabolic function and homeostatic set points, which leads to exacerbation the disease.[45] It is observed that TNF-α levels in mice were increased during the advancement of obesity, and when TNF-α was neutralized, there is improvement in insulin sensitivity.[17,46]

Tumor necrosis factor-α decreases insulin receptor (IR) activity by serine phosphorylation of insulin receptor substrate-1 (IRS1), a signaling protein downstream of the IR and thus linking adipose tissue inflammation with insulin resistance. Normally, binding of insulin to the IR leads to production of triacylglycerols from diet derived fatty acid and glucose-derived glycerol 3-phosphate.[47] Thus, insulin promotes uptake of lipids and glucose simultaneously into adipose tissue in vivo. Insulin resistance and subsequent impairment of insulin signaling, will lead to abundance of circulating glucose and free fatty acids, as in T2DM.[18]

Inflammation

Macrophage accumulation in obese adipose tissue, and subsequent secretion of proinflammatory cytokines, alter adipose tissue glucose and lipid metabolism. These macrophage-derived TNF-α and IL-6 leads to impaired lipoprotein lipase activity and subsequent increased blood triacylglycerol concentration. TNF-α causes enhanced hormone-sensitive lipase activity in adipose tissue and subsequent release of free fatty acid into the blood, and simultaneously reduces insulin stimulated glucose uptake through impaired insulin signaling.[48] Increased plasma concentrations of free fatty acid and ceramide link nutrient metabolism and inflammation. Ceramide induce IL-1 secretion from macrophages in obese individuals and HFD-fed animals,[49] while free fatty acid activate the NOD-like receptor family and NLRP3 (pyrin domain containing 3) inflammasome in hematopoietic cells and promote insulin resistance.[50] A recent study has also shown that activation of the macrophage inflammasome via islet amyloid polypeptide (IAPP) was dependent on altered glucose and fatty acid metabolism, and subsequent production of inflammatory cytokines IL-1 and IL-18.[51]

Infiltrating Macrophages

There are two different polarization states of macrophages, M1 (proinflammatory) and M2 (anti-inflammatory). The proinflammatory M1 form is activated by proinflammatory mediators like LPS, TNF-α, and interferon-gamma (IFN-γ), and secrete TNF-α, IL-1, and IL-6, thus enhancing the inflammatory response. The anti-inflammatory M2 secrete anti-inflammatory cytokines, like, IL-10. It is shown that ingestion of HFD causes polarization of Kupffer cells of the liver toward the proinflammatory M1 phenotype, and this polarization was implicated in the pathogenesis of obesity-induced insulin resistance and hepatic steatosis. TNF-α production by M1 macrophages in the liver leads to increased hepatic glucose production through gluconeogenesis and through inhibition of intracellular lipases enhances lipid production and storage. Therefore, increased TNF-α in the obese liver leads to hyperglycemia and hepatic steatosis.[52] Kupffer cells, in liver, via c-Jun N-terminal protein kinase 1 (JNK1) activation and lowering of heat shock protein (HSP) pathways, which are anti-inflammatory leads to insulin resistance, hepatic steatosis, and steatohepatitis.[53]

These finding suggested that the excessive nutrient flux in T2DM leads to activation of circulating macrophages that subsequently lead to chronic low-grade Inflammation, which is a pathognomonic of obesity and T2DM.

Impaired Insulin Signaling

Insulin resistance is a hallmark of pathogenesis and progression of chronic metabolic diseases, like obesity and T2DM. Insulin resistance is defined as impairment in insulin mediated signaling cascade in insulin sensitive tissues, like liver, skeletal muscle, and adipose tissue, leading to impaired glucose uptake and increased hepatic glucose production.[54] Insulin resistance is associated with serine phosphorylation of IRS proteins and subsequent, decreased interaction of IRS with phosphoinositide 3-kinase (PI3K). Adipose tissue expansion leads to enhanced proinflammatory cytokines synthesis and secretion, and subsequent activation of proinflammatory signaling proteins, like TNF-α and JNK1, induce serine phosphorylation in IRS1 and insulin resistance.[47]

Beta-cell Dysfunction

Insulin resistance is associated with deposition of amyloid in the islets via activation of NLRP3 inflammasome in resident macrophages and subsequent, processing and release of IL-1. Recently, it has been reported that the saturated fatty acid palmitate can activate the innate immunity via TLR4 in islet cells, and subsequent macrophage infiltration and chronic inflammation. Activation of proapoptotic proinflammatory transcription factors like NF-κB and the signal transducer and activator of transcription-1 in β-cells, leads to apoptosis of β-cells. IL-1 also promotes NF-κB dependent activation of the inducible nitric oxide synthase (iNOS), leading to β-cell death and dysfunction.[55] Normally, NF-κB is present in the cytoplasm, in inactive form, bound to inhibitory κB (IκB) proteins. IκB is phosphorylated by an IκB kinase complex (IKK), by IL-1R stimulation leading to degradation of IκB by the ubiquitin-proteasome system (UPS), and NF-κB is released and translocate into the nucleus, and bind target genes promoter regions. Activation of NF-κB also regulates iNOS and anti- and proapoptotic members of the Bcl-2 family.[56] iNOS expression leads to increased nitric oxide (NO) synthesis and subsequent β-cell secretory dysfunction and apoptosis.[57]

CONCLUSION

Chronic low-grade inflammation in pancreatic islets in T1DM is mediated by TLR2 and TLR4. Under conditions of excessive nutrition influx and obesity, TLR4 mediates sustained inflammation in pancreatic islet cells. The complex interaction between the microbiota and TLRs can induce chronic inflammation and subsequent insulin resistance. Increased IL-1β is tightly associated with the development of insulin resistance and consequent obesity and T2DM. Activation of the NLRP3 inflammasome in various tissues like adipose tissues, liver and pancreatic islets leads to development of obesity and T2DM. Thus, targeting the NLRP3 inflammasome may be a potential therapeutic approach in prevention or halting progression of DM.

REFERENCES

1. International Diabetes Federation. IDF Diabetes Atlas, 8th edition. Brussels, Belgium: 2018.
2. Wada J, Makino H. Inflammation and the pathogenesis of diabetic nephropathy. Clin Sci. 2013;124:139-52.
3. Murphy K, Travers P, Walport M, et al. Janeway's Immunobiology, 8th edition. St. Louis, USA: Garland Science; 2012.
4. Mogensen TH. Pathogen recognition and inflammatory signaling in innate immune defenses. Clin Microbiol Rev. 2009;22:240-73.
5. Dowling JK, O'Neill LA. Biochemical regulation of the inflammasome. Crit Rev Biochem Mol Biol. 2012;47:424-43.
6. Medzhitov R, Janeway CA Jr. Innate immunity: the virtues of a nonclonal system of recognition. Cell. 1997;91:295-8.
7. Medzhitov R. Pattern recognition theory and the launch of modern innate immunity. J Immunol. 2013;191:4473-4.
8. Spadoni I, Zagato E, Bertocchi A, et al. A gut-vascular barrier controls the systemic dissemination of bacteria. Science. 2015;350:830-4.
9. Bouziat R, Jabri B. IMMUNOLOGY. Breaching the gut-vascular barrier. Science. 2015;350:742.
10. Hinde K, Lewis ZT. MICROBIOTA. Mother's littlest helpers. Science. 2015;348:1427-8.
11. Lynch SV, Pedersen O. The Human Intestinal Microbiome in Health and Disease. N Engl J Med. 2016;375:2369-79.
12. Takeda K, Akira S. Toll-like receptors in innate immunity. Int Immunol. 2005;17:1-14.
13. Song DH, Lee JO. Sensing of microbial molecular patterns by Toll-like receptors. Immunol Rev. 2012;250:216-29.
14. Nakamura N, Lill JR, Phung Q, et al. Endosomes are specialized platforms for bacterial sensing and NOD2 signalling. Nature. 2014;509:240-4.
15. Lamkanfi M, Dixit VM. Inflammasomes: guardians of cytosolic sanctity. Immunol Rev. 2009;227:95-105.
16. Caruso R, Warner N, Inohara N, et al. NOD1 and NOD2: signaling, host defense, and inflammatory disease. Immunity. 2014;41:898-908.
17. Zipris D. Innate immunity and its role in type 1 diabetes. Curr Opin Endocrinol Diabetes Obes. 2008;15:326-31.
18. Li M, Song L, Gao X, et al. Toll-like receptor 4 on islet β cells senses expression changes in high-mobility group BOX 1 and contributes to the initiation of type 1 diabetes. Exp Mol Med. 2012;44:260-7.
19. Kruger B, Yin N, Zhang N, et al. Islet-expressed TLR2 and TLR4 sense injury and mediate early graft failure after transplantation. Eur J Immunol. 2010;40:2914-24.
20. Sarkar SA, Kutlu B, Velmurugan K, et al. Cytokine-mediated induction of anti-apoptotic genes that are linked to nuclear factor κ-B (NF-κB) signalling in human islets and in a mouse β cell line. Diabetologia. 2009;52: 1092-101.
21. Moran A, Bundy B, Becker DJ, et al. Interleukin-1 antagonism in type 1 diabetes of recent onset: two multicentre, randomised, double-blind, placebo-controlled trials. Lancet. 2013;381:1905-15.
22. Motta VN, Markle JG, Gulban O, et al. Identification of the inflammasome Nlrp1b as the candidate gene conferring diabetes risk at the Idd4.1 locus in the nonobese diabetic mouse. J Immunol. 2015;194:5663-73.
23. Fresno M, Alvarez R, Cuesta N. Toll-like receptors, inflammation, metabolism and obesity. Arch Physiol Biochem. 2011;117:151-64.
24. Tanti JF, Ceppo F, Jager J, et al. Implication of inflammatory signaling pathways in obesity-induced insulin resistance. Front Endocrinol. 2012;3:181.
25. Apostolopoulos V, de Courten MP, Stojanovska L et al. The complex immunological and inflammatory network of adipose tissue in obesity. Mol Nutr Food Res. 2016;60(1):43-57. [online] Available from http://dx.doi.org/10.1002/ mnfr.201500272.

26. Himes RW, Smith CW. Tlr2 is critical for diet-induced metabolic syndrome in a murine model. FASEB J. 2010;24:731-9.
27. Kuo LH, Tsai PJ, Jiang MJ, et al. Toll-like receptor 2 deficiency improves insulin sensitivity and hepatic insulin signalling in the mouse. Diabetologia. 2011;54:168-79.
28. Vitseva OI, Tanriverdi K, Tchkonia TT, et al. Inducible Toll-like receptor and NF-κB regulatory pathway expression in human adipose tissue. Obesity. 2008;16:932-7.
29. Velloso LA, Folli F, Saad MJ. TLR4 at the crossroads of nutrients, gut microbiota, and metabolic inflammation. Endocrine Rev. 2015;36:245-71.
30. Tsukumo DM, Carvalho-Filho MA, Carvalheira JB, et al. Loss-of-function mutation in Toll-like receptor 4 prevents diet-induced obesity and insulin resistance. Diabetes. 2007;56:1986-98.
31. Saberi M, Woods NB, de Luca C, et al. Hematopoietic cell-specific deletion of toll-like receptor 4 ameliorates hepatic and adipose tissue insulin resistance in high-fat-fed mice. Cell Metab. 2009;10:419-29.
32. Jia L, Vianna CR, Fukuda M, et al. Hepatocyte Toll-like receptor 4 regulates obesity-induced inflammation and insulin resistance. Nat Comm. 2014;5:3878.
33. Kiely A, Robinson A, McClenaghan NH, et al. Toll-like receptor agonist induced changes in clonal rat BRIN-BD11 -cell insulin secretion and signal transduction. J Endocrinol. 2009;202:365-73.
34. Hardy OT, Kim A, Ciccarelli C, et al. Increased Toll-like receptor (TLR) mRNA expression in monocytes is a feature of metabolic syndrome in adolescents. Pediatr Obes. 2013;8:e19-e23.
35. Pal D, Dasgupta S, Kundu R, et al. Fetuin-A acts as an endogenous ligand of TLR4 to promote lipid-induced insulin resistance. Nat Med. 2012;18:1279-85.
36. Nagareddy PR, Kraakman M, Masters SL, et al. Adipose tissue macrophages promote myelopoiesis and monocytosis in obesity. Cell Metab. 2014;19:821-35.
37. Caricilli AM, Picardi PK, de Abreu LL, et al. Gut microbiota is a key modulator of insulin resistance in TLR 2 knockout mice. PLoS Biol. 2011;9:e1001212.
38. Kellermayer R, Dowd SE, Harris RA, et al. Colonic mucosal DNA methylation, immune response, and microbiome patterns in Toll-like receptor 2-knockout mice. FASEB J. 2011;25:1449-60.
39. Kim KA, Gu W, Lee IA, et al. High fat diet-induced gut microbiota exacerbates inflammation and obesity in mice via the TLR4 signaling pathway. PLoS ONE. 2012;7:e47713.
40. Vijay-Kumar M, Aitken JD, Carvalho FA, et al. Metabolic syndrome and altered gut microbiota in mice lacking Toll-like receptor 5. Science. 2010;328:228-31.
41. Leichtle A, Hernandez M, Pak K, et al. TLR4-mediated induction of TLR2 signaling is critical in the pathogenesis and resolution of otitis media. Innate Immun. 2009;15:205-15.
42. Coope A, Milanski M, Arruda AP, et al. Chaperone insufficiency links TLR4 protein signaling to endoplasmic reticulum stress. J Biol Chem. 2012;287:15580-89.
43. Okla M, Wang W, Kang I, et al. Activation of Toll-like receptor (TLR) 4 attenuates adaptive thermogenesis via endoplasmic reticulum stress. J Biol Chem. [online] Available from http://dx.doi.org/ 10.1074/jbc. M115.677724 [Accessed October, 2018].
44. Oslowski CM, Hara T, O'Sullivan-Murphy B, et al. Thioredoxin-interacting protein mediates ER stress-induced β cell death through initiation of the inflammasome. Cell Metab. 2012;16:265-73.
45. Newsholme P, de Bittencourt PI. The fat cell senescence hypothesis: a mechanism responsible for abrogating the resolution of inflammation in chronic disease. Curr Opin Clin Nutr Metab Care. 2014;17(4):295-305.
46. Hotamisligil GS, Shargill NS, Spiegelman BM. Adipose expression of tumor necrosis factor-α: direct role in obesity-linked insulin resistance. Science. 1993;259(5091):87-91.
47. Hotamisligil GS, Peraldi P, Budavari A, et al. IRS-1-mediated inhibition of insulin receptor tyrosine kinase activity in TNF-α- and obesity-induced insulin resistance. Science. 1996;271(5249):665-8.
48. Tateya S, Kim F, Tamori Y. Recent advances in obesity induced inflammation and insulin resistance. Front Endocrinol. 2013;4:93.
49. Vandanmagsar B, Youm Y-H, Ravussin A, et al. The NLRP3 inflammasome instigates obesity-induced inflammation and insulin resistance. Nat Med. 2011;17(2):179-88.
50. Wen H, Gris D, Lei Y, et al. Fatty acid-induced NLRP3-ASC inflammasome activation interferes with insulin signaling. Nature Immunol. 2011;12(5): 408-15.
51. Masters SL, Dunne A, Subramanian SL, et al. Activation of the NLRP3 inflammasome by islet amyloid polypeptide provides a mechanism for enhanced IL-1beta 2 in type 2 diabetes. Nature Immunol. 2010;11(10):897-904.
52. Gao D, Nong S, Huang X, et al. The effects of palmitate on hepatic insulin resistance are mediated by NADPH oxidase 3-derived reactive oxygen species through JNK and p38 MAPK pathways. J Biol Chem. 2010;285(39):29965-73.
53. di Naso FC, Porto R, Fillmann H, et al. Obesity depresses the anti-inflammatory HSP70 pathway, contributing to NAFLD progression. Obesity (Silver Spring). 2015;23(1):120-29.
54. Masters SL, Latz E, O'Neill LA. The inflammasome in atherosclerosis and type 2 diabetes. Science Translational Medicine. 2011;3(81):Article ID81ps17.
55. Eguchi K, Manabe I, Oishi-Tanaka Y, et al. Saturated fatty acid and TLR signaling link β cell dysfunction and islet inflammation. Cell Metabol. 2012;15(4):518-33.
56. Gurzov EN, Eizirik DL. Bcl-2 proteins in diabetes: mitochondrial pathways of beta-cell death and dysfunction. Trend Cell Biol. 2011;21(7):424-31.
57. Størling J, Binzer J, Andersson AK, et al. Nitric oxide contributes to cytokine-induced apoptosis in pancreatic beta cells via potentiation of JNK activity and inhibition of Akt. Diabetologia. 2005;48(10):2039-50.

Chapter 2

Heavy Metals, Diabetes and Cardiovascular Risk

Sanjiv Shah, Trupti Kulkarni, Vikrant Tari

INTRODUCTION

There is an epidemiological evidence that exposure to metal pollutants, such as arsenic, lead, cadmium and mercury, plays a role in the development of atherosclerosis and cardiovascular mortality, thus creating a new risk factor for cardiovascular disease (CVD).[1] Recently in a secondary prevention trial, a metal chelator had an unexpected positive result in reducing cardiovascular events, which created the relationship between metal exposure and CVD. This chapter focuses on the four toxic, xenobiotic metals listed in Toxic Substances and Disease Registry Priority List of Hazardous.

How does Human Get Exposed to Metals?

Heavy metals are found naturally in environment, which can make their way into the food we eat. To eliminate them entirely from our food is not possible because these metals are found in the air, water and soil. Heavy metal fumes and aerosols released into the atmosphere can return by way of precipitation and contaminate the soil and surface water. These residues can be directly taken up by the plants grown on the soil, or alternatively deposited on leaves and fruits and then consumed and absorbed.[2] There is a direct relationship between atmospheric metal deposition and elevated concentrations of heavy metals in plants and top soil. Hence, cultivation areas near highways have higher atmospheric pollution in the form of metal containing aerosols. The high burden of environmental pollution in developed countries is due to high level of resource consumption, while in developing country, like India, it is due to outdated technologies, overexploitation of natural resources, and weak environmental regulations and enforcement.

The toxic elements can also enter the human body, to a lesser extent by inhalation of polluted air, use of cosmetics like talcum powder, lipsticks, shampoos, "kajal" and hair colors, and even items like toys, which have paints containing lead.[3]

METAL EXPOSURE AND COMPLEMENTARY MEDICINE (HERBAL)

All clinicians have seen occasional patient in practice, detected to have arsenic or lead in blood samples. This kind of exposure through alternative drugs, poor-quality herbal formulations, particularly "Ayurveda/Siddha bhasmas" herbomineral preparations, folk remedies, and "Unani". These herbal medicines are prescribed by the respective specialists or self-medicated by patients. It is not infrequent to see the patients with acute enal injury (CKD) due to toxic metal exposure.[4]

IMPACT OF INDUSTRIALIZATION ON HUMAN METAL EXPOSURE

Industrialization is also responsible for heavy metal-induced injury to our system. Heavy metal depositions are associated with a wide range of sources such as small-scale industries, including battery production, metal products, metal smelting and cable-coating industries, brick kilns, vehicular emissions, resuspended road dust and diesel generator sets. Coal combustion also has high heavy metal contents. Lead exposure occurs through gasoline additives, food can solder, E-waste, coal-based thermal power plants, ceramic glazes, drinking water system, lead–acid batteries, bangle industry and battery/plastic recycling industry. With the use of unleaded petrol, however, the burden of lead has reduced.

The production of compact fluorescent lamp bulbs has increased 25-folds within a decade. Each bulb has 3–12 mg of mercury, with no system to recover these bulbs and process for its safe disposal; they enter the body through food in the form of methyl mercury. Dental fillings, fluorescent lamps, and hospital waste (damaged thermometers, barometers and sphygmomanometers) also contribute to mercury contamination of soil and water bodies, absorbed by fishes, thereby entering the human food chain.[6]

METALS AND TISSUE DAMAGE

Environmental exposure to heavy metals, e.g. lead, mercury, arsenic and cadmium, is potentially alarming and harmful for human health. These metals get deposited in tissues and are nondegradable. There is a threshold for tissues to tolerate certain amount of metals after which the tissues get damaged. These heavy metals react with certain proteins in the body and modify their functions and kinetics, more frequently by oxidative damage.[5] They induce β-cell damage and accelerate the process of atherosclerosis. Some of these toxic metals like nickel and arsenic are also classified as carcinogens.

MECHANISM OF DIABETES DUE TO HEAVY METALS

Heavy metals may increase risk of type 2 diabetes mellitus. Different toxic metals have different levels of toxicities in pancreatic islet cells and can lead to early apoptosis of β-cells.[6] Disturbance in balance between healthy trace metals and heavy metals may impact the pancreatic β-cell function.[7]

It is a well-known fact that heavy and toxic metals have the ability to induce oxidative stress through increase in production of reactive oxygen species (ROS) like superoxide radicals, hydrogen peroxide and nitric oxide, which are highly reactive in nature, and this increase in ROS generation can lead to β-cell death.[8] Toxic metal-induced oxidative stress can also decrease insulin gene promoter activity and insulin mRNA expression in pancreatic β-cells.[9] These pancreatic β-cells have high expression for metal transporters and low expression for antioxidants, resulting in a weak antioxidant defense system in β-cells, which results in higher sensitivity to heavy metals leading to β-cell dysfunction or death.[10] Lead toxicity can lead to diabetes by generation of ROS and derangement of antioxidant pathways or lead getting used instead of zinc, in presence of zinc deficiency.[10]

Cadmium in high concentration can downregulate glucose transporter 4 (GLUT-4) translocation by insulin and may cause pancreatic β-cell damage by degranulation of β-cells and decreasing β-cell viability.[11]

Frequent exposures of arsenic can disrupt glucose metabolism due to alteration in cell-signaling transduction factors like tumor necrosis factor-α and mitogen-activated protein kinase, which in turn can lead to arrest of GLUT-4 translocation and can lead to β-cell dysfunction.[11]

Mercury inhibits magnesium and zinc levels as well as inhibiting glucose transfer is other mechanism by which mercury and cadmium can cause metabolic syndrome and insulin resistance. Mercury also induces mitochondrial dysfunction with reduction in adenosine triphosphate, depletion of glutathione and increased lipid peroxidation, which then increases oxidative stress and promotes atherosclerosis and CVDs.[12]

LEAD AND CARDIOVASCULAR DISEASE

After entering the body, 99% of lead binds to red blood cells and 1% remains in the serum. The half-life of lead in the bloodstream is 36 days; while in bones, it is 20–30 years. Weisskopf et al. analyzed 868 male participants of the Veterans Affairs Normative Aging Study and showed the association between patella and tibia lead with mortality,[13] even after multivariable adjustments. The participants in the third tertile were more likely to die from all causes [hazard ratio (HR) 2.52, P = 0.02], from cardiovascular causes (HR 5.63, p = 0.003), and nearly ten times more likely to die from ischemic heart disease (HR 8.37, p = 0.01). The National Health and Nutrition Examination Survey II (NHANES II) reported increased circulatory mortality [relative risk (RR) 1.39] in subjects with blood lead levels of 20–29 μg/dL compared to those having levels below 10 μg/dL and increased prevalence of peripheral artery disease (PAD) in presence of higher lead level.

Menke et al. studied follow-up of 13,946 adults of the NHANES III survey for 12 years and showed higher risk of cardiovascular events in participants in higher tertile of lead level, compared with those in the lowest tertile. All-cause mortality was higher by 25% (HR 1.25), while cardiovascular mortality was higher (HR 1.55), mortality from myocardial infarction was higher (HR 1.89), and mortality from stroke was higher by more than twofold (HR 2.51).[14]

There is an association of lead exposure with slight increase in blood pressure. Meta-analyses of 60 studies showed that a doubling of blood lead was associated with a modest increase in systolic blood pressure (SBP) of 1.0–1.25 mm Hg and diastolic blood pressure (DBP) of 0.6 mm Hg.

Lead exposure has also been linked to dyslipidemia and atherosclerosis.[4] There is an association between lead exposure and aortic atherosclerotic plaque burden in human autopsy studies. The cardioprotective antioxidant activity of high-density lipoprotein (HDL) is partially mediated by paraoxonase, an enzyme closely bound to the HDL particle and involved in inhibition of low-density lipoprotein (LDL) oxidation. Lead and other metals, by inactivation of paraoxonase, promote LDL oxidation and atherosclerosis development.[12]

CADMIUM AND CARDIOVASCULAR DISEASE

Cadmium is associated with cardiovascular and all-cause mortality. Menke et al. reported increase in risk of cardiovascular mortality (HR 1.21) and coronary artery disease (CAD)-associated mortality (HR 1.36) with higher cadmium exposure. In a review by Tellez-Plaza et al., the pooled analysis of 12 studies, RRs for CVD, CAD, stroke, and PAD were 1.36, 1.30, 1.18 and 1.49, respectively.[15] Cadmium has also been associated with PAD in both men and women. Participants in the 90th percentile of blood cadmium distribution had 1–3 mm Hg higher SBP and DBP levels compared to participants in the 10th percentile of blood cadmium distribution.[15]

MERCURY AND CARDIOVASCULAR EFFECTS

The relationship between mercury exposure is confounded by fish consumption, where both have opposing risk impact on cardiovascular risk. In 1995, Salonen et al. reported an association between high levels of mercury exposure through fish consumption and risk of CVD (2.9), acute myocardial infarction (MI) (1.69), and all-cause mortality (2.3). The finding on relationship between mercury exposure and blood pressure changes was inconsistent.[16]

CHELATION PRACTICE IN TACT TRIAL

Pharmaceuticals that chelate metal ions are chelators, which mobilize the metals from tissues and eliminate in the urine or in the bile via liver.

Chelation in a landmark trial involved multiple administrations of an edetate disodium-based infusion with other components including vitamin C, vitamin B, heparin, electrolytes, and procaine. In addition, high doses of oral antioxidant vitamins and minerals were recommended to be taken with the intravenous chelation treatment.[17]

A total of 37% patients (633) in Trial to Assess Chelation Therapy (TACT) had diabetes, whose beneficial findings are described here. Edetate disodium treatment reduced the RR of the primary endpoint by 41% over 5 years. The principal secondary endpoint, cardiovascular death, or recurrent MI or stroke occurred in 17% of placebo and 11% of edetate disodium treated patients, a 40% relative reduction in risk (p = 0.017). There was a 52% relative reduction in the risk of recurrent MI among patients with diabetes (p = 0.015), and a 43% relative reduction in the risk of death from any cause in patients with diabetes (p = 0.011). There was no effect on glycemic control during the course of initial 30 infusions.[18] To investigate the chelating effect of edetate disodium, Waters et al. replicated an infusion of edetate disodium similar to that used in TACT trial, showed the 24-hour urinary excretion of lead over 2 days increased by 3,830% and of cadmium by 514%, by mobilizing lead and cadmium from their chronic tissue storage compartments into the urine.[19]

Another trial on chelators has been recently funded by National Institutes of Health.

REFERENCES

1. Solenkova NV, Newman JD, Berger JS, et al. Metal pollutants and cardiovascular disease: mechanisms and consequences of exposure. Am Heart J. 2014;168:812-22.
2. Vouts D, Grimanis A, Samara C. Trace elements in vegetables grown in an industrial area in relation to soil and air particulate matter. Environ Pollut. 1996;94:325-35.
3. Indian National Science Academy. (2001) Hazardous metals and mineral pollution in India: sources, toxicity and management., [online] Available from http://insaindia.res.in/pdf/Hazardous_Metals.pdf [Accessed September, 2018].
4. Lunyera J, Smith SR. Heavy metal nephropathy: considerations for exposure analysis. Kidney Int. 2017;92:548-50.
5. Stohs SJ, Bagchi D. Oxidative mechanisms in the toxicity of metal ions. Free Radic Biol Med. 1995;18(2):321-36.
6. Khan AR, Awan FR. Metals in the pathogenesis of type 2 diabetes. J Diabetes Metab Disord. 2014;13(1):16.
7. Siddiqui K, Bawazeer N, Joy SS. Variation in macro and trace elements in progression of type 2 diabetes. Scientific World Journal. 2014;2014: 461591.
8. Sharma B, Singh S, Siddiqi NJ. Biomedical implications of heavy metals induced imbalances in redox systems. Biomed Res Int. 2014;2014: 640754.
9. Valko M, Morris H, Cronin MT. Metals, toxicity and oxidative stress. Curr Med Chem. 2005;12(10):1161-208.

10. Afridi HI, Kazi TG, Kazi N, et al. Evaluation of status of toxic metals in biological samples of diabetes mellitus patients. Diabetes Res Clin Pract. 2008;80(2):280-8.
11. Chen YW, Yang CY, Huang CF, et al. Heavy metals, islet function and diabetes development. Islets. 2009;1(3):169-76.
12. Gonzalvo MC, Gil F, Hernandez AF, et al. Inhibition of paraoxonase activity in human liver microsomes by exposure to EDTA, metals and mercurials. Chem Biol Interact. 1997;105:169-79.
13. Weisskopf MG, Jain N, Nie H, et al. A prospective study of bone lead concentration and death from all causes, cardiovascular diseases, and cancer in the Department of Veterans Affairs Normative Aging Study. Circulation. 2009;120(12):1056-64.
14. Solenkova NV, Newman JD, Berger JS, et al. Metal Pollutants and Cardiovascular Disease: Mechanisms and Consequences of Exposure. Am Heart J. 2014;168(6):812-22.
15. Tellez-Plaza M, Jones MR, Dominguez-Lucas A, et al. Cadmium exposure and clinical cardiovascular disease: a systematic review. Curr Atheroscler Rep. 2013;15(10):356.
16. Salonen JT, Seppanen K, Nyyssonen K, et al. Intake of mercury from fish, lipid peroxidation, and the risk of myocardial infarction and coronary, cardiovascular, and any death in eastern Finnish men. Circulation. 1995;91(3):645-55.
17. Lamas GA, Goertz C, Boineau R, et al. Design of the Trial to Assess Chelation Therapy (TACT). Am Heart J. 2012;163:7-12.
18. Escolar E, Lamas GA, Mark DB, et al. The effect of an EDTA-based chelation regimen on patients with diabetes mellitus and prior myocardial infarction in the Trial to Assess Chelation Therapy (TACT). Circ Cardiovasc Qual Outcomes. 2014;7:15-24.
19. Waters RS, Bryden NA, Patterson KY, et al. EDTA chelation effects on urinary losses of cadmium, calcium, chromium, cobalt, copper, lead, magnesium, and zinc. Biol Trace Elem Res. 2001;83:207-221.

Chapter 3

Toll-like Receptor in Diabetic Vascular Endothelium Dysfunction

Santosh Kumar Yadav, Richik Tripathi, Kamlakar Tripathi

INTRODUCTION

Toll-like receptors (TLRs) are cell receptors which have significant role in innate immune response in regulating damage associated molecular patterns in type 2 diabetes mellitus (T2DM). Production of cytokines and expression of other adhesion molecules is closely link with its activation and tissue damage.[1] TLR-2 perform key role in the initiation of innate immune response through a myeloid differentiation factor primary responce 88 (MyD88)-dependent pathway. In last two decades enough evidences have confirmed the suppression role of TLR-2 and ligand interaction on immune response.[2]

Toll-like receptor activation in diabetes alters vascular endothelium and remodeling of diabetes induced endothelium damage of macro- and microvascular system. These molecular event prime antigen specific adaptive immune response. Since, cardiovascular system has been recognized as a low chronic inflammation state and in diabetes molecular interaction with proinflammatory cytokine play determinant role in vascular endothelial damage, TLR inhibition and agonist have emerged as a potential therapeutic agent for prevention and treatment vascular complication in diabetes.

STRUCTURE AND FUNCTION OF TOLL-LIKE RECEPTORS

Toll-like receptor was identified for the first time in *Drosophila melanogaster in 1985 by Christiane Nüsslein-Volhard and Eric Wieschaus,* where it was shown as mutant gene of "Toll receptor". The *Toll* gene word was coined from German word "Wow" and found to be closely related to human Toll receptor. This was identified with a different name of TLR4 and subsequently continued to be known as TLR. These receptors are class of pattern recognition receptors (PRRs) who are known to play crucial role in innate immune system. These are germ line encoded host sensors who detect molecules during pathogenesis of inflammation.

TABLE 1: Distribution of different mammalian ligands and genomes.

TLR Family	TLR gene having similar genomic structure
1	TLR1, TLR-2, TLR6, TLR10
3	TLR3
4	TLR4
5	TLR5
7	TLR7, TLR8, TLR9
11	mTLR11, mTLR12, mTLR13

(TLR: Toll-like receptor.)

Toll-like receptors are transmembrane glycoprotein comprising of an amino terminal N that contain leucine-rich repeat and ligand recognition in a domain extending to carboxyl terminal 'C'. There are ten *TLR* genes in human being reported which belongs to mammalian TLR families (Table 1) and further 11 and 12 have also been added in vascular endothelial damage.

Many peptidoglycan, lipopeptide, flagellin protein and profiling protein specifically bind their ligands on TLRs which is present on its intracellular surface of plasma membrane as shown in Figure 1.

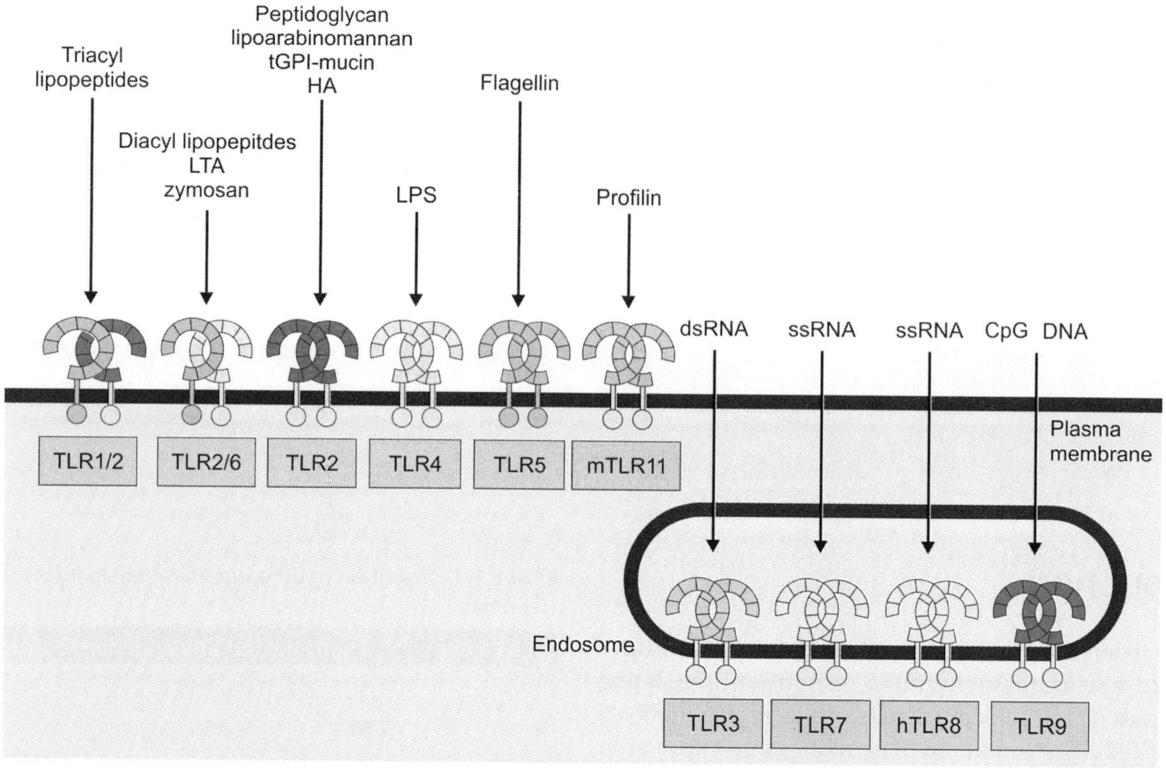

(DNA: deoxyribonucleic acid; dsRNA: double-stranded ribonucleic acid; HA: hemagglutinin; LPS: lipopolysaccharide; LTA: lipoteichoic acid; ssRNA: single-stranded ribonucleic acid; TLR: Toll-like receptor.)

Figure 1 Toll-like receptors and its intracellular surface with their ligands.

Toll-like Receptor 2

Toll-like receptor-2 mediated by cytokine CD282 was firstly discovered in 1998. The recognition of this cell receptor activated by MYD88-dependent pathway triggering signals nuclear factor kappa beta (NF-kβ) and mitogen-activated protein (MAP) kinase. It is located on short-arm of chromosome 4 (4p32) in *TLR* gene. This type 1 transmembrane protein has similar structure of extracellular leucine-rich repeat domain. TLR-2 is expressed in macrophage, dendritic cell, nonimmune cell type, epithelial cell line and hepatocyte.

The TLR-2 recognizes its ligands in lipopolysaccharide, lipoprotein, bacterial peptide glycan and glycoprotein. TLR-2 ligand interactions activate MYD88-dependent signaling pathways result activation of proinflammatory cytokine and subsequently reactivation of phosphorylation which induces the phosphoinositide 3-kinase (P13K)-pathway for up regulation of cytokine interleukin (IL) 10, resulting in modulation of immune responses by TLR-2.

There are several adaptor proteins and signaling molecule associated with TLR as shown in Figure 2.

Type 2 Diabetes and Toll-like Receptor-2

Zymogen activation of TLR-2 results into reactive oxygen species (ROS) production by neutrophils. This is dependent on TLR-2 nicotinamide adenine dinucleotide phosphate, (NADPH) oxidase but independent on mitogen-activated protein kinases (MAPK).[3] Hyperglycemia and chronic periodontitis also upregulate TLR-2 in the gingival tissue and initiate impaired glucose tolerance (IGT). It has been demonstrated that insulin suppresses the expression of TLR-2 by mitochondrial ribonucleic acid (mRNA) through down-regulation.[4] Kuzmicki et al. have shown that the gestational diabetic mothers had significantly higher TLR-2 expression than normal pregnant women.[5] Interestingly, TLR-2 was also found to be up-regulated in women who have normal glucose tolerance but later become diabetic when compared to the women having normoglycemia. Expression levels of TLR-2 were up-regulated in obese women who later developed diabetes individually. Ahamed et al. showed that obese type 2 diabetes patients had higher expressions of TLR-2 than obese patients without diabetes. Further diabetic patients were also found to have upregulated TLR-2.[6]

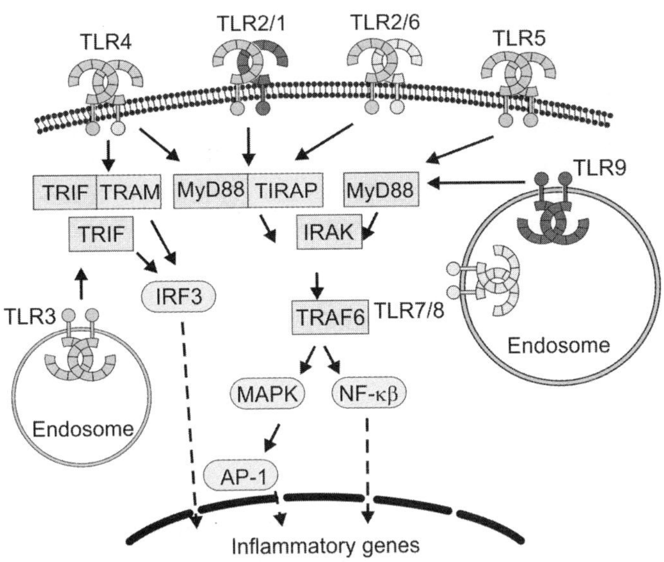

(AP1: activator protein-1; IRAK: interleukin-1 receptor-associated kinase; IRF3: interferon regulatory transcription factor; MAPK: mitogen-activated protein kinases; MyD88: myeloid differentiation factor 88; NF-kβ: nuclear factor kappa beta; TIRAP: Toll-like receptor adaptor protein; TLR: Toll-like receptor; TRIF: TIR-domain-containing adapter-inducing interferon-β; TRAM: TRIF-related adaptor molecule.)

Figure 2 Toll-like receptors, adapter proteins and signaling molecules.

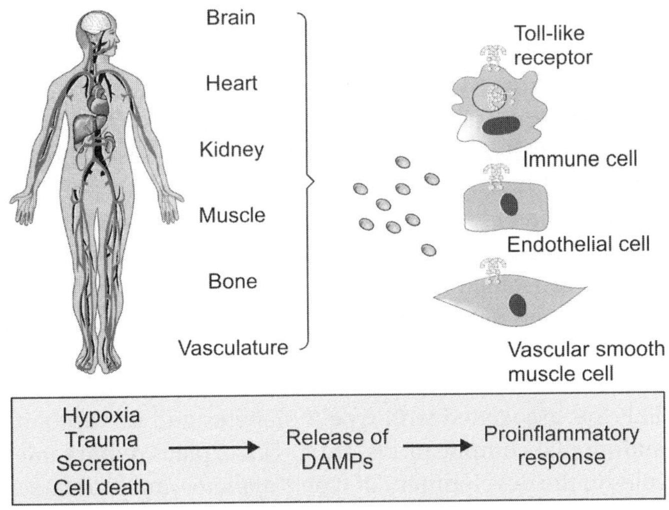

(DAMPs: damage-associated molecular patterns.)

Figure 3 Damage-associated molecular pattern-induced activation of Toll-like receptors.

Apart from regulating innate immune response, TLR-2 also participates in the development of type 2 diabetes and also involved in the pathogenesis of diabetes-related vascular complications.[7] Upregulation of IL-6 and osteopontin, TLR-2 induced impaired insulin-mediated brain activities is an early step in the development of type 2 diabetes.[8] In patients of chronic periodontitis higher level of mRNA of TLR-2 has been demonstrated than healthy individual having periodontal disease. Hence, TLR-2 is an established marker of T2DM in periodontitis patients. Free fatty acids and high glucose levels up-regulates the expression of TLR-2 and TLR-6, which enhances activity of coenocytes and production of superoxides, NF-kβ-dependent superoxide.[9] This is based upon damage-associated molecular pattern (DAMP) which is induced by TLR-2 receptor in diabetic patients which promoted proinflammatory response as shown in Figure 3.

Inflammation induced by free fatty acids has a significant role in the induction of inflammation in pancreatic beta-cells via TLR-2.[10] There are evidences that these receptors have not only been expressed on the immune cells of type 2 diabetes patients than on those of healthy subjects, but also at the levels of TLR-2 ligands, including hyaluronan, heat-shock protein 70 (HSP60), HSP70, high mobility group box 1 protein (HMGB1), and endotoxin.[11] TLR-2 antisense oligonucleotide leads to recovery of insulin sensitivity and signaling in muscle on mice that were fed a high-fat diet.[12] The oxidized low-density lipoprotein (LDL), which is produced during type 2 diabetes, induces expression of TLR-2 in macrophages and monocytes of obese women who showed higher expression on TLR-2.[13]

The TLR-2 recognizes pathogen-associated molecular patterns (PAMPs) such as exogenous microbial ligands, hence it is hypothesized that bacterial, viral and parasitic infections could play an important factors in the development of type 2 diabetes and may also participate in the pathogenesis of the disease. Ajuwon et al. demonstrated that peptidoglycan derived from *Staphylococcus aureus* resulted in the elevated TLR-2 expression on the 3T3-L1 adipocytes cell lines.[14] The treating agents who improve glycemic control have shown decreased expressions of TLR-2 and its related molecular signaling. There are evidences that decreased methylation is associated with higher expression of the gene, especially CpGs methylation in the promoter of the *TLR-2* gene which was decreased in type 2 diabetes patients.[15]

Other studies have verified that TLR-2 expression is decreased during type 2 diabetes. Cortez-Espinosa et al. showed that the percentage of TLR-2 positive monocytes is decreased in type 2 diabetes patients who have poor glycemic control than well-controlled patients. Although type 2 diabetes patients had higher serum levels of IL-6, the mRNA levels of TLR-2 have been found to be on lower side than in healthy subjects.[16] Thus, these invitro studies demonstrate that high glucose levels lead to reduced expression of TLR-2. Insulin in higher dose of more than 100 IU/mL may also increase IL-6 and decrease TLR-2 expression.[17] Thus, it has been shown that TLR-4 but not TLR-2 interaction with corresponded ligands leads to pancreatic beta-cell apoptosis.[18] The S6 kinase beta-1 (S6K1) has significant role in developing insulin resistance and pathogenesis of type 2 diabetes. Upregulation of S6K1 causes key role in reduction of NF-kβ and activating protein-1 activities by TLR-2 ligand interactions.[19] Maximum studies have reported that TLR-2 is associated with type 2 diabetes and its vascular endothelial complications. Thus, TLR-2 plays remarkable roles in the development of type 2 diabetes and its related complications. Modulating expression of TLR-2 and its related signaling molecules may result in innovation of developing novel approaches for the treatment of T2DM and prevention of macro- and microangiopathic complications.

Toll-like Receptor, Insulin Resistance and Atherothrombosis

In type 2 diabetes, insulin resistance plays an important role which develops in multiple organs, including skeletal muscle, liver, adipose tissue and heart. The onset of diabetes starts much earlier with beginning of insulin resistance and obesity plays a pivotal role in the phenomenon providing an important link between type 2 diabetes and fat deposition in liver, adipose tissue and skeletal muscle.

Type 2 diabetes with increased obesity has increased plasma levels of the inflammatory marker. Free fatty acid binds TLR activating NF-kβ through inhibitor of nuclear factor kappa-B (IKKB)-kinase. NF-kβ triggered inhibitory degradation complex lead to up-regulation of inflammatory gene *IL-6* and tumor necrosis factor (TNF).

Free fatty acids activating TLR leads to phosphorylation of insulin receptor substrate (IRS)-1 by amino-terminal kinase protein kinase C (PKC) and c-Jun N-terminal Kinase (JNK). It alters the ability to activate PI3K and down-regulation of the gene glucose transporter (*GLUT-4*) and insulin resistance initiate vascular dysfunction of type 2 diabetes. Downregulation of PI3K leads to nitric oxide synthase (NOS) inhibition and result in decreased nitric oxide (NO) production. Together with reducing NO synthesis, intracellular oxidation of stored free fatty acids generate ROS leading to vascular inflammation, age synthesis, reduced prostaglandin I2 (PGI2) synthase activity and PKC activation.

The alteration in vascular homeostasis due to endothelium and smooth muscle dysfunction is the main feature of diabetic vasculopathy favoring a proinflammatory state which ultimately leads to atherosclerosis. Early dysglycemia caused by obesity-related insulin resistance or impaired insulin secretion is responsible for the function and structural alteration of the vessel wall culminating with diabetic vascular complication.

CONCLUSION

Toll-like receptor-2 induces the creation of several molecules including ROS and proinflammatory cytokines, which contributes the pathogenesis of type 2 diabetes and related complications. The expression of TLR-2 directly correlates with elevated serum levels of free fatty acids and blood glucose in addition to obesity. Some exogenous and endogenous ligands induce the activation of immune cells and the dysfunction of pancreatic beta-cells in a TLR-2-initiated pathway-dependent manner. Different genetic variations and methylation play important roles in the up-regulation of TLR-2 in type 2 diabetes patients. Upregulation of insulin is an important mechanism that suppresses the expression of TLR. The activation of TLR-2-initiated pathways hypothesized that infection can be considered a key candidate for the development of type 2 diabetes and its related complications.

REFERENCES

1. Bhatelia K, Singh K, Singh R. TLRs: Linking inflammation and breast cancer. Cell Signal. 2014;26:2350-7.
2. Bagheri V, Askari A, Arababadi MK, et al. Can Toll-Like Receptor (TLR) 2 be considered as a new target for immunotherapy against hepatitis B infection? Hum Immunol. 2014;75:549-54.
3. Fagundes-Netto F, Anjos P, Volpe C, et al. The production of reactive oxygen species in TLR-stimulated granulocytes is not enhanced by hyperglycemia in diabetes. Int Immunopharm. 2013;17:924-9.
4. Ghanim H, Mohanty P, Deopurkar R, et al. Acute modulation of toll-like receptors by insulin. Diabetes Care. 2008;31:1827-31.
5. Kuzmicki M, Telejko B, Wawrusiewicz-Kurylonek N, et al. The expression of genes involved in NF-kB activation in peripheral blood mononuclear cells of patients with gestational diabetes. Eur J Endocrin. 2013;168:419-27.
6. Ahmad R, Al-Mass A, Atizado V, et al. Elevated expression of the Toll-like receptors 2 and 4 in obese individuals: its significance for obesity-induced inflammation. J Inflamm (Lond). 2012;9:48.
7. Jialal I, Kaur H. The role of toll-like receptors in diabetes-induced inflammation: implications for vascular complications. Curr Diab Rep. 2012;12:172-9.

8. Duarte PM, Szeremeske-Miranda T, Lima JA, et al. Expression of immune inflammatory markers in sites of chronic periodontitis in patients with type 2 diabetes. J Periodontol. 2012;83:426-34.
9. Dasu MR, Jialal I. Free fatty acids in the presence of high glucose amplify monocyte inflammation via Toll-like receptors. Am J Physio-Endocrinol Metab. 2011;300:E145-54.
10. Boni-Schnetzler M, Boller S, Debray S, et al. Free fatty acids induce a proinflammatory response in islets via the abundantly expressed interleukin-1 receptor I. Endocrinol. 2009;150:5218-29.
11. Dasu MR, Devaraj S, Park S, et al. Increased toll-like receptor (TLR) activation and TLR ligands in recently diagnosed type 2 diabetic subjects. Diabetes Care. 2010;33:861-8.
12. Caricilli AM, Nascimento PH, Pauli JR, et al. Inhibition of toll-like receptor 2 expression improves insulin sensitivity and signaling in muscle and white adipose tissue of mice fed a high-fat diet. J Endocrinol. 2008;199:399-406.
13. Holvoet P. Relations between metabolic syndrome, oxidative stress and inflammation and cardiovascular disease. Verhandelingen-Koninklijke Acad Geneeskunde Belgie. 2007;70:193-219.
14. Ajuwon KM, Banz W, Winters TA. Stimulation with Peptidoglycan induces interleukin 6 and TLR-2 expression and a concomitant down regulation of expression of adiponectin receptors 1 and 2 in 3 T3-L1 adipocytes. J Inflam. 2009;6:8.
15. Rozenberg JM, Tesfu DB, Musunuri S, et al. DNA methylation of a GC repressor element in the smooth muscle myosin heavy chain promoter facilitates binding of the notch-associated transcription factor, recombination signal binding protein for immunoglobulin k J Region/CSL1. Arterio Thromb Vasc Biol. 2014;34:2624-31.
16. Cortez-Espinosa N, Garcia-Hernandez MH, Reynaga-Hernandez E, et al. Abnormal expression and function of Dectin-1 receptor in type 2 diabetes mellitus patients with poor glycemic control (HbA1c > 8 %). Metabolism. 2012;61:1538-46.
17. Bernal-Lopez M, Llorente-Cortes V, Calleja F, et al. Effect of different degrees of impaired glucose metabolism on the expression of inflammatory markers in monocytes of patients with atherosclerosis. Acta Diabetol. 2013;50:553-62.
18. Lee SM, Choi SE, Lee JH, et al. Involvement of the TLR4 (Toll-like receptor4) signaling pathway in palmitate-induced INS-1 beta cell death. Mol Cell Biochem. 2011;354:207-17.
19. Kim SY, Baik KH, Baek KH, et al. S6K1 Negatively Regulates TAK1 Activity in the Toll-Like Receptor Signaling Pathway. Mol Cell Biol. 2014;34:510-21.

Chapter 4

Asian Phenotype and Diabetes Mellitus

Mala Dharmalingam, Ashish Reddy

INTRODUCTION

The differences in expression of disorders in health and diseases between Asians and non-Asians (Caucasians) are possibly what characterize the Asian phenotype. These differences are seen in expression of both the phenotype and the genotype across the whole life cycle and may be a continuum. This is a fallback of origin of the different races; the Asians were present in the earlier times, while the Caucasians are by far a newer race. This is particularly important as it has implications of management both in terms of prevention and management. It also opens realms of research to further science.[1] This along with the environmental and lifestyle changes has brought about an advent of disorders with long-reaching consequences.

Though there are many disorders unique to the Asian phenotype, disorders of insulin resistance (IR) with the risk of developing diabetes are the one most studied. This risk of developing type 2 diabetes mellitus (T2DM) has been noticed both in the native and migrant population of India and Southeast Asia. The most notable differences are the younger age of occurrence, lower body mass index (BMI), more visceral fat, the risk of coronary artery and cerebrovascular disease and renal complications. The risk is higher in Asians compared when compared with Caucasians counterparts even after adjusting for other variables.

EPIDEMIOLOGY

The intermediate distribution frame data puts the prevalence of diabetes at 451 million in 2017 with Southeast Asians contributing 83.6 million. The speculated increase in 2045 is 693 million, with Southeast Asians contributing around 155.6 million. The worrisome factor is that the steep increase is seen majorly in India, while the other regions do not show an increase or only a mild increase.[2] India contributes to 72.9 million which is second to China; however, this will almost double to 134.3 million by 2045 with a very small increase in China making India the world's capital of diabetes.

About 35.5 million diabetics are undiagnosed in India.[2] South Asian populations not only have a high prevalence of diabetes, but also of prediabetes and a more rapid progression to diabetes. Anjana et al. have shown the conversion to diabetes from prediabetes to be around 59% after a follow-up of 9.1 years.[3] The prevalence of gestational diabetes mellitus is also more in Asians, with a crude prevalence of 23.1%.[4]

Asians have higher risk for the development of diabetes for the same level of BMI or waist circumference than their Caucasian counterpart. The reasons attributed to this has been increased IR.[5] Even in relatively lean subjects, Asians are more insulin resistant than non-Asians with increased concentrations of free fatty acids (FFAs) and inflammatory markers.[6] The visceral fat is also much more. Asians exhibit higher glucose excursion during oral glucose challenge, suggesting lower β-cell function than non-Asians. These biological differences put Asians at high risk of developing diabetes in the presence of external stressors, such as obesity.[7] Some risk factors for T2DM have become of great concern among the developing countries in Asia. The increased prevalence of diabetes is related to changes in dietary pattern, sedentary behavior and obesity superimposed on a background of genetic/epigenetic susceptibility. Clinical features in Asian populations with diabetes are given in Box 1.[8]

Box 1: Clinical features in Asian populations.

- Low body mass index
- Increased body fat and especially visceral fat
- High rate of central obesity and metabolic syndrome
- Increased inflammatory markers such as TNF-α, IL-6 and CRP
- Insufficient β-cell response to counter insulin resistance
- Low rate of autoimmune type 1 diabetes
- High rates of young-onset type 2 diabetes
- High rate of childhood obesity
- High rate of gestational diabetes
- Higher triglycerides, small dense LDL and lower HDL levels
- Increased leptin and decreased adiponectin
- Increase risk of complications of diabetes

(CRP: C-reactive protein; HDL: high-density lipoprotein; IL6: interleukin 6; LDL: low-density lipoprotein; TNF: tumor necrosis factor.)

Genetic Factors

Diabetes is predominantly due to genetic factors. The prevalence of glucose intolerance in family members and siblings is commonly seen. In South Asians, the Pro12Ala polymorphism of the peroxisome proliferator activator g (*PPARg*) gene is present at the same frequency as Caucasians; however, the protective effect seen in Caucasians has not been uniformly observed in Asians and was not associated with a decreased risk of T2DM.[9] However, a study on Asian Indian Sikhs did see a protective effect of the polymorphism, suggesting that there might be differences between specific South Asian groups.[10]

In South Asians, the FTO polymorphism was found to be associated with T2DM, independently of BMI, implying that in South Asians, there may be a different relationship between BMI and T2DM.[11] Polymorphism in transcription factor-like protein which is associated with T2DM is also seen in Asians. The thrifty phenotype and thrifty genotype may also be responsible in Asians.

Insulin Resistance

South Asians have higher fasting insulin concentrations compared with other ethnic groups regardless of age, gender, or BMI, suggesting a higher rate of IR in this population.[12] Hyperinsulinemic euglycemic clamp studies performed in men and women of all age groups and relatively normal BMI show lower insulin sensitivity (up to almost 50%) in South Asians compared with different ethnic populations.[12] IR has been observed in childhood as well.

Diet and Exercise

The South Asian diet, characterized by high intake of carbohydrates, trans fats, and saturated fats, is associated with increased risk of development of T2DM.[13] Asians appear to have greater glycemic excursion to white rice compared with other populations.[14] STARCH study shows that total and complex carbohydrate (CHO) constitutes 64.1 % of total energy from diet in T2DM participants higher than that recommended in India.[15] Lack of physical activity is another risk factor for T2DM.Majority of South Asians were inactive during their leisure time.[16]

MARKERS OF INSULIN RESISTANCE

Body Mass Index

Asians develop diabetes at a considerably lower BMI compared with Europeans.[17] This is mainly because of increased visceral adiposity in Asian populations. As a result, in Asians, lower BMI cut-offs are being used to define obesity as well as lower waist circumference for defining central obesity. Criteria are a healthy BMI of 18.0–22.9 kg/m^2, an overweight BMI of 23.0–24.9 kg/m^2, and obesity ≥ 25 kg/m^2.

Waist Circumference

The healthy waist circumference limits are 90 cm for men and 80 cm for women as this has also been associated with more IR in Asians.

Body Composition and Fat Distribution

South Asians have a higher percentage of body fat for comparable levels of BMI compared with White Caucasians and are therefore referred to as "metabolically obese".[18] This was brought out very elegantly when Yagnik and Professor Yudkin of the same BMI were studied for visceral fat by dual-energy X-ray absorptiometry; Dr Yagnik had more visceral fat. This might be due to the Asian phenotype; however, lifestyle could also be a contributor. This has been called the Y-Y paradox.[19]

South Asian neonates exhibit the "thin-fat phenotype", described as low muscle mass with preserved subscapular (central) fat. Modi et al. showed that South Asian neonates have significantly increased abdominal adiposity compared with European babies. The "thin-fat phenotype" is also apparent in prepubertal Indian children who have greater adiposity than White UK children despite significantly lower BMIs.[20]

South Asians have high amounts of visceral adipose tissue (VAT) and that IR is correlated with total visceral and not with subcutaneous abdominal adipose tissue volume.[12] Sniderman et al. theorized in their "overflow hypothesis" that superficial subcutaneous adipose tissue (SAT) is the primary adipose tissue compartment, and deep SAT and VAT are secondary compartments, which have adverse metabolic consequences. They proposed that South Asians have a less developed primary compartment, resulting in earlier expansion of the secondary compartment, thereby leading to the increased risk of T2DM and cardiovascular disorders.[21]

Adipose Tissue Dysfunction and Inflammation

Adipose tissue not only stores fat but also secretes various cytokines like leptin, resistin and adiponectin. These are linked to metabolic disorders. South Asians have significantly increased subcutaneous adipocyte size. Hypertrophic adipocytes are considered dysfunctional and appear to be associated with IR in nondiabetic individuals independent of BMI and to be an independent predictor for the development of T2DM. Nondiabetic South Asians have higher fasting levels of FFAs compared with White Caucasians, even when adjusted for body fat content, and fail to completely suppress plasma FFA concentration during hyperinsulinemia induced by an oral glucose tolerance test. This suggests that in healthy South Asians, insulin is unable to sufficiently inhibit lipolysis, resulting in an excess efflux of FFA, which may play a role in the development of T2DM.

Plasma leptin levels were increased in South Asians as compared with White Caucasian subjects independent of overall or abdominal obesity. Leptin levels were found to be correlated with SAT and not with VAT.[22] South Asians exhibit lower levels of adiponectin compared with White Caucasians. Low adiponectin levels were found to be an independent predictor for T2DM development in South Asians.[23] Low adiponectin was correlated with high triglyceride and low high-density lipoprotein (HDL) levels. South Asians have higher levels of interleukin 6, tumor necrosis factor-α, C-reactive protein compared with Caucasians.

Dysfunctional adipose tissue and inflammation are likely to contribute to the South Asian phenotype of increased IR and T2DM.[24]

Brown Adipose Tissue

South Asians have lower resting energy expenditure, nonshivering thermogenesis, and decreased brown adipose tissue (BAT). This might be the underlying factor in their high susceptibility to metabolic disturbances, such as obesity and type 2 diabetes. The development of strategies to increase BAT volume and activity might help prevent and treat such disorders, particularly in South Asian individuals.[25]

Role of Skeletal Muscle

South Asians have less skeletal muscle mass and seem to have lower cardiorespiratory fitness and reduced capacity for fat oxidation during submaximal exercise, all correlating with their reduced whole-body insulin sensitivity, which is not reflected in reduced expression of oxidative and lipid metabolism genes in the skeletal muscle.[26]

Intrauterine Environment

In utero environment plays an important role in modifying development and physiology, thereby altering the risk of obesity, T2DM and other chronic diseases in adulthood.[27] Nutritional deprivation in utero may predispose an individual to T2DM in adult life. Early development issues and epigenetics may play an important role in the increasing burden of diabetes experienced in India.[28,29] The thrifty genotype and thrifty phenotype hypotheses seem to apply to Asian populations.

Micro-ribonucleic Acid

Paramasivam et al. analyzed the expression of circulating micro-ribonucleic acids (miRNAs) among the altered circulating miRNAs, miR-128 and miR-99b, appeared to be a "new lead" in Indians. It positively correlated with cholesterol both in prediabetic subjects and in diet-induced diabetic mice, suggesting that its increased level might be associated with the development of dyslipidemia associated with T2DM.[30] The miRNA was differentially expressed in Asians and was specific to gender.

COMPLICATIONS OF DIABETES

The World Health Organization Multinational Study of Vascular Disease in Diabetes had suggested comparatively high rates of albuminuria in Asian centers.[31] The prevalence of cardiovascular complications was also high in South Asians but in general was low in centers in China, Hong Kong and Japan.[32] The formation of unstable plaque is also more common in Indians.

South Asians and Chinese are more likely to suffer from proteinuric diabetic renal disease than from nonproteinuric diabetic renal disease.[33] A meta-analysis of studies on the prevalence of diabetic retinopathy noted that South Asians had the lowest prevalence.[34] A lower prevalence of peripheral sensory neuropathy was also reported in Asian patients in the Fremantle Diabetes Study in Australia compared with patients of European descent.[35] Risk of peripheral vascular disease have noted that South Asians are at lower risk of amputations than Europeans. This advantage may be nullified by bare foot walking. A diminished nitric oxide bioavailability in South Asians might be caused by both endothelial and HDL cholesterol dysfunction, and a factor in the increased incidence of T2DM and cardiovascular diseases in this ethnic group.[25]

In the Joint Asia Diabetes Evaluation program, among 41,029 patients recruited from across nine countries/regions in Asia, 18% had onset of T2DM below the age of 40, had longer disease duration, and had higher rates of retinopathy and end-stage renal disease than those with onset of diabetes after the age of 40.[36]

CONCLUSION

The prevalence of the Asian phenotype along with the lack of awareness of health issues results in high rates of smoking, consumption of energy-dense food, poor sleep hygiene and increased time on sedentary habits such as computer and television viewing. This can have very deleterious effects on the health of the individual. Chronic exposure to low-grade infections (e.g. hepatitis B infection) and environmental pollutants may result in abnormal neurohormonal responses resulting in obesity, metabolic syndrome and diabetes. This epidemic of diabetes and obesity can only be controlled when these factors are taken into consideration and preventive measures taken.

REFERENCES

1. Leow MK. Characterization of the Asian phenotype—an emerging paradigm with clinicopathological and human research implications. Int J Med Sci. 2017;14(7):639-47.
2. Cho NH, Shaw JE, Karuranga S, et al. IDF Diabetes Atlas: Global estimates of diabetes prevalence for 2017 and projections for 2045. Diabetes Res Clinc Pract. 2018;138:271-281.
3. Anjana RM, Shanthi Rani CS, Deepa M, et al. Incidence of diabetes and prediabetes and predictors of progression among Asian Indians: 10-year follow-up of the Chennai Urban Rural Epidemiology Study (CURES). Diabetes Care. 2015;38:1441-8.
4. Guariguata L, Linnenkamp U, Beagley J, et al. Global estimates of the prevalence of hyperglycemia in pregnancy. Diabetes Res Clin Pract. 2014;103:176-85.
5. Yoon KH, Lee JH, Kim JW, et al. Epidemic obesity and type 2 diabetes in Asia. Lancet. 2006;368:1681-8.
6. Misra A, Khurana L. Obesity and the metabolic syndrome in developing countries. J Clin Endocrinol Metab. 2008;93:S9-30.
7. King GL, McNeely MJ, Thorpe LE, et al. Understanding and addressing unique needs of diabetes in Asian Americans, native Hawaiians, and Pacific Islanders. Diabetes Care. 2012;35:1181-8.
8. Chan JC, Yeung R, Luk A. The Asian diabetes phenotypes: challenges and opportunities. Diabetes Res Clin Pract. 2014;105(1):135-9.
9. Radha V, Vimaleswaran KS, Babu HN, et al. Role of genetic polymorphism peroxisome proliferator-activatedreceptor-g2 Pro12Ala on ethnic susceptibility to diabetes in South-Asian and Caucasian subjects: evidence for heterogeneity. Diabetes Care. 2006;29:1046-51.
10. Sanghera DK, Demirci FY, Been L, et al. PPARG and DIPOQ gene polymorphisms increase type 2 diabetes mellitus risk in Asian Indian Sikhs: Pro12Ala still remains as the strongest predictor. Metabolism. 2010;59:492-501.
11. Li H, Kilpelainen TO, Liu C, et al. Association of genetic variation in FTO with risk of obesity and type 2 diabetes with data from 96,551 East and South Asians. Diabetologia. 2012;55:981-95.
12. Banerji MA, Faridi N, Atluri R, et al. Body composition, visceral fat, leptin, and insulin resistance in Asian Indian men. J Clin Endocrinol Metab. 1999;84:137-44.
13. Misra A, Khurana L, Isharwal S, et al. South Asian diets and insulin resistance. Br J Nutr. 2009;101:465-73.
14. Mohan V, Radhika G, Sathya RM, et al. Dietary carbohydrates, glycaemic load, food groups and newly detected type 2 diabetes among urban Asian Indian population in Chennai, India (Chennai Urban Rural Epidemiology Study 59). Br J Nutr. 2009;102:1498-506.
15. Joshi SR, Bhansali A, Bajaj S, et al. Results from a dietary survey in an Indian T2DM population: a STARCH study. BMJ open. 2014;4(10).
16. Ranasinghe CD, Ranasinghe P, Jayawardena R, et al. Physical activity patterns among South Asian adults: a systematic review. Int J Behav Nutr Phys Act. 2013;10:116.
17. Nyamdorj R, Pitk¨aniemi J, Tuomilehto J, et al. DECODA and DECODE study groups. Ethnic comparison of the association of undiagnosed diabetes with obesity. Int J Obes. 2010;34:332-9.
18. Rush EC, Freitas I, Plank LD. Body size, body composition and fat distribution: comparative analysis of European, Maori, Pacific Island and Asian Indian adults. Br J Nutr. 2009;102:632-41.
19. Yajnik CS, Yudkin JS. The Y-Y paradox. Lancet. 2004;363(9403):163.
20. Modi N, Thomas EL, Uthaya SN, et al. Whole body magnetic resonance imaging of healthy newborn infants demonstrates increased central adiposity in Asian Indians. Pediatr Res. 2009;65:584-7.
21. Sniderman AD, Bhopal R, Prabhakaran D, et al. Why might South Asians be so susceptible to central obesity and its atherogenic consequences? The adipose tissue overflow hypothesis. Int J Epidemiol. 2007;36:220-5.
22. Ramachandran A, Snehalatha C, Vijay V, et al. Plasma leptin in non-diabetic Asian Indians: association with abdominal adiposity. Diabet Med. 1997;14:937-41.
23. Bansal N, Anderson SG, Vyas A, et al. Adiponectin and lipid profiles compared with insulins in relation to early growth of British South Asian and European children: the Manchester children's growth and vascular health study. J Clin Endocrinol Metab. 2011;96:2567-74.
24. Donath MY, Shoelson SE. Type 2 diabetes as an inflammatory disease. Nat Rev Immunol. 2011;11:98-107.
25. Bakker LE, Boon MR, van der Linden RA, et al. Brown adipose tissue volume in healthy lean south Asian adults compared with white Caucasians: a prospective, case-controlled observational study. Lancet Diabetes Endocrinol. 2014;2(3):210-7.

26. Bakker LE, Sleddering MA, Schoones JW, et al. Pathogenesis of type 2 diabetes in South Asians. Eur J Endocrinol. 2013;169(5):R99-114.
27. Li Y, He Y, Qi L, et al. Exposure to the Chinese famine in early life and the risk of hyperglycemia and type 2 diabetes in adulthood. Diabetes. 2010;59:2400-6.
28. Yajnik CS. Nutrient-mediated teratogenesis and fuel-mediated teratogenesis: two pathways of intrauterine programming of diabetes. Int J Gynaecol Obstet. 2009;104(Suppl. 1):S27-31.
29. Nanditha A, Ma RC, Ramachandran A, et al. Diabetes in Asia and the Pacific: implications for the global epidemic. Diabetes Care. 2016;39(3):472-85.
30. Prabu P, Rome S, Sathishkumar C, et al. Circulating MiRNAs of 'Asian Indian Phenotype' identified in subjects with impaired glucose tolerance and patients with type 2 diabetes. PLoS One. 2015;10(5):e0128372.
31. Bennett PH, Lee ET, Lu M, et al. Increased urinary albumin excretion and its associations in the WHO Multinational Study of Vascular Disease in Diabetes. Diabetologia. 2001;44(Suppl. 2):S37-45.
32. Chi ZS, Lee ET, Lu M, et al. Vascular disease prevalence in diabetic patients in China: standardised comparison with the 14 centres in the WHO Multinational Study of Vascular Disease in Diabetes. Diabetologia. 2001;44(Suppl. 2):S82-6.
33. Bhalla V, Zhao B, Azar KM, et al. Racial/ethnic differences in the prevalence of proteinuric and nonproteinuric diabetic kidney disease. Diabetes Care. 2013;36:1215-21.
34. Yau JW, Rogers SL, Kawasaki R, et al. Meta-Analysis for Eye Disease (META-EYE) Study group. Global prevalence and major risk factors of diabetic retinopathy. Diabetes Care. 2012;35:556-64.
35. Tan ED, Davis WA, Davis TM. Changes in characteristics and management of Asian and Anglo-Celts with type 2 diabetes over a 15-year period in an urban Australian community: the Fremantle Diabetes Study. J Diabetes. 2016;8(1):139-47.
36. Yeung RO, Zhang Y, Luk A, et al. Metabolic profiles and treatment gaps in young-onset type 2 diabetes in Asia (the JADE programme): a cross-sectional study of a prospective cohort. Lancet Diabetes Endocrinol. 2014;2:935-43.

Chapter 5

Type 2 Diabetes Mellitus Originates in Liver

Rajesh Upadhyay, Anupam Prakash, Rashmi Rajput, Manshi Kashyap

INTRODUCTION

Liver is the largest metabolic organ of the human body. Liver like all vital organs, uses glucose as a fuel. Liver is the site for gluconeogenesis and is also the store house of glycogen. Therefore, in states of fasting or hypoglycemia, liver can release glucose in to the circulation by glycogenolysis and/or gluconeogenesis. It is a known fact, that total hepatectomy can result in death because of hypoglycemic shock.

LIVER AND PRANDIAL GLUCOSE EXCURSIONS

Liver also is believed to be the main organ which prevents rapid rise of blood glucose after ingesting food. Whatever glucose is absorbed from the intestines through the portal vein, almost all of it is retained by the liver. The rise in prandial plasma glucose reflects only a minor component of the absorbed glucose. It is pertinent to note that the first glycemic abnormality in type 2 diabetes mellitus (T2DM) is postprandial hyperglycemia, which may actually indicate insufficient trapping of glucose by the liver. It is believed that deficient meal-stimulated insulin release by the β-cells of pancreatic islets is the foremost abnormality resulting in postprandial hyperglycemia. However, it is possible that the trapping of all nutrients (including glucose) absorbed from the gut after a meal, which normally occurs in the liver, is actually dependent upon the effect of insulin. Whether the primary abnormality resulting in postprandial hyperglycemia is ineffective trapping of glucose by the liver, due to long-standing insulin resistance or due to reduced insulin release from the pancreatic β-cell islets or independent of insulin-effect, is a matter of conjecture. In fact, even hyperglucagonemia augments the hepatic glucose output by enhancing gluconeogenesis. However, it is universally known that insulin resistance is the primary abnormality which exists for a variable period of time before any hyperglycemia sets in, followed by postprandial hyperglycemia and then fasting as well as postprandial hyperglycemia associated with progressive β-cell failure. If one has to fit the role of liver in this pathogenetic pathway, keeping the aforementioned facts in mind, liver would be considered to be involved at the time of insulin resistance, which actually seems to antedate the stage of β-cell dysfunction.

GLUCOLIPOTOXICITY

Glucolipotoxicity refers to combined and deleterious effect of elevated levels of glucose and fatty acids on the functions and survival of pancreatic β-cells. Elevated levels of glucose (glucotoxicity) and elevated levels of fatty acids (lipotoxicity), both by themselves have a deleterious effect on β-cell functions, however when combined (glucolipotoxicity) can be synergistically harmful. At low glucose concentration, fatty acids via carnitine-palmitoyl transferase-1, are transported to mitochondria for beta oxidation. However, in presence of elevated glucose and fatty acids the action of carnitine-palmitoyl transferase-1 is inhibited and thus transport of fatty acids in mitochondria is reduced. Instead there is activation of esterification pathways that leads to cytosolic accumulation of signaling molecules derived from lipids like diglycerides, ceramide, phospholipids, triglycerides, that adversely affect β-cell functions. Prolonged exposure to elevated fatty acids in presence of elevated glucose levels may also impair insulin gene expression and β-cell death by apoptosis.

INCREASED HEPATIC GLUCOSE OUTPUT IN DIABETES

It is also well known that there is an increased hepatic glucose output in T2DM, which is a major contributor to fasting hyperglycemia. As increased free fatty acids inhibit the insulin action on liver itself, and insulin-induced suppression of glucagon is impaired, there is an increased hepatic glucose production. Excessive release of glucose from the liver is believed to occur early in the course of diabetes. Later in its course, β-cell dysfunction and reduced insulin secretion is a major contributor to the hyperglycemia observed.

HYPERINSULINEMIA AND THE LIVER

Hyperinsulinemia (as a consequence of insulin resistance) has several effects on various metabolic processes ongoing in the liver. First, it stimulates the enzyme hexokinase, which phosphorylates glucose. In addition, it also activates the enzymes phosphofructokinase and glycogen synthase, which are involved in glycogen synthesis. When glycogen stores are saturated, the excess glucose is then shunted to fatty acid synthesis.

DISORDERED FAT METABOLISM AND LIVER IN DIABETES

Absolute/relative insulin deficiency results in lipolysis in the adipose tissue, increased circulating levels of free fatty acids, resulting in increased fatty acid flux to the liver, where enhanced hepatic fat synthesis and beta oxidation of fat results in increased synthesis of triglycerides and a fatty liver, which further promotes insulin resistance. Insulin resistance and hyperinsulinemia also impair secretion of very low density lipoproteins (VLDL), which further exacerbates the accumulation of triglycerides in the liver and insulin resistance (lipotoxicity). Consequently, release of several cytokines and proinflammatory mediators from the liver (or fat accumulated in the liver) results in destruction of liver cells, as well as aggravates insulin resistance, since lipotoxicity also is detrimental to various other organs viz. pancreas, skeletal muscle and kidneys. In the liver per se, fat accumulation or steatosis may remain as such or progress to steatohepatitis and even cirrhosis, hepatocellular carcinoma and death.

THE LINK BETWEEN DIABETES MELLITUS AND FATTY LIVER

The last decade has seen a growing interest in the relationship between diabetes mellitus (DM) and chronic liver disease, particularly nonalcoholic fatty liver disease (NAFLD). With the growing incidence of metabolic diseases, incidence of NAFLD is also increasing worldwide. NAFLD is the most common cause of chronic liver disease in the United States and affects between 80 and 100 million individuals.[1] In India, a recent study cited the prevalence of NAFLD in patients who had DM to be 64%.[2] The common underlying mechanism for both T2DM and NAFLD is insulin resistance. Lipotoxicity, glucotoxicity and oxidative damage also play a role in its pathogenesis. However, this relationship between DM and liver disease is bidirectional, both supporting and accelerating the development of each other, as already discussed vide supra.

Fatty Liver

Day and colleagues had first proposed the Two Hit Hypothesis[3]—first hit being the hepatic steatosis (i.e. accumulation of triglycerides), while second hit being the oxidative stress that exacerbates the inflammation and progression to steatohepatitis and eventually fibrosis. But with further understanding of the molecular mechanisms involved, Tilg and Moschen have now cited "Multiple Parallel Hits" as the underlying pathogenetic mechanism.[4] The multiple hits include genetic influences, insulin resistance, systemic inflammation, dyslipidemia, glucotoxicity, lipotoxicity, oxidative stress as well as the role of intestinal microbiota, all of which are integral to and commonly found in T2DM.

Histologically, NAFLD progresses from a state of steatosis to steatohepatitis. Steatosis occurs as triglycerides accumulate as discussed earlier. The progression from simple steatosis to nonalcoholic steatohepatitis (NASH) is mediated by a combination of inflammation, circulating cytokines, oxidative stress and mitochondrial dysfunction. Finally, hepatocyte apoptosis, hepatic stellate cell activation and elaboration of fibrogenic growth factors leads to fibrosis.

It has been reported that the fat content of liver and not the peripheral adipose tissue fat content, is closely correlated to fasting insulin levels as well as to direct measures of hepatic insulin sensitivity.[5] Whether as a component of the extended definition of Metabolic syndrome or alone, various studies have reported that fatty liver is associated with an increased risk of developing type 2 diabetes, regardless of the presence of other cardiovascular risk factors.[6,7] NAFLD is associated with excess production of a number of known cardiovascular risk factors viz. VLDL, glucose, C-reactive protein (CRP), plasminogen activator inhibitor-1 (PAI-1), fibrinogen and coagulation factors.[8-10] Low serum adiponectin level, which is a characteristic feature in Metabolic syndrome, is also a predictor of advanced hepatic fibrosis in patients with NAFLD.[11]

Treatment of Fatty Liver can Ameliorate Insulin Resistance and Prevent Diabetes

In a rodent model, it was found that there was early development of hepatic insulin resistance without significant changes in insulin-stimulated glucose utilization or body weight in rodents fed with high fat diet.[12] In a study in T2DM patients subjected to a moderately hypocaloric and very low-fat diet, 81% reduction in intrahepatic fat content and improvement in basal and insulin-stimulated hepatic glucose metabolism was noted, however effects on insulin-stimulated peripheral glucose uptake were not significant.[13] So, dietary modification can improve hepatic insulin sensitivity. Weight loss interventions are also associated with improvement in liver histology and transaminases. Metformin an oral anti diabetic drug reduces plasma glucose via activation of AMP kinase, and reduces hepatic glucose synthesis. This enzyme also decreases lipid synthesis and enhances fat oxidation. Metformin treatment thus can improve insulin sensitivity and liver transaminases in patients with fatty liver disease. Thiazolidinediones are insulin sensitizers and can improve hepatic as well as peripheral insulin sensitivity. They can induce adipocyte differentiation, reduce free fatty acid levels and thus decrease their delivery to liver. They also increase adiponectin levels and can increase lipid oxidation of fatty acid in liver. They also reduce TNF-α and CRP which play a role in insulin resistance. Therefore, ample evidence indicates that targeting fatty liver has the potential to reduce insulin resistance.

SECONDARY DIABETES-RELATED TO LIVER

As liver is one of the major sites of action of insulin and other counter-regulatory hormones involved in glucose homeostasis, chronic liver disease from various causes are associated with impaired glucose tolerance and development of diabetes. Glucose intolerance can be seen in about 80% of patients, and diabetes in about 30–60% of patients[14,15] with chronic liver disease. Apart from fatty liver disease, other conditions like hemochromatosis, cystic fibrosis, chronic liver disease due to alcohol abuse, chronic hepatitis C, and glycogen storage disorders are also associated with development of diabetes.

Figure 1 diagrammatically depicts that liver is the central organ responsible for insulin resistance in T2DM.

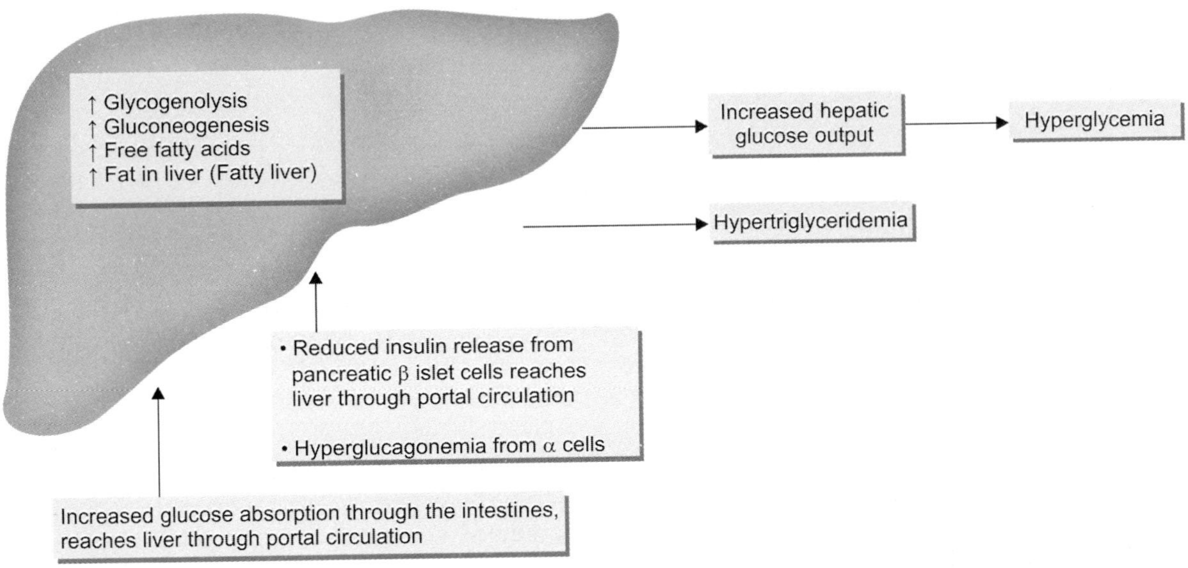

Figure 1 Liver: Seat of insulin resistance in diabetes.

CONCLUSION

The traditional triumvirate features in the pathogenesis of diabetes viz. insulin resistance, diminished insulin release from pancreatic islet β-cells and increased hepatic glucose output gave way to the ominous octet proposed by DeFronzo in his Banting Lecture a decade back.[16] However, it is imperative to note that the triumvirate features had the liver contributing to categorically two of the features and the third feature of pancreatic β-cell dysfunction may also be related to hepatic insulin resistance as has been discussed in this text. The octet may provide the treating physicians with different ways to tackle the treatment of diabetes, but it will be pertinent to understand that the liver-pancreas axis is involved in most of the features of the octet. Thus, apart from pancreas, liver is an important organ involved in glucose homeostasis and has a significant role in the pathogenesis of type 2 diabetes. In fact, reversal of fatty liver may help ameliorate insulin resistance and may aid in the prevention of development of type 2 diabetes.

REFERENCES

1. Loomba R, Sanyal AJ. The global NAFLD epidemic. Nat Rev Gastroenterol Hepatol. 2013;10:686-90.
2. Patel H, Verma YN. Prevalence of non-alcoholic fatty liver disease in type-2 diabetes mellitus patients. Int J Res Med Sci. 2018; 6:1322-6.
3. Day CP, James OF. Steatohepatitis: a tale of two "hits"? Gastroenterology. 1998;114:842-5.
4. Tilg H, Moschen AR. Evolution of inflammation in nonalcoholic fatty liver disease: the multiple parallel hits hypothesis. Hepatology. 2010;52: 1836-46.
5. Yki Järvinen H. Fat in the liver and insulin resistance. Ann Med. 2005; 37:347-56.
6. Tokita Y, Maejima Y, Shimomura K, et al. Non-alcoholic Fatty Liver Disease Is a Risk Factor for Type 2 Diabetes in Middle-aged Japanese Men and Women. Intern Med. 2017;56:763-71.
7. Lonardo A, Ballestri S, Guaraldi G, et al. Fatty liver is associated with an increased risk of diabetes and cardiovascular disease – Evidence from three different disease models: NAFLD, HCV and HIV. World J Gastroenterol. 2016;22:9674-93.
8. Priya MT, et al. A preliminary study of inflammatory markers in non-alcoholic steatohepatitis patients. Libyan J Med. 2010;5:5071.
9. Targher G, Chonchol M, Miele L, et al. Nonalcoholic fatty liver disease as a contributor to hypercoagulation and thrombophilia in the metabolic syndrome. Semin Thromb Hemost. 2009;35:277-87.
10. Thiruvagounder M, Khan S, Sheriff DS. Non-Alcoholic Fatty Liver Disease (NAFLD) - Is it an Emerging Risk Factor for Coronary Artery Disease?: Preliminary study in a local Indian population. Sultan Qaboos Univ Med J. 2010;10:221-6.
11. Savvidou S, Hytiroglou P, Orfanou-Koumerkeridou H et al. Low serum adiponectin levels are predictive of advanced hepatic fibrosis in patients with NAFLD. J Clin Gastroenterol. 2009;43:765-72.
12. Samuel VT, Liu ZX, Qu X, et al. Mechanism of hepatic insulin resistance in non-alcoholic fatty liver disease. J Biol Chem. 2004;279:32345-53.
13. Petersen KF, Dufour S, Befroy D, et al. Reversal of nonalcoholic hepatic steatosis, hepatic insulin resistance, and hyperglycemia by moderate weight reduction in patients with type 2 diabetes. Diabetes. 2005;54: 603-8.
14. Petrides AS. Liver disease and diabetes mellitus. Diabetes Rev. 1994; 2: 1-18.
15. García-Compean D, Jaquez-Quintana JO, Maldonado-Garza H. Hepatogenous diabetes: current views of an ancient problem. Ann Hepatol. 2009;8:13-20.
16. DeFronzo RA. From the triumvirate to the ominous octet: a new paradigm for the treatment of type 2 diabetes mellitus. Diabetes. 2009; 58:773-95.

Chapter 6

Nonalcoholic Fatty Liver Disease in Metabolically Healthy Obese

Naval K Vikram

INTRODUCTION

Nonalcoholic fatty liver disease (NAFLD) is the most prevalent form of asymptomatic chronic liver disease. It is wide spectrum of disorders ranging from simple steatosis, steatohepatitis, cirrhosis, and liver cancer seen in individuals who do not consume significant amount of alcohol, with increase in liver disease-related mortality.[1] Up to 3/4th of the individuals with obesity and type 2 diabetes mellitus (T2DM) have NAFLD suggesting a very close association. The prevalence of NAFLD is increasing worldwide and in all age groups. This may be a reflection of the increasing prevalence of obesity, particularly abdominal obesity in all age groups and all populations. Asian Indian population has been shown to be more prone to develop abdominal obesity and insulin resistance, and may be at increased risk of development of NAFLD. Increasing amount of evidence suggests close association of adiposity, insulin resistance, metabolic syndrome, and NAFLD.[2]

Obesity is associated with increase in all-cause mortality, as well as mortality associated with T2D, cardiovascular diseases (CVD), and malignancy. However, not all obese individuals have metabolic abnormalities and demonstrate increased risk of morbidity and mortality. Based on the presence of obesity and metabolic abnormalities, individuals may be characterized as 'metabolically healthy nonobese (MHNO)', 'metabolically healthy obese (MHO)', 'metabolically unhealthy nonobese (MUNO)', and 'metabolically unhealthy obese (MUO)'.[3] Increasing amount of evidence indicates that MHO may be a transient condition and these individuals may develop obesity-related metabolic complications in the course of time. It has been shown that about 30–40% of individuals with MHO converted to metabolically unhealthy status over a period of 6 years follow-up.[4] Therefore, there is need to understand the obesity-related metabolic health subtypes in appropriate management of obesity.

MHO AND NAFLD: CURRENT EVIDENCE

While obesity is a major determinant of increasing prevalence of NAFLD, the relationship between obesity and NAFLD is incompletely understood. Whether obesity per se, or presence of metabolic abnormalities is associated with risk of NAFLD, is not clear. There is limited data supporting each notion.

Association of obesity with hepatic steatosis and fibrosis was evaluated in a cross sectional study involving 2,198 Korean subjects.[5] These had less than two of the following abnormalities: elevated blood pressure, hypertriglyceridemia, low high-density lipoprotein cholesterol (HDL-C), and impaired fasting glucose. The study population was divided into MHNO, MUNO, MHO, MUO based on the presence of obesity and metabolic syndrome abnormalities. Hepatic steatosis and fibrosis progressively increased across these groups. There was significant interaction effect between obesity and metabolic health on measure of liver fibrosis and indicated by higher values of LSM in MHO group than MHNO group. In contrast, there was no difference in the LSM values among MHNO and MUNO groups. As compared to MHNO group, the odds of liver steatosis were observed to be 2.94 in MUNO, 4.62 in MHO and 12.02 in MUO, respectively. These observations suggest that obese individuals are at a higher risk of developing hepatic steatosis and fibrosis than those who are nonobese but metabolically unhealthy.

The association between body mass index (BMI) categories and development of NAFLD was evaluated in another prospective cohort study involving Korean subjects. This study included 77,425 individuals free from NAFLD and metabolic abnormalities at baseline, who were followed up for a mean duration of 4.5 years.[6] In multivariable adjusted analysis, the odds ratios for incidence of NAFLD were observed to be 2.15 and 3.55 in individuals who were overweight and obese at baseline, respectively, as compared to those who were normal weight at baseline. The association between BMI and incident NAFLD was observed to be strong and progressive across the whole range of BMI values.

In contrast to the studies mentioned earlier, some data suggests that metabolic health may be more important than obesity in the development of NAFLD. This was evaluated in a retrospective study involving 345 subjects without NAFLD at baseline who were followed up for years. The incidence of NAFLD was observed to be 10.5%, 31.4%, 23.3% and 42% in subjects who were MHNO, MHO, MUNO and MUO, respectively. The risk of developing NAFLD was observed to be consistently higher in subjects who were unhealthy both at baseline and at follow up compared to those who remained metabolically healthy throughout.

Some evidence also suggests that presence of NAFLD may increase the risk of developing metabolic abnormalities in nonobese individuals who are metabolically healthy. This was evaluated in a retrospective study involving Japanese subjects who were followed up for a period of about 5 years.[7] Subjects were divided into MHNO, metabolically healthy overweight (MHOW), and MHO. The hazard ratio (HR) of NAFLD on progression from metabolically healthy to unhealthy phenotype was observed to be 1.49 in MHNO, 1.37 in MHOW, and 1.38 in MHO, respectively, after adjusting for other conventional risk factors.

Increasing evidence indicates higher risk of CVD in patients with NAFLD. In a case-control study involving Asian Indians, higher carotid intima-media thickness (marker of preclinical atherosclerosis) and higher prevalence of abnormal flow-mediated dilatation (marker of endothelial dysfunction) was seen in NAFLD patients than controls.[8] Similar observations have been reported in other populations as well. A study involving Swedish subjects evaluated the relationship between NAFLD and measures of atherosclerotic CVD and how this is influenced by metabolic factors.[9] Prevalence of NAFLD was observed to be 10.4% of subjects and was strongly associated with obesity-related traits. Strong correlation was observed between NAFLD and coronary artery calcification scores, with the correlation being strongest in individuals with few metabolic risk factors. This suggests that presence of NAFLD may be a string predictor of increased coronary artery calcium score in metabolically healthy subjects.

The mechanism (s) by which obesity leads to development of NAFLD are not very clear. Expanded adipose tissue in obesity may be considered as the 'first hit' whereas metabolic abnormalities can be considered as the 'second hit' in the pathogenesis of NAFLD. Excess accumulation of fat in body and consequently in liver cells may increase the susceptibility of liver to the second hits such as oxidative stress and proinflammatory cytokines. The risk of hepatic steatosis with elevation in liver enzymes has also been shown to be higher in subjects with MHO than those who are MUNO. Further, the expression of proinflammatory genes was observed to be altered to a similar extent in MHO and MUO subjects.[10]

NAFLD is a marker of accumulation of ectopic fat and may indicate the reduced capacity of the adipose tissue of body to store fat. This may be seen more prominently in conditions such as lipodystrophies in which there is absence or marked decrease of subcutaneous adipose tissue. Excess accumulation fat in the visceral region in the absence of generalized obesity is also associated with NAFLD (the lean NAFLD) and metabolic abnormalities. The relationship between obesity and metabolic health with NAFLD is a complex and not clearly elucidated. A prospective investigation into this is likely to answer many of the questions.

REFERENCES

1. Marchesini G, Bugianesi E, Forlani G, et al. Nonalcoholic fatty liver, steatohepatitis, and the metabolic syndrome. Hepatol. 2003;37(4):917-23.
2. Bhatt SP, Misra A, Vikram NK. Non-alcoholic fatty liver disease in Asian Indians: relationship with insulin resistance, diabetes and cardiovascular risk. Curr Sci India. 2017;113(7):1303-10.
3. Samocha-Bonet D, Dixit VD, Kahn CR, et al. Metabolically healthy and unhealthy obese--the 2013 Stock Conference report. Obes Rev. 2014;15(9):697-708.
4. Soriguer F, Gutierrez-Repiso C, Rubio-Martin E, et al. Metabolically healthy but obese, a matter of time? Findings from the prospective Pizarra study. J Clin Endocrinol Metab. 2013;98(6):2318-25.
5. Huh JH, Kim KJ, Kim SU, et al. Obesity is more closely related with hepatic steatosis and fibrosis measured by transient elastography than metabolic health status. Metabolism. 2017;66:23-31.

6. Chang Y, Jung HS, Cho J, et al. Metabolically Healthy Obesity and the Development of Nonalcoholic Fatty Liver Disease. Am J Gastroenterol. 2016;111(8):1133-40.
7. Hashimoto Y, Hamaguchi M, Fukuda T, et al. Fatty liver as a risk factor for progression from metabolically healthy to metabolically abnormal in non-overweight individuals. Endocrine. 2017;57(1):89-97.
8. Thakur ML, Sharma S, Kumar A, et al. Nonalcoholic fatty liver disease is associated with subclinical atherosclerosis independent of obesity and metabolic syndrome in Asian Indians. Atherosclerosis. 2012;223(2):507-11.
9. Gummesson A, Stromberg U, Schmidt C, et al. Non-alcoholic fatty liver disease is a strong predictor of coronary artery calcification in metabolically healthy subjects: A cross-sectional, population-based study in middle-aged subjects. PLoS One. 2018;13(8):e0202666.
10. Gomez-Ambrosi J, Catalan V, Rodriguez A, et al. Increased cardio-metabolic risk factors and inflammation in adipose tissue in obese subjects classified as metabolically healthy. Diabetes Care. 2014;37(10):2813-21.

Chapter 7

Artificial Sweeteners in Diabetes: How Safe?

Sandeep Rai, Madhur Rai

INTRODUCTION

Artificial sweeteners (AS) are one of the most common food additives worldwide. By definition, AS, otherwise referred to as very low-calorie sweeteners, non-nutrient sweeteners, non-caloric sweeteners or intense sweeteners, have a greater intensity of sweetness than caloric sweeteners such as sucrose, corn syrups and fruit juice concentrates. As a sugar replacement, they are added in smaller quantities, hence, they provide no or only minimal calories. The Food and Drug Administration (FDA) has approved the use of six AS, which includes aspartame, sucralose, saccharin, advantame, neotame and acesulfame potassium (Ace-k), in food and beverages (Table 1). Federal regulations require that any food that contains aspartame bear this warning: "Phenylketonurics (PKU) Contains phenylalanine". This warning helps people with PKU avoid products that are a source of

TABLE 1: Artificial sweetener reference chart.

ARTIFICIAL SWEETENERS					
Generic name	**Brand name**	**Sweetness factor/ acceptable daily intake (ADI) mg of sweetener/ kg body weight/day**	**Uses**	**Additional facts/ metabolism**	**FDA approval**
Saccharin	Sweet'N Low, Sweet Twin, Necta Sweet, Sweetex	200–700 times sweeter than sugar ADI-5 mg/kg	Tabletop sweetener, beverages, baked goods, jams, gum	Heat stable/Metabolism-Nil bitter metallic after taste	2001
Aspartame	Nutrasweet/Equal	200 times sweeter than sugar ADI-50 mg/kg	In processed foods and beverages	Not heat stable/ metabolized to: Phenylalanine aspartic acid methanol	1981
Acesulfame-K	Sunett, Sweet One	200 times sweeter than sugar ADI-15 mg/kg	General purpose	Heat stable to 392 °F/ metabolism-Nil	1998
Sucralose	Splenda/Sugar Free Natura	600 times sweeter than sugar ADI- 5 mg/kg	General purpose	Can be used in home baking/metabolism-Nil	1998
Neotame	Newtame	8000 times sweeter than sugar ADI-18 mg/kg	General purpose/ metabolism by esterase	Similar to aspartame	2002

phenylalanine. Although AS are generally considered safe for human consumption, there is increasing controversy regarding their potential ability to promote metabolic derangements in humans.

ANY HEALTH RISKS OF USING ARTIFICIAL SWEETENERS?

This is still a highly controversial topic[1] AS have allegedly been linked to adverse effects such as cancer, weight gain, metabolic disorders, migraine, type-2 diabetes, vascular events, preterm delivery, hepatotoxicity, immune system disruptions and alteration of gut microbiota activity.[2] Although these potential health problems have long been studied, but a firm conclusion has yet to be reached on these allegations due to a lack of credible and consistent evidence. Some of these controversial areas are discussed below.

ARTIFICIAL SWEETENERS FUELING THE DIABESITY EPIDEMIC?

A statement from American Heart Association and American Diabetes Association in 2011 pointed out that non-nutritive sweetener may be good for health by reducing or controlling weight and can have other beneficial metabolic effects too.[3] However, recent concerns regarding the safety of AS have arisen from few studies in humans. In a large meta-analysis of prospective studies[4,5] (17 cohorts with 38,253 cases) it has been shown that AS were associated with the risk of type 2 diabetes mellitus (T2DM). Another similar study demonstrated that diets sweetened with either natural or artificial sugars are linked with an increase in type 2 diabetes.[6] In, a recently published study, which collected 10-year data from more than 10,000 women, who were consumers of AS as packet and tablets[7] showed an association between AS usage and risk of diabetes. More importantly they were also able to show a gradation of risk depending upon years of consumption and also the amount of AS consumed per day.

The explanation given for a probable association between AS and T2DM in observation studies is the reverse causation bias because of increase intake of AS is otherwise also seen among obese people.[8] Another convincing explanation is that an orosensory stimulus is silently generated by sweet foods, telling the body about the likely inflow of calories that is going to follow. This is followed by several gastrointestinal reflexes that finally relay in brain and intimate the hypothalamus through negative feedback signals to decrease hunger sensation and increase satiety feeling as body has already received calories, however when sweetness is sensed without inflow of calories (AS ingestion), gastrointestinal reflexes do not send signals to hypothalamus to decrease the hunger sensation (Fig. 1). The brain recalibrates and persons hunger sensation continues and this leads to increase in "total calories consumed". This ultimately leads to weight gain and consequently increases the risk of diabetes.

A study was conducted in the University of San Diego, California on volunteers who were given sips of water mixed with either sugar or sucralose. Functional magnetic resonance imaging scans of the brain were then recorded. Images showed that sugar activated areas of the brain which were involved in food reward, whereas sucralose did not have the same effect. These results proved that AS may not be effective in managing cravings for sweets.[9]

Another study was carried out on more than 3,000 individuals, which saw the impact of artificially sweetened drinks on the body weight. Results showed that those who consumed these drinks had a 47% higher increase in body mass index (BMI) than those who did not.[10] Another meta-analysis saw the effect of AS on body weight and cardio metabolic risk factors including.[7] Randomized controlled trials (RCTs) (1,003 participants; follow-up 6 months) and about 30 cohort studies (more than 400,000 participants; median follow-up 10 years) was critically analyzed. Evidence from RCTs does not support the benefits of AS for body weight management, and observational data suggest that routine intake of AS may be associated with increased BMI and cardiometabolic risk including coronary artery disease. In the cohort studies, it was found that consumption of AS was associated with increases in weight and waist circumference, and a higher incidence of obesity, metabolic syndrome, and type 2 diabetes.[11] However, publication bias was indicated for the studies with diabetes as an outcome.

ARTIFICIAL SWEETENER SAFE IN PREGNANCY?

Although many AS are considered safe during pregnancy, women with any form of diabetes must limit their use of these substitutes. According to a study saccharin has been shown to cause effects as anemia, iron and vitamin A deficiency, depressed growth and elevated vitamin E in rats. They are also linked with premature deliveries prompted by two observational studies published in 2010 and 2012. Therefore, at present time, till further large

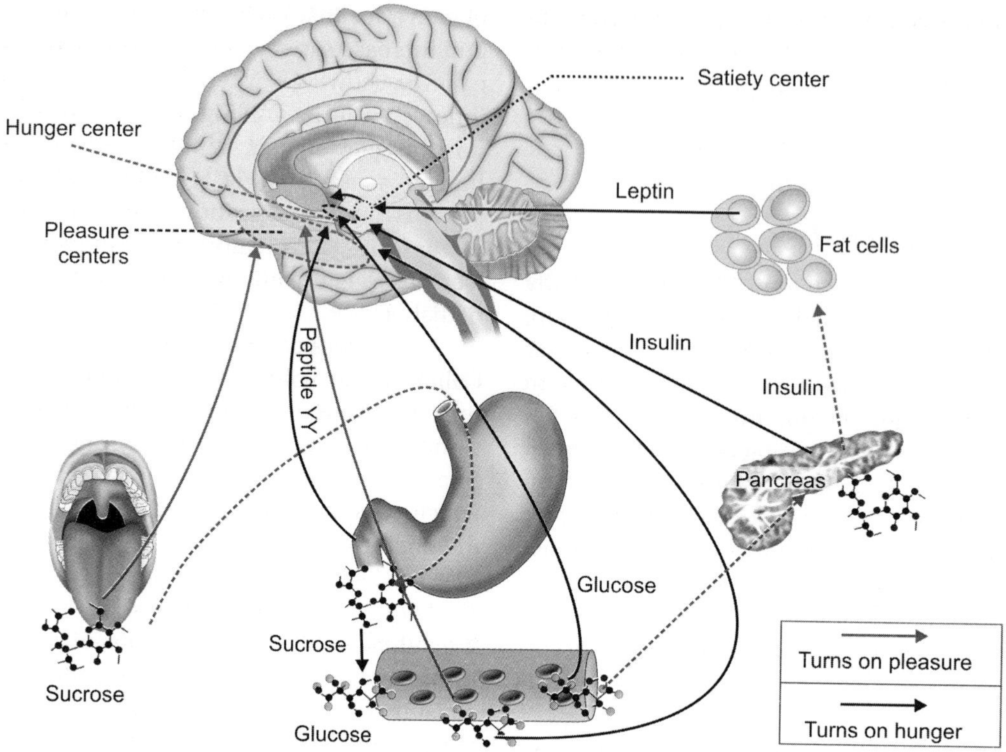

Figure 1 Sucrose ingestion leads to calorie inflow and activates multiple gastrointestinal (GI) negative feedback signals to hypothalamus to decrease hunger sensation, while artificial sweetener ingestion is followed by no calories and therefore no feedback inhibition of hunger sensation, leading to increase food intake and weight gain.

Source: Gabymichel, BruceBlaus, Mikael Haggstrom, Häggström, M (2014). "Medical gallery of Mikael Häggström 2014". *WikiJournal of Medicine* 1 (2)

scale studies are done, pregnant women must be advised to avoid these sweeteners.[12] It is also critical to investigate the effect of AS in other populations, such as infants and young children, lactating women, and those with metabolic diseases.

ARTIFICIAL SWEETENERS AND THE RISK OF CANCER?

In 1970, a research was conducted which showed the association of saccharin with bladder cancer in laboratory rats. Another study raised a needle of suspicion when it showed that aspartame intake is associated with malignancies like leukemia, lymphoma and multiple myeloma (in men).[13] However, this particular study was limited by inability to quantify exact consumption of aspartame because of variable presence of aspartame among the dietary sources. Another limitation of this study was the inability to explain the rationale behind male preponderance of carcinoma risk. Similarly, another study assessed the possible effects of five non-nutritive sweeteners on cell proliferation, morphology and cell's deoxyribonucleic acid (DNA). It was also seen that sodium saccharin and sucralose caused more DNA fragmentation in all cell lines than any other artificial sweetners.[14]

However, Weihrauch et al. after reviewing the literature meticulously, opined that there was no significant evidence of AS consumption and cancer risk with currently available AS.[15] Similar conclusions were also drawn by another large study which prospectively analyzed data from more than 400,000 men and women over a 5 years period and did not find any association between aspartame consumption and risk of hematopoietic or brain tumours.[16]

EFFECT OF ARTIFICIAL SWEETENERS ON GUT BIOME

Artificial sweeteners influence the microbial composition of the oral mucosa, and they are viewed positively by the dental community. It is therefore not surprising that AS have recently been shown to alter the gut microbiota, primarily in rodent models. Experimental evidence for -induced alterations in gut microbiota in humans is limited. AS exposure for 1 week was associated with changes in the gut microbiome and glucose metabolism in a small human sample.[17] Notably, several of the bacterial taxa that changed following AS consumption were previously associated with type 2 diabetes in humans,[18] including over-representation of Bacteroides and under-representation of Clostridiales. However, the lack of a control group makes these findings less interpretable. Nevertheless, further study in this area is warranted, given the emerging role of the gut microbiome in health and disease. In another study, the relative toxicity of six FDA-approved AS and that of ten sport supplements containing these AS were tested using genetically modified bioluminescent bacteria from *E. coli*. The bioluminescent bacteria, which luminescence when they detect toxicants, act as a sensing model representative of the complex microbial system. Both induced luminescent signals and bacterial growth were measured. Toxic effects were found when the bacteria were exposed to certain concentrations of the AS.[19]

NOVEL SWEETENERS

Novel sweeteners are hard to fit into a particular category because of what they're made from and how they're made. Stevia is extracted from the leaves of the plant species *Stevia rebaudiana*, native to Brazil and Paraguay. Stevia contains steviol glycosides, which are used as AS. FDA has not questioned the GRAS (generally, recognized as safe) status of certain high-purity steviol glycosides for use in food. However, stevia leaf and crude stevia extracts are not considered GRAS and do not have FDA approval for use in food. Tagatose is also considered a novel sweetener because of its chemical structure. Tagatose is a low-carbohydrate sweetener similar to fructose that occurs naturally but is manufactured from the lactose in dairy products. The FDA categorizes Tagatose as a GRAS substance.

ALTERNATIVES TO ARTIFICIAL SWEETENERS

Various natural sweeteners, which are safer, can be used instead of AS. Many of these include added benefits of being rich in minerals and vitamins. These include honey, coconut nectar, fruits, maple syrup, molasses, sugar alcohols, stevia, agave nectar, apple sauce and others. The key word here is alternatives meaning and they also contain sugar, but in less amount and should be used instead of refined sugar. Stevia is probably the healthiest option, is 100% natural, and contains zero calories, followed by xylitol, erythritol and yacon syrup. These contain less sugar compared to sucrose. Xylitol is a sugar alcohol that contains 40% fewer calories than sugar. Eating it may offer dental benefits. Erythritol is a sugar alcohol that tastes almost exactly like sugar, but it contains only 6% of the calories. It is an excellent sugar alternative. "Less bad" sugars like maple syrup, molasses and honey are slightly better than regular sugar, but should still be used sparingly. As with most things in nutrition, moderation is the key.

CONCLUSION

Artificial sweeteners are a ubiquitous part of modern life, especially of diabetes care. While it is nearly impossible to replicate "real-life" consumption in randomized controlled trials, epidemiological studies report positive associations with obesity and metabolic impairments. In contrast, human randomized controlled trials suggest that AS may be a useful, or at least neutral tool for weight management. Given the discrepancies in the available evidence, the extent to which AS are helpful or harmful for weight management and chronic disease prevention warrants further well designed, large scale studies. With all the evidence available till date, it is advisable that AS, if at all have to be used, should only be used occasionally and not chronically for long term, and that too, in a limited amount. Physicians who advise these AS to their obese or diabetic patients need to take a step back and re-evaluate their recommendations especially in light of the newer studies on various unfavorable metabolic effects that are emerging now. In fact, we may be dealing with a Wolf in a Sheep's clothing.

REFERENCES

1. Tandel KR. Sugar substitutes. Health controversy over perceived benefits. J. Pharmacol. Pharmacother. 2011;2:236-43.
2. Marinovich M, Galli CL, Bosetti C, et al. Aspartame, low-calorie sweeteners and disease. Regulatory safety and epidemiological issues. Food Chem Toxicol. 2013;60:109-15.
3. Gardner C, Wylie-Rosett J, Gidding SS, et al . Nonnutritive sweeteners: current use and health perspectives. A scientific statement from the American Heart Association and the American Diabetes Association. Diabetes Care. 2012;35:1798-1808.
4. Imamura F, O'Connor L, Ye Z, et al. Consumption of sugar sweetened beverages, artificially sweetened beverages, and fruit juice and incidence of type 2 diabetes: systematic review, meta-analysis, and estimation of population attributable fraction. BMJ. 2015;351:h3576.

5. Fagherazzi G, Gusto G, Affret A, et al. Chronic consumption of artificial sweetener in packets or tablets and type 2 diabetes risk, evidence from the E3N-European Prospective Investigation into cancer and nutrition study. Ann Nutr Metab. 2017;70:51-8.
6. Fagherazzi G, Vilier A, Saes Sartorelli D, et al. Consumption of artificially and sugar-sweetened beverages and incident type 2 diabetes. European Prospective Investigation into Cancer and Nutrition cohort. Am J Clin Nutr. 2013;97:517-23.
7. Anton SD, Martin CK, Han H, et al. Effects of stevia, aspartame, and sucrose on food intake, satiety, and postprandial glucose and insulin levels. Appetite. 2010;55:37-43.
8. Greenwood DC, Threapleton DE, Evans CE, et al. Association between sugar-sweetened and artificially sweetened soft drinks and type 2 diabetes: systematic review and dose-response meta-analysis of prospective studies. Br J Nutr. 2014;112(5):725-34.
9. Frank GK, Oberndorfer TA, Simmons AN, et al. Sucrose activates human taste pathways differently from artificial sweetener. Neuroimage. 2008;39:1559-69.
10. Fowler SP, Williams K, Resendez RG, Hunt KJ, Hazuda HP, Stern MP. Fueling the obesity epidemic? Artificially sweetened beverage use and long-term weight gain. Obesity. 2008;16:1894-900.
11. Azad MB, Ahmed M, Abou-Setta, et al. Nonnutritive sweeteners and cardiometabolic health: a systematic review and meta-analysis of randomized controlled trials and prospective cohort studies, CMAJ. 201;89(28):E929-39.
12. Englund-Ögge L, Brantsæter AL, Haugen M, et al. Association between intake of artificially sweetened and sugar-sweetened beverages and preterm delivery, a large prospective cohort study. Am J Clin Nutr. 2012;96:552-9.
13. Schernhammer ES, Bertrand KA, Birmann BM, et al. Consumption of artificial sweetener and sugar-containing soda and risk of lymphoma and leukemia in men and women. Am J ClinNutr. 2012;96:1419-28.
14. Van Eyk AD. The effect of five artificial sweeteners on Caco-2,HT-219 and HEK-293 cells. DrugChemToxicol. 2014;15:1-10.
15. Weihrauch MR, Diehl V. Artificial sweeteners—do they bear a carcinogenic risk? Ann Oncol. 2004;15(10):1460-5.
16. Lim U, Subar AF, Mouw T, et al. Consumption of aspartame-containing beverages and incidence of hematopoietic and brain malignancies. Cancer Epidemiol Biomark Prev. 2006;15(9):1654-9.
17. Suez J, Korem T, Zeevi D, et al. Artificial sweeteners induce glucose intolerance by altering the gut microbiota. Nature. 2014;514:181-6.
18. Qin J, Li Y, Cai Z, et al. A metagenome-wide association study of gut microbiota in type 2 diabetes. Nature, 2012;490:55-60.
19. Harpaz D, Yeo LP, Cecchini F, et al. Measuring Artificial Sweeteners Toxicity Using a Bioluminescent Bacterial Panel. Molecules. 2018;23(10):2454.

Chapter 8

Manipulating Macronutrients for Weight Reduction Important or Just Calorie Reduction

Kavita Gupta, Sunil Gupta

INTRODUCTION

Overweight [body mass index (BMI) 25–30 kg/m^2] and excessive fat accumulation result from a higher calorific intake than energy expenditure. Specific contributions of various etiological factors, such as the proportions of dietary macronutrients (fats, proteins and carbohydrates), the quantitative importance of physical activity patterns and the influence of genetic factors, are related to the rising levels of obesity (BMI >30 kg/m^2) observed in many countries worldwide, with a global increase in obesity from 28.8 to 36.9% in men and from 29.8 to 38% in women during the last 33 years. The excessive accumulation of body fat is associated with various health risks, most of which are linked to increased all-cause mortality.[1] It is unclear as to what extent individuals should be held accountable for the macronutrient composition of their diet.[1]

Last decade, a few narrative reviews addressed the role of diet in prevention of weight gain. Systematic reviews and meta-analysis have focused on specific issues, like the role of sugar-sweetened beverages.[2] The associations of dietary macronutrients, food intake and dietary patterns versus change in weight or waist circumference (WC) in adult populations is being evaluated.[2] The focus is on unraveling the optimal macronutrient distribution for achievement of sustainable weight loss using both energy-restricted and unrestricted diets. Systematic reviews of the literature and meta-analysis are also being conducted to ascertain the singular role of different macronutrients (Table 1).[1]

CARBOHYDRATES

A Cochrane review evaluated the outcomes of 202 overweight or obese participants showing low-glycemic index diet resulted in a significant weight reduction of 1.1 kg versus following the control diet. The researchers concluded that reducing glycemic load is advisable to facilitate weight loss.[3] About 94 studies were identified, comprising 3,268 adult participants reported a trend toward increased weight loss for diets with reduced carbohydrate content.[4] Exchanging dietary sugars for complex carbohydrates with a similar energy content did not result in a significant change in body weight.[5] A trial with 129 overweight or obese young adults were randomly assigned to one of four different diets over 12 weeks, the high-protein, low-glycemic-index diet specifically promoted body fat reduction, whereas the high-carbohydrate, low-glycemic-index diet elicited a clinically relevant cardiovascular risk reduction.[6]

FATS

A meta-analysis of data from 57,735 participants in these trials revealed that a low total dietary fat intake is linked to a reduction in body weight (–1.6 kg) versus a normal fat intake.[7] Total 1,224 participants from the PREDIMED multicenter trial showed no differences in body weight between Mediterranean diets containing fats and control diet.[8]

PROTEINS

In eight of the 15 trials, high-protein diets led to greater weight loss than low-protein diets. However, protein content had a neutral effect on weight loss in the remaining seven trials. The authors of this analysis concluded that high dietary protein intake was associated with increased thermogenesis and decreased appetite.[9]

LOW CARBOHYDRATE—HIGH PROTEIN DIETS

A meta-analysis with 447 participants from six trials, showed individuals on low-carbohydrate diets had

TABLE 1: Key trials* investigating the role of macronutrients in weight management.[1]

Reference	Participants	Comparison	Duration	Outcomes
Bravata et al. (2003)	3,268 overweight or obese adults	Systematic review of low-carbohydrate diet (<60 g daily) vs. control	Average 50–73 days	3.6 kg (95% CI, 1.2–6.0 kg) weight loss in low-carbohydrate group vs. 2.1 kg (95% CI, 1.6–2.7 kg) in control group
Halton and Hu (2004)	720 overweight or obese adults	Critical review of high dietary protein intake vs. control (meta-analysis)	7 days–6 months	Significant improvement in weight loss with high-protein diets in 7 of 15 trials. Other trials reported no significant differences
Nordmann et al. (2006)	447 obese adults	Meta-analysis of low-fat (<30% of total energy intake) vs. low carbohydrate (<60 g daily) diets	6–12 months	Low-carbohydrate diets resulted in a weight loss of 3.3 kg (95% CI, –5.3 to –1.4 kg) relative to low-fat diets at 6 months
Thomas et al. (2007)	202 overweight or obese adults	Cochrane review of low-glycemic-index vs. high-glycemic-index diets	5 weeks–6 months	Low-glycemic-index diets produced on average 1.1 kg more weight loss (95% CI, –2.0 to –0.2 kg, p <0.05)
Hooper et al. (2012)	73,589 normal, overweight or obese adults	Systematic review and meta-analysis of reduced fat intake vs. normal fat intake	6 months–7.5 years	Diets with reduced fat intake produced an additional 1.57 kg (95% CI, –2.0 to –1.2 kg) weight loss relative to normal fat intake
Wycherley et al. (2012)	1,063 adults, BMI status not specified	Systematic review and meta-analysis of high (27–35% total energy intake) vs. standard protein (16–21% total energy intake) low-fat diets	>12 weeks	High-protein diets result in 0.79 kg (95% CI, –1.5 to –0.08 kg) more weight loss after 12 or more weeks
Ajala et al. (2013)	3,073 normal weight, overweight or obese adults with or without diabetes	Systematic review and meta-analysis comparing low-carbohydrate, low-glycemic index, Mediterranean and high-protein diets	>6 months	Low-carbohydrate diets (–0.69 kg, p = 0.21) and Mediterranean diets (–1.84 kg, p <0.00001) gave greater weight loss relative to high-protein diets
Te Morenga et al. (2013)	1,286 adults	Meta-analysis of reduced dietary free sugars intake	10 weeks–8 months	Reduced sugar intake led to 0.80 kg (95% CI, 0.39–1.21 kg, p<0.001) of weight loss
Te Morenga et al. (2013)	138 normal weight, overweight and obese adults	Meta-analysis of isocaloric diets high and low in free sugars	2 weeks–6 months	No significant changes in body weight after isoenergetic exchanges of free sugars with other macronutrients
Clifton et al. (2014)	3,492 overweight and obese adults	Systematic review and meta-analysis of high protein (>25% total energy intake) vs. control	>1 year	Differences of 5% in protein intake led to nearly 1 kg reduction in fat mass compared to normal protein intake (p = 0.038)

*Systematic reviews, meta-analysis of randomized controlled trials, and cohort studies.

more substantial weight loss than those on low-fat diets.[10] Meta-analysis of 24 randomized trials involving 1,063 adult participants with an average intervention of 12 weeks, showed diets with the highest protein content significantly produced the most favorable reductions from baseline in body weight (–0.79 kg).[11]

MIXED DIETARY RESTRICTIONS

Two calorie-restricted diets high in either protein, carbohydrate, both with moderate fat content (30%, 55%, 30% of total calorific intake respectively) were compared in obese women (BMI >30 kg/m^2) over a 10-week study period showed individuals in the high-protein group lost significantly more weight than those in the high-carbohydrate group (a difference of 4.4 kg), which was mainly due to increased loss of fat (3.7 kg of the total) since losses of lean mass were similar in both groups.[12] Reducing calorie intake include to regulate appetite, increase satiety, or reduce portion size.[13] It has been claimed that "portion size is a modifiable determinant of energy intake that should be addressed in connection with the prevention and treatment of obesity".[13]

REDUCING THE SIZE OF MEALS

In relevant studies calories were removed from the diet without knowledge to the subjects. Any lost weight tends to be regained rapidly.[14] It is difficult to find studies that had covertly reduced energy consumption and monitored subsequent calorie intake as the majority of studies either had added calories or were not blind (Table 2).

TABLE 2: Energy compensation following covert reductions in the energy content of the diet.[13]

Study	Sample	Treatment	Energy substituted	Duration	Food available	Outcome
Porikos, Booth and van Itallie (1977)	8 obese adults	Metabolic ward with sugar or aspartame foods	850 and 897 kcal during two periods	9 days sucrose and 6 days aspartame	Prescribed by stage of study	50% energy compensation
Porikos, Hesser and van Itallie (1982)	6 normal-weight males	Metabolic ward with sugar or aspartame foods; days 7–18 the caloric content reduced by 25%	900 kcal	24 days	Prescribed by stage of study	40% energy compensation after 4–6 days on low-calorie diet then 85% energy for rest low-calorie period
Foltin, Fischman, Emurian and Rachlinski (1988)	6 normal-weight males	Metabolic ward with third of food low calorie on days 6–11	500 kcal	14 days	Apart from periods of lowcalorie foods a free choice	Days 6–11 100% energy compensation; days 12–14 with regular foods available failed to compensate for increased caloric intake
Louis-Sylvestre, Tornier, Verger, Chabert and Delorme (1989)	17 normal-weight males 15–17 years	Normal or low-energy snack (artificial sweeteners + fat) consumed for 5 days	200 kcal	6 days	Dinner provided 1 hour after snack on days 1 and 6	Day 1 snack was not compensated at dinner; day 6 there was precise energy compensation
Foltin, Fischman, Moran, Rolls, and Kelly (1990)	6 normal-weight males	Four lunches differing in fat and carbohydrate	Lunch offered 431 or 844 kcal	4 × 3 days	Apart from lunch freely chosen	76% energy compensation
Foltin et al. (1992)	6 normal-weight males	Metabolic ward with meals varying in fat and sugar/aspartame	Energy varied from 700 to 1,700 kcal	4 × 3 days	Foods varied in energy content in 4 stages of study	16% energy compensation
Naismith and Rhodes (1995)	10 normal-weight Males	Lunch sweetened with sucrose and then sweeteners	500 kcal	10 days	Freely chosen but foods varied in composition	42% energy compensation but varied from 0 to 90%
Lavin, French and Read (1997)	14 female restrained eaters of normal weight	4 × 330 mL sweetened sugar/aspartame: half informed of nature of drink although did not influence energy intake	330 kcal	2 days	High-carbohydrate and high-fat snacks available with drink; day 2 freely chosen	Over 2 days more energy consumed after aspartame drinks 111% compensation

Continued

Continued

Study	Sample	Treatment	Energy substituted	Duration	Food available	Outcome
Reid and Hammersley (1998)	14 normal-weight males and 13 females	Existing soft drinks replaced with those containing sucrose or aspartame	200–400 kcal	7 days	Freely chosen diet	Day 1 less carbohydrate consumed when aspartame consumed; by day 2, there were no differences in intake, that is, energy compensation had taken place

THE LONGER-TERM REGULATION OF ENERGY CONSUMPTION

Dieting

Diet may produce a short-term gain but it is at a long-term cost. One year after dieting, the levels of leptin, peptide YY, cholecystokinin, insulin, ghrelin, gastric inhibitory polypeptide and pancreatic polypeptide have been found to differ from baseline values.[15] A review concluded that "diet-induced weight loss results in long-term changes in appetite gut hormones, postulated to favor increased appetite and weight regain".[16] In long-term dieting does not work; any lost weight tends not to be maintained. An examination of the long-term consequences of low calorie diets found that between one-third and two-thirds of dieters regained more weight than they lost initially.[17] It is important to drive the attention to maintenance of weight loss which is unlikely than reduction of food intake.

Weight Fluctuation

The body has as short-term goals the smoothing out of energy intake and maintaining the existing body weight. Over a period of months large amounts of energy are consumed, over time there are often relatively small variations in body weight. The evidence that weight changes gradually over long periods may be misleading. Weight may not increase gradually, but rather stay stable for long periods,[18] with weight gain occurring at times of excessive intake such as festivals and holidays.[19] This observation of periods of weight stability suggests an ability to balance energy intake and expenditure. If for much of the time the body is able to generate energy balance, this would again argue against the expectation that reducing the caloric content of food will decrease body weight.

Maintaining a loss of weight is the key to reduce the weight. Of those who lose 10% of their weight, only 20% will maintain this loss for at least a year.[20] Thus in the short term it is possible to maintain weight loss, although very few will maintain that loss for 5 years and to increase this percentage and to understand the factors that prevent the regaining of weight.

CONCLUSION

A successful approach to controlling weight needs to take a wider and longer-term approach than studying the intake of calories. There is evidence of physiological mechanisms that monitor intake. On the other hand, most trials investigating dietary macronutrient content, distribution and restriction emphasize the beneficial role of protein and the type as well as proportion of carbohydrates over that of lipids as important factors in weight management.

REFERENCES

1. Martinez JA, Navas-Carretero S, Saris WH, et al. Personalized weight loss strategies—the role of macronutrient distribution. Nat Rev Endocrinol. 2014;10(12):749-60.
2. Fogelholm M, Anderssen S, Gunnarsdottir I, et al. Dietary macronutrients and food consumption as determinants of long-term weight change in adult populations: a systematic literature review. Food Nutr Res. 2012; 56.
3. Hu FB. Resolved: there is sufficient scientific evidence that decreasing sugar-sweetened beverage consumption will reduce the prevalence of obesity and obesity-related diseases. Obes Rev. 2013;14:606-19.
4. Bravata DM, Sanders L, Huang J, et al. Efficacy and safety of low-carbohydrate diets: a systematic review. JAMA. 2003;289:1837-50.
5. Saris WH, Astrup A, Prentice AM, et al. Randomized controlled trial of changes in dietary carbohydrate/fat ratio and simple vs complex carbohydrates on body weight and blood lipids: the CARMEN study. The Carbohydrate Ratio Management in European National diets. Int J Obes Relat Metab Disord. 2000;24:1310-18.

TABLE 1: **Drinks and its calories.**

Drink (ABV)	Measure	Calories (kcal)	Units
Beer/Lager (4%)	1 Pint (568 mL)	182	2.3
Beer/Lager (5%)	1 Pint (568 mL)	244	2.8
Beer/Lager (5%)	1 Bottle (330 mL)	142	1.6
Cider (4.5%)	1 Pint (568 mL)	216	2.6
Stout (4.1%)	1 Pint (568 mL)	210	2.3
Alcopop (4%)	Bottle (275 mL)	170	1.1
Champagne (12%)	Flute (125 mL)	89	1.5
Wine (13%)	Small (125 mL)	114	1.6
	Regular (175 mL)	159	2.3
	Large (250 mL)	228	3.2
Port/Sherry (18%)	Standard (50 mL)	65	0.9
Cream Liqueur (17%)	Standard (50 mL)	175	0.8
Spirit (40%)	Single (25 mL)	61	1.0
Dark spirit e.g. rum/ whisky (40%) + mixer	Large (50 mL) spirit	167	2.0
Light spirit e.g. vodka/gin (37.5%) + energy drink	Large (50 mL) spirit	170	1.9
Light spirit e.g. vodka/gin (37.5%) + diet mixer	Small (25 mL) spirit	54	0.9

(ABV: alcohol by volume)

Source: The information in this chart is taken from Drinkaware using average industry data

esophagus, liver, colon, rectum and female breast.[9] All these cancers showed evidence of a dose-response relationship; i.e. the risk of cancer increases steadily with greater volumes of drinking.[10]

Alcohol Diabetes and Glycemia

Acute intake of alcohol has been shown to improve postprandial controls and can even produce delayed hypoglycemia, since hepatic metabolism of alcohol hampers gluconeogenesis. This fact and nonconsumption of carbohydrates during alcohol intake can easily precipitate serious outcomes. The combination of alcohol-induced hypoglycemia, hypoglycemic unawareness, and delayed recovery from hypoglycemia can lead to deleterious health consequences.

Hypoglycemia is common in diabetic nephropathy due to diabetic medication. However, spontaneous hypoglycemia may also be seen in nondiabetics with chronic kidney disease (CKD).[11] Alcohol taken regularly in moderate quantities (1–2 drinks) a day, can cause improved insulin resistance and can reduce incidence of diabetes type 2.[12]

Alcohol and Cardiovascular Disease Risk

A popular notion is that although high doses of alcohol are harmful to the heart (sudden cardiac deaths, cardiomyopathy, arrhythmias and hypertension), mild-to-moderate alcohol consumption has been associated with reductions in coronary artery disease and even total mortality. The medical literature is full of publications which clearly indicate that a J-shaped curve wherein 1–2 alcoholic drinks a day can be protective for CV events, coronary heart disease (CHD), heart failure (HF) and even congestive heart failure (CHF) markers, CHF hospitalizations and HF mortality. A regular daily intake of such quantities is recommended by some enthusiasts.

Moderate drinking, however, was associated with a lower risk of initially presenting with stable angina in contrast with nondrinking.[13] Findings for alcohol consumption and unheralded coronary death, an outcome of major importance to public health, showing that both nondrinkers and heavy drinkers were more likely than moderate drinkers to present with coronary death with no previous symptomatic presentations have been reported. It was shown that heavy drinkers are more likely to initially present with peripheral arterial disease.[14]

GENETICS HAS A ROLE

There is also some evidence that genes influence how alcohol affects the CV system. An enzyme called alcohol dehydrogenase helps metabolize alcohol. One variant of this enzyme, called alcohol dehydrogenase type 1C (ADH1C), comes in two "flavors." One quickly breaks down alcohol; the other does it more slowly. Moderate drinkers who have two copies of the gene for the slow-acting enzyme are at much lower risk for CV disease than moderate drinkers who have two genes for the fast-acting enzyme.[15] Those with one gene for the slow-acting enzyme and one for the faster enzyme fall in between.

Alcohol and Stroke

Light and moderate alcohol consumption was found to be inversely associated with ischemic stroke, while heavy drinking increased risk of all stroke types, more so of hemorrhagic strokes.[16]

Alcohol and Psychosocial Issues

Aggression, bad judgment, risk taking behavior, antisocial behavior mental depression and psychosis are well-known health issues. Diabetics are known to be vulnerable to psychoaffective disorders and depression.[16]

Alcohol has been identified as one barrier to such limited adherence. In a study of college students with type 1 diabetes, glycemic control was impaired by alcohol use. Similarly, alcohol use was significantly associated with poor diabetes adherence among a sample of Finnish adolescents with insulin-dependent diabetes.[17] Genetics has a role here also.

ALCOHOL AS A FACILITATOR OF CARCINOGENESIS

The accumulation of evidence supporting the relationship between ethanol and cancers led the International agency for research on cancer (IARC) to recognize the cancer-inducing potential (i.e., carcinogenicity) of ethanol in animal models and to conclude that alcoholic beverages are carcinogenic to humans (IARC 2008). Specifically, the Global Burden of Disease (GBD) study found that alcohol increased the risk of cancers of the upper digestive tract (i.e. mouth and oropharynx, esophagus and larynx), the lower digestive tract (i.e. colon, rectum, and liver) and the female breast. More up-to-date systematic reviews and meta-analysis on alcohol consumption and the risk of developing cancer have been published for colorectal cancer[18] for esophageal squamous cell carcinoma, for laryngeal cancer[19] and for oral and pharyngeal cancers.[20,21]

Alcohol and Neuropsychiatric Illnesses

Neuropathy, higher mental functions and dementia are all believed to be exacerbated by acute or chronic intake of alcohol and more so in diabetics. When it comes to evidence base we do not find enough evidence to isolate alcohol consumption as sole factor or a strong contributor to diabetic neuropathy or dementia. However, a strong clinical correlationship of deteriorating neuropathic symptoms and dementia with alcohol intake cannot be negated. On the other hand, suppressing nocturnal neuropathic pains with alcohol are known to induce addictions.[22]

CONCLUSION

Despite clear and strong CV benefits, we as responsible clinicians can certainly not recommend alcohol to our patients. For those who are regularly consuming, a detailed counseling on hypoglycemia and all possible ill-effects is an obligation on part of the treating physician. While nutritional plans and calorie count must never be forgotten, discouraging binge drinking and heavy drinking is equally important. Moderate drinking of 1-2 drinks per day with background understanding of all acute and chronic issues related to alcohol can be a balanced recommendation for those who cannot abandon alcohol. Needless to state, a responsible drinking behavior must be encouraged.

REFERENCES

1. Shield KD, Parry C, Rehm J. Chronic diseases and conditions related to alcohol use. Alcohol Res. 2014;35(2):155-71.
2. Collins SE. Associations between socioeconomic factors and alcohol outcomes. Alcohol Res. 2016;38(1):83-94.
3. Gold MS, Adamec C. Benjamin rush and his views on alcoholism. Alcoholism Alcohol Abuse. 2011.
4. Hasin DS, Stinson FS, Ogburn E, et al. Prevalence, correlates, disability, and comorbidity of DSM-IV alcohol abuse and dependence in the United States: results from the National Epidemiologic Survey on Alcohol and Related Conditions. Arch Gen Psychiatry. 2007;64:830-42.
5. Bouchery EE, Harwood HJ, Sacks JJ, et al. Economic costs of excessive alcohol consumption in the U.S., 2006. Am J Prev Med. 2011;41:516-24.
6. Aston ER, Liguori A. Self-estimation of blood alcohol concentration: A review. Addict Behav. 2013;38(4):1944-51.
7. Bois C, Vogel-Sprott M. Discrimination of low blood alcohol levels and self-titration skills in social drinkers. Quarterly J Stud Alcohol. 1974;35(1):86-97.
8. Anderson P, Baumberg B (2006). Alcohol in Europe. A public health perspective. London, Institute of Alcohol Studies [online] Available from: http://ec.europa.eu/health-eu/doc/alcoholineu_content_en.pdf. [Accessed October 2018].
9. Scoccianti C, Lauby-Secretan B, Bello PY, et al. Female breast cancer and alcohol consumption: a review of the literature. Am J Prev Med. 2014;46 (Suppl 1):S16-25.
10. Rehm J, Gmel GE Sr, Gmel G, et al. The relationship between different dimensions of alcohol use and the burden of disease—an update. Addiction. 2017;112(6):968-1001.
11. Gouranga S, Roy D. A study on etiological spectrum of hypoglycemia in nondiabetic patients in a rural medical teaching institution. Int J Health Allied Sci. 2018;7(2):83-8.
12. Schrieks IC, Heil ALJ, Hendriks HFJ, et al. The effect of alcohol consumption on insulin sensitivity andglycemic status: A systematic review and meta-analysis of intervention studies. Diabetes Care. 2015;38:723-32.
13. Bell S, Daskalopoulou M, Rapsomaniki E, et al. Association between clinically recorded alcohol consumption and initial presentation of 12 cardiovascular diseases: population based cohort study using linked health records. BMJ. 2017;356:j909.

14. Camargo CA Jr, Stampfer MJ, Glynn RJ, et al. Moderate alcohol consumption and risk for angina pectoris or myocardial infarction in U.S. male physicians. Ann Intern Med. 1997;126:372-5.
15. Hines LM, Stampfer MJ, Ma J, et al. Genetic variation in alcohol dehydrogenase and the beneficial effect of moderate alcohol consumption on myocardial infarction. New Engl J Med. 2001;344(8):549-55.
16. Larsson SC, Wallin A, Wolk A, et al. Differing association of alcohol consumption with different stroke types: a systematic review and meta-analysis. BMC Med. 2016;14:178.
17. Engler PA, Ramsey SE, Smith RJ. Alcohol use of diabetes patients: The need for assessment and intervention. Acta Diabetol. 2013;50(2):93-9.
18. Kyngas H. Compliance of adolescents with chronic disease. J Clin Nurs. 2000;9:549-56.
19. Fedriko V, Tramacere I, Bagnardi V, et al. Alcohol drinking and colorectal cancer risk: an overall and dose-response meta-analysis of published studies. Annals of Oncol. 2011;22(9):1958-72.
20. Islami F, Fedirko V, Tramacere I, et al. Alcohol drinking and esophageal squamous cell carcinoma with focus on light-drinkers and never-smokers: a systematic review and meta-analysis. Int J Cancer. 2011;129(10):2473-84.
21. Islami F, Tramacere I, Rota M, et al. Alcohol drinking and laryngeal cancer: overall and dose-risk relation—a systematic review and meta-analysis. Oral Oncol. 2010;6(11):802-10.
22. Zeng L, Alongkronrusmee D, van Rijn RM, et al. An integrated perspective on diabetic, alcoholic, and drug-induced neuropathy, etiology, and treatment in the US. J Pain Res. 2017;10:219-28.

Chapter 12

Cultural Backgrounds of Nutrition: Impact on Diabetes Mellitus

Debaleena Mukherjee, Jotideb Mukhopadhyay

INTRODUCTION

Nutrition therapy plays a pivotal role in the management of diabetes. The role of diet in the etiology of diabetes mellitus came to the forefront when it was observed that the disease was flourishing in the higher socioeconomic strata, which correlating with the excessive consumptions of oil, flour, and sugar.[1] Interestingly during the first and second World Wars, food shortage and famines were documented to have led to a decline in the diabetes related mortality rates.

According to World Health Organization (WHO) and International Diabetes Federation (IDF) the diabetic population in India could rise to 70 million by 2025 and is expected to escalate to as high as 80 million by 2030.[2] India has a rich and highly varied cuisine, and the various dietary patterns are strongly related to socioeconomic status, cultural factors, local agricultural practices, and food availability.[3,4] The impact of diversity in diet reflects well on the anthropometric indices and incidence of obesity and diabetes mellitus and other metabolic diseases.[4]

"NO ONE SIZE FITS ALL" the basis behind planning nutrition therapy in diabetic patients holds true especially with respect to the cultural and dietary diversity. Today's world emphasizes on evidence-based medical practices to achieve maximum positive outcomes. The same applies to the role of nutrition in diabetes management. Medical nutrition therapy is defined as "nutritional diagnostic, therapy, and counseling services for the purpose of disease management, which are furnished by a registered dietician or nutrition professional pursuant to a referral by a physician."[5] Lack of definite guidelines in India and urgent need for evidence-based nutrition practice guidelines (EBNPG) led to the "Diabetes in India Nutrition Guidelines Study" (DINGS) conducted amongst the various states of India from 2012 to 2013.[6]

Traditional food choices are largely dependent on regional preferences. Studies suggest that 30% of Indians are vegetarian.[3,7] The concept of an "average diet" of India is difficult and majorly irrelevant owing to the geographical and cultural diversity. Religion and religious festivals in all groups in India contribute toward food inclusions and avoidances.[7]

Looking briefly at the common dietary preferences in the various zones of India:[3]

- North and West: Predominantly wheat- based diets including breads (roti and naan).Rice- based dishes include vegetables, meat, and legumes. Dairy products such as paneer, yoghurt, butter, ghee, are used extensively
- *South and East*: Predominantly rice-eating regions. A variety of dal and vegetables are popular. Coconut is used in cooking mainly in the Southern states. Southern states also prefer dairy mainly in the form of plain and unsweetened yoghurt.

Some of the common aspects are as follows:

- Meat (chicken or goat) is popular all over India. Beef is consumed mainly by Christians and Muslims, and pork by Christians. Fish is largely consumed in the coastal areas
- Fruits are consumed all over without significant regional variation
- Desserts made from milk, sugar, rice, dal, ghee, nuts, and spices are popularly consumed during special occasions
- Ghee, a popular flavor enhancer is widely used in several households

- Sesame, peanut, and other vegetable oils are generally used in cooking
- Pickles and pappadams are often used.

Green et al. identified 41 dietary patterns in India in a systematic review.[3] Twenty nine dietary patterns were predominantly vegetarian food groups, indicating that vegetarian diets are the predominant diet patterns in India.

As per the review, sweets and snacks were more popular in the East and South, while fruits, vegetables, rice, and pulses were more common in the North and West.[3] Dietary patterns from the East and South showed greater meat or fish consumption than those from the North and West.[3] No significant difference in the most common food groups of dietary patterns were noted with relation to sex or age. There is also a dearth of studies based on nutrition amongst children. Diets also appeared to be changing overtime to provide more energy, and contained larger proportions of potentially less healthy foods, high in sugar.

The following Table 1 are from the systematic review by Green et al. showing predominant dietary patterns with respect to different geographical regions of India.

Associations were reported between the dietary patterns and nutrition and health outcomes, the most common outcomes studied being body size [body mass index (BMI), abdominal adiposity, or waist circumference].[3] Other studies reported associations with diabetes, hypertension, and cholesterol (Table 2).

Presence of snacks as a major dietary component is posing as a major risk factor. Snacks in India are high-fat, high-salt fried foods often high in trans fats.[7] Diets rich in fruits, vegetables, pulses, and nuts are associated with lower cholesterol levels and better risk profile.[8]

Satija et al. identified three main dietary patterns:

1. "Cereals-savoury foods" (rice or rice-based dishes, grains, snacks, soups, spices, and nuts)
2. "Fruit-veg-sweets-snacks" (cereals, vegetables, fruits, cooked milk products, snacks, sugars, and sweets) and

TABLE 1: Dietary patterns with respect to different parts of the country. Dietary patterns in India : a systematic review.[3]

Model no.	Dietary pattern no.	Region	Foods used to define pattern	Variance explained
1	1	East	Snacks, sweets, fruit	14
	2		Fish, soft drinks	12
	3		Ghee, butter	11
	4		Fresh vegetables	10
	5		Dairy products	9
2	1	North	Fruit, dairy products, snacks	–
	2		Vegetables, pulses	–
3	1	West	Pulses, rice	–
	2		Sweets snacks	–
4	1	South	Fruit, vegetables	–
	2		Snacks, meat	–
5	1	East	Vegetables, sweets, fruit, pulses, nuts, poultry eggs	11
	2		Butter, oil, ghee	8
	3		Red meat, dairy products, cereals	8
6	1	South	Fruit, snacks, meat	9
	2		Rice, millet, dairy products	8
7	1	All	Meat, eggs, vegetables	9
	2		Pulses, eggs, leafy vegetables, dairy products	7
	3		Vegetables, meat	7
	4		Fruit, vegetables, dairy products, pulses	5
	5		Vegetables	5

Continued

Continued

Model no.	Dietary pattern no.	Region	Foods used to define pattern	Variance explained
8	1	All	Rice, nuts	–
	2		Other cereals, vegetables, fruit, dairy products, snacks, sweets	–
	3		Red meat, poultry, fish, eggs	–
9	1	West	Rice, pulses	–
	2		Snacks, fruit	–
	3		Wheat, dairy products, sprouts	–
	4		Millet, sprouts, leafy vegetables	–
	5		Sorghum, leafy vegetables	–
10	1	East	Dairy products, sugar	15
	2		Cereals, roots, vegetables, oils	10
	3		Cereals, pulses, nuts, seeds	9
	4		Cereals, leafy vegetables, fruit	8
	5		Fish, oils	8
	6		Meat, poultry	8
11	1	East	Dairy products, sugar	14
	2		Roots, vegetables	10
	3		Cereals, pulses, nuts, seeds	9
	4		Fish, oils	9
	5		Leafy vegetables, fruit	8
	6		Meat, poultry	8
TOTAL	41			

TABLE 2: Statistically significant relationship between dietary patterns and nutrition or health outcomes. Dietary patterns in India : a systematic review[3]

Nutrition/health outcome	Model no.	Dietary pattern no.	Foods used to define pattern	Direction of relationship
Body size (body mass index, abdominal adiposity or waist circumference)	2	1	Fruit, dairy products, snacks	+
	3	2	Sweets, snacks	+
	4	2	Snacks, meat	+
	5	2	Butter, oil, ghee	+
	6	1	Fruit, snacks, meat	–
	8	3	Red meat, poultry, fish, eggs	+
Hypertension	2	1	Fruit, dairy products, snacks	+
	4	1	Fruit, vegetables	–
Diabetes (or prediabetes)	3	1	Pulses, rice	–
	3	2	Sweets, snacks	+
Cholesterol	5	1	Vegetables, sweets, fruits, pulses, nuts, poultry, eggs	–

"animal-food" (red meat, poultry, fish or seafood, and eggs)[8]

3. "Animal food"(red meat,poultry, fish/seafood,eggs)

Positive associations were found between the "animal-food" pattern and obesity. "Cereals-savoury foods" pattern was associated with reduced incidence of obesity and central obesity.[8]

Diets rich in cereals, fruits, vegetables, adequate amount of protein, and low in trans fat improved insulin sensitivity and better glycemic and metabolic control. Whole grains contain fiber, starch, antioxidants, phenolic compounds, and lignin, which are again associated with reduced risk of insulin resistance, obesity, dyslipidemia, diabetes, and cardiovascular disease (CVD).[9] India went through a nutrition transition, shifting from diets rich in cereals and fiber to diets high in sugar, fats, and animal-source foods with consequent rise in obesity and diabetes.[10]

A review of national surveys on diet and nutrition in India found that between 1975 and 1995, along with a progressive reduction in cereal grain consumption, there was an increase in intake of milk and milk products, animal products and fats and oils. There is a strong positive association between an "animal-food" dietary pattern and obesity and diabetes in India.[11,12]

Beyond India, some studies in the United Kingdom have found vegetarian and vegan diets are associated with lower BMI and lesser weight gain compared to "omnivorous", or meat and fish based diets.[13]

In Saudi Arabia study of food choices revealed many Saudis are becoming more obese with quickly escalating diabetes incidence because of fast foods and consumption of high-sugar drinks.[14]

In Indonesia, a study of dietary practices among diabetic patients elaborated that the Indonesian people preferred to consume high-fat foods leading to an increased risk of CVD.[15] The trending norm of skipping breakfast has dramatically increased over the past 10 years amongst children, adolescents, and adults. It has been found to have strong correlation with obesity.[16] Frequent eating or snacking may also increase the body weight and risk of metabolic diseases.[17]

CONCLUSION

India is a nation with rich cultural diversity, which reflects well on the dietary choices of its people. With vegetarian diet being the predominant pattern, there is large regional variation and changing patterns over time. There is currently limited evidence of associations between dietary patterns and impact on diabetes but strong correlations do exist between consumption of animal and animal products rich food and snacks or fast food rich in Trans fat with obesity and diabetes. This brings up the need for EBPNG for implementation of medical nutrition therapy for management of diabetes, modified as per regional variation.

REFERENCES

1. Seidell JC. Dietary fat and obesity: an epidemiologic perspective. Am J Clin Nutr. 1998; 67(3 Suppl):546S-50S.
2. Wild S, Roglic G, Green A, et al. Global prevalence of diabetes: estimates for the year 2000 and projections for 2030. Diabetes Care. 2004;27(5):1047-53.
3. Green R, Milner J, Joy EJ, et al. Dietary patterns in India: a systematic review. Br J Nutr. 2016;116(1):142-8.
4. Subramanyam MA, Kawachi I, Berkman LF, et al. Socioeconomic inequalities in childhood undernutrition in India: analyzing trends between 1992 and 2005. PLoS One. 2010;5(6):e11392.
5. Centers for Medicare & Medicaid Services. Decision Memo for Medical Nutrition Therapy Benefit for Diabetes & ESRD (CAG-00097N). Washington, DC: Centers for Medicare & Medicaid Services; 2002.
6. Myers EF, Trostler N, Varsha V, et al. Insights From the Diabetes in India Nutrition Guidelines Study Adopting Innovations Using a Knowledge Transfer Model. Top Clin Nutr. 2017;32(1):69-86.
7. Misra A, Singhal N, Sivakumar B, et al. Nutrition transition in India: secular trends in dietary intake and their relationship to diet-related non-communicable diseases. J Diabetes. 2011;3(4):278-92.
8. Satija A, Hu FB, Bowen L, et al. Dietary patterns in India and their association with obesity and central obesity. Public Health Nutr. 2015;18(16):3031-41.
9. Vecchio MG, Paramesh EC, Paramesh H, et al. Types of food and nutrient intake in India: a literature review. Indian J Pediatr. 2014;81(Suppl 1):17-22.
10. Shetty PS. Nutrition transition in India. Public Health Nutr. 2002; 5(1A):175-82.
11. Habib F, Durrani AM. Impact of Dietary Pattern on Glycemic Level Among Type 2 Diabetic Patients. Curr Res Nutr Food Sci. 2018;6(1).
12. Patro S, Adhya AK, Pal P, et al. "Study of dietary patterns and risk profile among the patients of Diabetes Mellitus in Bhubaneswar"-an Original Research article. Int J Drug Devlop & Res. 2014;6(4):124-32.
13. Savoca M, Miller C. Food selection and eating patterns: themes found among people with type 2 diabetes mellitus. J Nutr Educ. 2001;33(4):224-33.
14. Badran M, Laher I. Obesity in arabic-speaking countries. J Obes. 2011; 2011:686430.
15. Persell SD, Keating NL, Landrum MB, et al. Relationship of diabetes-specific knowledge to self-management activities, ambulatory preventive care, and metabolic outcomes. Prev Med. 2004; 39(4):746-52.
16. Siega-Riz AM, Popkin BM, Carson T. Trends in breakfast consumption for children in the United States from 1965-1991. Am J Clin Nutr. 1998;67(4):748S-56S.
17. McCrory MA, Campbell WW. Effects of eating frequency, snacking, and breakfast skipping on energy regulation: symposium overview. J Nutr. 2011;141(1):144-7.

Chapter 13

Diet and Medications for Young Onset Diabetes—What is New?

Nitin Kapoor, Leepica Dahiya, Nihal Thomas

INTRODUCTION

The global prevalence of diabetes in children, adolescents and younger adults is rising.[1] Young onset diabetes is a chronic condition with implications not only limited to the affected patient, but also involves the whole family. These patients often have multiple queries regarding their disease, which need to be addressed by their healthcare provider (Fig. 1). To appropriately answer these questions and manage a given patient with young onset diabetes, it is essential for clinicians to characterize and identify the specific type of diabetes that may have manifested at an early age.[2] It is also imperative for the treating physicians to be abreast with the latest developments in the field and thereby provide the most updated evidence-based treatment to their patients. This chapter will highlight the most recent updates about the newer medications and dietary aspects for individuals with young onset diabetes.

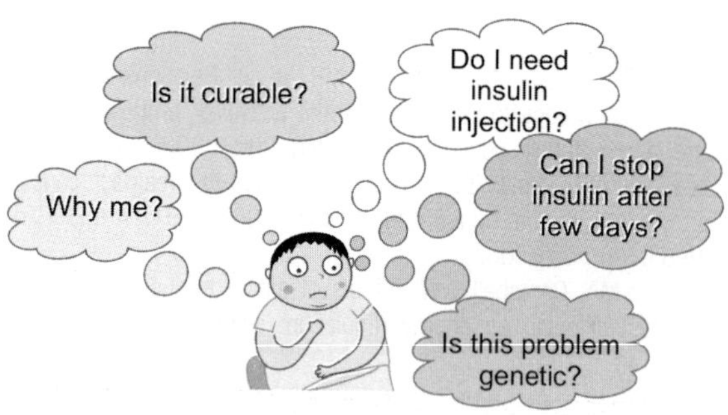

Figure 1 A newly diagnosed patient with young onset diabetes—a patients perspective.

ETIOLOGY OF YOUNG ONSET DIABETES

Though type 1 diabetes (T1D) is classically known to occur at a younger age, those presenting without its classical phenotype may have other types of diabetes manifesting at an early age. With the increasing prevalence of obesity, the quoted prevalence of young onset type 2 diabetes (T2D) is about 15–20% in the Indian population.[3] However, this may vary from different studies based on the age cutoff, limited etiological work up and also due to under diagnosis of less commonly thought but more prevalent forms of diabetes like the fibrocalcific pancreatic diabetes (FCPD) and maturity onset diabetes of the young (MODY).[4,5]

A comprehensive list of the various types of diabetes that occur at a young age is summarized in Box 1.[6] It is essential to gather detailed clinical information about the age of onset, initial symptoms, body weight changes, presence of ketosis, a three generation family history of diabetes, features of secondary diabetes and clinical markers of insulin resistance to make an appropriate clinical diagnosis of the type of diabetes in these individuals. This may further be confirmed by biochemical, radiological, and genetic testing, if available.[7,8]

MANAGEMENT OF YOUNG ONSET DIABETES

The main goals of managing diabetes in younger individuals include adequate glycemic control while avoiding hypoglycemia, assessment and regulation of normal growth and puberty, prevent diabetic ketoacidosis, and to coordinate the treatment regime with the patient's lifestyle and work or study pattern.

Box 1: Differential diagnosis for a patient with young onset diabetes.

I. Type 1 diabetes (β-cell destruction ultimately leading to complete insulin deficiency)
- Immune mediated
- Idiopathic

II. Type 2 diabetes (variable combination of insulin resistance and insulin deficiency)
- Typical
- Atypical

III. Genetic defects of β-cell function
- Maturity onset of the young (MODY) syndromes
- Mitochondrial DNA mutations (includes one form of wolfram syndrome; p Pearson syndrome; Kearns-Sayre syndrome, diabetes mellitus with deafness)
- Wolfram syndrome–DIDMOAD (diabetes insipidus, diabetes mellitus, optic atrophy and deafness): WFS1-Wolframin–chromosome 4p
  - Wolframin locus 2–chromosome 4q22–24
  - Wolframin mitochondrial
- Thiamine responsive megaloblastic anemia (Rogers syndrome)

IV. Drug or chemical induced diabetes

V. Diseases of exocrine pancreas

VI. Infections

VII. Variants of type 2 diabetes
- Genetic defects of insulin action
  - Rabson–Mendenhall syndrome
  - Leprechaunism
  - Lipoatrophic diabetes syndromes
  - Type A insulin resistance–acanthosis
- Acquired defects of insulin action
  - Endocrine tumors Pheochromocytoma cushing
  - Others
  - Anti-insulin receptor antibodies

VIII. Genetic syndromes with diabetes and insulin resistance/insulin deficiency
- Prader-Willi syndrome, chromosome 15
- Down syndrome, chromosome 21
- Turner syndrome
- Klinefelter syndroms
- Other
  - Bardet-Biedl syndrome
  - Alström syndrome
  - Werner syndrome

IX. Gestational diabetes

X. Neonatal diabetes
- Transient–chromosome 6q24, KCNJ11, ABCC8
- Permanent–agenesis of pancreas–glucokinase deficiency (homozygous) and KCNJ11, ABCC8, FOXP3, EIFAK3, IPF1 mutations

In a study published last month by Pinto et al. among individuals with young onset diabetes from the United States, it was shown that majority of these patients were treated with either Insulin (30.8%) or metformin (70.4%) and the usage of thiazolidinediones have declined significantly over the last decade. However, in about 65% of these individuals the glycated hemoglobin (HbA1c) goal (<7%) was not met even 7 years after diagnosis.[9]

Specific issues pertaining to diabetes in a young individual involve to manage the glycemic variability during the growth spurt and insulin resistance induced by the hormonal changes of puberty, to address the psychosocial impact of the diagnosis on the patient and the family, to monitor therapy based on changes in weight and to also account for irregular meal timings, exercise schedule, poor treatment adherence, peer group pressure and academic and professional stress.

A clinical approach to a patient with young diabetes is summarized in the algorithm below (Flowchart. 1).[6] As mentioned before, it is essential to establish the etiology of young onset diabetes prior to embarking on any therapy, as the natural history, therapeutic response and long-term complications would depend on the etiology.[5]

RECENT UPDATES

The primary modality of treatment for any type of diabetes would include lifestyle modifications, which include both physical activity and dietary related interventions. The exercise potential and response of a young individual may depend on several genetic and environmental factors including their birth weight.[10]

Dietary Interventions

Dietary interventions are the cornerstone in the management of Indian patients with young onset diabetes who predominantly consume a carbohydrate and fat-rich diet leading to an increase in body weight and subsequent insulin resistance.[11] The standard dietary recommendations for patients with young onset diabetes are summarized elsewhere[6] and the more recent updates are presented below.

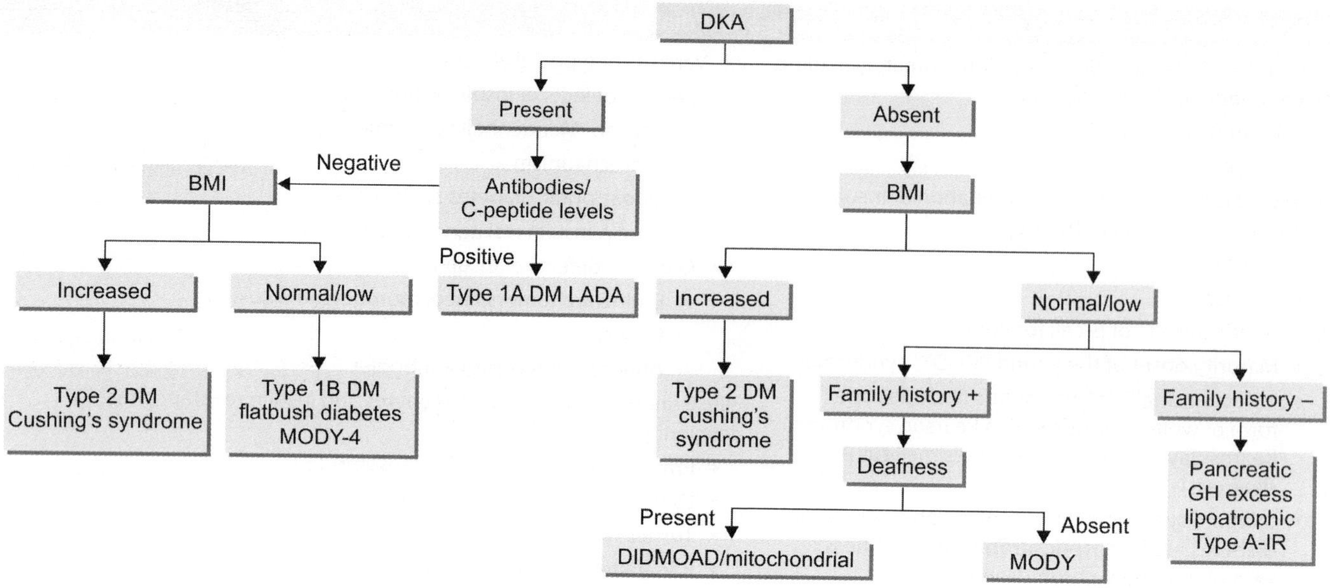

(BMI: body mass index; DIDMOAD: diabetes insipidus, diabetes mellitus, optic atrophy and deafness; DKA: diabetic ketoacidosis; DM: diabetes mellitus; LADA: latent autoimmune diabetes of the adult; MODY: maturity onset diabetes of the young.)

Flowchart 1 A clinical approach to a patients with young onset diabetes.

A recently conducted study in South Indian patients with T1D revealed that the overall nutrient intake, meal composition and meal frequency were inadequate in these patients. There was a deficit of approximately 250–300 calories in the daily diet, when compared to recommended dietary allowance (RDA) according to Indian Council for Medical Research 2010. The percent intake of macronutrients was not in line with the RDA for those with diabetes (carbohydrates 50–60%; proteins 15–20%; and fats 25–30%). The consumption of carbohydrates was 10% higher coupled with an inadequate intake of proteins. The intake of dietary fiber was poor in >50% of the patient population. Univariate regression analysis indicated that a higher percentage of carbohydrates in diet [p = 0.046; confidence interval (CI) = 0.000, 0.157] with a low protein intake (p = 0.045; CI = –1.664, –0.018) and lower meal frequency (p = 0.004; CI = –0.876, –0.170) was significantly associated with higher HbA1c levels.[12] On the basis of this study, it is recommended that adequate protein intake and appropriate meal frequency would help attain a better glycemic control in patients with T1D.

In another recently published study to identify the major barriers to good nutrition practices among young adults (18–45 years of age) with T1DM revealed that time constraints related to work and study responsibilities were the major hindrance to dietary compliance in this young adult population (53%). Lack of proper awareness (17%) about the importance of nutritional principles in diabetes was also a significant hindrance to the treatment process. Other issues faced by a minority of patients include a lack of support from the family, work colleagues and peers (15%), while affordability was an issue in a small number of these patients (14%). Lack of confidence and a low self-esteem was a barrier in following the general dietary advice imparted at the clinic in a proportion of the study population (15%).[13] The key message from this study was to emphasize on the coordination of meal pattern and timings with the work schedule of T1DM patients. There is also a need to enhance the availability of cost-effective, easy-to-prepare and nutrient-rich foods especially when eating out. The importance of meal-dependent insulin dose adjustments should be reinforced at every hospital visit.

It has also been identified that eating disorders are frequently observed in patients with young onset diabetes. A cross-sectional study conducted on 113 patients with T1DM and age gender-matched healthy controls revealed that patients with T1D had a high risk of developing eating disorder (screened using the Eating Attitude Test-26, a validated and standardized tool) when compared to those without diabetes (OR = 38.5 with 95% CI 8.7, 170.7; p <0.001). The risk of developing eating disorder increased with the duration of diabetes though did not correlate with glycemic control.[14]

More recently published work by Anoop Misra et al. has also emphasized the important role of incorporating nuts like almonds, cashews and pistachio nuts in Indian diets, which may lead to multiple beneficial effects on body composition, glycemic parameters and cardiovascular disease (CVD) risk factors in young Indian patients with type 2 diabetes mellitus (T2DM).[15]

Medications

The choice of medications that is used in patients with young onset diabetes predominantly depends on the type of diabetes in these individuals. While it has been possible to treat patients with T1DM after the discovery of insulin, its optimal management necessitates a team effort involving the patient, their family and the healthcare providers to ensure prevention of long-term complications and a high quality of life.[12]

The currently available insulins in the Indian market are summarized in Table 1. The concentrated insulins like glargine U300 that have been recently introduced tend to improve the delivery of insulin when very large doses are needed. This may sometimes be useful in young onset diabetes secondary to various subtypes of lipodystrophy. High dose insulin sensitizers like thiazolidinediones and metformin may also help to reduce the insulin dose in these individuals.[16]

Also the faster insulin aspart has been recently introduced, which has small modifications in its structure by addition of niacinamide, which is an absorption modifier and L-arginine which has been added for stability may be of more utility in individuals who may have brittle diabetes.

Among the oral antidiabetic agents, several oral antidiabetic agents have been recently tested in patients with young onset diabetes and have shown some success and may become future adjuncts in the management of patients with young onset diabetes.

Sulfonylureas are important modalities of treatment in certain younger individuals with monogenic forms of diabetes.[17] This is important as more recently, with the availability of cost effective genetic diagnostic platforms, it is now possible to confirm the molecular diagnosis in the index case and also screen other family members.[4] Given the fact that MODY is often misdiagnosed as either type 1 or type 2 diabetes, many patients end up receiving insulin, along with the complications of insulin therapy and manage to achieve only suboptimal glycemic control. This can be avoided, and treatment can be streamlined if the genetic subtype is known via molecular genetic methods.[8]

Metformin is known for its pleiotropic effects that improve several metabolic parameters. In patients with T1D its role has been suggested to reduce the insulin requirement in those patients with T1D who may have an additional component of insulin resistance. In a recently published paper about use of metformin in these patients, it was shown to be useful in the prevention of CV complications in adolescent patients with T1D. However, not all current literature confirm its usefulness and further studies are necessary.[18]

More recent trials involving sodium-glucose cotransporter-2 (SGLT2) inhibitors like dapagliflozin and sotagliflozin (oral SGLT1 and 2 inhibitor) in subjects with young onset T1D reveal evidence which may support their use as useful adjuncts to insulin in future management of T1D.[19,20]

Another study examined the role of sitagliptin (dipeptidyl peptidase-4 inhibitor) for reduction of postprandial glucose concentrations in young patients with T1D. The authors stated that sitagliptin may be considered as an adjunct therapy in a closed-loop setting.[18]

ANCILLARY MANAGEMENT STRATEGIES—THAT WORK

Role of Diabetes Educators

The role of diabetes educator cannot be under estimated in the management of young onset diabetes of any etiology. Any dietary intervention or drug therapy cannot reach its full potential without having gone through several sessions with the diabetes educator. The initial education session should happen as soon as child and family stabilizes and should comprise of explaining the physiology of glycemic control and talking about practical components in using insulin injections, dose adjustments, storage. It should also cover diet planning, exercise and blood glucose testing, which is customized to an individual patient. Hypoglycemia recognition and management and sick day care can often be lifesaving. Regular review and reinforcement are essential and key to success in the management of young onset diabetes.

Role of Support Groups

Diabetes support groups work well in all types of diabetes but in particular those who have young onset diabetes. Young individuals with diabetes feel often isolated, and often feel uncomfortable talking about it with their peers. Bringing patients with diabetes together to discuss common social problems and health related issues

TABLE 1: Profile of insulins available in the Indian market

Name	Type	Onset	Peak	Duration
Conventional Insulins				
Regular Insulin	Short acting	30–60 min	2–3 h	5–8 h
Biphasic 30/70 Insulin	Premixed	30–60 min	Dual	10–16 h
Biphasic 50/50 Insulin	Premixed	30–60 min	Dual	10–16 h
Neutral protamine hagedorn	Intermediate	120–240 min	4–10 h	10–16 h
Modern insulin				
Aspart	Rapid acting	5–15 min	0.5–1.5 h	<5 h
Lispro	Rapid acting	5–15 min	0.5–1.5 h	<5 h
Glulisine	Rapid acting	20 min	1.5 h	5.3 h
Fast Asp	Very rapid	5 min	20–30 min	4 h
Biphasic Aspart (BIAsp)	Premixed	5–15 min	Dual	10–16 h
Lispro Mix 25/75	Premixed	5–15 min	Dual	10–16 h
Lispro Mix 50/50	Premixed	5–15 min	Dual	10–16 h
Glargine	Long acting	120–240 min	Not pronounced	Up to 24 h
Detemir	Long acting	48–120 min	Not pronounced	Up to 24 h
Degludec	Ultra long acting	30–90 min	Peakless	>42 h
Degludec/Aspart (IDegAsp)	Coformulation	5–15 min	0.5–1.5 h	>24 h
Glargine U300	Long acting	120–240 min	No peak	Upto 36 h

provide them an opportunity to interact and share their experiences. This also provides a common platform for education, social and emotional support for each other. The confidence that a young patient gets seeing another similar aged patient handling his disease well can never match the confidence instilled by a healthcare provider.

CONCLUSION

Diabetes in young is becoming an increasingly prevalent disorder, which is driven by genetic and familial factors, fetal environmental factors, particularly maternal gestational diabetes and intrauterine growth retardation, lack of physical activity and poor dietary choices during childhood and adolescence. Therapeutic options are determined by the etiology of diabetes in a given patient and often require periodic review and reinforcement. It is important for the treating physician to be aware of the recent research on the dietary aspects and newer medications available in the field to be able to provide the most updated evidence-based treatment to their patients.

REFERENCES

1. Cho NH, Shaw JE, Karuranga S, et al. IDF Diabetes Atlas: Global estimates of diabetes prevalence for 2017 and projections for 2045. Diabetes Res Clin Pract. 2018;138:271-81.
2. Gupta RD, Ramachandran R, Gangadhara P, et al. Clinical characteristics, beta-cell dysfunction and treatment outcomes in patients with A-beta+ Ketosis-Prone Diabetes (KPD): The first identified cohort amongst Asian Indians. J Diabetes Complications. 2017;31(9):1401-7.
3. Thomas N, Asha HS, Spurgeon R, et al. Type 2 diabetes in rural India--new paradigms in its epidemiology and evolution. J Indian Med Assoc. 2009;107(11):785-6.
4. Chapla A, Mruthyunjaya MD, Asha HS, et al. Maturity onset diabetes of the young in India - a distinctive mutation pattern identified through targeted next-generation sequencing. Clin Endocrinol (Oxf). 2015;82(4):533-42.
5. Cherian KE, Shetty S, Kapoor N, et al. Carcinoma pancreas and fibrocalcific pancreatic diabetes: a dual association for weight loss. BMJ case rep. 2015;2015.
6. Thomas N, Kapoor N, Velavan J, et al. A Practical Guide to Diabetes Mellitus. New Delhi: Jaypee Brothers Medical Publishers Pvt. Limited; 2018.
7. Kapoor N, Fleming JJ, Ramakrishna B, et al. An unusual cause for weight loss and diabetes. Hong Kong Med J. 2011;17(6):505-6.
8. Nair VV, Chapla A, Arulappan N, et al. Molecular diagnosis of maturity onset diabetes of the young in India. Indian J Endocrinol Metab. 2013;17(3): 430-41.
9. Pinto CA, Stafford JM, Wang T, et al. Changes in diabetes medication regimens and glycemic control in adolescents and young adults with

youth-onset type 2 diabetes: The SEARCH for diabetes in youth study. Pediatr Diabetes. 2018.

10. Thomas N, Bygbjerg IB. Does being born low birth weight affect the ability to exercise? Indian J Endocrinol Metab. 2016;20(6):741-3.
11. Joseph M, Kapoor N, Ramasamy S, et al. Nutritional profile of the morbidly obese patients attending a bariatric clinic in a South Indian tertiary care centre. Obesity and metabolism. 2017;14(2):41-7.
12. Joseph M, Shyamasunder AH, Gupta RD, et al. Demographic details, clinical features, and nutritional characteristics of young adults with Type 1 diabetes mellitus - A South Indian tertiary center experience. Indian J Endocrinol Metab. 2016;20(6):799-804.
13. Joseph M, Gupta RD, Gangadhara P. Barriers to nutritional practices and dietary education in patients with type 1 diabetes mellitus in India. J Global Diabetes Clin Metabol. 2017;6:2.
14. Joseph M, Shyamasunder AH, Mammen P, et al. Type 1 diabetes mellitus and eating disorders. Int J Diabetes Developing Countries. 2017;37(4):502-6.
15. Gulati S, Misra A, Pandey RM. Effect of Almond Supplementation on Glycemia and Cardiovascular Risk Factors in Asian Indians in North India with Type 2 Diabetes Mellitus: A 24–Week Study. Metab Syndr Relat Disord. 2017;15(2):98-105.
16. Shetty S, Chapla A, Kapoor N, et al. A novel variant of the AGPAT2 mutation in generalized congenital lipodystrophy, detected by next generation sequencing. Australasian Med J (Online). 2016;9(6):164.
17. Heuvel-Borsboom H, de Valk HW, Losekoot M, et al. Maturity onset diabetes of the young: Seek and you will find. Net J Med. 2016;74(5):193-200.
18. Otto-Buczkowska E, Jainta N. Pharmacological Treatment in Diabetes Mellitus Type 1 – Insulin and What Else? Int J Endocrinol Metabol. 2018;16(1):e13008.
19. Dandona P, Mathieu C, Phillip M, et al. Efficacy and safety of dapagliflozin in patients with inadequately controlled type 1 diabetes (DEPICT-1): 24 week results from a multicentre, double-blind, phase 3, randomised controlled trial. Lancet Diabetes Endocrinol. 2017;5(11):864-76.
20. Garg SK, Henry RR, Banks P, et al. Effects of sotagliflozin added to insulin in patients with type 1 diabetes. New Engl J Med. 2017;377(24):2337-48.

Chapter 14

Pollution and Diabetes: The Link

NK Singh, Leena Singh, Richa Manaswita, Vaibhav Agnihotri

INTRODUCTION

In last few decades there has been an explosion in the prevalence of diabetes which cannot be fully explained only by the changes of classical lifestyle-related risk factors. There is limited evidence to suggest that decrease in physical exercise and increase in food intake are of large enough magnitude to explain this speed of epidemic of type 2 diabetes (T2D) in the present time. Recently, the role of other nontraditional risk factors is emerging. An increasing number of high to low quality studies indicates that persistent organic pollutants (POPs), air pollution and noise pollution could provide answer to unexplained explosive rise in diabetes prevalence (Flowcharts 1 and 2).[1]

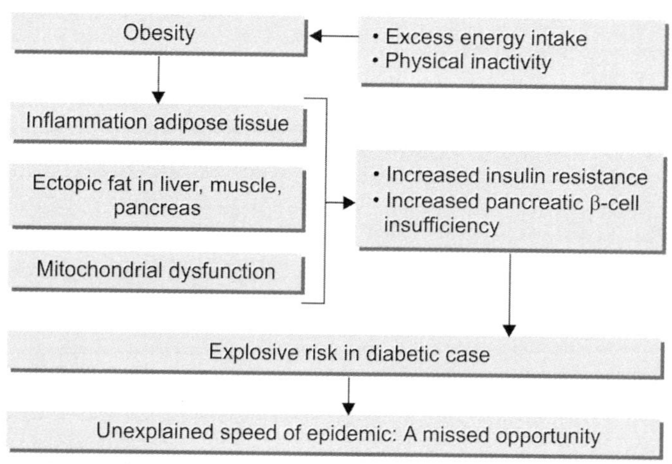

Flowchart 1 Traditional risk factors insufficient to explain explosive speed of diabetes prevalence.

PERSISTENT ORGANIC POLLUTANTS: WHAT ARE THEY (BOX 1)?

Persistent organic pollutants are organic compounds which have become part and parcel of modern lifestyle. These are resistant to environmental degradation and persist in the environment, these bioaccumulate in human and animal tissue and also in food chain. These act as endocrine-disrupting chemicals (EDCs) and thus interfere with the production, release, transport, metabolism, binding, action or elimination of natural hormones. Further, these lead to negative interference of hormonal regulation of adipocyte metabolism, molecular disruption and promote diabetogenesis. Mechanistic studies in animals have shown that these contaminants influence insulin secretion, induce pancreatic cell death, downregulate glucose transporters and lead to insulin resistance.

Evidence with Endocrine Disruptors

Epidemiological, longitudinal and prospective studies are in abundance to point the role of POPs in diabetogenesis (Fig. 1 and Flowchart 3). In 2006, DH Lee et al. for the first time significantly related the role of six different POPs, including polychlorinated biphenyls (PCBs), dioxins and organic pesticides in causation of diabetes by a landmark cross sectional study using USA National Health and Nutrition Examination Survey (NHANES).[2] Following this over 40 cross sectional studies have been published linking POPs and diabetes in different countries. The overall evidence is sufficient for a positive association of some organochlorine POPs. The strongest correlation of diabetes and POPs link has been shown with dichlorodiphenyldichloroethylene

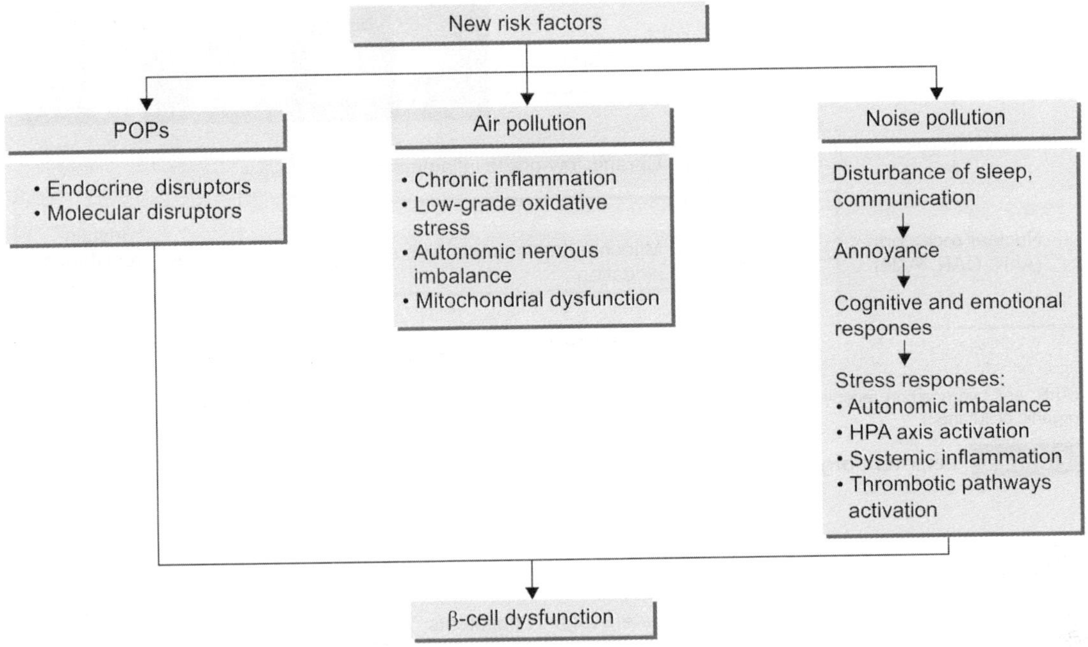

(HPA: hypothalamic-pituitary-adrenal; POPs: persistent organic pollutants.)

Flowchart 2 Nontraditional risk factors.

Box 1: Common chemical pollutants.

Organochlorine Compounds:

- Polychlorinated biphenyls (PCBs):
  - Used as coolants and insulating fluids for transformers and capacitors, as well as plasticizers in paints and cements
- Organochlorine pesticides:
  - DDT, heptachlor, chlordane, aldrin, dieldrin, and mirex
  - Used as herbicides, fungicides or insecticides
- Dioxins:
  - Many different compounds (TCDD)
  - Used as herbicides, fungicides or insecticides

Nonorganochlorine compounds:

- Polybrominated diphenyl ethers (PBDEs):
  - 209 possible compounds
  - Used as flame retardants
- Perfluorinated chemicals (PFCs):
  - Used to make everyday products more resistant to stains, to make clothes more waterproof

Others:

- Bishenol A and phthalates:
  - Used to make certain plastics and resins, lubricating oils, toys, food packaging, detergents etc.

(DDT: dichlorodiphenyltrichloroethane; TCDD: Tetrachlorodibenzo-p-dioxin.)

(DDE), transnonachlor, PCBs, dioxins and dioxin-like compounds.[3] We get strongest evidence for environmental exposures to contribute to the development of diabetes from longitudinal studies. Prospective studies especially by Lee DH et al. (2010), Wu et al. (2013), and Suarez-Lopez et al., (2015) showed significant link with different POPs with diabetes.[4–6] Some high quality animal studies do substantiate the link of POPs with insulin resistance. It has been shown by Ruzzin J et al. that rats fed with POP laden crude salmon oil developed insulin resistance, abdominal obesity and hepatosteatosis.[7] Another significant animal study by Ibrahim et al. showed that mice fed either with contaminated high fat or the western diet exaggerated insulin resistance, visceral fat accumulation, glucose intolerance and a reduction in muscle glucose uptake in response to insulin. Mice fed with the same diet, but with the reduced-POP salmon showed much better insulin sensitivity and glucose tolerance.[8]

Bisphenol A or Phthalates

Major controversy surrounds the roles of bisphenol A (BPA) and phthalates, which are daily used items in our life today. It has been well-shown that these induce the impairment of insulin and glucagon secretion, trigger inhibition of cell growth, and apoptosis and also insulin

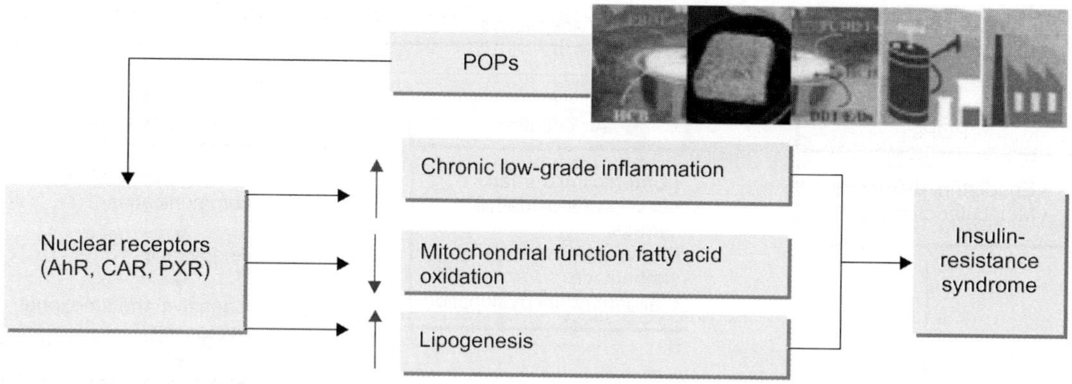

(AhR: aryl hydrocarbon receptor; CAR: constitutive androstane/activated receptor; PXR: pregnane X receptor; POPs: persistent organic pollutants.)

Figure 1 Persistent organic pollutants as molecular disruptors.

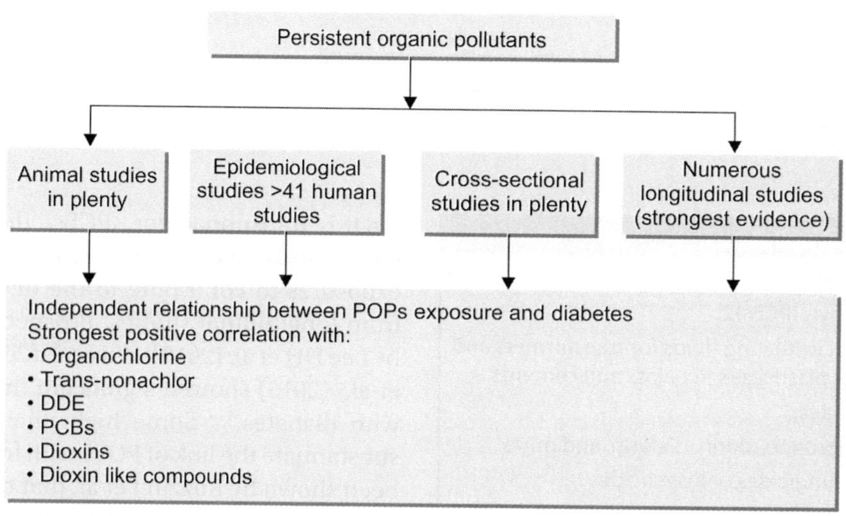

(DDE: dichlorodiphenyldichloroethylene; PCBs: polychlorinated biphenyls; POPs: persistent organic pollutants.)

Flowchart 3 Scientific evidence with persistent organic pollutants.

resistance. One recent study by Stojanoska MM et al. (2017), shows confirmed role of certain phthalates and BPA in diabetogenesis.[9] But as the data are rather inconsistent, we need well-designed prospective studies. Braun JM in a 2017 review concluded that short-lived, less lipophilic EDCs, prenatal exposure to phthalates and BPA (plastic-related chemicals) were not consistently associated with increased future weight. But most studies of perfluoroalkyl (and polyfluoroalkyl substances) have shown a relationship in the same context. The best evidence for EDCs inducing obesity is present for pesticide dichlorodiphenyltrichloroethane, (DDT) which is banned in India too but still being used.[10] A meta analysis of cross sectional and prospective studies by Sony T, Chou EL et al. in 2016, concluded that in the cross sectional studies significant association exists between levels of dioxins, PCBs, organochlorine pesticides and BPA and diabetes but relationship for phthalates was of borderline significance.[3]

In nutshell, it can be appreciated that prospective associations between background exposures to PCBs and organochlorine pesticides with incident diabetes exists.

Many recent prospective studies are in tune with results from a large number of cross sectional studies. A causal relationship between DDT, DDE exposure and diabetes development by experimental studies is very strong. It can be firmly said that many of the EDCs have shown to impair insulin secretion and sensitivity in both human and experimental studies. It is important to understand that, if we want a very high degree of evidence, randomized trials will be needed but it will be never possible to do in the field of EDC research due to practical reasons. An ideal study in this field will take 60–70 years to accomplish and chemicals used in day-to-day life keep changing. In practice we need to rely on results of available studies.

The role of contaminants as potential obesogenic factor is also evident from studies. It is well-known that lipophilic POPs, such as dioxins and organochlorine pesticides, accumulate in adipose tissues to a major degree.[11]

As take home message, it can be said that several epidemiological studies firmly link EDCs to diabetes and this appears enough to ensure high level of protection of human health by regulatory authorities. We have today moderate evidence for an association between EDCs and diabetes.

AIR POLLUTION AND DIABETES

Now air pollution has been shown to a significant risk for diabetes. A number of biological pathways can cause oxidative and endoplasmic reticulum stress, systemic and visceral adipose tissue inflammation and endothelial and mitochondrial dysfunction, which lead to abnormal insulin signaling and insulin resistance. Most of the studies have been derived from outdoor air pollution which also holds true for indoor air pollution.[12]

Traffic-related air pollution from cars, trucks and diesel exhaust is the most studied one in relation to diabetes. More than six published epidemiological studies in relation to diabetes show some degree of association. Although sample size was small, the overall trend of the point estimates was positive. A meta-analysis by Zhao et al. in 2016 suggested that residential proximity to major roadways could significantly increase risk of T2D as independent risk factor.[13] In a recent study by Trenton Honda et al. in USA, particulate matter (PM) 2.5 mm and nitrogen dioxide (NO_2) exposures were significantly associated with prevalence of diabetes and increased hemoglobin A1c (HbA1c) levels among both nondiabetic and diabetic participants. It has been suggested that long-term exposure on PM2.5 would be more likely to develop T2D.[14] These data have been supported by prospective panel studies too.

Taken together though not all findings from every study were positive, the majority of epidemiological studies support an association between air pollution and diabetes. But it must be appreciated that not all aspects of this relationship have been strongly elucidated at this time.

NOISE POLLUTION AND DIABETES RISK

Modern society has become exposed to dangerous noise levels due to faulty festivity and rapid urbanization. Recent studies have raised the concern for the plague-spreading pattern of noise as a risk factor of diabetes. Noise has been classified as a nonspecific environmental stressor. Recently, multiple observational and experimental studies have shown that noise exposure leads to arousal of the autonomic nervous system and endocrine system. The stress of noise elevates circulating cortisol and catecholamine level which leads to insulin resistance and development of T2D. So far no direct evidence has been found to establish the potential causative relationship between noise exposure and the onset of T2D. Sorensen et al., conducted an over 10-year prospective epidemiological study in a Danish cohort and found that each 10 dB increase in average road traffic noise at the current residence was found to be associated with a statistically significant 11% increased risk of incident diabetes and this risk was stronger for higher level exposure and slightly stronger for long-term exposure.[15] Kyoung-Bok Min et al. (2017) showed that first trimester exposure to night time noise was significantly associated with an increased risk for gestational diabetes mellitus (GDM).[16]

In a Danish cohort study no association between railway noise and diabetes was found. In contrast, road traffic noise was associated with diabetes. Interestingly in a recent study, Babisch et al. have shown that aircraft noise exposure during night-time can induce endothelial dysfunction in healthy subjects and is even more pronounced in coronary artery disease patients.[17] Recently by Dzhambov AM et al., a meta-analysis of nine relevant studies was done which showed that people exposed to roughly > 60 dB had 22% higher risk for T2D in comparison to those exposed to < 64 dB (4 dB "grey area"). When studies reporting contentious exposure were excluded there was still 19% risk for 60–70 dB versus less than 60 dB. These risks referred to residential noise exposure.[18]

Taken together, these studies do tell us to further explore the association between noise and diabetes as quality of the evidence till date is low enough to substantiate.

Box 2: How to prevent nontraditional risk factors?

What is urgently needed?

How to educate public?

- Wash fruits and vegetables in running water for at least 3 min
- Use a solution of vinegar or salt and soak fruits, vegetables in it for 5 min
- If possible, peel-off the skin of the fruit or vegetable that you are consuming
- Smaller farm produce is typically pesticide free. Try not to go to larger-sized vegetables or fruits produce
- Buy organic, biological pest control
- Use time honored materials such as glass and stainless steel rather than ubiquitous plastics (BPA-free bottles available)
- Awareness on air quality and noise regulation

(BPA: bisphenol A.)

CONCLUSION

Time has come to look beyond gluttony and laziness in causation of T2D (Box 2). Link with POPs and diabetes is of moderate grade. Among prospective data, most show positive results but results are not consistent across different POPs. An association between organochlorine exposure and T2D exists which includes also DDE, heptachlor, hexachlorobenzene (HCB), DDT and trans-nonachlor. Mechanistic studies do support this link. It is a serious public health issue which is so far not in limelight. Preventive measures exist to check POPs exposure but due to lack of awareness, nothing significant is being done. The role of air pollution is underestimated. Not all of human studies of air pollution and T2D show positive associations, the clear majority do, although there is high risk of bias. Noise pollution and diabetes is also not a fairy tale. Recent studies are alarming though the quality of association between traffic noise and diabetes is low.

REFERENCES

1. Mc Allister EJ, Dhurandhar NV, Keith SW, et al. Ten putative causes of obesity. Crit Rev Food Sci Nutr. 2009;48:868-913.
2. Lee DH, Lee IK, Song K, et al. A strong dose response relation between serum concentrations of persistent organic pollutants and diabetes: results from the national health and examination survey 1999-2002. Diabetes Care. 2006;29:1638-44.
3. Song Y, Chou EL, Baecker A, et al. Endocrine-Disrupting chemicals, risk of type 2 diabetes, and diabetes-related metabolic traits: a systematic review and meta-analysis. J Diabetes. 2016;8:516-32.
4. Hong Kyu Lee. Persistent organic pollutants and epidemic of diabetes and metabolic syndrome. Diabetes Investig. 2010;1(4):121-2.
5. Wu H, Bertrand KA, Choi AL, et al. Persistent organic pollutants and type 2 diabetes: a prospective analysis in the nurses' health study and meta-analysis. Environ Health Perspect. 2013;121(2):153-61
6. Suarez-Lopez JR, Lee DH, Porta M, et al. Persistent organic pollutants in young adults and changes in glucose related metabolism over a 23-year follow-up. Enivron Res. 2015;137:485-94.
7. Ruzzin J, Petersen R, Meugnier E, et al. Persistent organic pollutant exposure leads to insulin resistance syndrome. Environ Health Perspect. 2010;118:465-71.
8. Ibrahim MM, Fjaere E, Lock EJ, et al. Chronic consumption of farmed salmon containing persistent organic pollutant causes insulin resistance and obesity in mice. PLoS One. 2011;6:e25170.
9. Stojanoska MM, Milosevic N, Milic N, et al. The influence of phthalates and bisphenol A on the obesity development and glucose metabolism disorders. Endocrine. 2017;55(3):666-81.
10. Braun JM. Early-life exposure to EDCs: role in childhood obesity and neuro development. Nat Rev Endocrinol. 2017;13:161-73.
11. Lind PM, Lind L. Endocrine-disrupting chemicals and risk of diabetes: an evidence- based review. Diabetologia. 2018;61:1495-502.
12. Rajagopalan S, Brook RD. Air Pollution and Type 2 diabetes mechanistic insights. Diabetes. 2012;61(12):3037-45.
13. Zhao Z, Lin F, Wang B, et al. Residential proximity to major roadways and risk of type 2 diabetes mellitus: A meta-analysis. Int J Environ Res Public Health. 2016;14(1). pii: E3.
14. Honda T, Pun VC, Manjourides J, et al. Associations between long-term exposure to air pollution, glycosylated hemoglobin and diabetes. Int J Hyg Environ Health. 2017:220(7):1124-32.
15. Sorensen M, Andersen ZJ, Nordsborg RB, et al. Long-term exposure to road traffic noise and incident diabetes: A cohort study mette. Environ Health Perpect. 2013;121:217-22.
16. Kyoung-Bok M, Jin-Young M. Noise exposure during the first trimester and the risk of gestational diabetes mellitus. Environ Res Lett. 2017;12:074015.
17. Babisch W. Cardiovascular effects of noise. Noise Health. 2011;13:201-4.
18. Dzhambov AM. Long-term noise exposure and the risk for type 2 diabetes: A meta-analysis. Noise Health. 2015;17(74):23-33.

Chapter 15

Obstructive Sleep Apnea and Diabetes—The Link

Anil Bhoraskar, Jaydeep Khalpada

INTRODUCTION

Obstructive sleep apnea (OSA) is defined as repeated obstructions of upper airway, which may be partial or complete during sleep.[1] The prevalence of OSA has been reported to be between 4 and 26% in males and 2 and 28% in females.[2,3] The variation in prevalence rates amongst several studies is likely due to selection of different sample population in these studies, diagnostic method used in the study, and the criteria used to diagnose OSA in these studies (e.g. oxygen desaturation index, apnea-hypopnea index (AHI), reference daily intake). The prevalence of OSA is on the rise in recent years, which may be attributable to increased prevalence of risk factors for OSA, particularly obesity and also to increased awareness of this condition amongst medical professionals as well as patients in recent years.[2,3]

Obstructive sleep apnea and type 2 diabetes (T2D) share some common risk factors such as obesity and often coexist in patient population.[3,4] The prevalence of OSA is high in T2D patients with a prevalence of 14.1% for mild OSA, 21% for moderate OSA and 28.9% for severe OSA compared to 6.6% in patients without diabetes.[5] The prevalence of T2D is also found to be higher in patients with OSA with studies reporting a prevalence of 15–30%.[6] As a result to these factors, the International Diabetes Federation (IDF)[7] has recommended that patients with OSA shall be screened for metabolic syndrome and a practical approach for T2D patients with classical symptoms of OSA such as witnessed apneas, heavy snoring, or excessive daytime sleepiness (EDS) to be evaluated for OSA in a two-stage screening approach. The first stage is to use a standard questionnaire for sleep apnea such as STOP-Bang questionnaire[8] to establish pretest probability for OSA, and the patients at high risk shall then be advised to undergo a full-night evaluation for sleep apnea using portable monitoring device. However, despite the IDF statement, a majority of diabetes healthcare professionals are unaware of these recommendations and only a few practice screening for OSA in T2D population.

One possible explanation to the lack of OSA screening in patients with T2D could be the lack of awareness about associations between the two conditions amongst diabetes healthcare professionals. Other practical challenge is lack of clear practicing guidelines on when, how, whom and how often to screen for OSA. Overlapping symptoms between OSA and T2D make it difficult to assess whether the symptom is attributable to OSA or T2D, which may further add to the skepticism. The clinical evidence related to clinical, metabolic and economic benefit of treating OSA in T2D patients is scarce. The cost-effectiveness of screening and treatment of OSA in T2D patients is not well established, and the evidence on impact of OSA treatment on diabetes-related outcomes is also limited. The above issues may be the reason routine screening for OSA in T2D patients is difficult to practice by diabetes healthcare professionals.

OBSTRUCTIVE SLEEP APNEA OVERVIEW

Obstructive sleep apnea is the most common type of sleep disordered breathing characterized by repeated partial or complete blockage of upper airway during sleep. Partial blockage of upper airway leads to partial reduction in airflow—hypopnea, and complete blockage of upper airway results in complete cessation of airflow—apnea.[1] These events are often associated with increased negative intrathoracic swings in pressure as the patient attempts to breathe against a collapsed upper airway with increased breathing effort.[2] The lack of airflow leads to a decrease in oxygen saturation, which in conjunction with increased breathing effort may lead to a brief awakening termed as microarousal that often restores the upper airway patency owing to restoration of dilator pharyngeal muscle tone clearing the obstruction.[9] The above sequence of events often repeat itself every few minutes, which results in recurrent episodes of oxygen desaturations and microarousals disrupting the physiological sleep architecture.[10] Such patients usually are deprived of Stage 3 of non-rapid eye movement sleep (NREM sleep) (N3 or deep sleep or slow-wave sleep) and rapid eye movement (REM) sleep and spend most part of their sleep in stages Wake (W), Stage 1 of NREM sleep (N1), and Stage 2 of NREM sleep (N2). Such a sleep architecture is termed as fragmented sleep pattern, which is characteristic of OSA.[10] The lack of N3 and REM contributes to the classical symptom of EDS observed in a vast majority of OSA patients.[2] The above-mentioned series of apnea/hypopnea events in OSA patient also subjects them to cyclical changes in blood pressure (BP), heart rate (HR) and sympathetic tone.[1,2]

Obstructive sleep apnea is diagnosed using a full-night monitoring of various channels attached to the body.[10] The type 1 diagnostic study—a hospital sleep laboratory based attended polysomnography consisting usually of >24 channels along with audiovisual recording of the complete study is the gold standard test for diagnosis of OSA.[10] Since, the type 1 study is usually costly, cumbersome, requires hospital stay for one night and requires a resource-rich setup to conduct the study, alternative type 3 devices—home-based cardiorespiratory monitoring diagnostic devices with fewer number of channels (four to seven channels)—are increasingly used in practice as well as research and their use is supported by the American Association of Sleep Medicine[11] as well as IDF.[7] Modern-day type 3 devices have the sensitivity of 87–96% and specificity of 60–76% for AHI ≥5 events per hour, and sensitivity of 49–92%, specificity of 79–95% for OSA diagnosed as AHI ≥15 events per hour.[12]

Clinically, OSA is often associated with several signs and symptoms most common of which include snoring, witnessed apneas, EDS, insomnia, nocturia, night sweats, morning headache, irritability and concentration difficulty, sexual dysfunction, irregular HR and irregular breathing during sleep.[1,7,11,13-15] Snoring is usually the most common symptom present in as high as 95% of patients, but positive predictive value of this symptom is less owing to high prevalence of snorers without OSA.[11] It is difficult for diabetes practitioners to suspect OSA based on above signs and symptoms, as many of them can also be attributed to diabetes-related cause such as hypo- or hyperglycemia, comorbid cardiovascular disease (CVD), and diabetes complications such as nephropathy or neuropathy.

Some of the comorbidities of OSA include increased risk of motor vehicle accidents, increased risk of hypertension and nondipper phenotype (lack of nocturnal BP drop), increased inflammation, dyslipidemia, higher risk of several CVD including atrial fibrillation and sudden cardiac death, erectile dysfunction and reduced quality of life (QoL).[2,3,10,15-20]

The gold standard treatment of OSA is implementation of continuous positive airway pressure (CPAP) during sleep via a noninvasive vented mask.[21] CPAP treatment has been shown to reduce road traffic accidents, reduce AHI, Epworth Sleepiness Scale, diurnal systolic and diastolic BP, improvement in cognitive function poststroke and improvement in QoL.[10,13,17,22] Some of the other treatment options for OSA include dietary interventions, weight loss, use of mandibular advancement devices, bariatric surgery, and some upper airway surgeries for select group of patients.[4,12] CPAP in conjunction with weight loss is shown to have a greater impact on some cardiovascular risk factors in comparison to CPAP alone.[4]

Obstructive Sleep Apnea and Type 2 Diabetes: What causes What?

It is proven beyond doubt that OSA and T2D coexist; however, is there a causative hypothesis between these two conditions? And if so, which one comes first? There is enough evidence focused on analyzing the impact of OSA on incident T2D. A number of studies including longitudinal studies and meta-analysis have shown that OSA is a risk factor for T2D independent of obesity and other risk factors (Flowchart 1).[23-25] Several studies have shown that OSA contributes to β-cell dysfunction, leading to insulin resistance (IR) through several neurohormonal and inflammatory mechanisms, and elevated oxidative stress.[16,23,24] The severity of OSA is a contributor of degree of IR. The causal relationship between OSA severity and IR appears to be linear.[26,27] The effect of CPAP on IR has been studied in several trials, and early evidence suggests that CPAP treatment has a beneficial effect on IR in both diabetic and nondiabetic individuals.[21,28,29] A few studies,

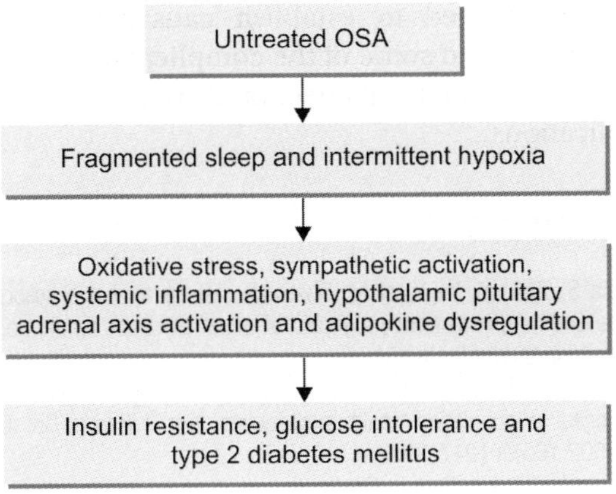

(OSA: obstructive sleep apnea.)

Flowchart 1 Pathogenesis of type 2 diabetes in untreated obstructive sleep apnea.

which did not show a beneficial effect had reduced compliance to CPAP in the study population, which shows that CPAP adherence and compliance play a key role in improvement of IR.[30] This beneficial effect of CPAP on IR and β-cell dysfunction may be due to reduction in oxidative stress, sympathetic activity, hypothalamic–pituitary–adrenal axis and inflammatory mediators.[23]

Whether T2D is a causative factor of OSA or is contributory toward worsening of pre-existing OSA is a plausible and requires more evidence to be confirmed. A meta-analysis has confirmed that moderate-to-severe OSA is associated with a greater risk of diabetes [relative risk 1.63; 95% confidence interval: 1.09–2.45] when compared with the absence of OSA.[24] One study has shown that baseline homa model assessment-estimated IR level is independent predictor of incident witnessed apneas.[31] Other possible causative mechanisms may be common risk factors such as waist circumference, smoking, and abnormal lipid profile.[31] T2D patients tend to gain weight, which has been shown to cause OSA or worsen preexisting OSA, and weight loss in T2D patients helps reduce the AHI.[32] Another possible explanation of development of OSA in T2D may be development of autonomic neuropathy, which can potentially impact upper airway innervation, thereby influencing the collapsibility, impact ventilatory drive, and have an effect on the response of respiratory centers in brain to hypercapnia all of which can lead to incident OSA.[33]

The relationship between OSA and T2D appears to be bidirectional—T2D is a risk factor for OSA, and OSA is a risk factor for T2D.[27] It is interesting that both OSA and T2D are associated with similar comorbidities, some of which include hypertension, CVD, dyslipidemia and chronic kidney disease (CKD).[2,18] Many of the ongoing trials are focusing on whether having both OSA and T2D is associated with greater severity of comorbid conditions compared to either of OSA or T2D alone.

Effect of Obstructive Sleep Apnea on Glycemic Control in Type 2 Diabetes

Several cross-sectional studies have demonstrated a link between OSA and poor glycemic measures like glycated hemoglobin (HbA1c), fasting glucose levels in plasma, and variation in plasma glucose levels following adjustments for several confounding factors.[5,6,26] However, to confirm the causal relationship between OSA and poor glycemic measures, more longitudinal studies would be required. OSA is an independent risk factor for development of T2D as confirmed by a recent meta-analysis.[24] The impact of OSA on glycemic control measured using HbA1c levels ranged between 0.72 and 3.69%, which may be attributable to variations in methodology of the trials and difference in OSA parameters assessed in these studies.[5,34]

Some randomized controlled trials have shown a beneficial effect of CPAP on glycemic controls while other trials did not show a statistically significant benefit.[35-37] These conflicting results could be related to multiple factors such as CPAP compliance in the study group, baseline parameters of glycemic control such as HbA1c and the β-cell function reserve. These finding reinforces the importance of CPAP compliance of its potential benefits on glycemic controls.[30]

Effect of Obstructive Sleep Apnea on Complications of Type 2 Diabetes

Obstructive Sleep Apnea and Hypertension in Type 2 Diabetes

Obstructive sleep apnea is an independent risk factor for hypertension and nondipper phenotype of BP.[23] In T2D patients, OSA treatment with CPAP has been shown to reduce the mean arterial pressure, systolic BP and diastolic BP.[22]

Obstructive Sleep Apnea and Comorbid Cardiovascular Disease in Type 2 Diabetes

Presence of OSA is shown to increase the risk of stroke, coronary artery disease, myocardial infarction and heart failure.[1,18] It is unclear, if treatment of OSA with CPAP alters the outcome of CVD once established; however,

CPAP has been shown to delay or prevent the occurrence of CVD.[1,38,39]

Obstructive Sleep Apnea Microvascular Complications—Retinopathy, Chronic Kidney Disease, Neuropathy

Obstructive sleep apnea can potentially worsen the microvascular complications of T2D as OSA can result in similar mechanisms involved in pathogenesis of microvascular complications of T2D such as oxidative stress and elevated advanced glycated end-products, poly (adenosine diphosphateri bose) polymerase activation, activation of protein kinase C pathway, endothelial dysfunction and inflammation in patients with and without T2D.[9,40]

With limited studies in T2D patients analyzing relationship between OSA and diabetic retinopathy (DR), early evidence indicates an association between OSA and more advanced DR such as preproliferative DR, proliferative DR and maculopathy.[9]

Obstructive sleep apnea is associated with CKD in patients with T2D where OSA leads to a decline in estimated glomerular filtration rate (eGFR) and treatment of OSA with CPAP has a beneficial effect on eGFR.[41]

Early evidence on effect of OSA on diabetic neuropathy shows that OSA is associated with lower intraepidermal nerve fiber density, foot insensitivity, and diabetic peripheral neuropathy. T2D patients with OSA often have history foot ulcers, and treatment of OSA with CPAP may contribute to better management of foot ulcers in such patients.[40]

SUMMARY

The prevalence of OSA in general population is high, and that in T2D population is even higher. Complications of untreated OSA are severe, which include EDS, increased motor vehicular accidents, several cardiovascular, metabolic and behavioral complications. OSA worsens the QoL and is a cause of mortality. Obstructive sleep apnea contributes to poor glycemic control in T2D patients and worsens their hypertension, CVD and other complications of T2D such as neuropathy, nephropathy and retinopathy. Early evidence has shown some promise that treatment of OSA with CPAP in T2D patients improves their glycemic control, BP and can potentially delay or reduce the severity of T2D complications, while definitely benefiting the patients for OSA complications such as EDS and motor vehicular accidents. More longitudinal studies would be needed to establish causative relationship between OSA and some of the complications of T2D, and the definitive beneficial effect of CPAP treatment on T2D complications.

REFERENCES

1. Jia S, Zhou Y, Yu Y, et al. Obstructive sleep apnea is associated with severity and long-term prognosis of acute coronary syndrome. J Geriatr Cardiol. 2018;15:146-52.
2. Young T, Peppard PE, Gottlieb DJ. Epidemiology of obstructive sleep apnea: a population health perspective. Am J Respir Crit Care Med. 2002;165(9):1217-39.
3. Franklin KA, Lindberg E. Obstructive sleep apnea is a common disorder in the population—a review on the epidemiology of sleep apnea. J Thorac Dis. 2015;7(8):1311-22.
4. Joosten SA, Hamilton GS, Naughton MT. Impact of weight loss management in OSA. Chest.2017;152(1):194-203.
5. Kent BD, Grote L, Ryan S, et al. Diabetes mellitus prevalence and control in sleep-disordered breathing: The European Sleep Apnea Cohort (ESADA) study. Chest. 2014;146(4):982-90.
6. Aronsohn RS, Whitmore H, Van Cauter E, et al. Impact of untreated obstructive sleep apnea on glucose control in type 2 diabetes. Am J Respir Crit Care Med. 2010;181(5):507-13.
7. International Diabetes Federation. The IDF consensus statement on sleep apnoea and type 2 diabetes. Belgium: International Diabetes Federation; 2008.pp.1-24.
8. Chung F, Abdullah HR, Liao P. STOP-Bang questionnaire: a practical approach to screen for obstructive sleep apnea. Chest. 2016;149(3):631-8.
9. Tahrani AA. Obstructive sleep apnoea and vascular disease in patients with type 2 diabetes. Eur Endocrinol. 2015;11(2):81-9.
10. Kapur VK, Auckley DH, Chowdhuri S, et al. Clinical practice guideline for diagnostic testing for adult obstructive sleep apnea: an American Academy of Sleep Medicine clinical practice guideline. J Clin Sleep Med. 2017;13(3):479-504.
11. Rosen IM, Kirsch DB, Chervin RD, et al. Clinical use of a home sleep apnea test: an American Academy of Sleep Medicine position statement. J Clin Sleep Med. 2017;13(10):1205-7.
12. McNellis RJ, Thomas S. Screening for obstructive sleep apnea in adults. Am Fam Physician. 2017;96(2):123-4.
13. Miyazaki T, Kojima S, Yamamuro M, et al. Nocturia in patients with sleep-disordered breathing and cardiovascular disease. Circ J. 2015;79(12):2632-40.
14. Tan NYQ, Chew M, Tham YC, et al. Associations between sleep duration, sleep quality and diabetic retinopathy. PLoS One. 2018;13(5):1-14.
15. Abumuamar AM, Dorian P, Newman D, et al. The prevalence of obstructive sleep apnea in patients with atrial fibrillation. Clin Cardiol. 2018;41(5):601-7.
16. Shen H, Zhao J, Liu Y, et al. Interactions between and shared molecular mechanisms of diabetic peripheral neuropathy and obstructive sleep apnea in type 2 diabetes patients. J Diabetes Res. 2018;2018:3458615.
17. Labarca G, Reyes T, Jorquera J, et al. CPAP in patients with obstructive sleep apnea and type 2 diabetes mellitus: systematic review and meta-analysis. Clin Respir J. 2018;12(8):2361-8.
18. Shpilsky D, Erqou S, Patel SR, et al. Association of obstructive sleep apnea with microvascular endothelial dysfunction and subclinical coronary artery disease in a community-based population. Vasc Med. 2018;23(4):331-9.
19. Wang X, Fan JY, Zhang Y, et al. Association of obstructive sleep apnea with cardiovascular outcomes after percutaneous coronary intervention: a systematic review and meta-analysis. Medicine (Baltimore). 2018;97(17):e0621.

20. Pascual M, de Batlle J, Barbé F, et al. Erectile dysfunction in obstructive sleep apnea patients: a randomized trial on the effects of continuous positive airway pressure (CPAP). PLoS One. 2018;13(8):1-13.
21. Chen L, Kuang J, Pei JH, et al. Continuous positive airway pressure and diabetes risk in sleep apnea patients: a systemic review and meta-analysis. Eur J Intern Med. 2017;39:39-50.
22. Joyeux-Faure M, Baguet JP, Barone-Rochette G, et al. Continuous positive airway pressure reduces night-time blood pressure and heart rate in patients with obstructive sleep apnea and resistant hypertension: the RHOOSAS randomized controlled trial. Front Neurol. 2018;9:318.
23. Tahrani AA. Chapter 22: Diabetes and sleep apnea. International textbook of diabetes mellitus. Sussex: John Wiley & Sons; 2015. pp. 316-36.
24. Wang X, Bi Y, Zhang Q, et al. Obstructive sleep apnoea and the risk of type 2 diabetes: a meta-analysis of prospective cohort studies. Respirology. 2013;18(1):140-6.
25. Anothaisintawee T, Reutrakul S, Van Cauter E, et al. Sleep disturbances compared to traditional risk factors for diabetes development: systematic review and meta-analysis. Sleep Med Rev. 2016;30:11-24.
26. Punjabi NM, Shahar E, Redline S, et al. Sleep-disordered breathing, glucose intolerance, and insulin resistance: the sleep heart health study. Am J Epidemiol. 2004;160(6):521-30.
27. Aurora RN, Punjabi NM. Obstructive sleep apnoea and type 2 diabetes mellitus: a bidirectional association. Lancet Respir Med. 2013;1(4):329-38.
28. Iftikhar IH, Khan MF, Das A, et al. Meta-analysis: continuous positive airway pressure improves insulin resistance in patients with sleep apnea without diabetes. Ann Am Thorac Soc. 2013;10(2):115-20.
29. Baburao A, Souza GD. Insulin resistance in moderate to severe obstructive sleep apnea in nondiabetics and its response to continuous positive airway pressure treatment. N Am J Med Sci. 2014;6(10):500-4.
30. Zhu B, Ma C, Chaiard J, et al. Effect of continuous positive airway pressure on glucose metabolism in adults with type 2 diabetes: a systematic review and meta-analysis of randomized controlled trials. Sleep Breath. 2018;22(2):287-95.
31. Balkau B, Vol S, Loko S, et al. High baseline insulin levels associated with 6-year incident observed sleep apnea. Diabetes Care. 2010;33(5):1044-9.
32. Kline CE, Burke LE, Sereika SM, et al. Bidirectional relationships between weight change and sleep apnea in a behavioral weight loss intervention. Mayo Clin Proc. 2018;93(9):1290-8.
33. Tantucci C, Scionti L, Bottini P, et al. Influence of autonomic neuropathy of different severities on the hypercapnic drive to breathing in diabetic patients. Chest. 1997;112(1):145-53.
34. Appleton S, Gill T, Taylor A, et al. Influence of gender on associations of obstructive sleep apnea symptoms with chronic conditions and quality of life. Int J Environ Res Public Health. 2018;15(5). pii: E930.
35. West SD, Nicoll DJ, Wallace TM, et al. Effect of CPAP on insulin resistance and HbA1c in men with obstructive sleep apnoea and type 2 diabetes. Thorax. 2007;62(11):969-74.
36. Dawson A, Abel SL, Loving RT, et al. CPAP therapy of obstructive sleep apnea in type 2 diabetics improves glycemic control during sleep. J Clin Sleep Med. 2008;4(6):538.
37. Martínez-Cerón E, Barquiel B, Bezos AM, et al. Effect of continuous positive airway pressure on glycemic control in patients with obstructive sleep apnea and type 2 diabetes. A randomized clinical trial.Am J Respir Crit Care Med. 2016;194(4):476-85.
38. Marin JM, Carrizo SJ, Vicente E, et al. Long-term cardiovascular outcomes in men with obstructive sleep apnoea–hypopnoea with or without treatment with continuous positive airway pressure: an observational study. Lancet. 2005;365(9464):1046-53.
39. Campos-Rodriguez F, Martinez-Garcia MA, Reyes-Nuñez N, et al. Role of sleep apnea and continuous positive airway pressure therapy in the incidence of stroke or coronary heart disease in women. Am J Respir Crit Care Med. 2014;189(12):1544-50.
40. Altaf QAA, Ali A, Piya MK, et al. The relationship between obstructive sleep apnea and intra-epidermal nerve fiber density, PARP activation and foot ulceration in patients with type 2 diabetes. J Diabetes Complications. 2016;30(7):1315-20.
41. Marrone O, Cibella F, Pépin JL, et al. Fixed but not autoadjusting positive airway pressure attenuates the time-dependent decline in glomerular filtration rate in patients with OSA. Chest. 2018;154(2):326-34.

Chapter 16

Driving Issues in Diabetes

Navneet Agrawal

INTRODUCTION

Driving is a skill of life required by many people for either professional or personal reasons. As the prevalence of diabetes is increasing worldwide, many of the driving license seekers might be suffering from diabetes.[1] Diabetes and its associated complication can affect the driving in many ways like hypoglycemia can impaired the cognitive functions; impairment of sensory and motor function due to retinopathy, neuropathy and peripheral vascular disease.[2] Though the driving is considered as light physical activity, but it has been shown by driving simulator studies that driving requires complex psychomotor skills and has increase metabolic demand. The people with diabetes who wish to drive should be assessed on the individual basis before granting driving license and should be revaluated at regular intervals.[3]

RISK OF DRIVING IN DIABETICS

Previous studies have shown that presence of diabetes in commercial or personal driving is associated with increased but acceptable risk of road traffic accidents as compared to nondiabetic drivers.[4] As per the meta-analysis of 15 studies the relative risk of having a motor vehicle accident in diabetics as compared with the general population range between 1.126 and 1.19, a 12–19% increased risk. Some other studies showed that type 1 diabetic drivers had slightly higher risk of motor vehicle accident though it was not confirmed by some other studies.[2]

Some studies have reported that road traffic accidents (RTAs) rates appear to be higher in drivers with diabetes whereas other studies found no increase.[5] The largest study that examined RTA risk in drivers with diabetes analyzed data from the entire adult Norwegian population (3.1 million) for slightly over 2 years; just over 170,000 were taking antidiabetes medications.[6] People with insulin-treated diabetes had a modestly increased risk of RTAs compared with the population as a whole, with an odds ratio of 1.4 (1.2–1.6). Those taking medication for peptic ulcers or gastroesophageal reflux (neither of which are thought to influence driving performance) had a similar elevation in risk with an odds ratio of 1.3 (1.2–1.4). A meta-analysis of data from all these studies failed to show a significantly higher accident rate, with a nonsignificant risk ratio of 1.26.[7]

The various ways by which the diabetes impacts safe driving are unrecognized hypoglycemia which impairs cogitative functions; retinopathy or cataract which impairs the vision; neuropathy or foot amputation which affect the use of foot pedal and effect of other associated medical condition like sleep apnea. However, the prevalence of these complications is not that extensive to justify restricting all diabetics from driving. The person with diabetes on insulin therapy are often considered for driving restrictions, but when the diabetes is controlled insulin therapy per se has not been found to be associated with increased risk.[8]

An important single factor associated with road traffic accident in drivers with diabetes was recent history of severe hypoglycemia, irrespective of the type of diabetes or the treatment used. In multicentric prospective study of 452 drivers with type 1 diabetes, who were followed for a year, 41% reported 503 episodes of moderate hypoglycemia, where driver could treat him/herself but could no longer drive safely, whereas 5% reported severe hypoglycemia where driver was unable to treat him/herself while driving.[9] Though the hyperglycemia may affect cognitive, motor and perceptual functions, but no significant data is available on the effect of hyperglycemia on driving.

ROLE OF HEALTHCARE PROVIDER

Healthcare provider has an important responsibility of educating people with diabetes on the effect of diabetes on driving. Many of times health professional are not discussing the driving issues with their patients. In a Scottish study, only 62% of healthcare professionals suggested that insulin-treated drivers should test their blood glucose before driving; 13% thought it to be safe to drive with blood glucose of 72 mg/dL, and 8% did not know that impaired awareness of hypoglycemia might be a contraindication to driving.[10]

In patients whose diabetes may pose a risk to safe driving must be assessed and evaluated at the time of giving license and at fixed interval thereafter. The medical examination should include an assessment of glycemic control; frequency and severity of hypoglycemia; symptomatic awareness of hypoglycemia; and the presence of retinopathy, neuropathy, nephropathy, amputation and cardiovascular disease, to identify whether any of these factors could significantly increase the risk of a motor vehicle accident. There should be a focus on various strategies to reduce the risk of hypoglycemia while driving and regular monitoring in patients on insulin or secret gauges. The commercial drivers stay on road for many hours continuously and away from home, should be advised to carry a glucometer and supplies of rapidly absorbed carbohydrate within easy reach.

RESPONSIBILITY OF DRIVER WITH DIABETES

The major responsibility of safe motor vehicle driving lies with the diabetic people who should assess their own fitness to drive and report to their physician if find any condition which can impair their ability of driving. Various studies have shown that majority of the patients do not follow recommendations for safe driving. In a large international study, nearly half of drivers with type 1 diabetes and three-quarters of those with type 2 diabetes had never discussed driving guidelines with their physician.[11] The person should report to the treating physician of any episode of hypoglycemia, any problems in visual acuity and any form of sensory or motor impairment in the limbs. Should not drive when their blood glucose (BG) level is <70 mg/dL. If the BG level is <70 mg/dL, they should not drive until atleast 40 minutes after successful treatment of hypoglycemia. They should avoid driving if feel any symptoms suggestive of hypoglycemia.

CURRENT SCENARIO IN INDIA

Driving in India is risky; at least 400 people are killed in road accidents every day. There are 18 cars per 1,000 people in India. India is also home to about 67 million people with diabetes. Therefore, the likelihood of the occurrence of such an accident is high.[12]

CONCLUSION

Risk of hypoglycemia among drivers with diabetes is high as driving requires complex psychomotor skills and has increase metabolic demand. Regular self-monitoring of blood glucose and strict consultation with health care professionals regarding the various strategies to be adopted to reduce the risk of hypoglycemia is required by the drivers with diabetes.

REFERENCES

1. American Diabetes Association. Defining and reporting hypoglycemia in diabetes: a report from the American Diabetes Association Workgroup on Hypoglycemia. Diabetes Care. 2005;28:1245-9.
2. Frier BM. Living with hypoglycaemia. In: Frier BM, Heller SR, McCrimmon RJ, editors. Hypoglycaemia in Clinical Diabetes. 3rd ed. Chichester: John Wiley & Sons; 2014;369-8.
3. Frier BM, Matthews DM, Steel JM, et al. Driving and insulin-dependent diabetes. Lancet. 1980;315:1232-4.
4. Kerr D, Olateju T. Driving with Diabetes in the Future: In-Vehicle Medical Monitoring. J Diabetes Sci Technol. March 2010;4(2):464-9.
5. Cox DJ, Ford D, Gonder-Frederick LG, et al. Driving mishaps among individuals with type 1 diabetes: a prospective study. Diabetes Care. 2009;32:2177-80.
6. Skurtveit S, Strom H, Skrivarhaug T, et al. Road traffic accident risk in patients with diabetes mellitus receiving blood glucose-lowering drugs. Prospective follow-up study. Diabet Med. 2009;26:404-408.
7. Bieber-Tregear M, Funmilayo D, Amana A, et al. Diabetes and commercial motor vehicle safety. Department of Transportation's Federal Motor Carrier Safety Administration. 2011.
8. Ainsworth BE, Haskell WL, Herrmann SD, et al. Compendium of Physical Activities: a second update of codes and MET values. Med Sci Sports Exerc. 2011;43:1575-81.
9. Graveling AJ, Deary IJ, Frier BM. Acute hypoglycemia impairs executive cognitive function in adults with and without type 1 diabetes. Diabetes Care. 2013;36:3240-6.
10. Watson WA, Currie T, Lemon JS, et al. Driving and insulin-treated diabetes: who knows the rules and recommendations? Pract Diabetes Int. 2004;24:201-6.
11. Harsch IA, Stocker S, Radespiel-Tröger M, et al. Traffic hypoglycemias and accidents in patients with diabetes mellitus treated with different antidiabetic regimens. J Intern Med 2002;252:352-60.
12. Diabetes care. Problems and recommendations for safe driving for people with diabetes. http://www.diabetacare.com/blog/problems-recommendations-safe-driving-people-diabetes/. [Accessed on 1 Nov 2018.]

Chapter 17

Shift Work Associated Metabolic and Genetic Dysregulation among Indians

SV Madhu, K Kiranmala

INTRODUCTION

Alteration of circadian rhythm among shift workers leads to increased cardiometabolic risk. Many hypotheses have been put forward to explain the underlying mechanism and pathogenesis of shift work related metabolic disorders without much success. Shift work causes circadian misalignment leading to alterations in pancreatic β-cell responses and abnormal glucose and lipid metabolism.[1,2] Factors that can cause circadian dysregulation include current lifestyle such as eating or working at night, artificial light exposure at night and change in sleeping schedules. Emerging evidence from many studies suggests that alteration in circadian gene expression particularly in response to one or more of these factors plays a significant role in the development of metabolic disease.

CARDIOMETABOLIC RISK AMONG SHIFT WORKERS

Several studies have shown increase in cardiovascular diseases (CVDs),[1,3] diabetes,[2] metabolic syndrome,[4] obesity[5] and dyslipidemia[6] (including hypertriglyceridemia) among shift workers. Knutsson et al. conducted a 15 years follow-up study and found that the relative risk (RR) of ischemic heart disease was directly proportional to the duration of exposure to shift work.[3]

A recent study in 290 nurses of our hospital at Delhi by our group found a high prevalence of obesity, central adiposity and dyslipidemia.[7] It was found that 80% were overweight or obese and over 82% had central obesity and >30% had hypertriglyceridemia. This indicates a significantly high cardiometabolic risk among nursing personnel. Whether these cardiometabolic abnormalities among nurses are related to shift work need further investigation.

In a prospective study conducted in a cohort of 79,109 women aged 42 to 67 years old from the Nurses' Health Study a higher age-adjusted relative risk of coronary heart disease was found in women who reported ever doing shift work compared with those who had never done so.[1] It was also reported in 2014 in a similar large cohort of nurses from the Nurses' Health Study that all-cause and CVD mortality were significantly increased among women with ≥5 years of rotating night shift work, compared to women who never worked night shifts.[8] Geliebter et al. found that nurses reported weight gain once they started shift work apparently due to changes in dietary habits and exercise patterns.[9]

Katherine Parks studied how shift patterns (day shifts versus day–night rotational shifts) interacted with age and years of shift work exposure in predicting body mass index (BMI). The findings were that age predicted BMI for day-shift workers, but for day–night shift workers, the major predictor of BMI was duration of exposure to day–night shift work.[10] In Belgium, a population-based cohort study followed 1,529 subjects with rotating shift work for 6.6 years and found that rotating shift increased the risk of metabolic syndrome.[4] Rotating shift work resulted in an increased risk of metabolic syndrome in the Taiwanese population.[11] Workers who initially had one or two risk factors for metabolic disease were 4.6 and 12.7 times respectively, more likely to develop metabolic syndrome if they were also engaged in rotating shift work.

Two prospective cohort studies involving shift workers of population on size 69,269 women aged 42–67 in Nurses' Health Study (NHS) I and 10,791 women aged 25–42 years in NHS II with 18 to 20 years of follow-up found an increased risk of type 2 diabetes mellitus (T2DM) in both cohorts.[2]

CIRCADIAN RHYTHMICITY OF GLUCOSE AND LIPID METABOLISM

Alteration in circadian rhythm has been shown to lead to changes in lipid metabolism.[12] Night-shift workers have higher levels of triglycerides in comparison to matched day workers.[13] Under experimental conditions, abrupt changes in timing of sleep and work is followed by significantly altered postprandial glucose, insulin secretion and lipid tolerance enough to lead to atherosclerosis and hence CVD.[12]

A simulated phase shift can significantly alter pancreatic β-cell responses and postprandial glucose and lipid metabolism[12] particularly postprandial triglyceride metabolism. In 2001, a British Antarctic Survey team studied the hormonal and metabolic responses to standard test meals given at three different days and found that subjects displayed altered metabolic responses in the form of glucose, insulin and triglycerides responses to meals after night shifts which returned to baseline 2 days after they returned to day work but triglycerides remain elevated.[14]

Postprandial Lipemia (PPL), particularly postprandial triglyceridemia, has been shown to be a significant independent risk factor for atherosclerosis notably in diabetic subjects.[15] Besides, its possible role in atherosclerosis, PPL particularly postprandial hypertriglyceridemia has also been recognized as a risk factor in insulin resistance. Recent studies including studies from our institution also suggest that high post prandial triglycerides may precede the onset of diabetes and may be associated with development of insulin resistance and diabetes.[16]

Altered lipid metabolism particularly of postprandial triglycerides could be an important intermediate step in cardiometabolic risks associated with shift workers. We assessed the postprandial triglyceride response after an oral fat challenge in doctors, nurses and other health care workers involved in shift work in order to ascertain if these responses are abnormal and could contribute to their cardiometabolic risk profile. Although our study did not find significant differences in postprandial triglyceride levels in health care shift workers when compared with non-shift workers there was a significant positive correlation of postprandial triglyceridemia with measures of insulin resistance in health care shift workers but not in non-shift workers indicating that altered post prandial triglyceride metabolism could be contributing significantly to cardiometabolic risk among health care shift workers.[17]

PATHOGENESIS OF CARDIOMETABOLIC DISORDERS AMONG SHIFT WORKERS

There have been recent advances in understanding the mechanisms and pathogenesis of cardiometabolic disorders among shift workers. Many hypotheses have been postulated to explain this association between shift work and cardiometabolic risk in the past decade. It is notable that chronic circadian misalignment has been proposed to be the underlying mechanism for the adverse metabolic and cardiovascular health effects of shift work.[14] The endogenous circadian timing system regulates much of our physiology and behavior across the 24-h day when it is properly aligned with the sleep/wake cycle. However, there is chronic misalignment between the endogenous circadian timing system and the behavioral cycles, including sleep/wake and fasting/feeding cycles in shift work.

Circadian Rhythm: Genetic and Molecular Mechanisms

All organisms exhibit circadian rhythm that is controlled by molecular circadian clocks. The suprachiasmatic nucleus (SCN) of the hypothalamus is the master circadian clock for the entire body in mammals. In addition there are self-sustained circadian clocks in every cell of tissues throughout the body which are called peripheral clocks.[18]

Genetic Regulation of the Molecular Circadian Clock

The molecular clock is present in all cell types, including pancreatic islets. The central clock is located in the hypothalamic suprachiasmatic nucleus (SCN), which functions as the pacemaker by synchronizing all peripheral clocks via neurohumoral pathways. Light is the primary signal regulating the central clock. In addition, other signals include activity, temperature and food.

Circadian clocks are closely linked to food intake and metabolism. It has been shown that loss-of-function of the circadian locomotor output cycles kaput (*CLOCK*) gene, brain and muscle Arnt-like 1 (BMAL1), in pancreatic β-cells can lead to hypoinsulinemia and diabetes.[19]

Moreover, *CLOCK* genes control many key enzymes in metabolically relevant tissues like liver, adipose tissues and pancreas. Therefore, clock disruption by genetic or behavioral means can lead to severe metabolic derangements including obesity, insulin resistance and metabolic syndrome.[20]

CLOCK gene expression of the central and peripherals clocks is regulated by several interconnected feedback loops.[18] These include both positive and negative autoregulatory feedback loops. The positive regulators are the heterodimers BMAL1/ CLOCK and BMAL1/NPAS2 and the negative regulators are (period) PER1, PER2, PER3, CRY1 (cryptochrome) and CRY2. PER and CRY proteins translocate into the nucleus and form a complex to inhibit transcriptional activity of BMAL1/CLOCK or BMAL1/NPAS2 in a negative feedback loop.

Recent advances have been made on circadian regulation of lipid homeostasis, lipid mobilization and storage in white adipose tissue, development of adiposity and its complications. Studies have shown rhythmicity of *CLOCK* genes expression in adipose tissue of mice and man[21,22] and modulate adipogenesis. It is not fully understood how circadian disruption in human shift workers and in various *CLOCK* gene mutant mice leads to increased adipose tissue deposition and obesity.

CLOCK Genes, Metabolic Syndrome and Type 2 Diabetes Mellitus

In humans, variants of the *CLOCK* gene have been associated with increased predisposition to total energy intake, obesity and metabolic syndrome[23] confirming a link between *CLOCK* genes and metabolism. *BMAL1* gene has been linked to type 2 diabetes and regulates many b-cell genes and affects insulin secretion.[24] The minor allele T of BMAL1-rs11022775 has been shown to be associated with a higher risk of T2DM than allele C in Asian populations.

Several animal studies support a link between *CLOCK* genes and endocrine pancreatic function. However, further research will be required to support their role in humans. Similarly, *CLOCK* gene expression in adipose tissue and in peripheral mononuclear blood cells have been studied by our group among shift workers and suggest that they may have a role in insulin resistance, glucose and lipid metabolism. These emerging evidences suggest that altered circadian gene expression may explain the underlying mechanism and pathogenesis for the adverse metabolic and cardiovascular health effects of shift work.[20]

CONCLUSION

Shift work related cardiometabolic disorders are becoming extremely important in the context of modern day work environments particularly among health care workers. The dysregulation of circadian genes are being increasingly understood and provide the basis for pathogenesis of these disorders. Studies in Indians including those from our group which are focusing on some of these important aspects of circadian gene expression are unraveling important links between circadian genes and metabolic disorders.

REFERENCES

1. Kawachi I, Colditz GA, Stampfer MJ, et al. Prospective study of shift work and risk of coronary heart disease in women. Circulation. 1995;92(11):3178-82.
2. Pan A, Schernhammer ES, Sun Q, et al. Rotating night shift work and risk of type 2 diabetes: two prospective cohort studies in women. PLoS Med. 2011;8(12):e1001141.
3. Knutsson A, Jonsson B, Akerstedt T, et al. Increased risk of ischaemic heart disease in shift workers. Lancet. 1986;328(8498):89-92.
4. Bacquer DD, Risseghem MV, Clays E, et al. Rotating shift work and the metabolic syndrome: a prospective study. Int J Epidemiol. 2009;38(3):848-54.
5. Antunes LC, Levandovski R, Dantas G, et al. Obesity and shift work: chronobiological aspects. Nutr Res Rev. 2010;23(01):155-68.
6. Knutsson A, Bøggild H. Shiftwork and cardiovascular disease: review of disease mechanisms. Rev Environ Health. 2011;15(4):359-72.
7. Aslam M, Siddiqui AA, Sandeep G, et al High prevalence of obesity among nursing personnel working in tertiary care hospital. Diabetes Metab Syndr. 2018;12(3):313-6.
8. Gu F, Han J, Laden F, et al. Total and cause-specific mortality of U.S. nurses working rotating night shifts. Am J Prev Med. 2015;48(3):241-52.
9. Geliebter A, Gluck ME, Tanowitz M, et al. Work-shift period and weight change. Nutrition. 2000;16(1):27-9.
10. Parkes KR. Shift work and age as interactive predictors of body mass index among offshore workers. Scand J Work Environ Health. 2002;28(1):64-71.
11. Lin YC, Hsiao TJ, Chen PC. Persistent rotating shift-work exposure accelerates development of metabolic syndrome among middle-aged female employees: a five-year follow-up. Chronobiol Int. 2009;26:740-55.
12. Hampton SM, Morgan LM, Lawrence N, et al. Postprandial hormone and metabolic responses in simulated shift work. J Endocrinol. 1996;151(2):259-67.
13. Morgan L, Hampton S, Gibbs M, et al. Circadian aspects of postprandial metabolism. Chronobiol Int. 2003;20(5):795-808.
14. Lund J, Arendt J, Hampton SM, et al. Postprandial hormone and metabolic responses amongst shift workers in Antarctica. J Endocrinol. 2001;171(3):557-64.
15. Ginsberg HN, Illingworth DR. Postprandial dyslipidemia: an atherogenic disorder common in patients with diabetes mellitus. Am J Cardiol. 2001;88(6A):9-15.

16. Aslam M, Aggarwal S, Sharma KK, et al. Postprandial hypertriglyceridemia predicts development of insulin resistance glucose intolerance and type 2 diabetes. PloS One. 2016;11(1):e0145730.
17 Kiranmala K, Aslam M, Brijesh M, et al. Postprandial triglycerides in health care shift workers : A pilot study. MD Thesis University of Delhi 2016 .
18. Ko CH, Takahashi JS. Molecular components of the mammalian circadian clock. Hum Mol Genet. 2006;15:271-7.
19. Marcheva B, Ramsey KM, Buhr ED, et al. Disruption of the clock components CLOCK and BMAL1 leads to hypoinsulinaemia and diabetes. Nature. 2010;466(7306):627-31.
20. Bass J, Takahashi JS. Circadian integration of metabolism and energetics. Science. 2010;330(6009):1349-54.
21. Ando H, Yanagihara H, Hayashi Y, et al. Rhythmic messenger ribonucleic acid expression of clock genes and adipocytokines in mouse visceral adipose tissue. Endocrinology. 2005;146(12):5631-6.
22. Otway DT, Mäntele S, Bretschneider S, et al. Rhythmic diurnal gene expression in human adipose tissue from individuals who are lean, overweight, and type 2 diabetic. Diabetes. 2011;60(5):1577-81.
23 Garaulet M, Lee YC, Shen J, et al. CLOCK genetic variation and metabolic syndrome risk: modulation by monounsaturated fatty acids. Am J Clin Nutr. 2009;90:1466-75.
24. Woon PY, Kaisaki PJ, Braganca J, et al. Aryl hydrocarbon receptor nuclear translocator-like (BMAL1) is associated with susceptibility to hypertension and type 2 diabetes. Proc Natl Acad Sci U S A. 2007;104(36): 14412-7.

Chapter 18

Noninsulin-based Therapies in Type 1 Diabetes Mellitus—What a Clinician Needs to Know

Kingshuk Bhattacharjee, Sujoy Ghosh

INTRODUCTION

As per the International Diabetes Federation (IDF) 2017 atlas, India ranks second after United States in type 1 diabetes mellitus (T1DM) with an estimated prevalence of 1,28,000. Earlier Indian studies have reported a prevalence varying from 3.8 cases to 17.93 cases per 100,000 populations.[1,2] Though insulin is the most efficacious agent and main stay of treatment in T1DM, it as many drawbacks. The need of four pricks in the basal-bolus treatment regimen on a life- long basis may have a detrimental effect on the overall health related quality of life in T1DM patients. Furthermore, insulin therapy comes with an inherent property of weight gain and hypoglycemia. The injectable nature and other side-effects of insulin therapy have generated a lot of interest for the use of other non-injectable therapies in T1DM. The purpose of this chapter is to review the latest evidence available with regards to the usage of non-insulin pharmacological agents in the management of T1DM.

BIGUANIDE IN TYPE 1 DIABETES MELLITUS

Metformin is the only biguanide currently in use and is the first line pharmacological agent in the treatment of type 2 diabetes mellitus (T2DM). With the increase in the prevalence of overweight (up to 47%) and obesity in T1DM (by 7-folds), the utility of insulin sensitizer like metformin in ever growing.[3] A variety of research papers has been published on the usage of metformin in T1DM. In 2010, Vella et al. had conducted a systematic review and meta-analysis of 197 published studies including clinical trials, database search and observational studies to evaluate the effect of metformin on HbA1c, body weight, insulin dose requirement and side-effect profile. Despite the heterogeneity in study design, metformin dosage, age of the study subjects and duration of study, the authors concluded that metformin causes reduction in the daily insulin dosage by 5.7–10.1 units, reduces HbA1c by 0.6–0.9% and reduced weight somewhere between 1.7–6.0 kg. The results were confirmed in a subsequent meta-analysis of eight controlled trials by Liu et al. where they found metformin to reduce the daily insulin dosage, body weight and lipid levels in T1DM without increasing the incidence of hypoglycemia and ketoacidosis.[4] However, the same authors in a subsequent meta-analysis though confirmed the same results of metformin in reducing HbA1c, body weight and insulin dosage, but suggested better outcomes in the effects of metformin in the overweight/obese versus non-obese adolescents. The risk of GI adverse event and severe hypoglycemia were also found to be increased with metformin treatment.[5] Nevertheless, the recently published double-blind randomised placebo controlled study (removal) to evaluate the CV and metabolic effect of metformin in T1DM subjects suggested that metformin may offer some atherosclerosis protection for patients with type 1 diabetes (T1D) but does not appear to improve glycaemic control.[6,7]

Thiazolidinedione

Insulin resistance (IR) have been documented even in lean T1DM patients.[6] Although a placebo controlled double blind study evaluating 4 mg rosiglitazone twice daily in overweight T1DM subjects have recommended the usage of thiazolidinedione in T1DM demonstrating a 11% reduction insulin dose and improvement in BP, with maximal benefit being observed in the cohort with greatest IR.[8] However, a more recent study by Stone et al. have reported a reduced insulin dose reduction versus placebo and no benefit in HbA1c reduction.[9] Accordingly in the package insert, the US Food and Drug Administration (USFDA) clearly mentioned rosiglitazone not to be used in T1DM patients.[10] A 6-month usage of 30 mg pioglitazone in T1D has resulted in a modest relative reduction of HbA1c by 0.2% versus placebo. Similarly, pioglitazone and rosiglitazone showed no benefit in IR adolescents with regards to insulin dosage and glycaemic control but caused weight gain.[9,11] Hence, the benefits of thiazolidinedione treatment are minimal and when weighed against the potential risk of oedema and anaemia, a glitazone as an add-on to insulin cannot be considered as a potential treatment of patients with T1DM. Furthermore, concerns exist about bone metabolism, bladder cancer and cardiovascular function with these agents and hence many nations have prohibited its usage and combination with insulin is often contraindicated by the label in the package insert.[12,13]

SULFONYLUREAS

Potentiation of insulin secretion from the pancreatic β-cell is the mode of action of Sus and hence, no benefit in glycaemic control and insulin dose reduction is anticipated in T1DM patients with negligible β-cell function. Two studies have reported betterment in glycaemic control and higher remission rate in new-onset adult T1DM patients with endogenous β-cell function.[14,15]

AMYLIN

Pramlintide is an injectable amylin analogue approved by USFDA for treatment of T1DM since 2005. The recommended starting dose in T1DM is 30 µg 3–4 times per day before main meals or an evening snack which can be up-titrated by 15 µg every 3–7 days reaching a maximal dose of 60 µg. It has no effect on fasting plasma glucose levels and doesn't alter the counter-regulatory response to hypoglycemia and glycaemic recovery time. However, it should never be used in patients with gastroparesis, recurrent hypoglycemic episodes and patients not adhering to SMPG.[16]

Three double-blind, placebo-controlled, randomized controlled trials (two 52 weeks and one 29 weeks) have evaluated pramlintide with placebo as adjuncts to either intensive insulin therapy in T1DM subjects. The 29 weeks study found no difference in HbA1c reduction versus placebo whereas the two 52 weeks reported improvement in HbA1c levels with pramlintide than placebo at 26 and 52 weeks, with between-group differences in HbA1c of 0.2% and 0.3%, respectively.[17-19] Mild-to-moderate nausea, vomiting, anorexia and severe hypoglycemia (during the first four weeks in the dose titration phase) were the most commonly reported adverse events in these clinical trials, numerically higher than placebo. One of these trials evaluated the patient-reported outcomes and reported overall greater satisfaction with pramlintide treatment than placebo.[20]

INCRETIN-BASED THERAPIES

The rationale behind incretin-based therapies in T1DM is based on the animal models and in-vitro studies which demonstrated these agents to have the potential to expand β-cell mass, promote proliferation of β-cells, islet cell neo-genesis and differentiation of β-cells precursors.

Glucagon-like Peptide-1 Receptor Agonists

Unlike T2DM, Glucagon-like peptide-1 (GLP-1) levels are in normal range in T1DM patients; however therapeutic response can only be attained by supraphysiological concentration of GLP-1 which demonstrated these agents have the potential to expand β-cell mass, proliferation of β-cells, islet cell neo-genesis and promote differentiation of β-cell precursors. Three randomized double blind studies of GLP-1 therapy in T1DM have yielded conflicting results. While the first two trials demonstrated no improvement in HbA1c reduction after 3–6 months with addition of liraglutide to insulin, the third study reported a significant HbA1c reduction with liraglutide as compared to placebo. Furthermore, six clinical studies have evaluated glycaemic variability and excursion with GLP-1 RAs. Two studies by Dejgaard et al. and Harrison et al. found no difference in glycaemic variability with liraglutide.[21] On the contrary, Varanasi et al. and Kudawai et al. found glycaemic variability to be significantly improved with time spent in hyperglycaemia is less and more in normoglycaemia but no change in hypoglycaemia.[22,23] Nevertheless, Keilgast et al. had reported the time spent in hypoglycemia to be significantly reduced in patients with preserved β-cell function when liraglutide was added to insulin but no effect in the insulin alone arm.[24] The effect of GLP-1 therapy on weight loss in T1DM subjects is robust and unequivocal with reductions from baseline ranging from -2.2% to -6.6%. The maximal weight loss occurred in the first 12 weeks which stabilised thereafter.

Dipeptidyl Peptidase-4 Inhibitors

Theoretically, the use of Dipeptidyl Peptidase-4 (DPP-4) is in T1DM makes sense in the setting of hyperglucagonemia and in the presence of residual β-cell function in some T1DM patients. Till date, six trials have evaluated this class of agents (Vildagliptin/Sitagliptin) in T1DM. Three placebo controlled studies demonstrated significant reduction in HbA1c ranging somewhere from 0.27% to 0.34% after 4–20 weeks of treatment.[25-27] However, a 52 weeks study with add-on sitagliptin to insulin resulted in no significant HbA1c reduction compared to insulin alone in newly diagnosed T1DM patients.[28] Two studies have demonstrated effective suppression of post-prandial glucagon secretion with vildagliptin but not with sitagliptin.[26,27] It is noteworthy that the counter-regulatory glucagon response in hypoglycemia was found to be intact with DPP-4is.[29] A 20 week placebo-controlled randomised trial with add-on sitagliptin to insulin demonstrated no benefit with regards to changes in body weight and insulin dose requirement versus insulin alone. The more the duration of diabetes, the less the benefits of DPP-4 are in reducing the insulin dose requirement.

SGLT2 Inhibitors and Dual of SGLT1/SGLT2 Inhibitors

The Sodium-glucose cotransporter-2 (SGLT2) inhibitor reduces renal glucose reabsorption and SGLT1 inhibitors decreases intestinal absorption of glucose. Currently, three SGLT-2 inhibitors namely empagliflozin, canagliflozin and dapagliflozin are approved in the treatment of T2DM only. Perkins and colleagues have evaluated 25 mg empagliflozin in an open label design among 40 long-standing T1DM patients over a period of 8 weeks. They reported a small reduction in HbA1c (0.4%), weight reduction by 2.6 kgs and insulin dose reduction by around 9 units. The incidence of hypoglycemia was reduced by 0.08 events per person per day. Two patients had to stop the treatment due to ketoacisosis.[30] In a double-blind, placebo-controlled, dose ranging study of dapagliflozin (n = 70), the 24 hours daily blood glucose concentration was found to be diminished by 2·3 mmol/L from baseline with dapagliflozin 10 mg once per day compared with a reduction of 1·13 mmol/L with placebo. Furthermore, glycosuria was also found to be significantly increased significantly with dapagliflozin compared to the placebo arm (p = 0·007).[31] Henry and associates carried out 18-week RCT of 100 mg or 300 mg canagliflozin once per day compared with placebo in 351 T1DM patients. Modest placebo-adjusted reductions in HbA1c of –0·29% and 0.25% were reported with 100 mg and 300 mg canagliflozin when used once per day. The total insulin dose was significantly reduced by –2·5 U/day and –6·0 U/day, with 100 mg and 300 mg canagliflozin respectively, compared with an increase of 1·6 U/day in the placebo arm. Both doses of canagliflozin reported significant weight loss. No difference in the frequency of hypoglycaemia, noted between canagliflozin and placebo groups. However, the incidence of diabetic ketoacidosis was significantly heightened with both doses of canagliflozin as 4·3% and 6% respectively.[32] In the EASD 2018, the results of the EASE programme evaluating empagliflozin in T1D as adjunct to insulin therapy was presented. EASE included two phase 3 trials with one trial including a new low dose, 2.5 mg, namely EASE-2: 52 weeks (10/25 mg) and EASE-3: 26 weeks (2.5/10/25 mg) respectively. Empagliflozin 2.5 mg as adjunct to insulin showed superior glycaemic control and significant body weight reduction vs placebo without increased risk of diabetic ketoacidosis. Empagliflozin 10 and 25 mg significantly increased risk of diabetic ketoacidosis (DKA), and one fatality occurred in the 25 mg group. Empagliflozin did not reduce the risk of severe hypoglycemia despite lower insulin dose. New 52-week data from the TANDEM programme of dual SGLT1/2 inhibitor sotagliflozin as adjunct to insulin in T1D was also presented in EASD 2018. It demonstrated HbA1c reduction attenuated at week 52 versus week 24 sustained body weight reductions and decreased in insulin dose (mainly bolus) but an increased risk of diabetic ketoacidosis (DKA) and diarrhea. In the similar lines, the new phase 3 data from the DEPICT programme on dapagliflozin in T1D also confirmed attenuated HbA1c reductions with time and increased risk of DKA. It is worth mentioning that both sotagliflozin and dapagliflozin have both confirmed increased risk of DKA, when used at the same doses as approved in T2D. Sotagliflozin and Dapagliflozin are under review in the EU, while in the US so far only sotagliflozin has been filed.[33,34]

CONCLUSION

The role of non-insulin pharmacological agents seems to be fascinating with regards to improving the overall quality of life of T1DM patients by the potential benefit of reducing body weight, lowering glycemic variability and insulin dose requirement. Development of longer acting pramlintide analogues or a dual or triple peptide agonist or antagonist compounds (i.e. GLP-1 combined with GIP and glucagon or PYY) or novel pump devices with the capability to give insulin, glucagon, and gut-derived peptides (i.e. GLP-1, PYY, or GIP) are interesting avenues to be explored in patients with type 1 diabetes.[35]

REFERENCES

1. Asha BP, Murthy BN, Chellamariappan M, et al. Prevalence of known diabetes in Chennai City. J Assoc Physicians India. 2001;49:974-81.
2. Kumar P, Krishna P, Reddy SC, et al. Incidence of type 1 diabetes mellitus and associated complications among children and young adults: Results from Karnataka Diabetes Registry 1995-2008. J Indian Med Assoc. 2008;106:708-11.
3. Conway B, Miller RG, Costacou T, et al. Temporal patterns in overweight and obesity in Type 1 diabetes. Diabet Med. 2010;27(4):398-404.
4. Liu C, Wu D, Zheng X, et al. Efficacy and safety of metformin for patients with type 1 diabetes mellitus: a meta-analysis. Diabetes Technol Ther. 2015;17(2):142-8.
5. Liu W, Yang X-J. The Effect of Metformin on Adolescents with Type 1 Diabetes: A Systematic Review and Meta-Analysis of Randomized Controlled Trials. Int J Endocrinol. 2016;3854071.
6. Petrie JR, Chaturvedi N, Ford I, et al. Cardiovascular and metabolic effects of metformin in patients with type 1 diabetes (REMOVAL): a double-blind, randomised, placebo-controlled trial. Lancet Diabetes Endocrinol. 2017;5(8):597-609
7. Del Prato S, Nosadini R, Tiengo A, et al. Insulin-mediated glucose disposal in type 1 diabetes: evidence for insulin resistance. J Clin Endocrinol Metab. 1983;57:904-10.
8. Gabbay Mde A. Adjunctive therapies to glycaemic control of type 1 diabetes mellitus. Arq Bras Endocrinol Metabol. 2008;52:279-87.
9. Stone ML, Walker JL, Chisholm D, et al. The addition of rosiglitazone to insulin in adolescents with type 1 diabetes and poor glycaemic control: A randomized controlled trial. Pediatr Diab. 2008;9:326-34.
10. Highlights of Prescribing Information: Avandia. Available from: https://www.accessdata.fda.gov/drugsatfda_docs/label/2007/021071s031lbl.pdf[Last Accessed on 2018 June 25]
11. Zdravkovic V, Hamilton JK, Daneman D, et al. Pioglitazone as adjunctive therapy in adolescents with type 1 diabetes. J Pediatr. 2006;149:845-49.
12. Grey A, Bolland M, Gamble G et al. The peroxisome proliferator-activated receptor-gamma agonist rosiglitazone decreases bone formation and bone mineral density in healthy postmenopausal women: a randomized, controlled trial. J Clin Endocrinol Metab 2007;92:1305-10.
13. Nissen SE, Wolski K. Effect of rosiglitazone on the risk of myocardial infarction and death from cardiovascular causes. N Engl J Med. 2007;356:2457-71.
14. Selam JL, Woertz L, Lozano J, et al. The use of glipizide combined with intensive insulin treatment for the induction of remissions in new onset adult type I diabetes. Autoimmunity. 1993;16:281-88.
15. Fallucca F, Sciullo E, Maldonato A. Combined therapy with insulin and sulfonylurea for the treatment of new-onset insulin-dependent diabetes mellitus. Horm Metab Res. 1996;28:86-88.
16. Chapman I, Parker B, Doran S, et al. Eff ect of pramlintide on satiety and food intake in obese subjects and subjects with type 2 diabetes. Diabetologia. 2005;48:838-48.
17. Edelman S, Garg S, Frias J, et al. A Double-Blind, Placebo-Controlled Trial Assessing Pramlintide Treatment in the Setting of Intensive Insulin Therapy in Type 1 Diabetes. Diabetes Care. 2006;29:2189-95.
18. Whitehouse F, Kruger DF, Fineman M, et al. A Randomized Study and Open-Label Extension Evaluating the Long-Term Efficacy of Pramlintide as an Adjunct to Insulin Therapy in Type 1 Diabetes. Diab Care. 2002;25:724-30.
19. Ratner RE, Dickey R, Fineman M, et al. Amylin replacement with pramlintide as an adjunct to insulin therapy improves long-term glycaemic and weight control in Type 1 diabetes mellitus: A 1-year, randomized controlled trial. Diabet Med. 2004;21:1204-12.
20. Marrero DG, Crean J, Zhang B, et al. Effect of Adjunctive Pramlintide Treatment on Treatment Satisfaction in Patients With Type 1 Diabetes. Diab Care. 2007;30:210-16.
21. Harrison LB, Mora PF, Clark GO, et al. Type 1 diabetes treatment beyond insulin: role of GLP-1 analogs. J Investig Med. 2013;61:40-44.
22. Varanasi A, Bellini N, Rawal D, et al. Liraglutide as additional treatment for type 1 diabetes. Eur J Endocrinol. 2011;165:77-84.
23. Kuhadiya ND, Sandeep MA, Sandhu SM, et al. Liraglutide as additional treatment to insulin in patients with type 1 diabetes mellitus: a randomized clinical trial. 23rd Annual Meeting and Clinical Congress of the American Association of Clinical Endocrinologists (AACE). Abstract No. 295, 2014
24. Kielgast U, Holst JJ, Madsbad S. Antidiabetic actions of endogenous and exogenous GLP-1 in type 1 diabetic patients with and without residual β-cell function. Diabetes 2011;60:1599-607.
25. Ellis SL, Moser EG, Snell-Bergeon JK, et al. Effect of sitagliptin on glucose control in adult patients with Type 1 diabetes: a pilot, double-blind, randomized, crossover trial. Diabet Med 2011;28:1176-81.
26. Farngren J, Persson M, Schweizer A, et al. Vildagliptin reduces glucagon during hyperglycemia and sustains glucagon counter regulation during hypoglycemia in type 1 diabetes. J Clin Endocrinol Metab. 2012;97:3799-806.
27. Garg SK, Moser EG, Bode BW, et al. Effect of sitagliptin on post-prandial glucagon and GLP-1 levels in patients with type 1 diabetes: investigator-initiated, double-blind, randomized, placebo-controlled trial. Endocr Pract. 2013;19:19-28.
28. Hari Kumar KVS, Shaikh A, Prusty P. Addition of exenatide or sitagliptin to insulin in new onset type 1 diabetes: a randomized, open label study. Diabetes Res Clin Pract. 2013;100:e55-58.
29. Schopman JE, Hoekstra JBL, Frier BM, et al. Effects of sitagliptin on counter-regulatory and incretin hormones during acute hypoglycaemia in patients with type 1 diabetes: a randomized double-blind placebo-controlled crossover study. Diabetes Obes Metab. 2015;17:546-53.
30. Perkins BA, Cherney DZI, Partridge H, et al. Sodium-glucose cotransporter 2 inhibition and glycemic control in type 1 diabetes: results of an 8-week open-label proof-of-concept trial. Diab Care. 2014;37:1480-83.
31. Henry RR, Rosenstock J, Edelman S, et al. Exploring the potential of the SGLT2 inhibitor dapaglifl ozin in type 1 diabetes: a randomized, double-blind, placebo-controlled pilot study. Diab Care. 2015;38:412-19.
32. Henry RR, Thakkar P, Tong C, et al. Efficacy and safety of canagliflozin, a sodium glucose cotransporter 2 inhibitor, as add-on to insulin in patients with type 1 diabetes. Diab Care. 2015;38:dc151730.
33. Available at EASE programme symposium at EASD2018, NCT02414958, NCT02580591, Diabetes Care online publication, Lilly+BI press release dated 4 October 2018. Accessed on October 14, 2018.
34. Available at EASD2018 programme symposium at EASD2018. Depict: 612 and 613, in TANDEM: 112 and OP19 and 609; ADA2018, 212-OR and 1122-P (in TANDEM) and 213-OR (DEPICT). Accessed on October 14, 2018.
35. Frandsen CS, Dejgaard TF, Madsbad S. Non-insulin drugs to treat hyperglycaemia in type 1 diabetes mellitus. Lancet Diabetes Endocrinol. 2016;4(9):766-80.

Chapter 19

Simultaneous Pancreas and Kidney Transplantation in Type 1 Diabetes Mellitus

Ashish Sharma, Sanjay K Bhadada

INTRODUCTION

Diabetes mellitus (DM) is a major health problem worldwide. Type 2 DM is the most common cause of diabetes in adults. However, in pediatric age group type 1 diabetes is the most common cause of diabetes. Good glycemic control in diabetes is associated with reduced morbidity and mortality. Treatment of diabetes consists of lifestyle modification, oral and injectable antidiabetic agents. Newer preparations of insulin improved the quality of life, but still it is an associated problem of frequent injections and hypoglycemia. With advent of insulin pump, the frequency of pricks reduced drastically, but not abolished completely because frequent glucose estimation is still required to adjust insulin doses and to watch for hypoglycemia. New generation of insulin pumps are equipped with autosuspension of insulin delivery in state of hypoglycemia. All these treatment modalities help in glycemic control and reduces morbidities associated with hyperglycemia, but none is known to reverse the existing diabetes specific complication.[1]

Pancreas transplantation alone or simultaneous pancreas and kidney transplantation can reverse peripheral neuropathy[2] and diabetic retinopathy,[3] prevent recurrence of diabetic nephropathy[4] in the grafted kidney and improve patients' quality of life and life span.[5] Simultaneous pancreas and kidney transplantation is an addition in the management of therapeutic armamentarium of type 1 DM.

EMBRYOLOGY AND ANATOMY OF PANCREAS

At 5 weeks of gestation, the dorsal and ventral pancreatic outpouching arises from the endoderm in the region that forms the future duodenum. Each outpouching develops into major pancreatic ducts which arborize and join coalescing secondary ducts to form the pancreatic ductal system, while the endodermal cells in the wall of the ducts multiply to form the exocrine and endocrine components of the pancreatic parenchyma. As the embryonic pancreas develops into the exocrine cell clusters which form ducts and acini, endocrine cells develop at the edges of these cell clusters forming the pancreatic islets. The islets are more numerous toward the tail region as compared to the body and head of the pancreas. Although comprising only 1% of the pancreatic cell mass, islet activity is detectable between 10–15 weeks of gestation whereas the exocrine pancreatic function begins after birth. The ventral pancreas develops slightly later than the dorsal pancreas and in proximity to the developing liver and bile duct complex. With the clockwise rotation of the foregut the ventral pancreas migrates posteriorly to fuse below the much larger and earlier developing dorsal pancreas trapping the artery of the midgut, the superior mesenteric artery (SMA), in between. The ventral pancreas contributes part of the head of the pancreas and the uncinate process while the dorsal pancreas forms the bulk of the pancreas by the head, body and tail of the pancreas. Being derived from the junction of the foregut and the midgut the pancreatic blood supply is derived from arteries of both regions of the gut, the celiac axis through the splenic artery and the SMA, with collateralization of both arterial trees around the head of the pancreas along the C loop of duodenum and within the pancreas body.[6]

ETIOLOGY AND PATHOGENESIS OF TYPE 1 DIABETES

Type 1 DM is an autoimmune disease which results in the destruction of β-cells within the pancreatic islets. The etiology is poorly understood and both genetic and environmental factors are implicated. Twin studies and studies on families with type 1 DM have revealed associations with specific areas on various chromosomes. The most prominent of these is locus 1 on chromosome 6 which also contains the human leukocyte antigen (*HLA*) genes related to the human immune system.[7] Although, the genetic factors are important, environmental triggers too contribute to the development of this disease as shown studies on twins where there is only 50% risk of type 1 DM in the other twin if one of them is affected. Similarly, where a parent or a sibling is affected, the risk of developing type 1 DM is less than 10%, but much higher than in the general population implying that environmental factors probably trigger the disease onset only when there exist a genetic predisposition. HLA-DR3 and DR4 alleles are associated with predisposition to the disease. Once triggered, the pathology results in both the cellular and humoral autoimmunity against the β-cells, detectable as anti-islet autoantibodies to targets such as insulin, glutamic acid decarboxylase (GAD) and islet antigen 2 (IA-2).

Autoimmune destruction of the pancreatic islets results in insulin deficiency. The resulting elevation in blood glucose levels accelerates the nonenzymatic covalent bonding of glucose to proteins and lipids which form advanced glycation end products. This alteration of structure affects the conformation, function and turnover of a wide variety of proteins and lipids, and triggers altered gene expression, chronic oxidative stress and immune dysregulation by binding to specific receptors of advanced glycated end products. The multiple levels of interference in myriad basic biological processes results in the constellation of disorders that characterizes DM. Autoantibodies may decrease by the time a patient comes for transplantation others such as anti-GAD may persist into the post-transplant period and may sometimes result in recurrence of autoimmune diabetes contributing to pancreas graft loss. Over the years, the pancreas becomes progressively fibrosed, small in size and there is loss of β-cells with prominence of α-cells. In early cases, lymphocytic infiltration may be seen in these areas suggesting that autoimmune response to β-cells is responsible for the disease.

INDICATIONS PANCREAS TRANSPLANTATION FROM DECEASED DONOR PANCREAS

Following are the indications of pancreas transplantation:

- Simultaneous pancreas-kidney (SPK) transplant, in which the pancreas and kidney are transplanted at the same time from the same deceased donor
- Pancreas after kidney transplant (PAK) where deceased, donor pancreas transplant is performed after a previous kidney transplant from a living or a different deceased donor
- Pancreas transplant alone (PTA) for a patient with type 1 diabetes who has brittle diabetes with severe, frequent or life threatening hypoglycemic episodes and hypoglycemic unawareness, but preserved kidney function.

It is being performed by conventional open approach although occasional cases have been reported in the literature with robotic assistance. The donor source is usually from deceased donors, but living donor pancreas transplantation has been also reported.

ISSUES WITH PANCREAS TRANSPLANTATION CLINICAL FEATURES

The patients will have a longstanding history of diabetes and will be on the multiple injections of insulin. Patients requiring SPK will have features of advanced or end stage renal disease. Patients for PAK would have undergone renal transplant for diabetic nephropathy and those with for PTA will have history of brittle diabetes with frequent hypoglycemic episodes. Patients often have received treatment for diabetic retinopathy which is nearly universal in patients with end-stage renal disease due to type 1 diabetes. Gastroparesis is an important problem in these patients as it may affect tolerance to immunosuppressive drugs which are required for successful functioning of transplanted organs. Involvement of the autonomic nervous system may also result in orthostatic hypotension, cystopathy with high post void residual urine. Nearly half of the patients presenting with diabetic nephropathy may have significant involvement of coronary arteries as well and careful evaluation of cardiac status should be carried out. These patients may not exhibit classical features of angina due to underlying neuropathy. Whenever possible, these lesions should be corrected before proceeding with transplant. Many patients will be in a state of fluid overload as ongoing proteinuria leads to lot of accumulation of third space fluid. Therefore, patients should be put on a high protein diet, while on dialysis and efforts should be made to improve the serum albumin. The long duration of diabetes puts these patients at an increased risk of peripheral vascular disease which sometimes may nearly obliterate the lumen of iliac artery and should be screened before transplant. Presence of obliterative vascular disease along diabetic neuropathy may result in non-healing foot ulcers which becomes a contraindication to perform organ transplant. Similarly, patients may also have history of stroke or transient ischemic attack.

ASSESSMENT OF THE POTENTIAL PANCREAS TRANSPLANT RECIPIENT

The patient for pancreas transplantation is one of the sickest patients with multisystemic involvement and the assessment for a successful outcome should include a thorough evaluation of all the clinical features mentioned above. The patient should have a detailed cardiac, neurologic and vascular evaluation apart from the regular evaluation for a kidney transplant patient. Patients would undergo ECG, echocardiography and stress thallium to evaluate the cardiac condition. Any abnormality in these would merit coronary angiography. Doppler of iliac vessels may be required if there is evidence of advanced vascular disease or weak femoral pulsations. It is important to measure C-peptide to confirm absence of insulin and to measure the glycated hemoglobin to know the control of blood glucose. Other routine investigations like blood counts, liver function tests and chest X ray are performed.

Other Nonsurgical Treatment

Advanced insulin pumps can deliver insulin throughout the day and patients can be kept on dialysis but the quality of life is much better after transplant as compared to the nonsurgical treatment.

Contraindications

Apart from the usual contraindications for transplant like presence of active infections, malignancy or other terminal organ failure, poor cardiac status and advanced vascular disease are contraindications for pancreatic transplantation.

EARLY SURGICAL PREPARATION OF RECIPIENT

On being informed of a potential donor, the surgical team should review prospective recipients. Although the prospective recipients may have been under periodic follow up in readiness for a pancreas transplant, the physiologic status is often labile and may have deteriorated in the interim period. Consent and information on possible complications, including outcomes, frequency of repeat surgeries and prolonged in hospital treatment should be reviewed with the patient. Preparation for surgery includes administration of the first dose of immunosuppression and 375 mg aspirin.

DONOR SURGERY

All steps of the surgery should be executed with utmost care to maintain hemostasis, maintain dissection planes and avoid unnecessary injury to the organs being retrieved. Usually, pancreas donor will be a multi-organ donor and all abdominal organs are retrieved together. Donor age should preferably be between 10–45 years and BMI should be less than 30 kg/m^2. The donor should not have any history of glucose intolerance or diabetes. Hyperglycemia at the time of brain death is not a contraindication to proceed with pancreas donation. Donors with history of prolonged ICU stay or hypotension with high ionotropic requirement should be approached with caution for pancreas donation.

INCISION

The donor surgery begins with a wide exposure of the abdomen through a midline incision extending from the suprasternal notch to the pubic symphysis in the midline. Occasionally as in obese donors, extending the incision crosswise across the umbilicus to beyond the rectus muscle on both sides helps to improve the exposure but it is not recommended as a routine in view of worse cosmetic outcome. The extension of incision upwards with a sternotomy greatly facilitates exposure of the upper abdomen, avoids a cruciate abdominal incision and allows access to the thoracic aorta for cross clamping should the surgeon be inclined to do so while adding, at most, a few minutes to the overall surgical duration. A sternal retractor and optionally a self-retaining retractor for the abdominal wall are placed. A quick and thorough examination of the abdominal and thoracic organs is performed before proceeding further. Injuries and pathologies must be noted for later reference.

MEDIAL ROTATION OF VISCERA

Once the abdominal cavity is opened, the bowel is retracted toward the left upper quadrant while the posterior peritoneum over the right iliac vessels is incised and reflected toward the aortic bifurcation exposing the distal inferior vena cava (IVC) and aorta both of which are isolated with vascular slings. Dissection is continued upwards staying close to the ascending colon and sweeping it and the duodenum off the Gerota's fascia and the great vessels till one reaches the left lateral edge of the aorta. During this medial rotation of the right viscera, the inferior mesenteric artery will be encountered arising off the aorta and is divided between ligatures. Accessory renal arteries may arise from the aorta and occasionally from the iliac arteries therefore, any artery arising and travelling laterally needs to be identified and preserved. This dissection is continued upwards till the level of the left renal vein and to the left till almost at the ligament of Treitz. At this point above the junction of the left renal vein with the IVC the SMA may be palpated through a thick mass of lymphatic tissue, arising anteriorly from aorta and coursing anteriorly. The left colon may be mobilized at this stage to assist in surface cooling of the kidney or else may be left until dissection during the cold phase.

Exposure of the Supra Celiac Aorta

The exposure of the supra celiac aorta begins with the division of the left triangular ligament which procedure allows the left lobe of liver to be folded downward. The gastrohepatic ligament is examined for an aberrant left hepatic artery before incising to expose the diaphragmatic crura. Keeping the esophagus to one side the diaphragmatic crura are divided transversely to expose the aorta. Careful palpation of the aortic pulsation helps to ensure that the plane of dissection is correct. The aorta is isolated with vascular slings to assist in cross clamping. The pancreas can be examined for suitability at this stage before proceeding further. Presence of fat infiltrating into its parenchyma or a fibrotic pancreas will preclude its use for transplantation.

EXPOSURE OF THE PORTA HEPATIS STRUCTURES

Between the duodenum and the gallbladder, the common bile duct (CBD) runs on the right, the common hepatic artery on the left and the portal vein posteriorly. An aberrant or accessory right hepatic artery may be palpated on the right of the porta hepatis structures traveling in the free edge of gastrohepatic ligament. The porta hepatis structures are carefully visualized with limited dissection revealing the common hepatic artery which, once identified, is traced to the origin from the celiac axis. During this dissection, the origins of the gastroduodenal artery, splenic artery and left gastric artery are noted. The gastroduodenal artery is ligated and the splenic artery is marked either by a suture or by slinging it. This vascular dissection can also be carried out in the cold phase after perfusion when there is no bleeding. However, identification is often easier before perfusion and dissection during cold phase is much faster if the vessels have already been identified during the warm phase. The CBD is then ligated distally and cut. The gallbladder fundus is nicked and the bile within the gall bladder is flushed out with copious irrigation till the effluent runs clear. Meanwhile, a nasogastric tube is advanced beyond the pylorus and 200 mL of 5% betadine with 50 mg of amphotericin is delivered into the duodenum.

The portal vein is also identified at this stage and a sling can be passed around the portal vein too. Similarly, the SMA can also be dissected out and a sling passed around it. The pancreas is removed along with a loop of duodenum and a window is made in the mesentery of duodenojejunal (DJ) flexure and the pyloric region where ligatures may pass and loosely tied to aid in identification and passage of stapler in the cold phase.

In case there is an accessory right hepatic artery arising from the SMA, pancreas retrieval may have to be abandoned especially if this artery arises intrapancreatic portion and the liver team wants the origin of SMA. But most liver transplant surgeons are well versed with handling these situations and a bench reconstruction can allow the pancreas donation to take place.

CROSS-CLAMPING

Twenty-five thousand units of heparin are injected 5 minutes prior to cross clamping of aorta. Aorta is cannulated at this stage just above the aortic bifurcation using a 20 F straight perfusion cannula. The supraceliac aorta is cross clamped and cold perfusion is begun through the aortic cannula using either University of Wisconsin (UW) solution or histidine-tryptophan-ketoglutarate (HTK) solution. The IVC is ligated just above its formation. Four to ten liters of cold perfusion fluid are infused via the aortic cannula depending on the type of fluid used till the abdominal organs become pale and perfused. Sometimes, during multiorgan retrieval, perfusion is also performed through the inferior mesenteric vein (IMV) especially in donors with marginal livers but has to be avoided at all costs while pancreas retrieval is being planned. Perfusion of IMV leads to edema of the pancreas because of increased pressures in its outflow tract. Once the perfusion is started, the abdominal cavity is packed with finely crushed ice slush ensuring that all organs are well covered with ice during the cold phase dissection. The IVC is opened up to vent blood out preferably just above the diaphragm where it enters into the right atrium. It can also be vented just above the ligation of infrarenal IVC if thorax has not been opened. Venting into thorax keeps the abdominal area free of blood and makes the dissection easier. Adequate flushing is confirmed by the cold and pale appearance of the liver and bowel, and lower poles of the kidney can be examined via a nick in the Gerota's fascia at the lateral border of the kidneys. At our center we use histidine tryptophan ketoglutarate (HTK) solution as perfusion fluid. The UW solution is more viscous and a lower volume may suffice.

COLD DISSECTION

Once the organs are assessed to be adequately perfused, the portal dissection is continued by completing the dissection of the common hepatic artery to the aorta where the celiac axis origin is taken off along with a cuff of aorta. The splenic artery is transected close to it sorigin and its distal cut end is marked with a suture for identification during the bench preparation of the pancreas. The portal vein is divided leaving 1–1.5 cm of portal vein with the pancreas graft. The drainage of coronary vein can be taken as a landmark to divide the portal vein so that reasonable length of portal vein remains with the pancreatic graft. The IVC is transected above its junction of right renal vein and a finger is placed in the IVC to complete below the diaphragm. The hepatic retrieval is completed by dividing the diaphragmatic attachments of the liver and IVC.

The pancreas retrieval begins by opening the lesser sac along the whole of the greater curve of the stomach from the pylorus to the spleen. This is followed by detaching the transverse mesocolon off the anterior surface of the pancreas and dividing the middle colic artery. At this stage, the transverse colon and left colon can be dissected and the bowel loops can be pushed out of the field after stapling and disconnecting DJ flexure and root of mesentery. A stapler is also fired across the duodenum just distal to the pylorus after withdrawing the nasogastric tube to leave the C loop of duodenum with the pancreas. The pancreas only remaining vascular attachment i.e. the SMA is now divided. After the vascular attachments have been divided, the stomach is separated from the pancreas and spleen by sharp dissection. The ligamentous attachments of the spleen are divided and the spleen is used as a handle to lift the pancreas and is held up to dissect pancreas off the posterior body wall. The donor team should remember to retrieve an arterial graft comprising of the common iliac bifurcation for arterial reconstruction of the pancreas graft.

Thereafter, retrieval of the kidneys is begun with identification of ureters at the pelvic brim where they are divided along with the accompanying gonadal veins. Care should be taken not to strip the periureteric tissue for fear of jeopardizing the ureteric blood supply. Both kidneys are now freed of their lateral attachments and rotated medially while dividing their posterior attachments till the IVC on the right side and the aorta on the left side. The anterior wall of aorta is incised with scissors after removing aortic cannula and the aortic lumen is inspected for the ostia of the renal arteries. This maneuver helps to identify the origins of any accessory renal arteries. The left renal vein is next incised just lateral to its insertion into IVC. Lastly, the posterior wall of aorta is incised with a knife in the midline to split the aorta into two half with each half having ostia to the corresponding kidney. The IVC and the split halves of the aorta are dissected off the vertebrae till the level of the SMA where transection of both vessels completes the kidney retrieval. The dissection of kidneys should remain posteriorly in the lumbar fascia and superiorly above the adrenal to avoid injuries to the vascular supply.

Once the organs have been retrieved and placed in ice slush for transportation the donor abdomen and chest are closed in two layers with the skin closed using a continuous watertight technique.

BENCH SURGERY

The pancreas is placed in a wide basin filled with slushed frozen Ringer's lactate fluid. Ice slush with both frozen and liquid phases maintains a steady temperature. Over the slush a thin sterile plastic sheet holds enough perfusion fluid to immerse the pancreas completely. It is important to keep the pancreas submerged in the cold perfusion fluid throughout the back bench surgery. The seating position should be comfortable as this phase of surgery may take time. The use of magnification is recommended. All tissue around the pancreas is tied meticulously otherwise troublesome bleeding will occur after reperfusion. This part of the dissection can also be carried out using vessel sealers which expedites the whole process. Direct handling of the pancreas should be minimized and care should be taken to support the whole of the pancreas whenever the need arises to manipulate the pancreas. A methodical and meticulous back bench preparation contributes significantly to the success of a pancreas transplant. Although efforts should be made to keep the ischemia as short as possible, a patient approach is the key to good back bench surgery.

ASSESSMENT OF DONOR PANCREAS

The pancreas is assessed for suitability for transplantation. An excessively fatty pancreas is a contraindication to transplantation and care should be taken to distinguish fat outside the pancreas capsule from interlobular fat within the pancreas. The pancreas should be very gently palpated for areas of fibrosis or tumors. Vessels should be checked for injury such as dissection, intimal damage, venous traction tears and thrombi. The splenic artery and SMA are flushed with perfusion fluid to check for collateral flow into the gastroduodenal artery. Injury to the pancreas parenchyma and the duodenum should be carefully ruled out.

DISSECTION

The pancreas is placed in its anatomical position. Stay sutures can be taken to spread out the duodenum, avoid taking suture bites from the pancreatic capsule/parenchyma. Dissection starts with removing fat from the superior and inferior borders of the pancreas up to the splenic hilum. One should be mindful of the tortuosity of the splenic artery and keep an adequate distance from the superior pancreas border proper to avoid injury to this vessel. Splenectomy with individual ligation of splenic artery and vein follows. The IMV is then identified posterior to the duodenum and ligated. The root of the mesentery is tackled next by overrunning the staples with 4-0 polypropylene and ligating the superior mesenteric vessels and its major branches including the middle colic artery. Alternatively, a vascular stapler may be used taking care not to include any part of pancreas parenchyma in the staple line. The duodenal staples need to be reapplied to remove the excess part of the C loop, taking care not to injure the vascular arcade connecting the superior and inferior pancreaticoduodenal vessels along the inside of the C loop of duodenum. The staple line is buried with a non absorbable suture line. The length of duodenal loop is kept around 10–12 cm for an enteric drained pancreas but needs to be kept shorter for a bladder drained pancreas. The lymphatic and ganglionic tissue around the SMA and splenic artery is ligated to decrease incidence of lymphatic collections. Thin veins running to the portal vein from the surrounding tissue are ligated with care.

VESSEL RECONSTRUCTION

The iliac bifurcation retrieved from the donor is used as a Y graft to the SMA and the splenic artery using 6-0 polypropylene sutures. The two limbs of the Y should be kept short especially the internal iliac which joins the splenic artery to ensure there is no kinking during the recipient surgery. The portal vein would not usually require any lengthening despite appearances. The vascular anastomoses as well as the ligatures of splenic artery and mesenteric root are checked by gentle perfusion for any leak before proceeding with implantation.

RECIPIENT SURGERY

Preparing the Pancreas Bed

The recipient surgery begins with a midline incision starting from pubic symphysis and extending about a hands breadth above the umbilicus. The bowel is retracted toward the left upper quadrant and the peritoneum above the right common iliac artery is incised and dissected upwards exposing the right common iliac vessels and the lower IVC and aorta. The lumbar veins draining into the IVC should be ligated with care as in the event as in the event of an injury these vessels retract along the vertebral bodies leading to troublesome bleeding. The surgeon should bear in mind that some patients may have significant vascular disease due to their diabetes thereby being prone to complications such as intimal dissection. The kidney is implanted first in the left iliac fossa, while the benching of pancreas is performed. The renal allograft is implanted on the recipient's left external iliac vessels. If the cold ischemia time of pancreas is prolonged for any reason, consideration should be given to implant the pancreas first as kidney tolerates ischemia much better than pancreas.

Implanting the Pancreas

The pancreas is positioned "head-up", with the C loop of the duodenum toward the liver and the tail toward the pelvis, and the stem of the iliac vessel interposition graft anastomosed end to side with the common iliac artery. The position of the pancreas and the lie of the common iliac artery dictate the angle at which this anastomosis is made. If the iliac interposition graft is too long or the angle of the anastomosis too acute there is a possibility of a kink at the splenic artery of the graft which needs to be avoided. The IVC is side clamped and the portal vein is anastomosed end to side with it. The portal vein may appear short as it retracts into the pancreas, but the first few sutures of the anastomosis will coax out an adequate length of vein for a tension free suture line. Although portal vein extension has been described by using interposition graft of iliac vein, it is not recommended as it may increase the chances of venous thrombosis.

On declamping the pancreas and duodenum should "pink up" all over and arterial pulsations should be easily palpable over all the main vessels. The pancreas often oozes blood from minute vessels on its surface and any significant bleed should be controlled at this stage. After confirming good perfusion of the graft duodenum, it is anastomosed side to side with the recipient jejunum across a mesocolic window in the right mesocolon. The anastomosis can be hand sewn or stapled with equivalent result. The jejunum is then secured to the mesocolic window as a safeguard against a possible internal hernia. Pliable soft drains are placed in the pelvis and above the pancreas. The abdomen is closed in a single layer in continuous fashion using nonabsorbable sutures. The duodenum can also be anastomosed to the bladder dome which can be of help in monitoring rejection in patients undergoing pancreas transplant alone. Bladder drainage has now been mostly abandoned given the high incidence of complications requiring conversion to enteric drainage in up to one-third of the patients.

Postoperative Care

Soon after restoration of blood flow to the pancreas, the blood sugars may fall precipitously and should be monitored at frequent intervals and titrated using dextrose infusion to maintain between 120 and 180 mg%. Functioning pancreas grafts do not require additional insulin to maintain blood glucose within this range and requirement of higher doses of insulin to control blood sugars is an indication to assess pancreas vascularity. Some surgeons like to keep insulin infusion for the first few days to give rest to the pancreas. Serial Doppler assessments are useful to assess pancreas vascularity and the threshold for a computed tomography (CT) imaging should be low.

Anticoagulation is initiated once adequate hemostasis is confirmed and low dose heparin 300–500 units per hour is continued till the patient resumes oral diet when it is substituted with low dose aspirin. Oral feeds are started as soon as accepted by the patient. Antibiotic prophylaxis is administered as per hospital policy.

Most units will use induction therapy with either anti-thymocyte globulin, Campath or basiliximab. Immunosuppression is continued post operatively with triple drug regimen of tacrolimus, mycophenolate and steroid with steroid withdrawal by end of first week. Valganciclovir and cotrimoxazole prophylaxis is continued till 3 and 6 months respectively.

Long-term Follow-up

After discharge patients are followed up frequently for the first few months and the interval between visits is increased as time passes. The kidney is a convenient surrogate for pancreas rejection too and the biopsies should be done whenever there is graft dysfunction. The metabolic side effects of immunosuppression are many and require multidisciplinary follow-up.

Outcome

One-year patient survival now exceeds 95% and recent five-year survival was reported to be 78.2% for PTA, 89.6% for SPK, and 91.1% for PAK, respectively.[8] The current half-life of SPK is now approximately 14 years with 5-year graft survival exceeding 80%.[9] SPK offers a significant patient and graft survival advantage over kidney transplant alone in patients with type 1 diabetes beyond the first year and the differences in survival keep on widening with each passing year.[5]

Complications

The complexity of pancreas transplantation surgery means that a higher than usual rate of complications seems to be the norm than the exception. However, with advancement in techniques many units now report a fairly low incidence of complications but the exact incidence still varies a lot depending upon the available expertise. In addition to the usual suspects of transplantation complications, infection and rejection, pancreas transplantation has a host of unique complications. Most early complications are related to the grafted pancreas itself and reoperation rates may be high. The physiology of the exocrine pancreas, ischemic insult, low flow resting state compared to most other organ transplants and the need for a bowel anastomosis are probably factors in the occurrence of complications. Complications of the grafted pancreas range from mild localized pancreatitis and necrosis to severe graft pancreatitis with life threatening systemic manifestations.

Some degree of graft pancreatitis often accompanies a pancreas transplant. It does not require any specific treatment and is expected to improve in most patients over the first week after transplantation. Some patients have a severe form of pancreatitis associated with hemodynamic instability. The clinical picture dictates the course of further action more than the outcomes of investigations and early decision to perform graft pancreatectomy is a lifesaving procedure in patients who continue to worsen clinically.

Vascular Complications

Hemorrhage requiring re-exploration is not uncommon, especially in patients who are given aggressive anticoagulation. Vascular complications are one of the major causes of graft loss after pancreas transplantation and can involve either venous or arterial systems. These usually present in the first week after transplant. Venous thrombosis is the more common than arterial and present with worsening blood glucose control and pain around the graft site. Venous congestion may also lead to hemorrhagic drain output. Arterial thrombi usually present with deranged blood glucose along with unexplained fever and minimal local findings. While sequential ultrasound examinations can offer rapid and early evaluation for vascular thrombosis, a contrast enhanced CT is essential in defining the exact lesion and pancreas perfusion. Large thrombi will require graft pancreatectomy to prevent septic complications. Segmental thrombi with preservation of perfusion of majority of the pancreas can be managed with therapeutic anticoagulation.

Pseudoaneurysm involving the arterial anastomosis or the Y graft is a rare but life threatening condition. These usually result from infection (bacterial or fungal) and present with sudden hypotension in the second week after transplantation. Most cases will require graft nephrectomy although occasional cases have been salvaged by revision of vascular anastomosis. It is important to identify the organism and give appropriate antibiotics.

Bowel anastomotic leaks are the third major group of complications unique to pancreas transplantation. Bowel leaks occur most often at the anastomosis or from the duodenal stump and sometimes at sites of unrecognized bowel injury. The size of leak and the health of the surrounding tissue determine course of action. Whereas, primary repairs may be attempted sometimes for circumscribed leaks, graft excision may also be required for large uncontrolled leaks with extensive inflammation. Most of the contained leaks can however be managed by adequate drainage and sometimes may take months to heal.[10] A Roux-en-Y conversion of the anastomosis allows to continue enteral nutrition while waiting for the leak to heal.

Infections are a major cause of morbidity and mortality. Predisposition to infections results from immunosuppression, donor derived infections, latent infections harbored in the recipient, multiple interventions, prolonged hospital stay, tissue injury and fluid collections related to the graft pancreas and the complications related to the bowel anastomosis. The choice of prophylactic antibiotic varies across different hospitals. Antibiotic prophylaxis should cover gram positive and gram-negative bacteria and fungi. Immunosuppression may need to be decreased or withheld when dealing with severe or life threatening infections.

Rejection of the grafted pancreas presents as a loss of glycemic control, sometimes associated with a spike in serum amylase levels with elevation of creatinine in the simultaneous pancreas kidney transplant recipient. Severe rejections may present with fever and progress to vascular thrombosis. A high index of suspicion and early intervention is required to manage such rejections. A kidney biopsy may serve as a surrogate marker for pancreas rejection in such cases.

Postoperative fluid collections around the grafted pancreas are common. The abundance of lymphatic tissue around the pancreas vascular pedicle, localized pancreatic inflammation and necrosis, rich network of vessels are possible factors contributing to the formation of such collections. While some fluid collections may be amenable to percutaneous drainage other will require a repeat laparotomy for draining out. Once infected, these fluid collections can rapidly progress to severe sepsis.

Indian Experience of Simultaneous Pancreas-Kidney

The first pancreas transplant of India was performed at IKD, Ahmedabad in 1990, but it was unsuccessful and the patient died shortly thereafter. The first successful SPK transplant was reported from the AIIMS in 2004 and the patient remained dialysis and insulin free for the next 10 years.[11] There is no other published series so far from India. Analysis of state deceased donor registries reveal that less than 50 such transplants have taken place across India till 2016. The maximum numbers (21) of these transplants have been reported from Tamil Nadu and 18 SPK transplants have been performed at PGIMER, Chandigarh so far with seven patients achieving insulin independence and normal kidney function. Two out of eleven patients required graft pancreatectomy for thrombotic complications and one for a pseudoaneurysm involving the vascular allograft. All three patients were discharged with a normal kidney function. There was one early mortality possibly due to donor derived infection. Overall outcomes have been mixed but other individual centers have also conveyed successful outcomes in different patients.

CONCLUSION

Simultaneous pancreas and kidney transplantation is recent addition in management of type1 DM. Successful simultaneous pancreas and kidney transplantation improves quality of life. However, in India facility for SPK is limited to few centers.

REFERENCES

1. Orlando G, Stratta RJ, Light J. Pancreas transplantation for type 2 diabetes mellitus. Curr Opin Organ Transplant. 2011;16:110-5.
2. Navarro X, Sutherland DE, Kennedy WR. Long-term effects of pancreatic transplantation on diabetic neuropathy. Ann Neurol. 1997;42(5):727-36.
3. Giannarelli R, Coppelli A, Sartini MS, et al. Pancreas transplant alone has beneficial effects on retinopathy in type 1 diabetic patients. Diabetologia. 2006;49:2977-82.
4. Fioretto P, Steffes MW, Sutherland DE, et al. Reversal of lesions of diabetic nephropathy after pancreas transplantation. N Engl J Med. 1998;339(2):69-75.
5. Mohan P, Safi K, Little DM, et al. Improved patient survival in recipients of simultaneous pancreas–kidney transplant compared with kidney transplant alone in patients with type 1 diabetes mellitus and end-stage renal disease. Br J Surg. 2003;90:1137-41
6. https://embryology.med.unsw.edu.au/embryology/index.php/Endocrine-Pancreas Development (assessed on 1st October 2017)
7. https://www.omim.org/entry/222100(assessed on 1st October 2017
8. Kandaswamy R, Stock PG, Gustafson SK, et al. 2015. OPTN/SRTR Annual Data Report: Pancreas. Am J Transplant. 2017;17(Suppl 1):117-73.
9. Gruessner RW, Gruessner AC. The current state of pancreas transplantation. Nat Rev Endocrinol. 2013;9:555-562.
10. Kumar S, Singh S, Kenwar DB, et al. Management of Graft Duodenal Leak in Simultaneous Pancreas Kidney Transplant— A Case Report from India and Review of Literature. The Indian Journal of Surgery. 2016;78(5):402-06.
11. Guleria S, Aggarwal S, Bansal VK, et al. The first successful simultaneous pancreas-kidney transplant in India. Natl Med J India. 2005;18(1):18-9.

Chapter 20

Nonglycemic Effects of Glucagon-like Peptide-1 Analogs

SK Sharma

INTRODUCTION

Glucagon-like peptides-1 (GLP-1) agonists represents a novel class of antihyperglycemic agents that have cause increase in the insulin and decrease in the glucagon, thereby improving hyperglycemia. GLP-1 analogs improve the health and survival of β-cells, improve insulin resistance (modest effect) and influence energy intake (augment satiety signal) with minimal, if at all, any side effects (weight neutral and nonhypoglycemic). The GLP-1-based therapy addresses most of the proposed pathogenetic mechanisms that are involved in the development of type 2 diabetes mellitus (T2DM).

Glucagon-like peptide-1 agonists have shown to have a cardiac-friendly profile, preserve neuronal cells and safeguard from neuronal degeneration, improve hepatic inflammation and hepatosteatosis, improve insulin resistance, promote weight loss and induce satiety. There is growing evidence that they may also be renoprotective and help with wound healing.[1]

INCRETIN-BASED THERAPY—GLUCAGON-LIKE PEPTIDE-1 ANALOGS

Glucagon-like peptide-1 is secreted by L-cells present in distal small intestine. The half-life of circulating native bioactive GLP-1 is <2 minutes. Incretin mimetics (exenatide, liraglutide) work by stimulating the GLP-1 receptor (GLP-1R) directly. Glucose-dependent insulinotropic polypeptide (GIP) is secreted by neuroendocrine K-cells present in stomach and proximal small intestine and has a half-life of approximately seven minutes in healthy individuals and 5 minutes in patients with T2DM, being degraded by dipeptidyl peptidase-4 (DPP-4) also. GIP is rapidly cleared through the kidney. GLP-1 has a wide tissue distribution and acts through the GLP-1R.

The GLP-1 receptors have been identified in pancreas, lung, heart, vascular smooth muscle cells, endothelial cells, macrophages and monocytes, kidney, gastrointestinal tract, central nervous system and peripheral nervous system. In the brain, the GLP-1R is found only on neurons and not on glial cells. It is present mainly on the large output neurons such as pyramidal neurons, dentate granule neurons and Purkinje cells. In the brainstem, GLP-1R is mostly distributed in the brainstem nucleus and hypothalamus.[2]

INCRETIN MIMETICS

"Amongst all the currently available antidiabetic agents, GLP-1 receptor agonists (GLP-1 RAs) address most of the 'pathogenetic octet' components of T2DM, as proposed by Ralf Defranzo".[2]

Glucagon-like peptide-1 receptor agonists occupying a unique position in the management of T2DM based on the fact that they are weight reducing and free of hypoglycemia (Table 1). For this very reason, they are commonly advised as second-line therapy along with an insulin sensitizer like metformin. They are indicated and approved for the use as follows:

- Second line as add-on therapy to pre-existing monotherapy [metformin, sulphonylureas (SU), thiazolidinediones (TZD), alpha-glucosidase inhibitor, meglitinide] for uncontrolled T2DM with HbA1c >7%. Caution is advised along with the use of SU, as it may potentiate its action and cause hypoglycemia.[3,4]

TABLE1: Glucagon-like peptide-1 receptor agonists.

GLP-1 RAs	Brand name	Administration	Duration of action
Exenatide	Byetta®	Twice daily	Short acting
Exenatide-LAR	Bydureon®	Once weekly	Long acting
Lixisenatide	Lyxumia®	Once daily	Short acting
Liraglutide	Victoza®	Once daily	Long acting
Albiglutide	Eperzan®	Once weekly	Long acting
Dulaglutide	Trulicity®	Once weekly	Long acting

(GLP-1 RAs: glucagon-like peptide-1 receptor agonists.)

Dose titration of SU (reduce to half-existing dose) is recommended when used along with GLP-1 analog

- Third line as add-on therapy to pre-existing dual combination therapy (metformin, SU, TZD, alpha-glucosidase inhibitor, meglitinide).[4]

PLEIOTROPIC EFFECTS OF GLUCAGON-LIKE PEPTIDE-1-BASED THERAPY

Cytoprotection

Glucagon-like peptide-1 receptor stimulation has been associated with cytoprotection and anti-apoptosis in all tissue types bearing the receptor. The trophic actions are probably mediated through protein kinase A (PKA) and phosphoinositide 3-kinase (PI3K) signaling.

Pancreas, brain and heart have been shown to express exactly the same GLP-1R type and it would only be appropriate to suggest that the cytoprotective benefit would in least extend to these tissue types as they bear the same receptor type.

Cardiovascular Effects

Glucagon-like Peptide Analogs and Cardiovascular System

The GLP-1 analogs have shown to exert a positive effect on myocardial contractility, hypertension (natriuretic/diuretic effect), endothelium (antiatherosclerotic) and lipid profile.

The human heart usually uses fats as a metabolic fuel in the normoxic state. When acutely stressed (ischemic), it switches from lipid metabolism to carbohydrate oxidation, which is although adaptive initially, eventually leads to insulin resistance and a loss of metabolic flexibility, which is detrimental to the heart. GLP-1R stimulation helps improve insulin sensitivity and shifts cardiac metabolism in favor of cardioprotection.

Glucagon-like peptide-1 has shown to decrease pyruvate and lactate concentrations both in normoxic and ischemic conditions of the heart, suggesting cardioprotective effects.[5]

POTENTIAL BENEFITS

- *Ionotropic*: The GLP-1 agonists have shown to limit infarct size and improve left ventricular (LV) function
- *Blood pressure*: In humans, the use of GLP-1 analogs (exenatide and liraglutide) has shown a significant reduction in both systolic and diastolic blood pressure when compared with placebo. The main mechanism for this antihypertensive effect, however, seems to be related to weight loss. In addition, GLP therapy has shown to have a natriuretic/diuretic effect (inhibiting sodium reabsorption in the proximal tubule and angiotensin II), peripheral vasodilatory effect and endothelial function stabilizing effect in preclinical studies, all shown to contribute to improvements in blood pressure
- *Vascular endothelium*: The GLP-1R agonists have shown to inhibit monocyte/macrophage accumulation in the arterial wall, inhibit expression of inflammatory marker
- *Dyslipidemia*: Glucagon-like peptide-1 agonists have been shown to increase high-density lipoprotein (HDL) and reduce triglyceride, apolipoprotein B-48 (apoB-48, a component of chylomicrons, rich in triacylglycerol, produced after fat ingestion)
- *Weight loss:* The GLP-1 agonists cause weight loss, probably by decreasing appetite, improving satiety and by reducing gastric emptying.

CARDIOVASCULAR BENEFITS: POSSIBLE MECHANISMS

The Role of Glucagon-like Peptide-1 Analogs in Cardiovascular Disease—A Clinical Study

Glucagon-like peptide-1 analogs are a class of injectable diabetic drugs that activate the endogenous GLP-1R. They promote glucose dependent insulin release, inhibit glucagon secretion and delay gastric emptying (Fig. 1).

It is apparent from the results of the published trials that the benefits of GLP-1 analogs may not be a class effect. While LEADER and SUSTAIN-6 were able to demonstrate cardiovascular (CV) event reduction, the results of ELIXA were not as encouraging and EXSCEL showed borderline beneficial effects.

The positive results of the LEADER shows that liraglutide is noninferior to placebo, it was superior in reducing the primary composite outcome of CV death, myocardial infarction (MI) and stroke (13% vs. 14.9% in placebo; p = 0.01). The reduction in the primary end point was driven by significantly lower CV mortality (4.7% vs. 6%; p = 0.007). Liraglutide reduced all-cause mortality (8.2% vs. 9.6%; p = 0.02). While there was numerical reduction in MI and stroke rates, this did not reach statistical significance.

The SUSTAIN-6, also showed composite CV event reduction (6.6% vs. 8.9%; p = 0.02) with semaglutide (weekly injection), which was driven by a significant reduction in strokes (1.6% vs. 2.7%; p = 0.04) rather than CV mortality or MI.

Neither liraglutide nor semaglutide had a significant effect on heart failure (HF) admissions, suggesting a different mechanism of action than sodium-glucose cotransporter-2 inhibitors. Though not completely understood, it has been postulated that these drugs may have more of an anti-atherothrombotic effect. Other positive effects like blood pressure lowering, weight reduction and avoidance of hypoglycemia may contribute to improved CV outcomes. The FDA has approved specific labels for liraglutide to reduce the risk of CV death in adults with diabetes and cardiovascular disease (CVD).

Antiatherosclerotic Effects of the Glucagon-like Peptide-1

Glucagon-like peptide-1 receptor agonists, such as liraglutide/exenatide are found to be successful in providing

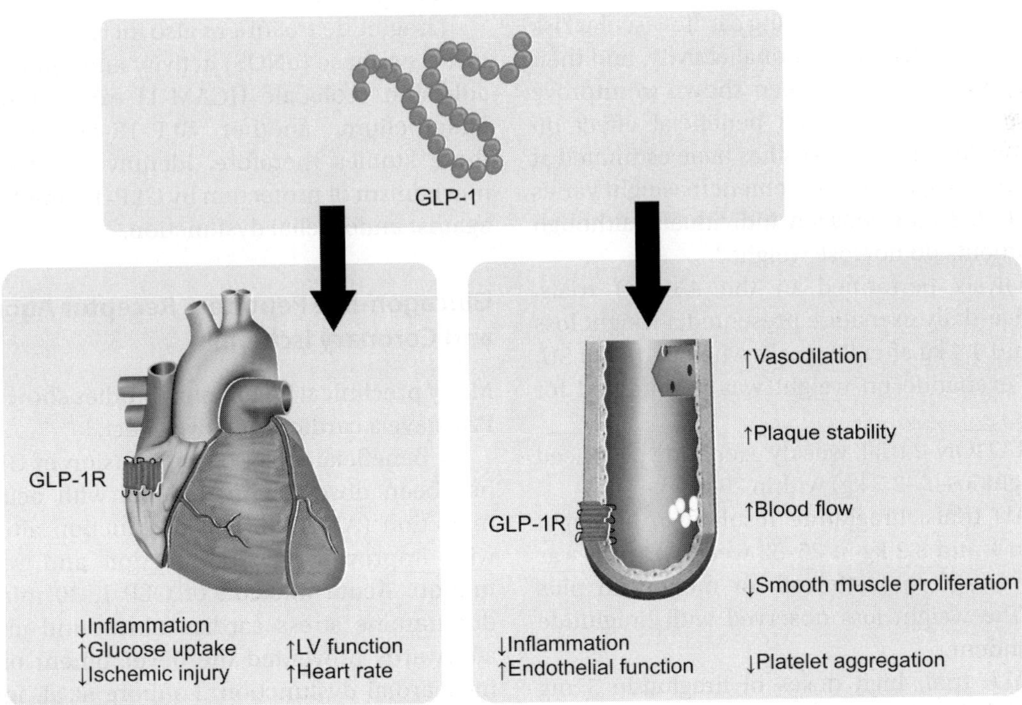

(GLP-1: glucagon-like peptide-1; GLP-1R: glucagon-like peptide-1 receptor; LV: left ventricular.)

Figure 1 CV benefits: Possible mechanisms.

supra-physiological levels of GLP-1. Preliminary evidence favor GLP-1 based therapies in providing beneficial effects against atherosclerosis as indicated by the significant reductions in atherosclerosis markers including B-type natriuretic peptide, plasminogen activator inhibitor-1 (PAI-1), and high-sensitivity C-reactive protein (CRP), besides statistically nonsignificant reductions in several other markers including intima-media thickness, flow-mediated dilation (FMD), interleukin-6 (IL-6) and tumor necrosis factor-alpha (TNF-α).

The GLP-1-based therapies were also associated with significant reductions in total cholesterol, LDL- cholesterol and triglycerides. GLP-1-based therapies significantly reduce CRP while statistically non-significantly reducing TNF-α and IL-6 levels. This is suggestive of the effects of GLP-1-based therapies on attenuating inflammatory processes that may cause atherosclerosis development. There is significant reduction in PAI-1 with GLP-1 based therapies in diabetic patients.

Weight Reduction by Glucagon-like Peptide-1 Analogs

Obesity contributes to the development of both T2DM and CVD. Modest weight losses of 5–10% have been found to contribute to changes in glycaemic control, number of medications for controlling cardiovascular risk factors (CVRF), the patient's functional activity, and their quality of life. GLP-1 RAs have been shown to improve glycaemic control with an added beneficial effect on weight reduction. Mean weight loss has been estimated at between 0.4 and 5.1 kg, this improvement in weight varies between GLP-1 RAs and between individuals, although up to 30% of patients do not lose weight.[6]

In the analysis performed in the AMIGO trials, patients on twice-daily exenatide presented a weight loss of between 4 and 4.4 kg after 82 weeks when added to SU; the impact of exenatide on weight was maintained for 3 years (–5.3 kg).

In the DURATION-2 trial, weekly exenatide produced significant weight loss (–2.3 kg) within 26 weeks.

In the LEAD trials, liraglutide resulted in a weight loss of between 1 and 3.2 kg in 26–52 weeks when it was used alone or added to metformin or metformin plus rosiglitazone. The weight loss observed with liraglutide was dose-dependent.

In the SCALE trial, high doses of liraglutide 3 mg resulted in a weight loss of 8.4 kg (8% of weight) at 56 weeks compared with placebo. Liraglutide 3mg subcutaneous injection per day is now used as a weight reducing drug (SAXENDA).

Glucagon-like Peptide-1 and Endothelial Function

Endothelial dysfunction is a pathological process that links diabetic macro- and microvascular disease. Studies conducted in humans observed that the infusion of native GLP-1 in healthy volunteers improved the blood flow in the forearm induced by the secretion of acetylcholine, as measured by plethysmography.

In fasting T2DM subjects with stable coronary artery disease (n = 12), a notable improvement was found in endothelial function after the infusion of GLP-1, as demonstrated by an increase in flow-mediated vasodilation of the brachial artery during a hyperinsulinemia clamp. Similarly, in an observational study of 20 diabetic subjects receiving metformin, exenatide treatment (twice daily) for 16 weeks improved flow-mediated vasodilation of the brachial artery after 5 minutes of ischemia, as determined by ultrasound, compared with patients receiving glimepiride.

Liraglutide attenuates induction of PAI-1 and vascular adhesion molecule (VAM) expression in human vascular endothelial cells (hVECs) in vitro. It may protect against endothelial dysfunction, an early abnormality in vascular disease in diabetic patients. In vitro studies demonstrated GLP-1R-mediated inhibition of PAI-1 and VAM expression.

Liraglutide treatment also increased endothelial nitric oxide synthase (eNOS) activity and reduced intercellular adhesion molecule (ICAM-1) expression in the aortic endothelium, another GLP-1R-dependent effect. All these studies therefore, identify a potential molecular mechanism of protection by GLP-1R-mediated liraglutide against endothelial dysfunction.

Glucagon-like Peptide-1 Receptor Agonists and Coronary Ischemia

Many preclinical and clinical studies show that the GLP-1 RAs have a cardioprotective effect.

A beneficial effect of the infusion of GLP-1 (for 72 h) has been observed in patients with acute myocardial infarction (AMI) and LV dysfunction after reperfusion, with improved ejection fraction and ventricular wall motion. Acute infusion of GLP-1, 30 minutes before a dobutamine stress cardiac ultrasound and 30 minutes afterwards prevented the development of postischemic myocardial dysfunction. Lønborg et al. investigated the effects of a 6-hour infusion of exenatide compared with placebo during the 15 minutes prior to reperfusion in patients about to undergo a coronary intervention to treat ST-segment elevation myocardial infarction (STEMI).[7]

Exenatide was effective in reducing the size of the infarct in relation to the ischemic area and increased the myocardial salvage index measured by cardiac magnetic resonance 90 days postinfusion. In contrast, patients treated with exenatide had no reduction in mortality or improvement in LV contractility.

Liraglutide also demonstrated cardioprotection in a trial with 96 patients with STEMI who underwent percutaneous coronary angioplasty. Liraglutide treatment (0.6 mg for 2 days, 1.2 mg for 2 days and 1.8 mg for 3 days) was compared with placebo, finding a better myocardial salvage index in the liraglutide treatment arm (0.66 ± 0.14 vs. 0.55 ± 0.15), smaller infarct size (15 ± 12 vs. 21 ± 15), and lower high-sensitivity CRP levels.

Glucagon-like Peptide-1 Receptor Agonists and Heart Failure (Fig. 2)

Meta-analyses of phase II/III clinical trials of exenatide, liraglutide, albiglutide and dulaglutide have shown that they do not increase the risk of hospitalization for HF, confirming the findings of CV safety trials.

The LEADER trial with liraglutide has showed a significant 12% reduction in the expanded composite outcome comprising the primary endpoint plus coronary revascularizations and hospitalizations for angina and HF. However, there was no significant benefit on HF admissions. For the moment, clinical data have demonstrated a neutral effect on the incidence of hospitalization for HF; nevertheless, this has to be explored as a primary objective in future trials.

Cardiovascular Outcome Trials on Glucagon-like Peptide-1 Receptor Agonists

ELIXA Study

Lixisenatide showed a neutral CV profile in patients with type 2 diabetes and a recent acute coronary syndrome.

LEADER Study

With respect to primary outcomes, the liraglutide group had a statistically significant lower risk of MACE compared with placebo [hazard ratio (HR) = 0.87, 95% confidence interval (CI), 0.78–0.97]. With respect to deaths from CV causes, the risk was also lower in the liraglutide group (HR = 0.78, 95% CI, 0.66– 0.93, p = 0.007). The risk of death

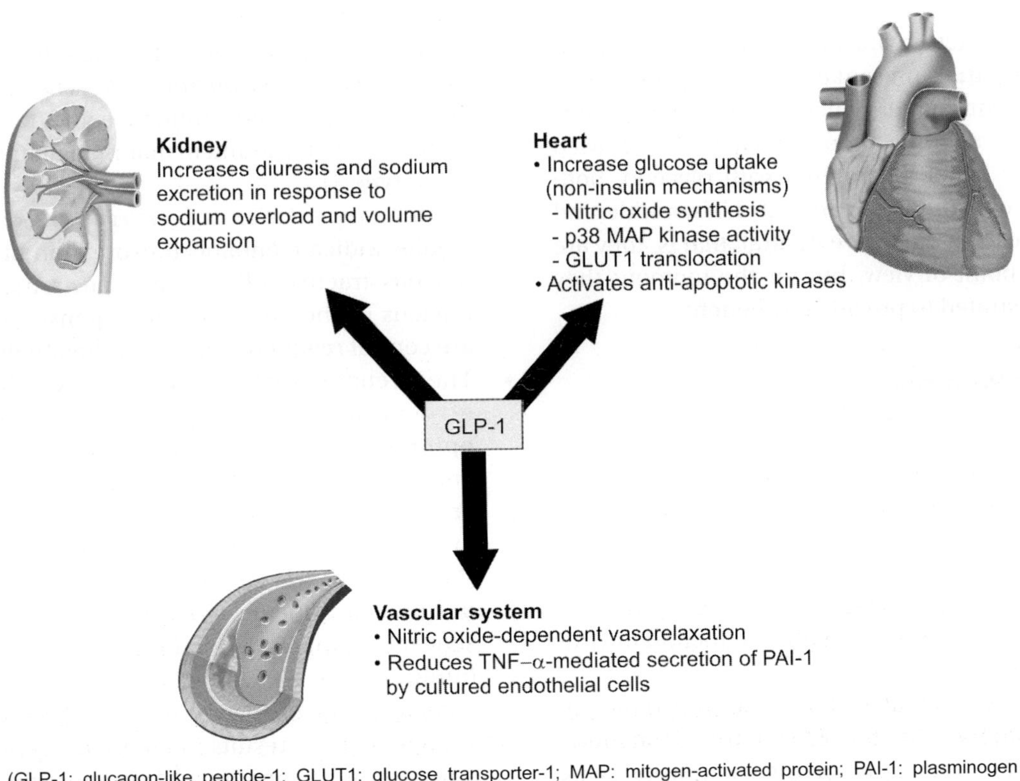

(GLP-1: glucagon-like peptide-1; GLUT1: glucose transporter-1; MAP: mitogen-activated protein; PAI-1: plasminogen activator inhibitor-1; TNF-α: tumor necrosis factor-alpha.)

Figure 2 Postulated effects of glucagon-like peptide-1 in the cardiovascular system.

from any cause was also lower in the liraglutide group (HR = 0.85; 95% CI, 0.74–0.97; p = 0.02), as was the risk of nonfatal MI and nonfatal stroke, but the results were not statistically significant.

SUSTAIN-6

Patients on semaglutide treatment had a 26% lower risk of developing the primary outcome. This lower risk is attributed above all to the significantly lower risk of developing nonfatal stroke (39%) and a nonsignificant reduction in the risk of developing a nonfatal MI (26%). Thus, semaglutide shows superiority as regards CV safety.[7]

EXSCEL

Weekly exenatide did not increase the incidence of the first episode of MACE (death from CV causes, nonfatal MI,, and nonfatal stroke) compared to placebo (HR = 0.91, 95% CI, 0.83–1.00; p <0.001 for noninferiority). Fewer episodes were observed with exenatide (839; 11.4%) than with placebo (905; 12.2%), but statistical significance was not reached to demonstrate superiority (p = 0.061).[7]

Summary

Clinical trials conducted with GLP-1 RAs and cardiovascular outcomes trials present considerable differences in design and enrolment which limits comparisons among them. Liraglutide and semaglutide showed superiority in CV benefit compared with placebo, both in the presence of standard treatment. Lixisenatide and extended-release exenatide were neutral, that is, they are safe from a CV point of view, but for the moment they have not demonstrated to provide any benefit.

Glucagon-like Peptide-1 in Diabetic Nephropathy

Accumulated evidence suggests that long term treatment with GLP-1 RA is associated with a reduction in measured glomerular filtration rate (GFR), preservation of renal function and/or a decrease in the incidence of CV events.

A small comparison of exenatide and glimepiride for 16 weeks showed a numerically higher reduction in UAE with exenatide.

Liraglutide was evaluated for renal outcomes in addition to CV endpoints in the LEADER trial. Liraglutide led to a significant reduction of the composite renal endpoint at 22%.[8]

This study shows the bias of a composite endpoint, as the effect was driven predominantly by a 26% reduction of persistent macroalbuminuria whereas, the other endpoints studied showed only minor effects. The risk for renal adverse events was not elevated. Lixisenatide reduces progression of urinary albumin-to-creatinine ratio (UACR) in macroalbuminuric patients, and is associated with a lower risk of new-onset macroalbuminuria after adjustment for baseline and on-trial HbA1c and other traditional renal risk factors.

Effects on the Nervous System: Neuroprotective Effects of Glucagon-like Peptide-1

Patients with T2DM are predisposed to the development of neurodegenerative disorders like Alzheimer's disease and the association has been referred to as type 3 diabetes mellitus. Desensitization of insulin receptors has been observed in the brains of patients with Alzheimer's disease, and any process (GLP-1 analogs or DPP-4 inhibitors) that can up-regulate the insulin receptors should theoretically have the potential to improve the clinical course. Augmentation of the incretin system has demonstrated the potential advantage of preservation of neuronal cells.

Glucagon-like peptide-1 inhibits eating responses (taste aversion, satiety) through its action on GLP-1R.

- *Modulation of peripheral taste sensation:* The GLP analogs can directly influence the taste receptors. Human GLP-1 is found in mammalian taste cells (type 2 and type 3)
- *Central modulation of energy intake:* Preclinical studies indicate enhanced expression of c-Fos in the nucleus tractus solitarii, area postrema and central nucleus of the amygdale in response to GLP, which are central regulators of energy metabolism
- The arcuate nucleus contains two distinct types of neurons, anorexigenic [neuropeptides pro-opiomelanocortin (POMC) and cocaine- and amphetamine-regulated transcript (CART)] and orexigenic [neuropeptide Y (NPY) and agouti-related protein (AgRP)]. There exist several NPY-receptors (NPY-R); NPYR1- and Y5-receptor activation appears to stimulate appetite, while NPYRY2- and Y4-receptor activation suppresses food intake through presynaptic inhibition of NPY release. GLP-1 has shown to antagonize the orexigenic effects of NPY. Central GLP-1 augmentation results in an anorexigenic effect with a reduction in appetite by 12% approximately for the subsequent meal.[8]

The incretins have numerous pleiotropic effects with clear benefits to the neuronal system. Central augmentation of the incretin system has been shown to protect neuronal cells (neuroprotection), influence neurobehavioral changes (enhanced learning, cognition, spatial orientation) and regulate food and energy intake (weight loss). This adds a new dimension to the use of GLP-1 augmenting therapies for patients with diabetes.

Gastrointestinal and Hepatobiliary Effects

Glucagon-like peptide-1 has shown to improve β-cell health and suppress glucagon, thereby improving postprandial and fasting hyperglycemia, respectively.

Potential Benefits

- Appetite suppression
- Delayed gastric emptying causing prandial satiety
- *Weight reduction/antiobesity*: This results from the cumulative effect of central appetite suppression, modulation of peripheral taste sensation and gastric slowing (prandial satiety)
- *Increased insulin secretion (improvement in β-cell health):* The GLP-1 analogs improve β-cell health and insulin secretion. Suggested mechanism includes anti-apoptosis with evidence of increased markers of cell proliferation (Ki67)
- *Suppression of glucagon:* The α-cells have been found to be dysfunctional (loss of glucose sensing mechanism) in T2DM. GLP-1 analogs suppress the secretion of glucagon from α-cells
- *Hepatosteatosis:* Hepatic insulin resistance contributes to ectopic fat deposition in the liver, resulting in hepatic steatosis known as nonalcoholic fatty liver disease (NAFLD). NAFLD can later progress to nonalcoholic steatohepatitis (NASH) and cirrhosis. GLP-1 has shown to attenuate weight gain and improve insulin resistance. Weight loss has been shown to reduce hepatic steatosis. It has also been demonstrated that GLP-1Rs are hepatoprotective. They can act directly on the hepatocytes and improve hepatic steatosis. In a meta-analysis of the LEAD program, liraglutide has shown to improve NAFLD fibrosis score, biochemical transaminitis/fatty liver independent of weight loss

Insulin Resistance

Insulin resistance is associated with an increased risk of metabolic abnormalities (dyslipidemia, T2DM). In one study, waist circumference and body mass index (BMI) were independently associated with CVD risk factors (such as hypertension, metabolic syndrome, and dyslipidemia) in both men and women. GLP-1 has shown to reduce insulin sensitivity through restoration of insulin signaling and by reduction of hepatic gluconeogenesis. Enhanced insulin secretion causes increased uptake of glucose in the muscle and adipocyte and reduced outpouring of glucose from the liver. Obesity is associated with insulin resistance.

The GLP analogs cause significant weight loss (reduce free fatty acids), improve insulin secretion and suppress glucagon. In addition, they directly enhance β-cell fatty acid oxidation promoting lipolysis within the β-cell.

Skeletal Effects

A growing body of evidence suggests that by augmenting the incretin system, bone health improves. A study has shown that GLP-1 promotes cellular proliferation and cytoprotection of progenitor bone forming mesenchymal cells. It also prevents these cells from differentiating into adipocytes. NPY has emerged as an important peptide in the regulation of bone remodeling. Central NPY over-expression decreases osteoblastic activity, while on the other hand, specific NYPR1 receptor deletion enhances bone mass. GLP-1 has shown to antagonize the effects of NYP, suggesting that it may help increase bone mass (trabecular and cortical). These effects seem to be dependent mostly on the NPYR1 receptor, with regulatory input from NYPR2 and 4 and the leptin system.

Wound Healing

The GLP-1 has shown to influence positively macrophage-mediated inflammation response and tissue remodeling, which may have benefits with regard to suppression of vascular inflammation and improvement in wound healing.

Glucagon-like Peptide-1 in Diabetic Nephropathy

The GLP-1 has shown to reduce albuminuria in a small pilot study, without affecting the GFR, most likely due to its beneficial effect on blood sugar, blood pressure and inflammation.

Accumulated evidence suggests that long term treatment with GLP-1 RA is associated with a reduction in measured GFR, preservation of renal function and/or a decrease in the incidence of CV events.

Liraglutide is evaluated for renal outcomes in addition to CV endpoints in the LEADER trial. Liraglutide led to a significant reduction of the composite renal endpoint at 22%.

Lixisenatide reduces progression of UACR in macro-albuminuric patients, and is associated with a lower risk of new-onset macroalbuminuria after adjustment for baseline and on-trial HbA1c and other traditional renal risk factors.

CONCLUSION

Augmentation of the incretin axis by the use of GLP-1 agonists represents a novel therapeutic concept that is not only antihyperglycemic but has substantial pleiotropic effects. Benefits extend to virtually every organ system, providing CV stability (anti-ischemic, anti-hypertensive, ionotropic, antiatherosclerotic) weight loss, neuronal-protection, liver and skeletal health and improvement in insulin resistance. Incretin agonism clearly represents the future of antidiabetes therapy given its impressive pleiotropic actions.

REFERENCES

1. Gupta V. Pleiotropic effects of incretins. Indian J Endocr Metab 2012;16:S47-56
2. Defronzo RA. Banting Lecture: From the triumvirate to the ominous octet: A new paradigm for the treatment of type 2 diabetes mellitus. Diabetes 2009;58:773-95.
3. Drucker DJ, Nauck MA. The incretin system: Glucagon-like peptide-1 receptor agonists and dipeptidyl peptidase-4 inhibitors in type 2 diabetes. Lancet 2006;368:1696-705.
4. Drucker DJ. The biology of incretin hormones. Cell Metab 2006;3:153-65.
5. Charbonnel B, Cariou B. Pharmacological management of type 2 diabetes: The potential of incretin-based therapies. Diabetes Obesit Metab. 2011;13:99-117.
6. Hossain P, Kawar B, El NM. Obesity and diabetes in the developing world—a growing challenge. N Engl J Med 2007;356:213–5.
7. Whelan RS, Kaplinskiy V, Kitsis RN. Cell death in the pathogenesis of heart disease: mechanisms and significance. Annu Rev Physiol 2010;72:19–44.
8. Tsimihodimos V, Elisaf M. Effects of incretin-based therapies on renal function. Eur J Pharmacol. 2018;5;818:103–109.La Barre J. Sur le possibilité d'un traitement du diabète par l'incrétine. Bull Acad R Med Belg. 1932;12:620-4.

Chapter 21

Fixed-dose Combinations in Type 2 Diabetes Mellitus Management: How Effective?

Mangesh Harihar Tiwaskar

INTRODUCTION

Diabetes mellitus (DM), one of the greatest health emergencies of the 21st century worldwide, affects 425 million adults, i.e. 1 in every 11 adults aged 20–79 years, according to the 8th Edition of the Atlas of International Diabetes Federation (IDF). By 2045, this number is expected to grow by 48% to 629 million,[1] with the greatest increase coming from India, where the number of diabetics has doubled in the last two decades, from 32.7 million in 2000[2] to 73 million in 2017 and is expected to further double to 134.3 million by 2045.[1] DM not only contributes to the burden of mortality,[3] with one death occurring every 8 seconds,[1] but also to disability, which has increased considerably since 1990.[3] According to The Global Burden of Diseases, Injuries and Risk Factors Study 2015, high fasting plasma glucose (FPG) with 143.1 million global disability-adjusted life years (DALYs) is the third largest contributor to global DALYs.[4] This burden of mortality and disability can be chiefly traced to the diabetic complications associated with DM.[2]

The Diabetes Control and Complications Trial (DCCT)[5] and the United Kingdom Prospective Diabetes Study (UKPDS),[6] the largest and longest studies in Type 1 DM (T1DM) and Type 2 DM (T2DM) respectively, showed that lowering blood glucose concentrations could slow or prevent the development of diabetic complications. Epidemiological analyses of the UKPDS data further showed that for every 1% drop in glycosylated hemoglobin (HbA1c), there was a 35% reduction in the risk of complications, a 25% reduction in diabetes-related deaths, a 7% reduction in all-cause mortality and an 18% reduction in combined fatal and nonfatal myocardial infarction (MI).[6] Furthermore, lowering of A1c from 7 to 6% was associated with a further decrease in the risk of microvascular complications, though the absolute reduction in risk turned out to be much smaller.[7]

Based on these important trials, various leading associations like the American Association of Clinical Endocrinologists (AACE),[8] the American Diabetes Association (ADA)[7] and Diabetes Canada[9] recommend a HbA1c goal of <6.5% to <7% (Table 1) in patients with DM. While monotherapy is recommended by these international bodies for the initial management of DM, there has been a recent favorable incline toward therapy initiation with a combination of drugs (Table 1).[10-14]

Given the progressive nature of the disease, is combination therapy the answer to achieve glycemic control? Is initial combination therapy actually more effective than monotherapy in terms of glycemic control and safety? Are single pill fixed-dose combinations (FDCs) the way to go to improve adherence and subsequently control? This chapter aims to answer these queries through meticulous analysis of available data.

COMBINATION THERAPY IN T2DM

Worldwide, average HbA1c levels range from 7.0 to 12.6%, indicating inadequate glycemic control.[15] The management of T2DM is challenging due to the progressive nature of the disease along with its many contributory physiological defects.[16] The UKPDS reported that the progressive deterioration of diabetes control was such that only ~50% and ~25% of patients achieved their therapeutic goals with monotherapy after 3 and 9 years, respectively.[17]

TABLE 1: Guideline recommended hemoglobin A1c (HbA1c) and treatment thresholds.

Guidelines	ADA[7]	Diabetes Canada[9-11]	AACE[8,12]	ADA EASD[13]	NICE[14]
Recommended goal					
HbA1c (%)	<7*	≤6.5 to ≤7$	≤6.5#	7	6.5–7^
FPG (mg/dL)	80–130*	72–126	<110	–	–
PPBG (mg/dL)	<180*	90–180	<140	–	–
Threshold HbA1c to initiate therapy					
For initial monotherapy (HbA1c %)	<9	6–6.4	<7.5	>7	>6.5
For initial combination (HbA1c %)	≥9	≥8–8.5	≥7.5	≥9	–

Note:

Values of mg/dL obtained from conversion of mmol/L using conversion factor: 1 mmol/L = 18 mg/dL.

* More or less stringent glycemic goals may be appropriate for individual patients. Goals should be individualized based on duration of diabetes, age/life expectancy, comorbid condition, known cardiovascular disease (CVD) or advanced microvascular complications, hypoglycemia unawareness and individual patient considerations.

$ A1c ≤7% should be targeted to reduce the risk of microvascular CV complication, if implemented early in the course of disease and ≤6.5% may be targeted to reduce the risk of chronic kidney disease (CKD) and retinopathy, if at low risk of hypoglycemia.

Closer to normal for healthy and less stringent for "less healthy".

^ 6.5% for adults with type 2 diabetes managed either by lifestyle and diet, or by lifestyle and diet combined with a single drug not associated with hypoglycemia and 7.0% for adults on a drug associated with hypoglycemia.

(AACE: American Association of Clinical Endocrinologist; ADA: American DiabetesAssociation; CVD: cardiovascular disease; EASD: European Association for the Study of Diabetes; FPG: fasting plasma glucose; HbA1c: glycosylated hemoglobin; NICE: National Institute of Care and Excellence; PPBG: postprandial blood glucose.)

In patients with metformin failure, compared to later use of oral add-on drug to metformin, early use increased the odds of glycemic goal attainment (HbA1c <7%) by 36% in those with HbA1c ≥7.5%, with the odds increasing to 53% in those with HbA1c >8% and by 2.6-fold in those with HbA1c >9%. Additionally, greater number of early add-on patients achieved their glycemic targets. One of the key reasons why patients do not achieve glycemic targets is the failure of therapy escalation, which is primarily attributed to clinical inertia.[18] Available evidence shows that, on an average, therapy intensification occurs only after HbA1c deteriorates to >9%. Moreover, addition of the second agent takes place after a period of nearly 30 months from the first time a HbA1c level of >8% is recorded.[15] In a United States (US) Database Study of 7,109 participants, only one-third of the study population (38%) with inadequate glycemic control (HbA1c >7%) demonstrated addition of a second antidiabetic medication to the primary metformin monotherapy.[19] In another retrospective United Kingdom study conducted on 105,477 individuals, when compared to those who received prompt (<1 year) treatment intensification, those who experienced a 1-year delay showed an enhanced risk of MI (67%), stroke (51%), heart failure (HF; 64%) and composite cardiovascular/macrovascular events (CVE; 62%).[20] Since intensification of therapy and achievement of glycemic goals are distinctly linked,[18] early initiation of combination therapy may help to delay the deterioration of glycemic control.[21] Combining metformin and an agent from another class with a different mechanism of action may help to preserve β-cell function and thereby to maintain a long-term glycemic efficacy or "durability" as opposed to a stepwise treatment approach.[22]

A network meta-analysis of 277 articles undertaken by Zintzaras E et al.[23] extrapolated data from >100,000 patients over 30 years with 69 treatments and 173 direct comparisons for efficacy and 71 treatments and 180 direct comparisons for tolerability. Metformin used in combination with either glucagon-like peptide-1 (GLP-1) agonists, sulfonylureas (SU), dipeptidyl peptidase-4 (DPP-4) inhibitors, thiazolidinediones (TZDs), meglitinide and α-glucosidase inhibitor (AGI) outperformed its monotherapy, with 3–11-fold greater odds of patients achieving the HbA1c goal. An indirect analysis across the two-drug regimens that superseded metformin monotherapy showed that five combinations (Met formin + GLP-1 agonists or SU or DPP-4 inhibitor or TZD / meglitinide) yielded similar results. In the tolerability analysis, compared to monotherapy, only the metformin + GLP-1 agonists combination was associated with a lower risk of hypoglycemia while all the other combinations demonstrated a 19% to 4-fold higher odds of hypoglycemia.[23]

Another systematic review and meta-analysis of 36 studies by Cai X et al.[24] suggests that, compared with monotherapy, all initial combination therapies resulted in significant HbA1c reduction. The risk of hypoglycemia though, was higher with the combination of metformin with SU or TZD and similar with the combination of metformin with sodium/glucose cotransporter-2 (SGLT2) inhibitors or DPP-4 inhibitors (Table 2).[24]

A smaller systematic review and meta-analysis of 15 randomized clinical trials involving 6,693 patients (48.4–62.7 years) with a mean baseline HbA1c of 7.2–9.9%, mean diabetes duration of 1.6–4.1 years and a median follow-up period of 6 months showed that combination therapy had a greater likelihood of attaining the HbA1c goal <7%. Compared to metformin monotherapy, combination therapy reduced FPG by 14.3 mg/dL, HbA1c by a further 0.43% and increased HbA1c goal attainment by 40%, but the risk of hypoglycemia increased by 56%. When SUs and glinides were excluded from the analysis, this increased risk of hypoglycemia was no longer significant. Some studies also reported greater improvement in insulin resistance among patients on initial combination therapy; one study specifically showed that combination therapy of metformin with DPP-4inhibitors improved β-cell function at week 18 compared with metformin monotherapy.[22]

The benefits of combination therapy are further enhanced by the addition of a third agent. The impact of adding a third antihyperglycemic drug when blood glucose control is not achieved with metformin + SU was evaluated in a network meta-analysis of 18 randomized, controlled trials with 4,535 participants. The mean trial duration was 31.3 weeks with mean baseline HbA1c level of 8.8%, mean baseline body mass index (BMI) of 28.8 kg/m^2 and diabetes duration of 8.9 years. The addition of a third agent such as acarbose, DPP-4 inhibitors, GLP-1 agonists, or TZDs to the existing therapy led to mean

TABLE 2: **Efficacy of initial combination therapy.**[24]

Initial combination	Comparator Monotherapy	Efficacy (WMD)				SAFETY (RR)					
		HbA1c (%)	FPG (mg/dL)	PPBG (mg/dL)	Body weight (kg)	AEs	Drug related AEs	Hypoglycemia	GI AEs	SAE	Discontinuation due to AE
DPP-4 inhibitors + Metformin	vs. Metformin	−0.44	−13.86	−29.7	0.38	0.92	0.97	1.15	0.91	0.71	0.88
	vs. DPP-4 inhibitors	−0.88	−28.98	−48.42	−1	1.07	1.73	1.84	2.19	0.7	0.77
SU/glinides + Metformin	vs. Metformin	−0.68	−15.66	−12.6	2.6	1.26	–	8.91	0.7	–	–
	vs. SU/glinide	−0.49	−11.88	−15.66	−0.1	0.98	–	0.63	1.42	–	–
TZDs + Metformin	vs. Metformin	−0.44	−15.84	–	1.93	1.06	–	1.6	0.87	0.98	1.06
	vs. TZD	−0.83	−22.5	–	−1.22	1.31	–	1.53	–	0.87	–
SGLT2 inhibitors + Metformin	vs. Metformin	−0.47	−24.84	–	−2	1.19	1.45	1.37	0.72	0.84	0.82
	vs. SGLT2 inhibitors	−0.64	−14.94	–	−0.66	1.16	1.13	2.23	1.99	0.62	0.83
DPP-4 inhibitors + TZD	vs. TZD	−0.54	−16.02	-35.46	0.96	0.94	1.06	1.08	0.86	1.31	0.8
	vs. DPP-4 inhibitors	−0.62	−25.38	–	3.51	1.09	1.4	0.84	–	1.31	–

Note: Values of mg/dL obtained from conversion of mmol/L using conversion factor: 1 mmol/L = 18 mg/dL.

(AE: adverse effects; DPP-4: dipeptidyl peptidase-4; FPG: fasting plasma glucose; GI: gastrointestinal; HbA1c: glycosylated hemoglobin; RR: relative risk; PPBG: postprandial blood glucose; SAE: serious adverse effect; SGLT2: sodium/glucose cotransporter-2; TZD: thiazolidinediones.)

HbA1c reductions of −0.60%, −0.89%, −1.04%, and −1.15%, respectively. While addition of acarbose and GLP-1 agonists had favorable effects on weight, TZDs were associated with weight gain. This analysis observed no significant difference in benefit between drug classes and concluded that the choice of the agents used for combination therapy should be customized as per the patient's clinical characteristics.[25]

A retrospective cohort analyses of 20,070 T2DM patients with a mean age of 59 years compared the time to treatment failure among patients on metformin + SU (n = 15,508), metformin + DPP-4 inhibitors (n = 3,080) and metformin + TZD (n = 1,482). The primary composite outcome was defined as the time to substitution or intensification of treatment with a third agent at HbA1c ≥7.5%. Secondary outcomes included glycemic effectiveness and body weight responses. The metformin + SU combination was associated with the highest reduction in HbA1c while metformin + DPP-4 inhibitors produced a significant 1.8 kg weight loss. However, second line use of TZDs had the best durability of glycemic control with the longest mean time to treatment failure (Table 3).[26]

These analyses suggest that initial combination therapy could have a beneficial impact on glycemic outcomes in diabetes compared to metformin monotherapy across a wide range of baseline HbA1c levels. However, a large retrospective analysis of 23,400 patients showed that multiple-drug regimens were associated with significantly poorer patient persistence and compliance than a single-drug regimen (Fig. 1).[27] It is well known that adherence (encompassing both compliance and persistence)[27] to oral anti diabetes drugs (OADs) helps to achieve glycemic control.[28] More adherent patients were found to have lower HbA1c levels compared to the less adherent ones (7.1% vs. 8.5%). Also, patients reaching HbA1c <7% have higher adherence rates compared to those who do not. Data from retrospective studies indicate that every 10% decrease in adherence is related to a 0.10–0.15% increase in HbA1c.[28]

Paradoxically, though initial combination therapy could help to achieve glycemic goals, it could be associated with lower adherence resulting in poorer control. The availability of FDCs of OADs may help to address this concern.

TABLE 3: **Comparison of primary and secondary outcomes with metformin + thiazolidinediones (TZD) or sulfonylurea (SU) or dipeptidyl peptidase-4 inhibitors.**

	Metformin + TZD	Metformin + SU	Metformin + DPP-4 inhibitors
HbA1c reduction (%)	−1.2	−1.3	−0.9
Weight gain (kg)	1.8	−0.2	−1.8
% patients needing add on or switch to other OADs	30	44	44
Mean time to treatment failure (years)	3.3	2.4	1.6
Dual therapy failure rates			
At 1 year (%)	8	15	23
At 2 years (%)	12	26	38

(DPP-4: dipeptidyl peptidase-4; HbA1c: glycosylated hemoglobin; OAD: oral antidiabetes drugs.)

FIXED-DOSE COMBINATIONS IN T2DM

Single-pill FDCs simplify the treatment regimen by reducing pill burden and improving tolerability leading to improved adherence,[29] better glycemic control,[30] and reduced healthcare costs, unlike the separate pills or loose-dose combinations (LDCs).

Effectiveness of Therapy

Thayer S et al.[30] in a retrospective database analysis, showed that subjects switching from LDCs to FDCs experienced a greater absolute reduction in A1c (−0.06% vs. −0.51%; p = 0.004). Moreover, the average percent reduction in A1c was larger for the FDC cohort compared

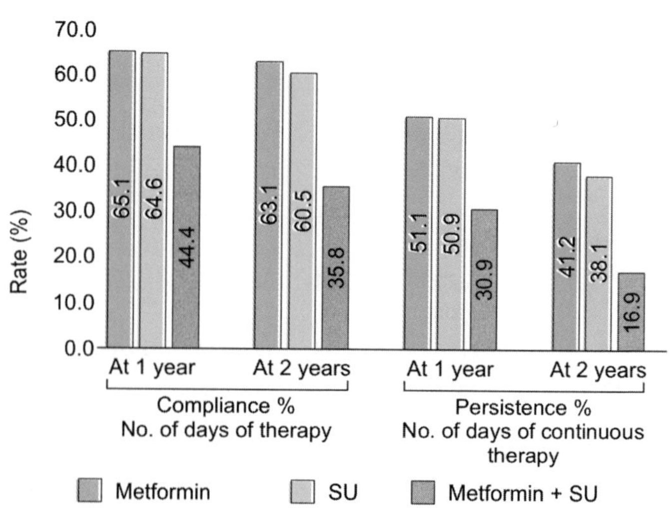

Figure 1 Compliance and persistence rates with monotherapy and combination therapy[27] (SU: sulfonylurea.)

with the LDC cohort (p = 0.05). Three studies evaluating the efficacy of SU + metformin FDC demonstrated 0.4–1% significantly greater reductions in HbA1c compared to monotherapy.[31]

Blonde L et al.[32] evaluated 1,421 patients receiving FDC (67%—glibenclamide + metformin) versus those receiving LDC (33%—glibenclamide coadministered with metformin), in a retrospective cohort study analysis. Compared to patients on LDC, 1.8-fold more patients on FDC achieved HbA1c of <7% with a 0.5% greater reduction in HbA1c overall and a significant 1% greater reduction in those with baseline HbA1c ≥8%. These benefits were also significant in those new to oral combination therapy (Table 4). Medication adherence was higher in the FDC group but was not a significant predictor of decrease in HbA1c. FDCs may thus be especially beneficial when baseline HbA1c is ≥8%.

Adherence to Therapy

Melikian C et al.[33] in a retrospective database analysis of pharmacy claims evaluated adherence rates among 6,502

TABLE 4: Efficacy and outcome evidence summary for fixed-dose combination (FDC) versus loose-dose combination (LDC).

Study	Characteristics and outcomes	Results		
		FDC	LDC	ST
Williams SA et al.[37] Type of study—retrospective claims database analysis Medication—Metformin/SU/TZD /DPP-4 inhibitor/AGI (LDC/ST) / Meglitinide derivatives (LDC/ST)/GLP-1 (ST only)	Number of patients	8,416	4,225	8,407
	Average changes in HbA1c	↓1.65	↓1.51	↓1.36
	Diabetes-related ambulatory visits (count)	2.7	3.2	3.7
	Diabetes-related inpatient visits (%)	1.7	2.6	2.7
	Diabetes-related ER visits (%)	1.4	1.7	2
	Adjusted all-cause total costs ($)	8,445	10,294	10,352
	Adjusted diabetes related costs ($)	1,713	1,925	2,005
Thayer S et al.[30] Type of study—retrospective database analysis Medication—rosiglitazone/glimepiride (FDC)/ SU and rosiglitazone (LDC)	Number of patients	543	2,518	–
	HbA1c reduction (%)	–1.08	–0.77	–
	MPR (%)	87	81	–
Blonde et al.[32] Type of study—retrospective cohort study analysis Medication—glibenclamide and metformin	Number of patients	950	471	–
	Mean fose/day	6 mg + 893 mg	10 mg and 1,297 mg	–
	↓ In HbA1c: All patients	↓2.02	↓1.49	–
	↓ In HbA1c: Baseline HbA1c ≥8%	↓2.93	↓1.92	–
	↓ In HbA1c: Baseline HbA1c <8%	↓0.54	↓0.23	–
	↓ In HbA1c: Patients previously on monotherapy	↓1.34	↓1.26	–
	↓ In HbA1c: Patients new to oral therapy	↓3.19	↓1.94	–
	↓ In HbA1c: Patients <60 years	↓2.31	↓1.67	–
	↓ In HbA1c: Patient ≥60 years	↓1.89	↓1.09	–
	% Patients achieving A1c of <7%	55.9	31.2	–
	% Patients adherent	84	76	
Cheong et al.[34] Type of study—retrospective cohort analysis using Rx claims Medication—metformin+glibenclamide or metformin + rosiglitazone or metformin + glipizide (given as FDC or LDC)	Number of patients	7,570	14,762	–
	MPR (%)	78.6	77.2	–
	MPR (%) in patients switching from LDC to FDC	81.7	72.7	–
	Odds ratio for regimen adherence rate vs. LDC	1.867	Reference	–

Continued

Continued

Study	Characteristics and outcomes	Results		
		FDC	LDC	ST
Lokhandwala T et al.[35] Type of study—retrospective cohort study Medication—meglitinides + biguanides, SUs + Biguanides, SUs + TZDs, TZDs + biguanides, Bile acid sequestrant combinations, AGI combinations	Number of patients	12,590	10,771	–
	Rate of non persistence to therapy (%)	67.9	73.4	–
	Rate of adherence to therapy (%)	57	50.7	–
	Time to non persistence (days)	207.1	186.3	–
	Patients who experienced hypoglycemia (%)	72	107	–
	Number of hypoglycemic events, rate per PY	8	16	–
	All-cause hospitalization (%)	7.4	10.1	–
	Emergency room visits (%)	15.4	19.9	–
	T2DM related hospitalization (%)	0.1	0.3	–
	T2DM related emergency room visits (%)	1.3	2.5	–
	Total predicted monthly all-cause costs ($)	1,008	1053	–
	Total predicted monthly T2DM-related costs ($)	142	155	–
Brook RA et al.[36] Type of study—retrospective analysis Medication—metformin or SU + TZD (pioglitazone/ Rosiglitazone) given as LDC or FDC	Number of patients	163	163	–
	Medication possession ratio (%)	65	50	–
	Medical cost ($)	2,285	2,666	–
	Prescription drug cost ($)	2,370	2,678	–
	Sick leave cost ($)	384	472	–
	Overall health cost expense ($)	5,360	6,173	–
Cugnardey N et al.[40] Type of study—peer-reviewed, published, validated computer simulation model Medication—metformin + glibenclamide (FDC), metformin + rosiglitazone (LDC)	Undiscounted life expectancy (years)	14.73	14.4	–
	Delay in diabetes-related complications vs. LDC (years)	0.3	–	–
	Treatment and complication costs vs. LDC ($/patient)	−5,605	Reference	–
Delea et al.[39] Type of study—retrospective longitudinal design Medication—rosiglitazone + metformin (FDC), rosiglitazone +metformin or SU (LDC)	Visits per quarter	0.76	0.82–0.86	–
	Risk of hospitalization (% per quarter)	7.1	8–9.1	–
	Cost ($ per quarter)	2,261	2,677–3,027	–
	Mean change in MPR (%)	−2	−9.3 to −11.2	
Duh MS et al.[38] Type of study—observational study Medication—rosiglitazone + metformin (FDC), metformin + SU (LDC)	Number of patients	1,507	1,255	–
	Frequency of inpatient visit vs. LDC (per pt per year)	↓0.36	Reference	–
	Frequency of outpatient visit vs. LDC (per pt per year)	↓3.32	Reference	–
	Number of hospital days vs. LDC (days per pt per year)	↓1.08	Reference	–
	Total direct cost ($ per pt per month)	−143	Reference	–
Patel BV et al.[41] Type of study—retrospective study Medication—TZD and metformin	Number of patients	729	19,440	–
	Odds ratio for regimen adherence vs. LDC	1.50	Reference	–

Continued

Continued

Study	Characteristics and outcomes	Results		
		FDC	LDC	ST
Melikian C et al.[33] Type of study—retrospective database analysis medication—metformin + glibenclamide (FDC)/metformin and glibenclamide (LDC)	Number of patients	105	1,815	–
	Adherence rate (%)	77	54	–

(AGI: alpha-glucosidase inhibitor; DPP-4: dipeptidyl peptidase-4; ER: emergency room; FDC: fixed-dose combination; LDC: loose dose combination; MPR: medication possession ratio; PY: person year; Pt : patient; Rx: prescription; ST: step therapy; SU: sulfonylurea; TZD: thiazolidinedione.)

newly treated patients receiving monotherapy, LDC, or FDC. Switching from monotherapy to FDC resulted in significantly greater adherence (77%) compared to those switched to LDC (54%). Adherence also significantly improved in patients switching from LDC (71%) to FDC (87%), p <0.001. This impact was confirmed by Cheong C et al.[34] who retrospectively evaluated patient adherence to the various antidiabetic regimens by analyzing prescription claims of 22,332 patients during a 12-month preindex and 12-month postindex period. The index date was defined as the date at which the first qualifying OAD prescription was filled. Adherence was measured using the medication possession ratio (MPR). Postindex, FDC users had a 1.8% higher MPR. FDC users were more likely to have higher regimen adherence rates than LDC users [odds ratio (OR) = 1.867; p <0.001). There was a 12.4% absolute change in MPR in those switched from LDC in the preindex period to FDC in the postindex period.

Lokhandwala et al.[35] analyzed 23,361 patients with T2DM and ≥1 additional oral antidiabetic prescription for persistence (no ≥30-day gap) and adherence (MPR ≥0.8) as primary endpoints and hypoglycemia, healthcare resource utilization, and costs as secondary endpoints. Compared to LDC patients, patients on FDC showed 21% lower odds for nonpersistence, 28% greater odds for adherence with a longer time to nonpersistence, i.e. 20.8 days. Total predicted all-cause monthly costs and T2DM-related costs were also lower in the FDC cohort (Table 4).

Brook RA et al.[36] in a retrospective claims analysis found that mean MPR was significantly higher for FDC (65%) than for LDC (50%). FDCs also showed a trend toward reduction in both direct (medical and prescription) and indirect (sick leave, short- and long-term disability, and workers' compensation) costs.

Cost-effectiveness of Therapy

The FDCs were found to be associated with lower costs and better healthcare resource use along with a greater likelihood of HbA1c goal attainment versus LDC or step treatment (ST) in an analysis by Williams SA et al.[37] which included 21,048 treatment-naïve T2DM patients. The date on which the first qualifying OAD prescription was filled—was deemed the index date and the 12-month period following this date was considered the postindex period. Metformin was the most commonly prescribed agent for all cohorts. SUs were commonly prescribed as part of LDC or ST, while TZD or DPP-4 inhibitor was often part of the FDC cohort. In the postindex period, the FDC group experienced a larger average drop in HbA1c and a higher achievement rate of HbA1c <7%. Compared to the FDC cohort, patients in the LDC cohort had 27% lower odds of achieving HbA1c goal and 26% higher odds of all-cause inpatient or emergency room (ER) visits. Moreover, the adjusted all-cause total costs and diabetes-related costs were 15% and 11% significantly lower in the FDC cohort compared to the LDC cohort.

Duh et al.[38] analyzed medical, pharmacy and disability claims data from 2001 to 2004 in 2,762 T2DM patients newly initiated on FDC or LDC with 60 days of uninterrupted treatment. Compared to the LDC group, the FDC group presented with significantly lesser inpatient visits [↓0.36 per patient per year (PPPY)], outpatient visits (↓3.32 PPPY) and number of hospital days (↓1.08 PPPY). Similarly, the total direct and indirect costs were also significantly lower in the FDC group [↓$172 per patient per month (PPPM)].

Delea et al.[39] employed a retrospective longitudinal design to demonstrate that FDCs improve outcomes and reduce costs compared to LDCs. Patients on FDCs had 7–12% fewer mean visits, 11–22% lower risk of hospitalization and 16–25% lower costs on a quarterly basis compared to those on LDCs. The mean reduction in MPR was significantly lower with FDC (–2.0%) than with LDC (–9.3 to –11.2%) therapy.

Cugnardey et al.[40] demonstrated that FDCs, in addition to a significantly greater lowering of HbA1c by 0.4%, enhanced quality-adjusted life expectancy by 0.18 years, delayed diabetes-related complications by 0.3 years and lowered direct costs (treatment and complications) by €5,605 per patient, compared to LDCs.

Data from real-world practice analyzed by Colombo GL et al.[42] showed that in 169,375 patients treated with OADs during 2008, FDCs were associated with lower average number of specialist examinations and a better adherence compared to LDCs. Average annual cost per patient with respect to medication cost and specialist and diagnostic care was also lower in the FDC group.

Treatment Satisfaction

Hutchins V et al.[43] reviewed five randomized controlled trials (RCTs) that included patient-reported outcomes. FDC regimens had greater treatment satisfaction compared to monotherapies, placebo and previous treatment. While improved efficacy was one of the reasons for greater treatment satisfaction, in one study where efficacy was similar, the satisfaction was higher due to the lesser hypoglycemia with the FDC regimen. In a 26-week open label RCT by Raskin et al.[44] patients inadequately controlled on monotherapy/LDC and randomized to FDC therapy were more satisfied with their current therapy compared to the previous therapeutic regimen.

Available evidence thus suggests that in patients with T2DM, FDCs offer excellent efficacy and a similar tolerability as LDCs. Lower doses of constituent drugs in FDCs may additionally improve tolerability.[16] However, use of FDCs minimizes the dosing flexibility compared to LDCs. In spite of this drawback, the pros of FDCs far outweigh their cons (Table 5).[45,46]

Which fixed-dose combination when?

Metformin is the preferred initial OAD while SUs, TZDs, DPP-4 inhibitors, SGLT2 inhibitors, AGIs, GLP-1 agonists and insulin are the major classes of antidiabetic agents that can be combined with metformin. The ADA recommends choosing any of the classes as an initial addition to metformin based on efficacy, safety, and costs. The AACE prioritizes combination of metformin with SGLT2 inhibitors, DPP-4 inhibitors, TZD, AGI and SU in that order.[47] While target achievement and reduced side effects are the major goals of combination therapy, the choice of agents needs careful assessment of potential risks and benefits[15] by considering several variables such as patient/drug characteristics, patient preferences, comorbidity and pharmacological costs.[47]

As an add-on to metformin, SUs offer excellent reductions in HbA1c, but their use is associated with increased risk of hypoglycemia,[48] while TZDs offer good glycemic durability but are associated with side effects like weight gain, edema and the risk of congestive heart failure.[49,50] A DPP-4 inhibitors added to metformin achieves good glycemic control with low risk of hypoglycemia and results in weight neutrality while combination of SGLT2 inhibitors with metformin enhances glycemic control and decreases body weight and blood pressure. However, both DPP-4 inhibitors and SGLT2 inhibitors may be associated with increased costs.[49] AGIs lower glucose through insulin-independent pathways and effectively lower postprandial hyperglycemia[31] but are associated with gastrointestinal (GI) side effects.[48]

As there is no clear consensus on which OAD should be used initially or which agent in a specific class should be preferred over the other, agent-specific information should be carefully assessed to ensure treatment is individualized to suit specific patient needs. Considerations for choice of various drug classes and their possible combinations are presented in Table 6.[51]

FIXED-DOSE COMBINATIONS IN THE INDIAN SCENARIO

The FDCs have not been without their fair share of controversy in India. Many FDCs, including some anti-diabetic FDCs, have been found to have no therapeutic

TABLE 5: **Advantages and disadvantages of fixed-dose combination (FDCs) in type 2 diabetes mellitus (T2DM).[45,46]**

Advantages	Disadvantages
Combination therapy helps to target several pathogenic mechanisms concurrently, preferably via complementary mechanisms of action	Makes assessment of efficacy/ side effects due to individual drugs more difficult
Aids in swifter and greater achievement of glycemic goals	Hampers dose titration
Reduces the patient's medication burden to the patient, since two drugs are combined into a single-dose form	Could interfere with the bioavailability of agents
Supports improvement of the adherence rates in T2DM patients	–
Potentially delays disease progression and assists in preservation of β-cell function	–
Reduces clinical inertia	–

TABLE 6: **Considerations for choice of various drug classes and their possible combinations[7,8,13,31,48,51].**

Drug class	Mode of action	Commonly used agents	Efficacy	Safety		Elderly patients	CV patients	CKD patients	Other considerations	Could be combined with
				Change in weight	Risk of hypo-glycemia					
Biguanides	↓ Hepatic glucose production	Metformin	High	Neutral	No	Benefit, avoid if there is intercurrent disorder (tissue hypoperfusion)	Potential benefit	Contraindicated in eGFR <30	• GI side effects common (diarrhea, nausea) • Potential for B12 deficiency	SUs, TZDs, DPP-4 inhibitor, AGIs, SGLT2 inhibitor
Sulfonylureas	↑ Insulin secretion	Glibenclamide, glipizide, glimepiride, gliclazide	High	Gain	Yes	Avoid	Neutral	Glibenclamide: Not recommended, glipizide and glimepiride: initiate conservatively, Gliclazide : No dose adjustment required	• FDA special warning on increased risk of CV mortality based on studies of an older SU (tolbutamide)	Biguanides, TZDs, DPP-4 inhibitor, AGIs, SGLT2inhibitor
TZDs	↑ Insulin sensitivity	Pioglitazone, Rosiglitazone	High	Gain	No	Can cause potential AE	Potential benefit	No dose adjustment required, Not recommended in renal impairment due to potential for fluid retention	• FDA Black Box: Congestive heart failure (pioglitazone, rosiglitazone) • Fluid retention, risk of bone fractures, • Bladder cancer (pioglitazone), ↑ LDL-C (rosiglitazone) • Benefit in NASH	Biguanides, SU, DPP-4 inhibitor, SGLT2 inhibitor
AGIs	Slows intestinal carbohydrate digestion/ absorption	Acarbose, miglitol, voglibose	Intermediate	Neutral	No	Effective, can cause adverse GI effects	Neutral	Avoid if GFR <25 mL/min or Cr >2 mg/dL, do not use in dialysis	• GI side effects	Biguanides, SU

Continued

Continued

Drug class	Mode of action	Commonly used agents	Efficacy	Safety		Elderly patients	CV patients	CKD patients	Other considerations	Could be combined with
				Change in weight	Risk of hypoglycemia					
DPP-4 inhibitor	↑ Insulin secretion (glucose dependent); ↓ Glucagon secretion (glucose dependent)	Sitagliptin, saxagliptin, linagliptin, alogliptin	Intermediate	Neutral	No	Benefit	Neutral	Dose adjustment required, except for linagliptin	• Potential risk of acute pancreatitis • Joint pain	Biguanides, TZD, SU, DPP-4 inhibitor
SGLT2 inhibitor	Blocks glucose reabsorption by the kidney, increasing glucosuria	Canagliflozin, dapagliflozin, empagliflozin	Intermediate	Loss	No	Can cause potential AE	Benefit	Canagliflozin: Not recommended with eGFR <45, Dapagliflozin: Not recommended with eGFR <60; Contraindicated with eGFR <30, Empagliflozin: Contraindicated with eGFR <30	• FDA Black Box: Risk of amputation (canagliflozin) • Risk of bone fractures (canagliflozin), genitourinary infections, risk of volume depletion, hypotension, ↑ LDL-C	Biguanides, TZD, SU, DPP-4 inhibitor

(SU: sulfonylurea; TZD: thiazolidinedione; AGI: alpha-glucosidase inhibitor; DPP-4: dipeptidyl peptidase-4; SGLT2: sodium/glucose cotransporter 2; CV: cardiovascular; CKD: chronic kidney disease; eGFR: estimated glomerular filtration rate; GI: gastrointestinal; FDA: Food and Drug Administration; AE: adverse effect; LDL-C: low-density lipoprotein cholesterol; NASH: nonalcoholic steatohepatitis, Cr: creatinine)

Source: Mode of action--ADA 2018. Iglesias P, Heras M, Díez JJ. Diabetes mellitus and kidney disease in the elderly. Nefrologia. 2014;34(3):285-92.

justification due to which the Government of India in a gazette notification, as recent as September 8, 2018, has banned the manufacture, sale and distribution of 328 FDCs with immediate effect with certain conditions placed on six others.[52] Banned FDCs include those containing pioglitazone in the smaller doses of 7.5 mg, metformin in smaller doses of 325 mg and 400 mg, the triple FDCs of voglibose with metformin and gliclazide or pioglitazone and those containing chromium picolinate/polynicotinate. Amongst triple FDCs of SU + metformin + TZD, only the following strengths have been recommended for treatment of T2DM when diet, exercise along with monotherapy, and dual therapy do not achieve the glycemic target: glimepiride (1/2 mg) + pioglitazone (15 mg) + metformin 500 mg (immediate or sustained or extended release) and glibenclamide 5 mg + metformin 500 mg sustained release (SR) + pioglitazone 15 mg.[53]

The FDCs have been a norm in India since almost the past 50 years, though they have only recently been recognized for their potential benefits and are being recommended as initial therapy in treatment guidelines.[54] According to an ecologic study by McGettigan P et al. most metformin FDC formulations in India have the approval of Central Drugs Standard Control Organization (CDSCO), the national regulator.[55] Thus, while some of the antidiabetic FDCs lack rationale or evidence and are associated with potential safety concerns, most of them are rational and have proven benefits.

CONCLUSION

Accumulating evidence encourages early intervention to slow the onset and progression of T2DM. In spite of the current OAD armamentarium, diabetes control is far from satisfactory, with Indian patients reporting at least a 2% higher HbA1c[56] than that recommended by guidelines. Initial combination treatment, specifically as a FDC, has several distinct advantages since it may help to avoid clinical inertia, achieve early lowering of HbA1c levels with more individuals achieving their glycemic goals, preserve β-cell function thereby offering durable glycemic control and cause fewer adverse events (AEs) due to the complementary mechanisms of action/lower doses of individual agents, besides lowering total and diabetes-related costs. FDCs, while not a panacea, have the definite potential to optimize the management of T2DM by improving control, increasing adherence, and reducing costs. In the larger public interest, proper regulation and prudent use of FDCs is the need of the hour.

REFERENCES

1. The International Diabetes Federation. (2017). IDF Diabetes Atlas, 8th edition. [online] Available from: http://diabetesatlas.org/resources/2017-atlas.html. [Accessed September, 2018].
2. Pradeepa R, Mohan V. Prevalence of type 2 diabetes and its complications in India and economic costs to the nation. Eur J Clin Nutr. 2017;71(7):816-24.
3. Zheng Y, Ley SH, Hu FB. Global aetiology and epidemiology of type 2 diabetes mellitus and its complications. Nat Rev Endocrinol. 2018;14(2):88-98.
4. GBD 2015 Risk Factors Collaborators. Global, regional, and national comparative risk assessment of 79 behavioural, environmental and occupational, and metabolic risks or clusters of risks, 1990-2015: a systematic analysis for the Global Burden of Disease Study 2015. Lancet. 2016;388(10053):1659-724.
5. American Diabetes Association. Implications of the diabetes control and complications trial. Diabetes Care. 2003;26 (Suppl 1):S25-7.
6. Genuth S, Eastman R, Kahn R, et al. American Diabetes Association. Implications of the United Kingdom prospective diabetes study. Diabetes Care. 2003;26 (Suppl 1):S28-32.
7. American Diabetes Association. (2018) Standards of Diabetes Care in Diabetes—2018 [online] Available from: https://diabetesed.net/wp-content/uploads/2017/12/2018-ADA-Standards-of-Care.pdf. [Accessed September, 2018].
8. Garber AJ, Abrahamson MJ, Barzilay JI, et al. Consensus statement by the American Association of Clinical Endocrinologists and American College of Endocrinology on The Comprehensive Type 2 Diabetes Management Algorithm—2018 Executive Summary. Endocr Pract. 2018;24(1):91-120.
9. Imran SA, Agarwal G, Bajaj HS, et al. Targets for Glycemic Control. Can J Diabetes. 2018;42 Suppl 1:S42-6.
10. Lipscombe L, Booth G, Butalia S, et al. Pharmacologic Glycemic Management of Type 2 Diabetes in Adults. Can J Diabetes. 2018;42 (Suppl 1):S88-103.
11. Prebtani APH, Bajaj HS, Goldenberg R, et al. Reducing the Risk of Developing Diabetes. Can J Diabetes. 2018;42 (Suppl 1):S20-6.
12. AACE Diabetes Resource Center (2018). Type 2 Diabetes Glucose Management Goals. [online] Available from: http://outpatient.aace.com/type-2-diabetes/management. [Accessed September, 2018].
13. Inzucchi SE, Bergenstal RM, Buse JB, et al. Management of hyperglycemia in type 2 diabetes, 2015: a patient-centered approach: update to a position statement of the American Diabetes Association and the European Association for the Study of Diabetes. Diabetes Care. 2015;38(1):140-9.
14. NICE guideline (2017). Type 2 diabetes in adults: management. [online] Available from: https://www.nice.org.uk/guidance/ng28 [Accessed September, 2018].
15. Zinman B. Initial combination therapy for type 2 diabetes mellitus: is it ready for prime time? Am J Med. 2011;124(1 Suppl):S19-34.
16. Harris SB. The power of two: an update on fixed-dose combinations for type 2 diabetes. Expert Rev Clin Pharmacol. 2016;9(11):1453-62.
17. Turner RC, Cull CA, Frighi V, et al. Glycemic control with diet, sulfonylurea, metformin, or insulin in patients with type 2 diabetes mellitus: progressive requirement for multiple therapies (UKPDS 49). UK Prospective Diabetes Study (UKPDS) Group. JAMA. 1999;281(21):2005-12.
18. Rajpathak SN, Rajgopalan S, Engel SS. Impact of time to treatment intensification on glycemic goal attainment among patients with type 2 diabetes failing Metformin monotherapy. J Diabetes Complications. 2014;28(6):831-5.
19. Yu S, Schwab P, Bian B, et al. Use of add-on Treatment to Metformin monotherapy for Patients with Type 2 Diabetes and Suboptimal Glycemic Control: A U.S. Database Study. J Manag Care Spec Pharm. 2016;22(3):272-80.

20. Paul SK, Klein K, Thorsted BL, et al. Delay in treatment intensification increases the risks of cardiovascular events in patients with type 2 diabetes. Cardiovasc Diabetol. 2015;14:100.
21. Cahn A, Cefalu WT. Clinical Considerations for Use of Initial Combination Therapy in Type 2 Diabetes. Diabetes Care. 2016;39 (Suppl 2):S137-45.
22. Phung OJ, Sobieraj DM, Engel SS, et al. Early combination therapy for the treatment of type 2 diabetes mellitus: systematic review and meta-analysis. Diabetes Obes Metab. 2014;16(5):410-7.
23. Zintzaras E, Miligkos M, Ziakas P, et al. Assessment of the relative effectiveness and tolerability of treatments of type 2 diabetes mellitus: a network meta-analysis. Clin Ther. 2014;36(10):1443-53.
24. Cai X, Gao X, Yang W, et al. Efficacy and Safety of Initial Combination Therapy in Treatment-Naïve Type 2 Diabetes Patients: A Systematic Review and Meta-analysis. Diabetes Ther. 2018;9(5):1995-2014.
25. Gross JL, Kramer CK, Leitão CB, et al. Effect of antihyperglycemic agents added to Metformin and a sulfonylurea on glycemic control and weight gain in type 2 diabetes: a network meta-analysis. Ann Intern Med. 2011;154(10):672-9.
26. Mamza J, Mehta R, Donnelly R, et al. Important differences in the durability of glycaemic response among second-line treatment options when added to Metformin in type 2 diabetes: a retrospective cohort study. Ann Med. 2016;48(4):224-34.
27. Dailey G, Kim MS, Lian JF. Patient compliance and persistence with anti-hyperglycemic therapy: evaluation of a population of type 2 diabetic patients. J Int Med Res. 2002;30(1):71-9.
28. Schernthaner G. Fixed-dose combination therapies in the management of hyperglycaemia in Type 2 diabetes: an opportunity to improve adherence and patient care. Diabet Med. 2010;27(7):739-43.
29. Blonde L, San Juan ZT, Bolton P. Fixed-dose combination therapy in type 2 diabetes mellitus. Endocr Pract. 2014;20(12):1322-32.
30. Thayer S, Arondekar B, Harley C, et al. Adherence to a fixed-dose combination of rosiglitazone/glimepiride in subjects switching from monotherapy or dual therapy with a thiazolidinedione and/or a sulfonylurea. Ann Pharmacother. 2010;44(5):791-9.
31. Mooradian A, Chehade JM, Mooradian AD. Advantages and pitfalls of antihyperglycemic combination pills as first-line therapy in the management of type 2 diabetes. Am J Ther. 2016;23(6):e1857-66.
32. Blonde L, Wogen J, Kreilick C, et al. Greater reductions in A1C in type 2 diabetic patients new to therapy with glyburide/Metformin tablets as compared to glyburide co-administered with metformin. Diabetes Obes Metab. 2003;5(6):424-31.
33. Melikian C, White TJ, Vanderplas A, et al. Adherence to oral antidiabetic therapy in a managed care organization: a comparison of monotherapy, combination therapy, and fixed-dose combination therapy. Clin Ther. 2002;24(3):460-7.
34. Cheong C, Barner JC, Lawson KA, et al. Patient adherence and reimbursement amount for antidiabetic fixed-dose combination products compared with dual therapy among Texas Medicaid recipients. Clin Ther. 2008;30(10):1893-907.
35. Lokhandwala T, Smith N, Sternhufvud C, et al. A retrospective study of persistence, adherence, and health economic outcomes of fixed-dose combination vs. loose-dose combination of oral anti-diabetes drugs. J Med Econ. 2016;19(3):203-12.
36. Brook RA, Kleinman NL, Wingenbach D, et al. Medication possession ratio and health benefit cost comparisons in type 2 diabetes patients using fixed- and loose-dose thiazolidinedione combination products [abstract]. Diabetes 2008;57:1214-P.
37. Williams SA, Buysman EK, Hulbert EM, et al. Hemoglobin A1c outcomes and health care resource use in type 2 diabetes mellitus patients treated with combination oral antidiabetic drugs through step therapy and loose-dose and fixed-dose combinations. Manag Care. 2012;21(7):40-8.
38. Duh MS, Gosselin A, Beaulieu N, et al. Comparison of resources utilization (RU) and costs in drug-naïve type 2 diabetes (T2D) patients (PTS) treated with rosiglitazone (RSG)/metformin (MET) as fixed-dose combination (FDC) vs. sulfonylurea (SU) plus Metformin (MET) as combination therapy (CT) [abstract]. Diabetes. 2007;56:2202-PO.
39. Delea T, Arondekar B, Kartashov A, et al. Add-on therapy with rosiglitazone (RSG)/Metformin (MET) as a fixed-dose combination (FDC) vs RSG plus met or RSG plus sulfonylurea (SU) as separate pills (SP): Retrospective study of outcomes and costs [abstract]. Diabetes. 2007;56:2200-PO.
40. Cugnardey N, Roze S, Palmer AJ, et al. Fixed combination metformin plus glibenclamide (Glucovance) is cost- and life-saving compared to metformin plus rosiglitazone in type 2 diabetes patients in France [abstract]. ISPOR 8th Annual European Congress; Florence, Italy: 2005. PDB25.
41. Patel BV, Leslie RS, Aranda GA. Retrospective comparison of compliance to fixed-dose combination versus single agent combination therapy for the treatment of diabetes [abstract]. ISPOR 12th Annual International Meeting: Arlington, VA, USA; 2008. PDB14.
42. Colombo GL, Rossi E, De Rosa M, et al. Antidiabetic therapy in real practice: indicators for adherence and treatment cost. Patient Prefer Adherence. 2012;6:653-61.
43. Hutchins V, Zhang B, Fleurence RL, et al. A systematic review of adherence, treatment satisfaction and costs, in fixed-dose combination regimens in type 2 diabetes. Curr Med Res Opin. 2011;27(6):1157-68.
44. Raskin P, Lewin A, Reinhardt R, et al. Repaglinide/Metformin Fixed-Dose Combination Study Group. Twice-daily and three-times-daily dosing of a repaglinide/Metformin fixed-dose combination tablet provide similar glycaemic control. Diabetes Obes Metab. 2009;11(10):947-52.
45. Cersosimo E, Johnson EL, Chovanes C, et al. Initiating therapy in patients newly diagnosed with type 2 diabetes: Combination therapy vs a stepwise approach. Diabetes Obes Metab. 2018;20(3):497-507.
46. Vijayakumar TM, Jayram J, Meghana Cheekireddy V, et al. Safety, Efficacy, and Bioavailability of Fixed-Dose Combinations in Type 2 Diabetes Mellitus: A Systematic Updated Review. Curr Ther Res Clin Exp. 2017;84:4-9.
47. Moon MK, Hur KY, Ko SH, et al. Combination Therapy of Oral Hypoglycemic Agents in Patients with Type 2 Diabetes Mellitus. Diabetes Metab J. 2017;41(5):357-66.
48. Harper W, Clement M, Goldenberg R, et al. Pharmacologic management of type 2 diabetes. Can J Diabetes. 2013;37 (Suppl 1):S61-8.
49. Lavernia F, Adkins SE, Shubrook JH. Use of oral combination therapy for type 2 diabetes in primary care: Meeting individualized patient goals. Postgrad Med. 2015;127(8):808-17.
50. Cavaiola TS, Pettus JH. (2017). Management of Type 2 Diabetes: Selecting Amongst Available Pharmacological Agents. In: De Groot LJ, Chrousos G, Dungan K, et al (Eds). Endotext [Internet]. South Dartmouth (MA): MDText.com, Inc.; 2000. [online] Available from: http://www.ncbi.nlm.nih.gov/books/NBK425702/. [Accessed September, 2018].
51. Iglesias P, Heras M, Díez JJ. Diabetes mellitus and kidney disease in the elderly. Nefrologia. 2014;34(3):285-92.
52. Ministry of Health and Family Welfare (2018). Health ministry bans 328 fixed dose combination drugs with immediate effect. [online] Available from: https://scroll.in/latest/894223/health-ministry-bans-328-fixed-dose-combination-drugs-with-immediate-effect. [Accessed September, 2018].
53. Ministry of Health and Family Welfare (2018). The Gazette of India. [online] Available from: http://www.cdsco.nic.in/writereaddata/2018_09_07_S_0_%204379(E)%20to.pdf. [Accessed September, 2018].
54. Balasubramanian J, Radhika N, Badarinath AV. The Crave of Fixed Dose Combination in Indian Market. Asian J Pharm Clin Res. 2004;7(4):106-10.
55. McGettigan P, Roderick P, Mahajan R, et al. Use of Fixed Dose Combination (FDC) Drugs in India: Central Regulatory Approval and Sales of FDCs Containing Non-Steroidal Anti-Inflammatory Drugs (NSAIDs), Metformin, or Psychotropic Drugs. PLoS Med. 2015;12(5):e1001826.
56. Joshi SR. Diabetes Care in India. Ann Glob Health. 2015;81(6):830-8.

Chapter 22

Emerging Injectable Therapies in Type 2 Diabetes Mellitus

DC Sharma

INTRODUCTION

As diabetes is a progressive disease, intensification of treatment is often needed to achieve and maintain glycemic control.[1] Many new injectable therapies including insulin analogs have been developed to improve the glycemic control and avoid adverse effects. This chapter aims to review the new and emerging short-acting insulins, longer-acting insulins/basal insulins, glucagon-like peptide (GLP)-1 receptor agonists and the available combinations of insulin plus GLP-1 analogs.

ULTRA-RAPID INSULINS

New ultra-short acting analog [e.g. fast-acting insulin aspart (FiAsp), a new formula of insulin aspart],[2] have a faster onset of action which enables more rapid correction of hyperglycemia and prevents and/or reduces postprandial glycemic excursions. FiAsp is produced by adding the excipient niacinamide (vitamin B3, to increase the speed of initial absorption) and L-arginine (as a stabilizing agent).[3] In a pooled analysis of six trials evaluating the pharmacokinetic and pharmacodynamic characteristics of FiAsp in adults with type 1 diabetes, FiAsp consistently demonstrated earlier onset of appearance, and greater early insulin exposure and glucose-lowering post-prandially than traditional insulin aspart across all trials.[3] In phase III trials, FiAsp was shown to improve postprandial glucose control compared with insulin aspart after a mixed meal tolerance testing in individuals with type 1 or type 2 diabetes.[2] The improved effect of FiAsp is also attributed to an earlier suppression of endogenous glucose.[4] Compatibility, efficacy, and safety of FIASP in continuous subcutaneous insulin infusion (CSII) was found to be comparable to insulin aspart, in addition to improved postprandial glucose (PPG) control.[2] Other ultra-rapid formulations of insulin lispro (Eli Lilly, Adocia) are under development and are likely to soon enter phase III trials in the near future.[2]

NEW AND EMERGING BASAL INSULINS

Table 1 compares some of the properties of these newest basal insulin preparations and compares them with those of the older basal insulin analogs (detemir U100 and glargine U100) and neutral protamine Hagedorn (NPH).

TABLE 1: **Select PK/PD parameters of recently approved insulin component agents and their existing comparator counterparts (long-acting).**

PK/PD Parameter	Degludec U100 and U200	Glargine U300	Glargine U100	Determir U100	NPH U100
Onset of action	30–90 min	Develops over 6 h	2–4 h	0.8–2 h	24 h
Duration of action	42 h	>30 h	Up to 24 h	Up to 24 h	10–16 h
Half-life	25 h	18–19 h	~12 h	5–7 h	6.6 h
Time to steady state	3–4 days	3–4 days	2–3 days	24 h	Not available

(PK: pharmacokinetic; PD: pharmacodynamic.)

A newer concentrated insulin glargine U300, once injected forms a compact subcutaneous depot with a smaller surface area to produce a more gradual and prolonged release of insulin than glargine U100. Glargine U300 maintained blood glucose control (≤105 mg/dL) for approximately 5 hours longer (median of 30 hours) when compared with glargine U100[5] and showed lower fluctuation and higher reproducibility in insulin exposure.

While the glucose-lowering effect of glargine U300 is comparable to that of glargine U100, lesser incidence of day-time and nocturnal confirmed (≤70 mg/dL) or severe hypoglycemia (that required assistance) is a distinct advantage of glargine U300 and has been found to be true in a broad range of patients.[6] In addition, weight gain (<1 kg) was low with glargine U300 in the patient-level meta-analysis of the EDITION 1, 2, and 3 studies and was statistically significantly lower than observed with glargine U100 ($p < 0.05$).[6]

American Association of Clinical Endocrinologists (AACE) recommendations[1] suggest starting with a basal insulin analog, if possible, when there is need for basal insulin. Insulin-naïve patients tend to do well when started on 10 units or 0.1–0.2 U/kg and then titrated upward until target fasting plasma glucose (FPG) levels are attained. Frequent monitoring of blood glucose levels is suggested during the early weeks of treatment.

Insulin degludec is an another new ultra-long acting basal insulin analog. Two dose formulations are available in the USA: U200 (pen device, with maximum dose of 160 units per injection [in 2 unit increments]) and U100 (pen device, with maximum dose of 80 units per injection [in 1 unit increments]). However, in India only U100 is available. It is also now available as a new premixed product with insulin aspart and in combination product with a glucagon-like peptide-1 receptors agonists (GLP-1 RA) (liraglutide). Insulin degludec forms soluble and stable dihexamers with the help of phenol and zinc, thus providing prolonged duration of action. Individual hexamers slowly disassemble from long hexamer chains releasing monomers, which are then absorbed from the depot into circulation. Degludec thus achieves steady-state concentrations with a half-life of more than 25 hours and duration of action of up to 42 hours. It was shown in patients with type 1 diabetes mellitus that insulin degludec had one-fourth the pharmacodynamic variability of insulin glargine U100.

A pre-planned meta-analysis of all of the phase 3 type 2 diabetes mellitus (T2DM) trials confirmed that lowering of A1c levels are similar with insulin degludec as are achievable with insulin glargine U100.[7] Rates of significant and confirmed nocturnal hypoglycemia among insulin-naïve T2DM subjects were significantly lower with insulin degludec in comparison to insulin glargine U100 (estimated rate ratio [RR]: 0.8 and RR: 0.64). Similar findings were also reported in the overall T2DM population.

The new premixed insulin degludec with insulin aspart offers stable daytime basal coverage, a lower rate of hypoglycemia, and some flexibility in injection timing compared with other premixed insulins.[8] The onset of action for the insulin aspart component is 14 minutes; the peak plasma time for aspart is 72 minutes, and that of insulin degludec is 9 hours. Steady state for insulin degludec occurs in 3–4 days. The half-life of insulin degludec is approximately 25 hours.

GLUCAGON- LIKE PEPTIDE-1 RECEPTOR AGONISTS

There is widespread reluctance to intensify insulin treatment, understandably due to fear of weight gain and hypoglycemia; these are both reduced with use of the GLP-1 RA.[9] GLP-1 is a naturally occurring hormone responsible for the incretin effect. The incretin effect is a response to release more insulin with oral meals or oral glucose as compared to intravenous glucose given the same rise in blood glucose. Studies suggest that patients with type 2 diabetes have an attenuated incretin effect, possibly because of reduced levels of active GLP-1. Evidence shows that GLP-1 regulates the expression of β-cell genes by inhibiting β-cell apoptosis, prevents β-cell gluco-lipotoxicity, improves β-cell function, and suppresses glucagon release and hepatic glucose output. GLP-1 also decreases the rate of gastric emptying and acid secretion, thereby reducing appetite and contributing to weight loss. GLP-1 is however rapidly degraded by dipeptidyl peptidase (DPP)-4, hence it has a very short half-life.[1] This has led to the development of analogs of GLP-1 RA.

Currently, 5 GLP-1 RA are FDA-approved for the treatment of patients with type 2 diabetes.[9] Their formulations vary from the twice-daily injection of exenatide to once-weekly formulations of Exenatide ER, Dulaglutide and Semaglutide. Several head-to-head comparison studies have compared the GLP RA. In DURATION-6, once-daily treatment with liraglutide 1.8 mg resulted in significantly greater reduction of A1c (difference, 0.21%) and greater weight loss (difference, 0.90 kg) in comparison with once-weekly exenatide 2 mg, although gastrointestinal (GI) adverse events occurred more often with patients taking liraglutide.[10] Similarly, in LEAD-6, liraglutide 1.8 mg had a significantly greater A1c reduction (difference, –0.33%) and less adverse effects, including hypoglycemia, than exenatide 10 mcg twice daily.[11] HARMONY-7 compared once-weekly albiglutide 50 mg with liraglutide 1.8 mg and showed greater A1c reduction with liraglutide (difference, 0.21%; non-inferior).[12] There were more injection-site reactions with albiglutide (difference, 7.5%), but more GI events with liraglutide (difference, 13.1%). AWARD-6 compared once-weekly dulaglutide 1.5 mg with liraglutide 1.8 mg, showing greater A1c reduction with dulaglutide (difference, –0.06%; non-inferior), although liraglutide had significantly greater weight loss (difference, 0.71 kg). No significant differences in the adverse-effect profile were noted in the study.[13]

GetGoal-X compared lixisenatide 20 mcg with exenatide 10 mcg twice daily and showed similar A1c reduction, although there was less hypoglycemia and nausea with lixisenatide. Lixisenatide is currently marketed mainly as a 5 mcg dose in combination with insulin glargine (Soliqua).[9]

Glucagon-like peptide-1 RA are indicated if patients are overweight or obese, have cardiovascular disease or renal disease, or are at high risk for hypoglycemia. Clinical trials demonstrate the superiority of GLP-1 RA to other antidiabetic drugs in A1c reduction, blood pressure reduction, and facilitating weight loss, without hypoglycemia risk. Unlike metformin, there is no contraindication to giving patients with renal disease a GLP-1 RA. As efficacy of the individual agents is generally comparable, choosing among the available GLP-1 RA will likely depend on patient preferences, reaction to adverse effects, and cost. Their use may be limited by GI adverse effects (AEs).[9]

Combination of Basal Insulin with GLP-1 Receptor Agonists

The combination of basal insulin and a GLP-1 RA offers several potential benefits to patients with type 2 diabetes in addition to providing complementary effects on glycemic control. While basal insulin targets fasting glucose, GLP-1 receptor agonists provide improvements in both PPG and FPG levels (Table 2). GLP-1 RA usually cause weight loss and have a low risk of hypoglycemia. Combining the two classes may allow patients to achieve glycemic control with lower doses, which could potentially result in fewer AEs than when the individual drugs are used independently. This combination also offers a potentially safer and easier approach to achieving glycemic control compared to adding prandial insulin.

The pharmacokinetics, pharmacodynamics, dosing, and clinical effects of GLP-1 RA differ among these agents. The shorter-acting agents (exenatide and lixisenatide) are associated with more significant delays in gastric emptying and more targeted reductions in PPG. Compared to short-acting GLP-1 RA, the longer-acting agents (dulaglutide, exenatide XR, and liraglutide) have less of an effect on gastric emptying and rely more on the insulin secretion mechanism, which leads to reductions in both FPG and PPG.[14,15] Of note, although liraglutide and lixisenatide both are dosed once daily, lixisenatide has a shorter half-life and primarily lowers PPG, whereas liraglutide has a longer half-life, thus lowering both PPG

TABLE 2: Complementary characteristics of basal insulin and glp1 receptor agonists.

	Basal insulin	GLP1 receptor agonists
Mechanism of action	• Augments basal insulin • Increases glucose disposal • Decreases hepatic glucose production	• Increases glucose-dependent insulin secretion from the pancreas • Decreases glucose-dependent secretion of glucagon • Slows gastric emptying • Increased satiety
Glucose profile effects	• Primarily lowers FPG	• Short-acting agents primarily lower PPG excursions • Longer-acting agents lower PPG and FPG
Effect on weight	• Increases weight	• Decreases weight
Main adverse effect	• Hypoglycemia	• GI issues (nausea, vomiting, diarrhea) • Low risk of hypoglycemia
Administration requirements	• Subcutaneous injection once or twice daily	• Subcutaneous injection once or twice daily or once weekly

(GLP: glucagon-like peptide; FPG: fasting plasma glucose; GI: gastrointestinal; PPG: postprandial glucose.)

and FPG.[16] These distinctions should be considered when selecting a specific GLP-1 RA to use in combination with basal insulin.

CONCLUSION

Exogenous preparations of insulin have been in constant evolution since its initial development in the 1920s. Since then, several new insulins have been developed to address the basal and prandial needs; and other injectable therapies like GLP1 analogues having additional benefits have also been developed to address some of the unmet needs in diabetic patients. These injectable formulations are emerging as promising therapies. The new basal insulin agents address some of the limitations of existing basal insulins, such as hypoglycemia (particularly nocturnal hypoglycemia), and to increase duration of action without peak activity, facilitating once-daily dosing. More concentrated formulations of existing insulins have been produced for patients who are very insulin resistant and require high doses/high volumes of insulin. A new premixed insulin having less variability and associated with reduced incidence of hypoglycemia is also available. GLP1 RAs alone or as titrable fixed ratio combinations with basal insulin may represent a promising option for prandial control or treatment intensification in patients with type 2 diabetic inadequately controlled on oral agents.

REFERENCES

1. Garber AL, Abrahamson MJ, Barziley JI, et al. Consensus statement by the American Association of Clinical Endocrinologists and American College of Endocrinology on the comprehensive type 2 diabetes management algorithm—2018 executive summary. EndocrPract. 2018;24(1):91-120.
2. Bailey TS, Walsh J, Stone JY. Stone. Emerging technologies for diabetes care. Diabetes Technol Ther. 2018;20(S2):S278-84.
3. Heise T, Pieber TR, Danne T, et al. A pooled analysis of clinical pharmacology trials investigating the pharmaco-kinetic and pharmacodynamic characteristics of fast-acting insulin aspart in adults with type 1 diabetes. Clin Pharmacokinet. 2017;56:551-559.
4. Basu A, Pieber TR, Hansen AK, et al. Greater early postprandial suppression of endogenous glucose production and higher initial glucose disappearance is achieved with fast-acting insulin aspart compared with insulin aspart. Diabetes Obes Metab. 2018;20(7):1615-22.
5. Becker RH, Dahmen R, Bergmann K, Lehmann A, Jax T, Heise T. New insulin glargine 300 Units·mL-1 provides a more even activity profile and prolonged glycemic control at steady state compared with insulin glargine 100 Units · mL-1. Diabetes Care. 2015;38(4):637-43.
6. Ritzel R, Roussel R, Bolli GB, et al. Patient-level meta-analysis of the EDITION 1, 2 and 3 studies: glycaemic control and hypoglycaemia with new insulin glargine 300 U/ml versus glargine 100 U/ml in people with type 2 diabetes. Diabetes Obes Metab. 2015;17(9):859-67.
7. Ratner RE, Gough SC, Mathieu C, et al. Hypoglycaemia risk with insulin degludec compared with insulin glargine in type 2 and type 1 diabetes: a pre-planned meta-analysis of phase 3 trials. Diabetes Obes Metab. 2013;15(2):175-84.
8. Kumar S, Jang HC, Demirağ NG, Skjøth TV, Endahl L, Bode B. Efficacy and safety of once-daily insulin degludec/insulin aspart compared with once-daily insulin glargine in participants with Type 2 diabetes: a randomized, treat-to-target study. Diabet Med. 2017;34(2):180-88.
9. Tran KL, Park YI, Pandya S, et al. Overview of Glucagon-like Peptide-1 Receptor Agonists for the Treatment of patients with Type 2 Diabetes. Am Health Drug Benefits. 2017;10(4):178-88.
10. Buse JB, Nauck M, Forst T, et al. Exenatide once weekly versus liraglutide once daily in patients with type 2 diabetes (DURATION-6): a randomised, open-label study. Lancet. 2013;381:17-24.
11. Buse JB, Rosenstock J, Sesti G, et al. Liraglutide once a day versus exenatide twice a day for type 2 diabetes: a 26-week randomised, parallel-group, multinational, open-label trial (LEAD-6). Lancet. 2009;374:39-47.
12. Pratley RE, Nauck MA, Barnett AH, et al; for the HARMONY 7 Study Group. Once-weekly albiglutide versus once-daily liraglutide in patients with type 2 diabetes inadequately controlled on oral drugs (HARMONY 7): a randomised, open-label, multicentre, non-inferiority phase 3 study. Lancet Diabetes Endocrinol. 2014;2:289-97.
13. Dungan KM, Povedano ST, Forst T, et al. Once-weekly dulaglutide versus once-daily liraglutide in metformin-treated patients with type 2 diabetes (AWARD-6): a randomised, open-label, phase 3, non-inferiority trial. Lancet. 2014;384:1349-57.
14. Meier JJ. GLP-1 receptor agonists for individualized treatment of type 2 diabetes mellitus. Nat Rev Endocrinol. 2012;8:728-42.
15. Meier JJ, Rosenstock J, Hincelin-Mery A, et al. Contrasting effects of lixisenatide and liraglutide on postprandial glycemic control, gastric emptying, and safety parameters in patients with type 2 diabetes on optimized insulin glargine with or without metformin: a randomized, open-label trial. Diabetes Care. 2015;38:1263-73.
16. Kapitza C, Forst T, Coester HV, et al. Pharmacodynamic characteristics of lixisenatide once daily versus liraglutide once daily in patients with type 2 diabetes insufficiently controlled on metformin. Diabetes Obes Metab. 2013;15:642-49.

Chapter 23

Metformin Revisited

Hemraj B Chandalia

INTRODUCTION

Metformin is an old oral glucose lowering agent. It is used in 70 countries, including India since 1950s. It was approved for use in the year 1994 in USA, which led to a resurgence of interest in this molecule. The extended release form was introduced in the year 2000. More recently, we have gained further insights into the mechanism of action of this drug, its pharmacokinetics, pharmacodynamics and mechanism of genesis of side effects. We have also discovered additional effects of this drug leading to its use in polycystic ovarian syndrome (PCOS) and diabetes with pregnancy. Very interestingly, the drug has shown some cancer protective effect.

PHARMACOLOGY OF METFORMIN AND GENESIS OF ITS SIDE EFFECTS

Metformin is predominantly absorbed from the small intestine although a "delayed form" of metformin is shown to be absorbed from the ileum. The drug uptake by the intestinal wall is a saturable, dose-dependent mechanism. Genetic polymorphism in transporters or a transporter-inhibiting drug can reduce absorption, thus attaining higher drug concentrations in the gastrointestinal (GI) lumen, which is responsible for the GI intolerance.[1] Genetic polymorphism of organic cation transporter-1 (OCT-1) has been described.[2] OCT-1 and OCT-3 are encoded by *SLC22A1* and *SCL22A3*, respectively. Polymorphism of these genes will affect the uptake of the drug by enterocytes or hepatocytes or its transport from lumen to serosal side.[3] Medications which cause inhibition of OCT-1 includes many commonly used drugs like tricyclic antidepressants, proton-pump inhibitors, verapamil, doxazosin, spironolactone, clopidogrel, and tramadol. Metformin is excreted in the bile by multidrug and toxin extrusion-1 (MATE-1), taken up by renal epithelial cells by transfer OCT-2 and excreted in the urine by transporter MATE-1 and MATE-2. Polymorphism of the genes encoding these transporters can affect the pharmacokinetics of the drug.

The mechanism of action of metformin has been expanded considerably. The primary action is increased glucose utilization by anaerobic glycolysis, inevitably leading to lactic acid production (Fig. 1). Metformin also suppresses hepatic glucose production and increases

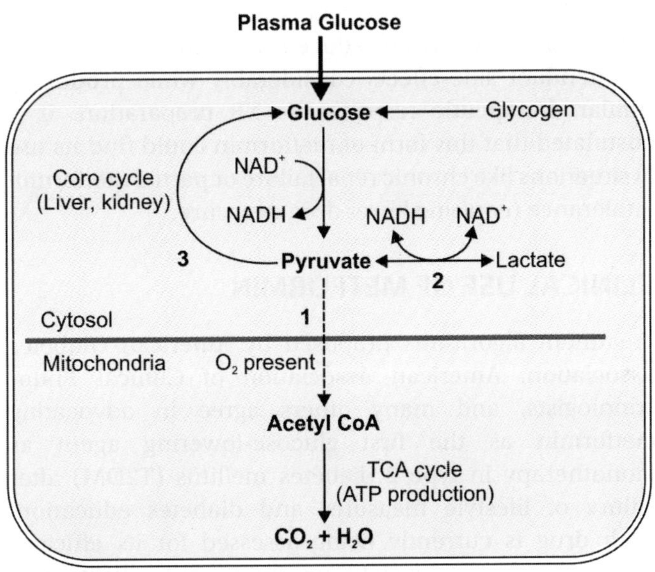

Figure 1 Biochemistry of Lactate production.

glucose utilization by muscle and fat. On a positron emission tomography-computed tomography (PET-CT), increased glucose utilization can be seen by diffusely increased fludeoxyglucose F 18 (^{18}F-FDG) uptake. Metformin reduces absorption of nutrients, including glucose and vitamin B12, shown by invitro studies done on everted intestinal loops. Metformin alters gut microbiota, so as to improve glucose tolerance. Metformin also increases active glucagon-like peptide 1 (GLP-1) levels[4] from the L-cells. However, it does not increase gastric inhibitory polypeptide (GIP) from K cells. It also increases expression of GLP-1 and GIP receptors in the beta cells of the pancreas. The mechanism involved in its insulin sensitizing effect is via a peroxisome proliferator-activated receptor α (PPAR-α)-dependent mechanism and not by increasing dipeptidyl peptidase-4 (DPP4) activity. Thus, the sensitizing effect of metformin is different from that of DPP4 inhibitors, which makes a metformin-DPP-4 inhibitor combination rational.[5]

IMMEDIATE RELEASE VERSUS EXTENDED RELEASE METFORMIN

Both immediate release (IR) and extended release (XR) metformin are in extensive use. The area under the curve of plasma concentration achieved by the same dose of both preparations is similar. The efficacy has been reported to be similar[6] or better with XR.[7] The GI side-effects as described by most authors are lesser with slow release form.[8] A delayed form of metformin has also been described which predominantly releases into the ileum, thereby stimulating GLP-1 and Peptide YY (PYY).[9] This form of metformin reduced the drug exposure and its attendant side-effects considerably while producing similar therapeutic response as XR preparation. It is postulated that this form of metformin could find its use in situations like chronic renal failure or partial metformin intolerance requiring lower drug exposure.

CLINICAL USE OF METFORMIN

Treatment algorithms proposed by American Diabetes Association, American Association of Clinical Endocrinologists, and many others agree in advocating metformin as the first glucose-lowering agent as monotherapy in type 2 diabetes mellitus (T2DM) after failure of lifestyle measures and diabetes education. Each drug is currently being assessed for its efficacy, hypoglycemia risk, weight neutrality, side-effects and cost. Metformin emerges as the drug of choice on all these counts. There is a debate whether two-drug therapy should be introduced as initial regime in patients having a high hemoglobin A1c (HbA1c) (10% or more). There is presently a new approach being considered where an alternative drug is proposed as initial monotherapy, which is usually Sodium-glucose cotransporter 2 inhibitor (SGLT2 i). In spite of all these contrarian views, metformin continues to occupy a place of pride in the initial monotherapy of T2DM. Metformin intolerance is rare, but rough estimates put it at 10% of population. In almost half of these individuals, the intolerance in the form of GI side-effect is serious enough to necessitate drug discontinuation. The mechanism of metformin intolerance has been discussed above. As the incidence of genetic polymorphism of various transporters may be different in varied populations, metformin intolerance may have different incidence in different communities. There are no accurate figures of the incidence of intolerance yet available.

Metformin is proposed to be used in tier-2 treatment algorithms in combination with one of the six treatment options—sulfonylureas, thiazolidinediones, DPP4 inhibitors, SGLT2 inhibitors, GLP-1 receptor agonists and basal insulin. Even in the tier-3 treatment algorithms, where triple drug therapy is proposed, metformin is an important ingredient. Furthermore, even when insulin therapy is initiated either as basal insulin or basal-bolus regime, metformin continues to be used as an insulin sensitizer. Thus, in vast majority of metformin-tolerant T2DM without any contraindication to metformin therapy, this drug will be used for most part of patient's life. This establishes the preeminence of this molecule in T2DM.

Metformin and Cardiovascular Disease

In the United Kingdom Prospective Diabetes Study (UKPDS), metformin was the only drug that showed a 32% reduction in diabetes-related end-point, 42% reduction in diabetes-related death, and 36% reduction in all cause mortality. Since UKPDS, there have been multiple studies examining this issue. Metformin modifies plasma lipids favorably.[10] It also promotes mild-to-moderate weight loss or facilitates the weight loss maintenance when used as monotherapy or reduces the weight gain in combination with other weight-enhancing modes of treatment like sulfonylureas and insulin.[11] These effects on cardiovascular (CV) risk factors are likely to be translated into CV benefits. A 5-year retrospective analysis of a cohort comparing metformin with lifestyle measures showed a 30% reduction in cardiovascular disease (CVD) events and all-cause mortality in the metformin group.[12] Comparison of metformin versus glipizide was made in a group of 150 subjects prospectively for 3 years. The hazard ratio for metformin was 0.54 [confidence interval (CI) 0.3–0.9, p = 0.026]. A meta-analysis of 13 trials which include UKPDS as the main study showed reduction of myocardial infarction, peripheral vascular disease (PVD) and all cause mortality, but it did not attain significance.[13] In patients of T2DM suffering from ST-segment elevation myocardial infarction, a propensity matched analysis did not reveal any cardio-protection by metformin.[14]

Metformin and Gut Microbiota

Metformin increases the bile acid pool in the intestinal tract. This affects the stool consistency, blood cholesterol levels and gut microbiome.[1] The altered microbiome may improve glucose tolerance, as it increases *Firmicutes* bacteria and decreases *Bacteroides*. On the other hand, some changes in microbiota may increase metformin intolerance. In a 2-week crossover study, metformin 500 mg daily was administered with or without a microbiome modulator, consisting of three prebiotics: (i) inulin (ii) beta-glucan and (iii) blueberry-derived polyphenols. The microbiome modulator treated subjects showed better tolerance to metformin and a lower fasting blood glucose.[15]

Box 1: Metformin: Indications and contraindications.

Indications:

- Type 2 diabetes:
  - Monotherapy in those uncontrolled on lifestyle measures
  - Two drug combination therapy with DPP4-i, SGLT2-i, Sulphonylureas, Thiazolidinediones, GLP-RA or Basal insulin
  - Triple drug combination: MF plus any 2 of the 6 treatment modalities listed above
  - With basal or basal plus or basal-bolus insulin therapy.
- Diabetes with Pregnancy
  - Gestational diabetes, previous GDM or Pregestational obese Type 2 diabetic, if required in combination with insulin therapy
- Polycystic ovarian syndrome

Contraindications:

- Broad Clinical contraindications:
  - Type 1 DM
  - Metformin intolerance
  - Undernutrition
- Specific Contraindications:
  - Impaired renal function
    - Safe to use in eGFR > 45 ml/min/1.73m2
    - Between eGFR 30-45 ml/min/1.73m2, use cautiously and reduce MF dose by 50-75%
  - Impaired hepatic function
  - Congestive heart failure
  - Hypoxia of any origin, poor tissue perfusion,
  - Respiratory failure
  - Proposed contrast studies
  - Acutely ill patients with dehydration, hypotension
  - Peri-operative period

CONTRAINDICATIONS TO METFORMIN THERAPY (BOX 1)

Metformin is contraindicated in type 1 diabetes mellitus (T1DM), except in T1DM adults who are excessively obese. Once fully insulinised, they may receive metformin to restore insulin sensitivity and promote peripheral glucose utilization. However, it is usually a taboo to use metformin in T1DM.

Most important contraindications include major organ dysfunction, hypoxic states, emergencies associated with poor tissue perfusion or dehydration and hypotension. Additionally, it should be avoided in situations that demand flexibility of treatment due to variable food intake. This excludes its use in most hospitalized patients and in the perioperative period in contrast to the fact that it is the most commonly used drug in ambulatory T2DM. Metformin therapy can be reinstated in hospitalized patients, only after full stabilization of basic disease or at the time of discharge from the hospital.

Metformin was contraindicated in renal failure until about a decade ago when its safety was proven with estimated glomerular filtration rate (eGFR) >45 mL/min/1.73 m^2. It is now well-accepted for use in this situation, although there is controversy in its use in eGFR 30–45 mL/min/1.73 m^2, where if used, a reduction in the dose by 50–75% is suggested.[16,17] Such recommendations are based on a stable eGFR, but in clinical settings, GFR can change rapidly. A patient with eGFR of 60 mL/min/1.73 m^2 may suddenly drop to 20 mL/min/1.73 m^2 with a bout of gastroenteritis and dehydration. Hence, for clinicians who work with the principle of "Primum non-nocere", metformin is rarely used with any degree of renal compromise. This approach is also based upon the fact that there are several alternative options available for the treatment of T2DM, hence incurring any degree of risk in this situation is not justified.

Metformin is contraindicated in hepatic dysfunction; however, there are exceptions to this rule. For example, in early chronic liver disease like cirrhosis due to nonalcoholic steatohepatitis, it may be used cautiously. Metformin is also one among a veritable type of drugs used in steatohepatitis with limited degree of success. In chronic liver disease, the fasting blood glucose tends to be low due to impaired gluconeogenesis and hence use of metformin in the evening to suppress basal glucose production is fraught with danger. However, some patients show severe postprandial blood glucose surge, which is difficult to control even with large doses of premeal, rapid acting insulin analogs. The therapeutic options to sensitize such a patient to insulin are severely limited and hence a small dose of metformin, like 250 mg TDS may be permissible if Child's score is <9. As the liver disease advances, metformin must be withdrawn.

Congestive heart failure (CHF), which now accounts for almost one-third of hospital admissions in diabetics with CVD is often associated with hypoglycemia and hyperlactatemia. Hence, metformin should be avoided in this setting. However, anecdotal case reports of diabetic patients suffering from CHF due to a cardiomyopathy of metabolic origin (poor glycemic control, lipid, and glycogen infiltration of myocardium) have appeared showing a successful outcome.

Proposed contrast studies in a diabetic with <60 mL/min/1.73 m^2 eGFR is an important contraindication to the use of metformin.[18] This is now an established practice to omit metformin 24 hours before the procedure and further for 72 hours after the injection of contrast medium, in order to ensure renal excretion of most of the contrast medium. This precaution is advisable even in diabetics with normal eGFR as case reports of such patients showing temporary advent of renal failure and emergence of lactic acidosis have been published.

It is important to reiterate that notwithstanding all above contraindications, metformin is rightfully used in vast majority of T2DM during major part of their diabetic lives.

METFORMIN AND LACTIC ACIDOSIS

Metformin promotes anaerobic glycolysis, thus leading to high lactate levels.[19] This has the potential to produce lactic acidosis (LA). The first biguanide to be used extensively in the US and many other countries was phenformin. The incidence of lactic acidosis described with its use was 0.23–0.60 per 1,000 person-years in various European countries.[20] The mortality reported was 67%. Phenformin is hydroxylated in the liver and excreted in the urine. Genetic polymorphism resulting in variable hydroxylation activity has been described. On the other hand, metformin is excreted by the kidney and feces unchanged. This accounts for the advent of LA in some of the patients treated with phenformin. Phenformin also binds more avidly to mitochondrial membrane while metformin does so poorly. LA with metformin has been described to be rare, 0.03–0.06 per 1,000 patient-years. A large number of patients (n = 50,048) taking metformin or sulfonylurea were compared.[21] It revealed no difference in the incidence of LA between metformin and sulfonylurea treated groups. A review of 347 trials and cohort studies compared LA in metformin users (70,490 patient-years) versus nonmetformin users (55,451 patient-years). LA was found to be similar in both groups.[21] As a part of pharmacovigilance in Italy, 650 cases of adverse drug reaction (ADR) to metformin were identified.[22] Of these, 59 patients had LA with a mortality of 25.4%. In 90% of patients, one risk factor for LA was identified. Predictors of death were low pH and absence of acute kidney injury, because those with acute kidney injury offered the possibility of reversal of kidney failure.

Prospective studies from India were reported to show a consistent elevation of blood lactic acid in phenformin-treated subjects, which settled down at a 6-month follow-up period, thus indicating a process of adaptation.[23,24] A well-documented case of LA in a 42-year old male without pre-existing renal disease was described.[25] In a group of patients with LA and severe septic shock, the mortality was lower in metformin users (56.8%) versus metformin nonusers (88.1%) (p <0.0001). Thus, presence of a reversible risk factor predicted better outcomes.

METFORMIN IN PREGNANCY WITH DIABETES

Our interest in this subject was kindled by the landmark studies of Rowan et al.[26] These authors treated 751 gestational diabetics diagnosed at 20–33 weeks of pregnancy, divided into two treatment arms—metformin with insulin versus insulin alone. The primary end-points were a composite of neonatal hypoglycemia, respiratory acidosis, need for phototherapy, birth trauma, prematurity and a 5-minute APGAR (appearance, pulse, grimace, activity, and respiration) score <7. The aim of the study was to rule out a 33% increase in the composite end-points with metformin use. Secondary end-points included anthropometric measurements of newborn, maternal glycemic control, postpartum glucose tolerance and acceptability of treatment. Of 363 patients randomized to metformin group, 42% received supplemental insulin in order to achieve good glycemic control. Primary composite end-points were similar in both groups [32% metformin group, 32.2% insulin group, relative risk (RR) 0.99, 95% CI 0.8–1.23], thus proving safety of metformin in pregnancy. There was no significant difference in secondary end-points except the acceptability of treatment (metformin 76.6%, insulin 27.2%, $p < 0.001$). Another study in GDM[27] showed significantly less maternal weight gain in the metformin group. A study on the first trimester in utero exposure to metformin,[28] did not reveal any increase in teratogenicity in the metformin group.

The evidence of metformin use in women with pregestational T2DM, impaired glucose tolerance, and previous GDM[29] with pregnancy continue to suffer from poor quality and bias. A meta-analysis of six studies on the metformin use in the prevention of GDM showed a reduction of GDM incidence without any effect on abortion, preterm delivery, neonatal death, gestational age at birth, or birth weight. Metformin in PCOS pregnancy reduced early pregnancy loss and preterm labor.[30] There was no evidence of teratogenicity, intrauterine deaths, or developmental delays.

Metformin in Polycystic Ovarian Syndrome

Metformin improved menstrual cyclicity and decreased body mass index (BMI). It reduces serum-free testosterone and LH levels, which reached a steady state at 6 months of treatment.[31] Metformin increases adipokine levels and decreases leptin, and C-reactive protein (CRP) levels.

A meta-analysis of four randomized controlled trials (RCTs) was made to compare effects of oral contraceptive pill (OCP) versus metformin in PCOS women.[32] OCP improved menstrual cycle frequency while metformin reduced BMI, dysglycemia and low-density lipoprotein cholesterol (LDL-C). The impact on hirsutism was similar by both agents. The quality of evidence was considered low. Eight weeks of metformin therapy reduced anti-Müllerian hormone levels, which was more noticeable in women with higher BMI.[33] Metformin improves invitro-fertilization (IVF) outcomes. In 102 obese PCOS patients studied, metformin reduced the number of retrieved oocytes but there was no difference in rate of fertilization, miscarriages and implantation. Metformin reduced ovulation by 77.9% of PCOS women with BMI >30 kg/m^2 thus reducing multiple follicular maturation.[34] In obese PCOS, metformin reduced vitamin B12 levels by 20–30% without any change in folic acid levels.[35] This appears to be a clinically relevant side-effect of the drug. Based upon above effects of metformin, the drug is commonly used in PCOS as a nonhormonal therapy, with improvement in several parameters of PCOS.

METFORMIN AND CANCER

Metformin down-regulates androgen receptor through activation of adenosine monophosphate-activated protein kinase (AMPK). This leads to reduction of mammalian target of rapamycin (mTOR) activity and decreased cellular proliferation and cancer genesis.[36] Biguanides inhibit angiogenesis in breast cancer cells both in vitro and in animal models.[37] A meta-analysis of prostate cancer in diabetes mellitus showed better recurrence prognosis in metformin users.[38] Metformin inhibits bladder cancer cells and a combination of simvastatin plus metformin reduced cell viability and metastatic properties of castration-resistant prostate cancer cells.[39]

The data on prostate, breast and other cancers in metformin users are attractive but better evidence is yet to be adduced. Presently, a diabetic with such cancers, if using metformin will be proactively continued on metformin therapy unless an important contraindication to metformin exists.

In summary, stated simply, metformin is one of the oldest and least expensive drugs that continues to undergo newer studies on its mechanism of action, genesis of its side effects and its newer action on seemingly unrelated diseases. Its potential for the production of lactic acidosis is very low and primarily occurs when other risk factors for such development coexist. Besides reigning supreme in the management of T2DM at all stages of the disease, the drug is being used in PCOS and gestational diabetes. Its role as an adjunct to anticancer therapy needs to be further documented.

REFERENCES

1. McCreight LJ, Bailey CJ, Pearson ER. Metformin and the gastrointestinal tract. Diabetologia. 2016;59:426-35.
2. Dujic T, Zhou K, Donnelly LA, et al. Association of organic cation transporter 1 with intolerance to metformin in Type 2 diabetes: A GoDARTS Study. Diabetes. 2015;64:1786-93.
3. Florez JC. The pharmacogenetics of metformin. Diabetologia. 2017;60: 1648-55.

4. Cho YM, Kieffer TJ. New aspects of an old drug: metformin as a glucagon-like peptide-1 (GLP-1) enhancer and sensitiser. Diabetologia. 2011;54:219-22.
5. Mulherin AJ, Oh AH, Kim H, et al. Mechanisms underlying metformin-induced secretion of glucagon-like peptide-1 from the intestinal L cell. Endocrinol. 2011;152:4610-9.
6. Bhansali A, Masoodi SR. Efficacy of once- or twice-daily extended release metformin compared with thrice-daily immediate release metformin in type 2 diabetes mellitus. J Assoc Physic India. 2005;53:441-5.
7. Derosa G, D'Angelo A, Romano D, et al. Effects of metformine xtended release compared to immediate release formula on glycemic control and glycemic variability in patients with type 2 diabetes. Drug Design Dev Ther. 2017;11:1481-8.
8. Ghorpade W, Hiray RS, Daswani BR, et al. Comparison of conventional and sustained-release formulation of metformin in type 2 diabetics. Int J Basic Clin Pharmacol. 2016;5:274-80.
9. DeFronzo RA, Buse JB, Kim T, et al. Once-daily delayed-release metformin lowers plasma glucose and enhances fasting and postprandial GLP-1 and PYY: results from two randomised trials. Diabetologia. 2016;59:1645-54.
10. Zhang Y, McCoy RG, Mason JE, et al. Second-line Agents for Glycemic Control for Type 2 Diabetes: Are Newer Agents Better?. Diabetes Care. 2014;D_131901.
11. Chandalia HB, Lamba PS, Chandalia SH, et al. Weight gain in Type 2 Diabetics with different treatment modalities. Metab Synd Rel Disord. 2005;3:130-6.
12. Fung CSC, Wan EYF, Wong CKH, et al. Effect of metformin monotherapy on cardiovascular diseases and mortality: a retrospective cohort study on Chinese type 2 diabetes mellitus patients. Cardiovasc Diabetol. 2015;14:137.
13. Griffin SJ, Leaver JK, Irving GJ. Impact of metformin on cardiovascular disease: a meta-analysis of randomised trials among people with type 2 diabetes. Diabetologia. 2017;60:1620-9.
14. Basnet S, Kozikowski A, Makaryus AN, et al. Metformin and myocardial injury in patients with diabetes and st-segment elevation myocardial infarction: A propensity score matched analysis. J Am Heart Assoc. 2018;4:1-7.
15. Burton JH, Johnson M, Johnson J, et al. Addition of a gastrointestinal microbiome modulator to metformin improves metformin tolerance and fasting glucose levels. J Diab Sci Technol. 2015;9:808-814.
16. Ekström N, Schiöler L, Svensson AM, et al. Effectiveness and safety of metformin in 51 675 patients with type 2 diabetes and different levels of renal function: a cohort study from the Swedish National Diabetes Register. BMJ Open. 2012;2(4):e001076.
17. Nathan DM, Buse JB, Davidson MB, et al. American Diabetes Association; European Association for Study of Diabetes. Medical management of hyperglycemia in type 2 diabetes: a consensus algorithm for the initiation and adjustment of therapy: a consensus statement of the American Diabetes Association and the European Association for the Study of Diabetes. Diabetes Care. 2009;32:193-203.
18. McCartney MM, Gilbert FJ, Murchison LE, et al. Metformin and contrast media--a dangerous combination?. Clin Radiol. 1999;54(1):29.
19. DeFronzo R, Fleming GA, Chen K, et al. Metformin-associated lactic acidosis: Current perspectives on causes and risk. Metab Clin Exp. 2015;65:20-9.
20. Berger W. Incidence of severe side effects during therapy with sulfonylureas and biguanides. Hormone and metabolic Research. Suppl Series. 1985;15:111-5.
21. Salpeter SR, Greyber E, Pasternak GA, et al. Risk of fatal and nonfatal lactic acidosis with metformin use in type 2 diabetes mellitus (Review). Coch Datab Syst Rev. 2010;4:CD002967.
22. Renda F, Mura P, Finco G, et al. Metformin-associated lactic acidosis requiring hospitalization. A national 10 year survey and a systematic literature review. Eur Rev Med Pharmacol Sci. 2013;17(Suppl 1):45-9.
23. Chandalia HB, Rangnath M. Biguanide-induced lactic acidosis. J Assoc Physic India.1990;38:620-2.
24. Chandalia HB, Sadikot S. Blood Lactic Acid Levels in Diabetics Treated with Phenformin - Evidence for a Process of Adaptation. In: JS Bajaj (Ed). Diabetes Mellitus in Developing Countries. Delhi: Interprint; 1984. pp. 337-9.
25. Chandalia HB. Metformin-induced acidosis. Bulletin of Jaslok Hospital. 1980;5:45.
26. Rowan JA, Hague WM, Gao W, et al. Metformin versus Insulin for the treatment of gestational diabetes. New Engl J Med. 2008;358:2003-2015.
27. Ainuddin JA, Karim N, Zaheer S, et al. Metformin treatment in type 2 diabetes in pregnancy: An active controlled, parallel-group, randomized, open label study in patients with type 2 diabetes in pregnancy. J Diabetes Res. 2015;2015:325851.
28. Diav-Citrin O, Steinmetz-Shoob S, Shechtman D, et al. In-utero exposure to metformin for type 2 diabetes or polycystic ovary syndrome: A prospective comparative observational study. Reproduct Toxicol. 2018;80:85-91.
29. Tieu J, McPhee AJ, Crowther CA, et al. Screening for gestational diabetes mellitus based on different risk profiles and settings for improving maternal and infant health. Coch Datab Syst Rev. 2017;21(6):854-8.
30. Lautatzis ME, Goulid DG, Vrontakis M. Efficacy and safety of metformin during pregnancy in women with gestational diabetes mellitus or polycystic ovary syndrome: a systematic review. Metabolism. 2013;62:1522-34.
31. Yang PK, Hsu CY, Chen MJ, et al. The Efficacy of 24-month metformin for improving menses, hormones, and metabolic profiles in polycystic ovary syndrome. J Clin Endocrinol Metab. 2018;103:890-9.
32. Al Khalifah RA, Florez ID, Dennis B, et al. Metformin or Oral contraceptives for adolescents with polycystic ovarian syndrome: A meta-analysis. pediatrics 2016;137(5):e20154089.
33. Fatemeh F, Mansooreh S, Kosar HA, et al. Effect of metformin on the anti-Müllerian hormone level in infertile women with polycystic ovarian syndrome. Electron Physic. 2017;9:5969-73.
34. Al-Ruthia YS, Al-Mandeel H, AlSanawi H, et al. Ovulation induction by metformin among obese versus non-obese women with polycystic ovary syndrome. Saudi Pharmaceut J. 2017;25:795-800.
35. Esmaeilzadeh S, Gholinezhad-Chari M, Ghadimi R. The effect of metformin treatment on the serum levels of homocysteine, folic acid, and vitamin B12 in patients with polycystic ovary syndrome. J Human Reprod Sci. 2017;10:95-101.
36. Demir U, Koehler A, Schneider R, et al. Metformin anti-tumor effect via disruption of the MID1 translational regulator complex and AR downregulation in prostate cancer cells. BMC Cancer. 2014;52.
37. Orecchioni S, Reggiani F, Talarico G, et al. The biguanides metformin and phenformin inhibit angiogenesis, local and metastatic growth of breast cancer by targeting both neoplastic and microenvironment cells. Int J Cancer. 2015;136:534-44.
38. Hwang IC, Park SM, Shin D, et al. Metformin association with lower prostate cancer recurrence in type 2 diabetes: a systematic review and meta-analysis. Asian Pacific J Cancer Prev. 2016;16:595-600.
39. Babcook MA, Shukla S, Fu P, et al. Synergistic simvastatin and metformin combination chemotherapy for osseous metastatic castration-resistant prostate cancer. Molecul Cancer Ther. 2014;13:2288-302.

Chapter 24

What Next After Metformin—A Million Dollar Question

CL Nawal, Amandeep Singh

INTRODUCTION

As the management of diabetes mellitus is advancing daily, the important thing is to achieve normal glucose levels in diabetic patients using various glucose-lowering agents available in our armamentarium. Initially, all patients are managed with changing life style but later on large number of people requires hypoglycemic drugs. Now the pathophysiology behind type 2 diabetes mellitus (T2DM) has been well-revealed, our approach toward keeping it under the control has been changed from being glucocentric to patient centric. Plenty of drugs to treat T2D are available with similar efficacy but with variable adverse effects.

Various guidelines available suggests that metformin is the first-line as glucose-lowering therapy; there is no definite status for the second-line agents as many of the drug classes are recommended.[1] Here we will discuss the best possible drugs which can be used as second-line agents after metformin failure based on the recent studies published (Table 1).[2]

TABLE 1: Evolution of therapy in type 2 diabetes mellitus management.[2]

1920–1930	Animal insulin preparations, isolation of insulin
1930–1940	NPH insulin
1940–1950	Sulfonylureas, metformin
1950–1960	Lente insulin series
1960–1970	First insulin analogs
1970–1980	United Kingdom Prospective Diabetes Study
1980–1990	Acarbose
1990–2000	Glinides, basal insulin analogs
2000–2010	Thiazolidinediones, GLP-1 receptor agonists, SGLT2 inhibitors
2010–2018	DPP4 inhibitors, long-acting GLP-1 receptor agonists, basal insulin with ultra-long duration of action

(DPP4: dipeptidyl peptidase-4; GLP-1: glucagon-like peptide-1; NPH: neutral protamine Hagedorn; SGLT2: sodium glucose cotransporter 2.)

Source: Khunti K, Chatterjee S, Gerstein HC, et al. Do sulphonylureas still have a place in clinical practice? Lancet Diabetes Endocrinol. 2018;6(10):821-32.

ALTERNATIVES WHEN METFORMIN FAILS

Flowchart 1 describes alternatives when metformin fails.

Sulfonylureas

These are the most commonly used second-line agents along with metformin or after failure of metformin (Table 2).[3] Sulfonylureas (SUs) have best efficacy and the cost is low but with common side effects of hypoglycemia and increase in weight.

The SUs act by rising the plasma insulin concentrations; thus, they are effective only when β-cells of pancreas are functioning. They block the flow of K^+ within the β-cell leading to depolarization of the cell membrane which increases the flow of calcium into β-cells causing excretion of large amount of insulin.[4,5] Fixed dose combination of SUs and metformin improves the patient's adherence to drugs and offers inexpensive option too.[1] As hypoglycemia is a common side effect of it, new generation SUs cause less hypoglycemia and its cost

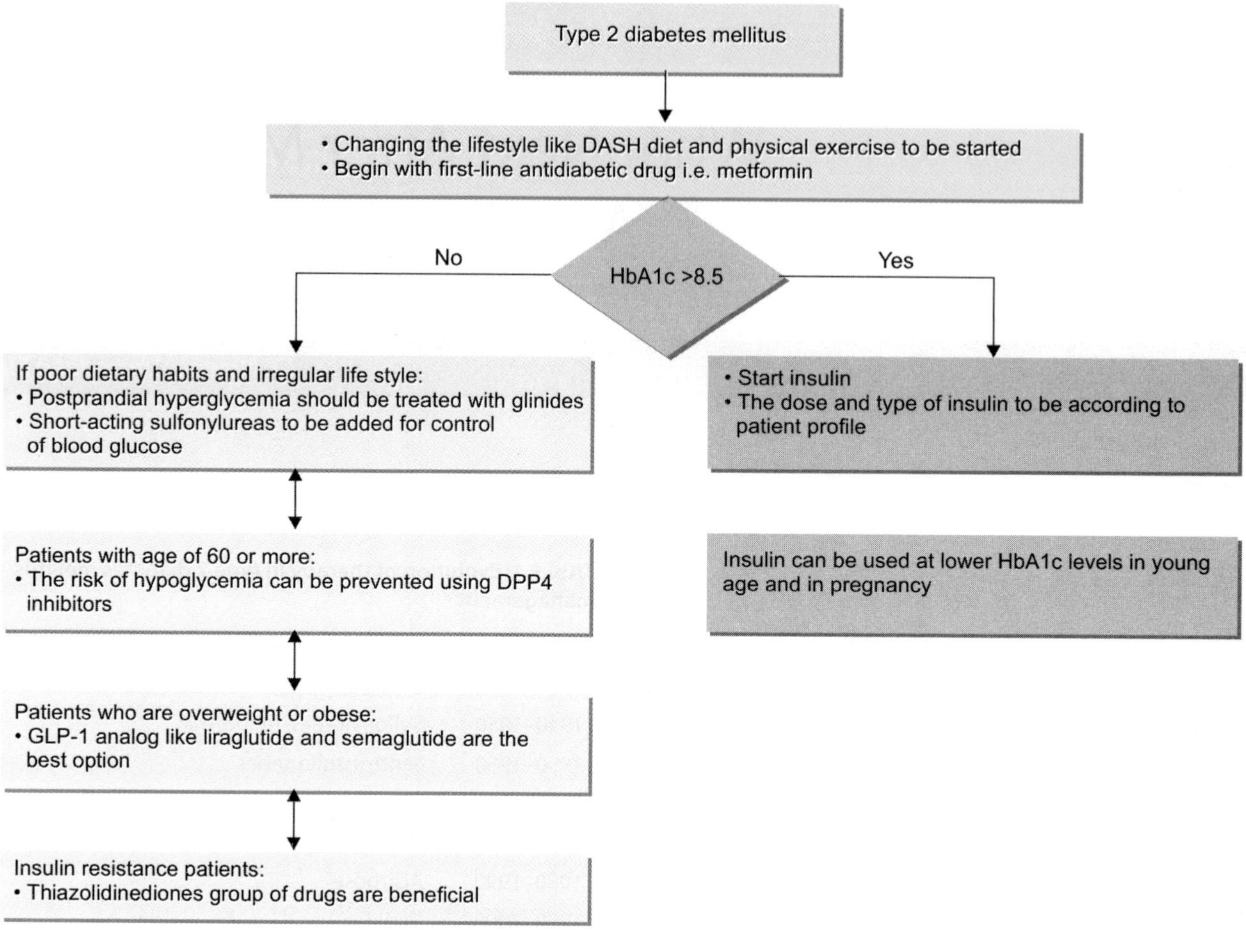

(DASH: dietary approaches to stop hypertension; DPP4: dipeptidyl peptidase-4; GLP-1: glucagon-like peptide-1; HbA1c: glycated hemoglobin.)

Flowchart 1 Treatment decision pathway, when metformin fails.
Source: Bollaerts K, Mathieu C. Managing type 2 diabetes in patients not controlled on metformin. 2007;2:55-9.

TABLE 2: **Classification of sulfonylureas.**[3]

Short acting	Tolbutamide
Intermediate acting	Glipizide, gliclazide, gliquidone
Long acting	Chlorpropamide, glibenclamide, glimepiride

effectiveness makes them easy affordability availability.[2] Recent cohort study has observed that the SUs, if used as a second-line therapy, increase the incidence of myocardial infarction when it is compared to metformin alone. It is also seen that it is safer to continue metformin and use SUs as add-on therapy rather than switching it.[6]

Dipeptidyl Peptidase-4 Inhibitors

Dipeptidyl peptidase-4 (DPP4, also called as CD26) is a glycoprotein which has gained attention recently due to its role in catalytic degradation of incretins.[7] Glucagon-like peptide-1 (GLP-1) and gastric inhibitory polypeptide (GIP), which are incretin peptides, modulate the blood glucose level after meals by increasing glucose secretion from β-cells of the pancreas and by its inhibitory effect on glucagon level. DPP4 rapidly causes inactivation of GLP-1 leading to their short time of action. Inhibition of DPP4 enzyme improves glucose tolerance.[8] Many DPP4 inhibitors available in the market are sitagliptin, alogliptin, linagliptin, saxagliptin, vildagliptin, omarigliptin, gemigliptin, trelagliptin, anagliptin and teneligliptin. Dutogliptin, gosogliptin, and evogliptin are in phase 3 trials.

Recent studies have suggested that, from cardiovascular (CV) perspective, DPP4 inhibitors are safe, whereas no improvement has been observed in various CV endpoints on T2DM patients with these hypoglycemic agents.[7] The risk of heart failure is negligible with these agents.[9] A recent study has shown that the baseline metformin status affects the CV outcome with DPP4 inhibitors use.[10,11] A recent study has proven that DPP4 inhibitors improve the functional outcome and decrease the disability after stroke. Linagliptin acts as a neuroprotective agent via the stromal cell-derived factor-*1* alpha/CXC receptor 4 (SDF-1α/CXCR4) pathway that regulates homeostasis of calcium ions and reduction of the calpain activity. The activity of calpain and the calcium ions present intracellularly regulates neurogranin and myelin basic protein detection.[12]

Merits of Dipeptidyl Peptidase-4 Inhibitors

- Glycated hemoglobin (HbA1c) reduction is at par with SUs
- Hypoglycemia is minimal with no change or slight reduction in the weight
- It has great pleiotropic effects and also prevents further destruction of β-cell.

Demerits of Dipeptidyl Peptidase-4 Inhibitors

- The cost of the drugs is high
- There are various possible off target effects with this class of drugs.[13]

Sodium-Glucose Cotransporter 2 Inhibitors

Sodium-glucose cotransporter 2 (SGLT2) inhibitors are new group of drugs that functions by promoting glucose excretion via urine. It blocks the reabsorption of glucose in the proximal tubules of kidneys. The overall effect of its mechanism is double as it is an insulin-independent glycemic control and also a mode of calorie loss.[11] Many new SGLT2 inhibitors are available, e.g. empagliflozin canagliflozin, dapagliflozin, ertugliflozin, luseogliflozin, ipragliflozin and tofogliflozin. The efficacy of the SGLT2 inhibitors have been well proven for treating T2DM.[14] There is well documentation of the safety and efficacy of SGLT2 inhibitors (including canagliflozin, dapagliflozin, and empagliflozin) for treating T2DM. As they have a great beneficial effect on the cardiac health, these are a useful drug as add-on therapy for diabetes treatment.[15] Two latest study Empagliflozin Cardiovascular Outcome Event Trial in Type 2 Diabetes Mellitus Patients (EMPA-REG OUTCOME) and Canagliflozin Cardiovascular Assessment Study (CANVAS) trials done with empagliflozin have proven that it significantly reduces CV events in diabetes patients and also in those who are suffering from CV illness.[16,17]

Glucagon-like Peptide-1 Analogs

Normally, intake of glucose increases the glucose secretion via incretins. GLP-1 acts as incretins and works similarly. Five approved GLP-1 analogs for treating both T2DM and obesity have been developed.[18]

These are classified on the basis of duration of action.[19]

- *Short-acting:*
  - Exenatide
  - Lixisenatide.
- *Long-acting:*
  - Albiglutide
  - Dulaglutide
  - Semaglutide
  - Liraglutide.

These are useful in both type 1 diabetes mellitus (T1DM) as well as T2DM. Along with the use in T2DM, these are also helpful in T1DM. It significantly decreases the levels of blood glucose along with weight reduction and daily insulin requirements. GLP-1 analogs have significant pleiotropic effects on every organ system.[20]

Thiazolidinediones

Thiazolidinediones (TZDs) are the group of drugs that increases the insulin sensitivity by activating an enzyme, i.e. peroxisome proliferator-activated receptor gamma (PPAR-γ). This enzyme regulates various metabolic parameters. Rosiglitazone and pioglitazone are the two drugs in this group. Due to the problems with the safety of these drugs (specifically the CV safety), its use has been questioned. It was the reason that rosiglitazone was removed from the market. In contrast, pioglitazone shows beneficial safety profile.[21] In the joint position statement for managing diabetes, the American Diabetes Association and the European Association for the Study of Diabetes has classified TZDs as a therapy of choice after metformin failures.[22]

Comparison between Sulfonylureas and Dipeptidyl Peptidase-4 Inhibitors

Which one should be preferred among SUs and DPP4 inhibitors is an important question. A recent study has observed that, although both of these drugs are equally efficacious in controlling blood glucose levels, DPP4 inhibitors are safer than SUs. It is true that SUs decrease the HbA1c in a small period but with this, these also pose eminent threat of hypoglycemia and weight gain. DPP4 inhibitors lead to slow reduction in glucose levels without causing hypoglycemia and thus preferred in patients in whom it would lead to great risk.[23] Long-term treatment with DPP4 inhibitors conferred better glycemic control compared with SUs in T2DM patients, which may reflect that DPP4 inhibitors better preserve islet β-cell function than do SUs.[24] A study done in the month of Ramadan has observed that the incidence of hypoglycemia was very less with sitagliptin in comparison to glipizide or glimepiride. These are specialized sample of population as these people remain on fast from dusk to dawn.[25]

Comparison between SGLT2 and DPP4 Inhibitors

Sodium glucose cotransporter 2 inhibitors are among the new modality of treatment of T2DM. A study comparing the effects of SGLT2 inhibitors with the DPP4 inhibitors have seen that the SGLT2 inhibitors have better control of blood glucose levels along with significant weight reduction. Both these drugs act similarly on lipids, although SGLT2 inhibitors are more effective in those patients who have low high-density lipoprotein cholesterol (HDL-C). Combination of both the drugs have beneficial effects on CV as well as renal problems along with controlling blood glucose.[26] Another study also concluded that SGLT2 inhibitor have greater beneficial effects on lipid profile in patients with low HDL-C.[27]

Comparison between GLP-1 Analogs and DPP4 Inhibitors

Glucagon-like peptide-1 analogs are more effective in decreasing HbA1c as well as weight in comparison to sitagliptin but both have equal effects on blood pressure and lipid profile. The gastrointestinal side effects are more with GLP-1 analogs.[28] Another study shows that GLP-1 analogs are superior to sitagliptin in controlling blood glucose levels as well as weight reduction. GLP-1 analogs, although parenteral, are easy to administer. Satisfaction data also suggests that patients are more satisfied with GLP-1 receptor agonist (GLP-1RA) than with sitagliptin.[29]

If we see α-glucosidase inhibitors, in a study it was seen that this group of drug reduces HbA1c levels by 0.8% when comparing with placebo, but it is less effective than the effects of SUs and metformin. Others than this, its effect on decreasing blood glucose level is not dose-dependent and if given in high doses, it may contribute to more side effects.[30] Insulin has high risk of hypoglycemia. It is more costly and not better than SUs in improving the quality of life of peoples.[31] As it is administered parenterally, it seems inconvenient regimen for the patients due to fear of needles as well as less information about its importance.[32,33]

CONCLUSION

Sulfonylureas would be the preferred drug as a second-line agent during metformin failure. Also, fixed dose combinations of these two classes target both insulin resistance as well as deal with deficiency of insulin. It is also cost effective than other options available.[1] Other than this, combination of metformin and pioglitazone or metformin and DPP4 inhibitor are better options and may have more beneficial effects.[34,35]

REFERENCES

1. Lim PC, Chong CP. What's next after metformin? Focus on sulphonylurea: add-on or combination therapy. Pharm Pract (Granada). 2015;13(3):606.
2. Khunti K, Chatterjee S, Gerstein HC, et al. Do sulphonylureas still have a place in clinical practice? Lancet Diabetes Endocrinol. 2018;6(10):821-32.
3. Kalra S, Bahendeka S, Sahay R. Consensus recommendations on sulfonylurea and sulfonylurea combinations in the management of type 2 diabetes mellitus: International Task Force. Indian J Endocrinol Metab. 2018;22(1):132-57.
4. Ramracheya R, Ward C, Shigeto M, et al. Membrane potential-dependent inactivation of voltage-gated ion channels in alpha-cells inhibits glucagon secretion from human islets. Diabetes. 2010;59:2198-208.
5. Braun M, Ramracheya R, Amisten S, et al. Somatostatin release, electrical activity, membrane currents and exocytosis in human pancreatic delta cells. Diabetologia. 2009;52:1566-78.
6. Douros A, Aniello SD, Oriana Hoi Yun Yu. Sulfonylureas as second line drugs in type 2 diabetes and the risk of cardiovascular and hypoglycaemic events: population based cohort study. BMJ. 2018;362:k2693.
7. Zhong J, Kankanala S, Rajagopalan S. DPP4 inhibition: Insights from the bench and recent clinical studies. Curr Opin Lipidol. 2016;27(5):484-92.
8. Marguet D, Baggio L, Kobayashi T, et al. Enhanced insulin secretion and improved glucose tolerance in mice lacking CD26. Proc Natl Acad Sci USA. 2000;97:6874-9.
9. Zhong J, Gong Q, Goud A. Recent advances in dipeptidyl-peptidase-4 inhibition therapy: Lessons from the bench and clinical trials. J Diabetes Research. 2015, Article ID 606031.

10. Crowley MJ, Williams JW, Kosinski AS, et al. Metformin use may moderate the effect of DPP-4 inhibitors on cardiovascular outcomes. Diabetes Care. 2017;40:1787-9.
11. Shiba K, Tsuchiya K, Komiya C, et al. Canagliflozin, an SGLT2 inhibitor, attenuates the development of hepatocellular carcinoma in a mouse model of human NASH. Sci Rep. 2018;8(1):2362.
12. Chiazza1 F, Tammen H, Pintana H. The effect of DPP-4 inhibition to improve functional outcome after stroke is mediated by the SDF-1α/CXCR4 pathway. Cardiovasc Diabetol. 2018;17:60.
13. Singh AK. Deciding oral drugs after metformin in type 2 diabetes: An evidence-based approach. Indian J Endocrinol Metabol. 2014;18(5):617-23.
14. Fujita Y, Inagaki N. Renal sodium glucose cotransporter 2 inhibitors as a novel therapeutic approach to treatment of type 2 diabetes: clinical data and mechanism of action. J Diabetes Investig. 2014;5:265-75.
15. Kalra S. Sodium-glucose cotransporter 2 (SGLT2) inhibitors and cardiovascular disease: A systematic review. Cardiol Ther. 2016;5(2):161-8.
16. Zinman B, Wanner C, Lachin JM, et al. Empagliflozin, cardiovascular outcomes, and mortality in type 2 diabetes. N Engl Med. 2015;373:2117-28.
17. Neal B, Perkovic V, Mahaffey KW, et al. Canagliflozin and cardiovascular and renal events in type 2 diabetes. N Engl J Med. 2017;377:644-57.
18. Taylor SI. GLP-1 receptor agonists: differentiation within the class. Lancet Diabetes Endocrinol. 2018;6(2):83-5.
19. Meier JJ. GLP-1 receptor agonists for individualized treatment of type 2 diabetes mellitus. Nat Rev Endocrinol. 2012;8:728-42.
20. Gupta V. Glucagon-like peptide-1 analogues: An overview. Indian J Endocrinol Metab. 2013;17(3):413-21.
21. Rizos CV, Kei A, Elisaf MS. The current role of thiazolidinediones in diabetes management. Arch Toxicol. 2016;90(8):1861-81.
22. Inzucchi SE, Bergenstal RM, Buse JB, et al. Management of hyperglycemia in type 2 diabetes, 2015: a patient-centered approach: update to a position statement of the American Diabetes Association and the European Association for the Study of Diabetes. Diabetes Care. 2015;38:140-9.
23. Mishriky BM, Cummings DM, Tanenberg RJ. The efficacy and safety of DPP4 inhibitors compared to sulfonylureas as add-on therapy to metformin in patients with type 2 diabetes: A systematic review and meta-analysis. Diabetes Res Clin Pract. 2015;109(2):378-88.
24. Chen K, Kang D, Yu M. Direct head-to-head comparison of glycaemic durability of dipeptidyl peptidase-4 inhibitors and sulphonylureas in patients with type 2 diabetes mellitus: A meta-analysis of long-term randomized controlled trials. Diabetes Obes Metab. 2018;20(4):1029-1033.
25. Al Sifri S, Basiounny A, Echtay A, et al. The incidence of hypoglycaemia in Muslim patients with type 2 diabetes treated with sitagliptin or a sulphonylurea during Ramadan: a randomised trial. Int J Clin Pract. 2011;65(11):1132-40.
26. Xourgia E, Papazafiropoulou AK, Karampousli E, et al. DPP-4 inhibitors vs. SGLT-2 inhibitors; cons and pros. Jour Ren Med. 2017;1(2):7.
27. Seon-Ah Cha, Yong-Moon Park, Jae-Seung Yun. A comparison of effects of DPP-4 inhibitor and SGLT2 inhibitor on lipid profile in patients with type 2 diabetes. Lipids Health Dis. 2017;16:58.
28. Tiansheng Wang, Zhuoyue Gou, Fei Wang. Comparison of GLP-1 analogues versus sitagliptin in the management of type 2 diabetes: Systematic review and meta-analysis of head-to-head studies. PLoS One. 2014;9(8):e103798.
29. Brunton S. GLP-1 receptor agonists vs. DPP-4 inhibitors for type 2 diabetes: is one approach more successful or preferable than the other? Int J Clin Pract. 2014;68(5):557-67.
30. Van de Laar FA, Lucassen PL, Akkermans RP, et al. Alpha-glucosidase inhibitors for type 2 diabetes mellitus. Cochrane Database Syst Rev. 2005;2:606.
31. Zhang Y, McCoy RG, Mason JE, et al. Second-line agents for glycemic control for type 2 diabetes: are newer agents better? Diabetes Care. 2014;37(5):1338-45.
32. Korytkowski M. When oral agents fail: practical barriers to starting insulin. Int J Obes Relat Metab Disord. 2002;26(Suppl 3):S18-S24.
33. Meece J. Dispelling myths and removing barriers about insulin in type 2 diabetes. Diabetes Educ. 2006;32(1 Suppl):9S-18S.
34. Morgan CL, Poole CD, Evans M. What next after metformin? A retrospective evaluation of the outcome of second-line, glucose-lowering therapies in people with type 2 diabetes. J Clin Endocrinol Metabol. 2012;97(12):4605-612.
35. Bollaerts K, Mathieu C. Managing type 2 diabetes in patients not controlled on metformin. 2007;2:55-9.

Chapter 25

Sulfonylureas Revisited

Rajesh K Marya

INTRODUCTION

Today, with the ever increasing knowledge about the underlying pathophysiological abnormalities in diabetes and availability of newer agents targeting specific abnormality, the physicians are spoilt for choice. Therapeutic decision making as far as choosing an agent is concerned has become more and more challenging. In such a scenario there seems to be an attempt to edge out the older agents in order to make place for the newer ones. Sulfonylureas (SUs) are the oldest oral agents available; aspersions are being cast on their efficacy, durability (β-cell exhaustion), side effects (hypoglycemia and weight gain), safety [cardiovascular (CV) outcomes, ischemic preconditioning, all causes mortality]. What is their status in the emerging scenario needs to be reviewed.

In 1937, synthetic sulphur compounds were found to cause hypoglycemia, five years later while treating typhoid patients with sulfonamide, hypoglycemia was observed. In 1946 aryl SU was shown to stimulate insulin secretion by Auguste laboratories. Tolbutamide was the first SU to be marketed in Germany followed by other first generation SUs like chlorpropamide, acetohexamide, and tolazamide. Second generation SU glipizide and glyburide were discovered in Italy, were approved in USA in 1984. This was followed by the introduction of glimepiride and gliclazide.[1]

MECHANISM OF ACTION

The SUs are insulin secretagogues. They act by binding to the pancreatic β-cell sulfonylurea receptor 1 (SUR1), resulting in closure of ATP-sensitive potassium (KATP) channel, thereby causing membrane depolarization, opening of voltage dependent calcium channel leading to influx of calcium ions, and subsequent release of insulin from storage.[2] KATP channel is hetro-octameric complex comprising of pore forming subunit Kir6.x having two isoforms Kir6.1 and Kir6.2 and a regulatory subunit SURx having three isoforms SUR1, SUR2A and SUR2B. The KATP channels are widely distributed all over the body and differ as far as their composition is concerned. Kir6.2 plus SUR1 constitutes pancreatic β-cell KATP channels, Kir6.2 plus SUR2A constitutes cardiac and skeletal muscle KATP channels. Kir6.2 plus SUR2B constitutes smooth muscle KATP channels and Kir6.1 plus SUR2B constitutes vascular smooth muscle KATP channels.[3] The affinity with which different SUs bind with SUR subunits of KATP channels is variable in different tissues.[4] Gliclazide and tolbutamide block SUR1 with higher affinity compared to SUR2 while glibenclamide and glimepiride block both receptors with similar affinity.[5] However the glimepiride, blocks SUR1 and preferentially the sarcolemmal SUR2 while sparing the mitochondrial SUR.[6]

A novel cyclic adenosine monophosphate (cAMP)-binding protein family, termed Epac (exchange protein activated by cAMP) has been identified. There are two members of the Epac family, Epacl and Epac2. Epac2 potentiates cAMP-dependent, PKA-independent insulin secretion.[7] All SUs other than gliclazide bind to Epac2 to augment their insulin secreting action. This may partially explain the lower potential for hypoglycaemia with gliclazide.[4]

EFFICACY

Whether used alone or in combination, SUs have demonstrated a robust effect on glycemia lowering. A systemic review and meta-analysis concluded that SU monotherapy lowered HbA1c by 1.51% more than placebo [95% confidence interval (CI), 1.25, 1.78).[8] A meta-analysis of 15 randomized controlled trials (RCTs) with 1,681 adult T2DM patients concluded that glimepiride was as effective in glycemia control as metformin.[9] A systematic review and meta-analysis of 31 trials with mean duration of 16 weeks demonstrated that SU as add on therapy further reduced HbA1c by 1.62%.[10] Fixed-dose combination of glimepiride/metformin was found to be more effective in glycemic control than metformin up titration, and was well tolerated in type 2 diabetic patients inadequately controlled by low-dose metformin monotherapy.[11]

BETA-CELL EXHAUSTION

There is a misconception that SUs being secretagogues make β-cell work more thus leading to their getting exhausted. The ADOPT study, demonstrated that as a monotherapy failure after 5 years of treatment was highest with glyburide 34%, followed by metformin 21%, and 15% for rosiglitazone. It was also demonstrated that β-cell function was similar in all groups 5 years later.[1] It has been seen that continuous exposure to high plasma levels SU impairs rather than improves therapeutic efficacy, probably due to downregulation of SUR. The dose-response curve of SU during chronic treatment is a bell-shaped and not sigmoidal, so using high doses of SU may not be effective in lowering hyperglycemia, with consequent therapeutic failure.[12] A 10-year observational study demonstrated that it was not long-term treatment with SUs, but poor glycemic control was associated with a decrease in β-cell function.[13] A RCT in 40 subjects with early T2D treated with exenatide, sitagliptin or the glimepiride for 6 months demonstrated that it was glimepiride but not exenatide or sitagliptin, that enhanced β-cell secretory capacity and functional β-cell mass.[14] Further, it has been suggested that β-cell failure in diabetes is due to β-cell de-differentiation rather than β-cell death.[15]

HYPOGLYCEMIA

Hypoglycemia with its associated risks of altered sensorium, falls, fractures and CVD complications, is a well-established limiting factor in our efforts to achieve a tight glycemic control. Risk of hypoglycemia is more in older patients, patients treated with polypharmacy, concomitant use of insulin and SU potentiating drugs, long acting SU (chlorpropamide and glibenclamide), renal and hepatic impairment. In a population-based study of health service resource use incidences of severe hypoglycemia on SU treated patients was 0.9% per 100 patient years.[16] Annual incidence of hypoglycemia was 17.7% in patients treated with SU compared to 36.5% in those treated on insulin in 10 years follow-up analysis of United Kingdom Prospective Diabetes Study (UKPDS).[17] A systemic review and meta-analysis showed a 52% higher risk of hypoglycemia secondary to glyburide, when compared with other secretagogues [relative risk 1.52 (95% CI, 1.21–1.92)].[18]

A significantly lower rates of confirmed hypoglycemia (blood glucose <3 mmol/L) with gliclazide modified release (MR) were reported in comparison to glimepiride (3.7% vs. 8.9%, p = 0.003) in GUIDE study. However, there were no episodes of severe hypoglycemia/hypoglycemia requiring external assistance in either arm.[19] In a prospective, population-based, 4-year study glimepiride was reported to be associated with fewer episodes of severe hypoglycemia than glibenclamide in routine clinical use (0.86/1000 person-years vs. 5.6/1000 person-years, respectively).[20]

WEIGHT GAIN

Weight gain is commonly seen with SUs. In UKPDS compared to conventionally treated group the intensively treated group showed a weight gain of 2.6 kg with chlorpropamide and 1.7 kg with glibenclamide.[21] Unlike the weight gain with insulin which is progressive, weight gain with SUs stabilizes after 3–4 years.[22] The newer SUs are not known to cause significant weight gain. Gliclazide MR did not cause any weight gain during the 5-year follow up in ADVANCE trial.[23] In another study gliclazide MR was associated with a similar weight loss as vildagliptin (–1.1 kg).[24] Glimepiride has been shown to provide equivalent glycemic control compared to glibenclamide but with significantly greater reduction in body weight and body mass index.[25]

EFFECT ON CARDIOVASCULAR OUTCOME AND MORTALITY

A recent systematic review and network meta-analysis concluded that gliclazide and glimepiride were associated with a lower risk of all-cause and CV-related mortality compared with glibenclamide.[26] A recent Cochrane systematic review and meta-analysis concluded that evidence suggests that, compared with metformin, second- and third-generation SU may not affect all-cause or CV mortality but may decrease the risk of nonfatal macrovascular outcomes among type 2 diabetes.[27] Another meta-analysis of 62 trials reporting major CV events with SUs versus various comparators has provided perhaps the best synthesis of data to date. An overall odds ratio (OR) for major CV events with SU treatment versus comparators of 1.08 (95% CI 0.86–1.36), thus detecting no signal for CV risk. Use of SU is not associated with any significant difference in the incidence of myocardial infarction with respect to comparators [OR: 0.88 (0.75–1.04)].[28] A retrospective cohort study in type 2 diabetes mellitus (n = 11,141) in those with documented CAD, demonstrated a trend toward increased overall mortality with glyburide versus glimepiride [hazard ratio (HR) 1.36] glipizide versus glimepiride (HR 1.39).[29]

ISCHEMIC PRECONDITIONING

Although, both the glibenclamide and glimepiride bind SUR2 receptor but in an experimental study with rat hearts, blocking of the protective ischemic effect was seen with glibenclamide but not with glimepiride. In the rat cardiomyocytes glimepiride blocked the sarcolemmal KATP channel opening but not the mitochondrial KATP channels opening.[30] A double blind placebo controlled demonstrated that compared to glibenclamide, glimepiride maintained myocardial preconditioning with fewer CV side effects as ($p = 0.01$ vs. $p = 0.34$, respectively).[31] Impact of type of preadmission SUs on mortality and CV outcomes in diabetic patients with acute MI was studied in a nationwide registry. It concluded that no hazard was associated with the use of SUs before the acute episode. Rather patient's previously receiving gliclazide or glimepiride had improved in-hospital outcomes, compared with those on glibenclamide.[32]

CONCLUSION

Sulfonylureas are time tested agents, corner stone of type 2 diabetes treatment since over 60 years and are likely to continue to be a reliable and effective treatment as monotherapy or in combination therapy. SU have an established long-term benefit with regard to decreased risk of micro- and macrovascular diabetes-related complications especially with modern SUs. Glimepiride and gliclazide MR exhibits lower risk of hypoglycemia and have neutral effect on weight, do not adversely affect ischemic preconditioning or CV outcome, can be safely used in renal impairment and are cost-effective and safe SU with good compliance.

REFERENCES

1. Guimarães J. Diabetes-Old Therapies Revisited. Endocrinol Metab Int J. 2016; 3(4): 00056.
2. Seino S. ATP-sensitive potassium channels: a model of heteromultimeric potassium channel/receptor assemblies. Annu Rev Physiol. 1999; 61: 337-362.
3. Seino S, Zhang C, Shibasaki T. Sulfonylurea action re-visited. J Diabetes Investig. 2010; 1(1–2): 37-39.
4. Kalra S, Aamir AH, Raza A, et al. Place of sulfonylureas in the management of type 2 diabetes mellitus in south Asia: A consensus statement. Indian J Endocrinol Metab. 2015;19:577-96.
5. Ashcroft FM, Gribble FM. Tissue-specific effects of sulfonylureas: Lessons from studies of cloned K (ATP) channels. J Diabetes Complications. 2000;14:192-6.
6. Ballagi-Pordány G, Németh M, Aranyi Z, et al. Effect of glimepiride on the electrical activity of isolated rabbit heart muscle. Arzneimittelforschung. 1992;42:111-3.
7. Zhang CL, Katoh M, Shibasaki T, et al. The cAMP sensor Epac2 is a direct target of antidiabetic sulfonylurea drugs. Science. 2009; 325(5940): 607-610.
8. Hirst JA, Farmer AJ, Dyar A, et al. Estimating the effect of sulfonylurea on HbA1c in diabetes: A systematic review and meta-analysis. Diabetologia. 2013;56:973-84.
9. Zhu H, Zhu S, Zhang X, et al. Comparative efficacy of glimepiride and metformin in monotherapy of type 2 diabetes mellitus: Meta-analysis of randomized controlled trials. Diabetol Metab Syndr. 2013;5:70.
10. Hirst JA, Farmer AJ, Dyar A, et al. Estimating the effect of sulfonylurea on HbA1c in diabetes: A systematic review and meta-analysis. Diabetologia. 2013;56:973-84.
11. Hye-soon Kim, Doo-man Kim, Bong-soo Cha, et al. Efficacy of glimepiride/metformin fixed-dose combination versus metformin uptitration in type 2 diabetic patients inadequately controlled on low-dose metformin monotherapy: A randomized, open label, parallel group, multicenter study in Korea. J Diabetes Invest. 2014; 5: 701-708.
12. Melander A. Kinetics-Effect Relations of Insulin-Releasing Drugs in Patients with Type 2 Diabetes Brief Overview. Diab. 2004; 53(Suppl 3): S151-5.
13. Nybäck-Nakell A, Bergström J, Adamson U, et al. Decreasing postprandial C-peptide levels over time are not associated with long-term use of sulphonylurea: An observational study. Diab Metab. 2010;36:375-80.
14. Gudipaty L, Rosenfeld NK, Fuller CS, et al. Effect of exenatide, sitagliptin, or glimepiride on ß-cell secretory capacity in early type 2 diabetes. Diab Care. 2014;37:2451-8.
15. Dor Y, Glaser B. β-cell dedifferentiation and type 2 diabetes. N Engl J Med. 2013;368:572-3.
16. Leese GP, Wang J, Broomhall J, et al. Frequency of severe hypoglycemia requiring emergency treatment in type 1 and type 2 diabetes: a population-based study of health service resource use. Diabetes Care. 2003; 26(4): 1176-80.
17. Intensive blood-glucose control with sulphonylureas or insulin compared with conventional treatment and risk of complications in patients with type 2 diabetes (UKPDS 33). UK Prospective Diabetes Study (UKPDS) Group. Lancet. 1998;352:837-53.

18. Gangji AS, Cukierman T, Gerstein HC, et al. A systematic review and meta-analysis of hypoglycemia and cardiovascular events: a comparison of glyburide with other secretagogues and with insulin. Diab Care. 2007; 30(2): 389-94.
19. Schernthaner G, Grimaldi A, Di Mario U, et al. GUIDE study: Double-blind comparison of once-daily gliclazide MR and glimepiride in type 2 diabetic patients. Eur J Clin Invest. 2004;34:535-42.
20. Holstein A, Plaschke A, Egberts EH. Lower incidence of severe hypoglycaemia in patients with type 2 diabetes treated with glimepiride versus glibenclamide. Diab Metab Res Rev. 2001;17:467-73.
21. Turner R. Intensive blood-glucose control with sulphonylureas or insulin compared with conventional treatment and risk of complications in patients with type 2 diabetes (UKPDS 33). Lancet. 1998;352:837-53.
22. Turner R, Cull C, Holman R. United Kingdom Prospective Diabetes Study 17: A 9-year update of a randomized, controlled trial on the effect of improved metabolic control on complications in non-insulin-dependent diabetes mellitus. Ann Intern Med 1996;124(1 Pt 2):136-45.
23. Zoungas S, Chalmers J, Neal B, et al. Follow-up of blood-pressure lowering and glucose control in type 2 diabetes. N Engl J Med. 2014;371:1392-406
24. Hassanein M, Abdallah K, Schweizer A. A double-blind, randomized trial, including frequent patient-physician contacts and Ramadan-focused advice, assessing vildagliptin and gliclazide in patients with type 2 diabetes fasting during Ramadan: The STEADFAST study. Vasc Health Risk Manag. 2014;10:319-26.
25. Martin S, Kolb H, Beuth J, et al. Change in patients body weight after 12 months of treatment with glimepiride or glibenclamide in Type 2 diabetes: A multicentre retrospective cohort study. Diabetologia. 2003;46:1611-7.
26. Simpson SH, Lee J, Choi S, Vandermeer B, Abdelmoneim AS, Featherstone TR. Mortality risk among sulfonylureas: A systematic review and network meta-analysis. Lancet Diabetes Endocrinol. 2015;3:43-51.
27. Hemmingsen B, Schroll JB, Wetterslev J, et al. Sulfonylurea versus metformin monotherapy in patients with type 2 diabetes: a Cochrane systematic review and meta-analysis of randomized clinical trials and trial sequential analysis. CMAJ Open. 2014 Jul 22; 2(3): E162-75
28. Monami M, Genovese S, Mannucci E. Cardiovascular safety of sulfonylureas: a meta-analysis of randomized clinical trials. Diabetes Obes Metab. 2013 Oct;15(10):938-53.
29. Pantalone KM, Kattan MW, Yu C, et al. The risk of overall mortality in patients with type 2 diabetes receiving glipizide, glyburide, or glimepiride monotherapy: a retrospective analysis. Diab Care. 2010;33:1224-9.
30. Mocanu MM, Maddock HL, Baxter GF et al. Glimepiride, a novel sulfonylurea, does not abolish myocardial protection afforded by either ischemic preconditioning or diazoxide. Circulation. 2001;103:3111-6.
31. Klepzig H, Kober G, Matter C, et al. Sulfonylureas and ischaemic preconditioning; a double-blind, placebo-controlled evaluation of glimepiride and glibenclamide. Eur Heart J. 1999;20:439-46.
32. Zeller M, Danchin N, Simon D, et al. Impact of type of preadmission sulfonylureas on mortality and cardiovascular outcomes in diabetic patients with acute myocardial infarction. J Clin Endocrinol Metab. 2010;95:4993-5002.

Chapter 26

Cancer and Antidiabetic Drugs

Girish Mathur, Ashutosh Chaturvedi

INTRODUCTION

Diabetes mellitus is one of the fastest growing public health concerns worldwide. As per International Diabetes Federation Atlas, worldwide there were around 366 million people with diabetes in 2011 which is expected to grow up to 552 million by 2030.[1] The complications of diabetes are diverse and serious. Apart from increased risk of kidney disease, heart disease, blindness, cerebrovascular accidents and amputations, emerging data has shown association of diabetes with an increased risk of many types of cancer.[2] With diabetes on rise continuously, this deadly diabetes-cancer duo has warranted research to generate further evidences regarding their serious association.

THE LINK BETWEEN DIABETES AND CANCER

Type 2 diabetes (T2D) and cancer share many pathophysiologic mechanisms and risk factors. Modifiable risk factors are lower socioeconomic status, alcohol consumption and obesity whereas nonmodifiable risk factors include advanced age, ethnicity, male sex and family history.[3] All these risk factors finally cause insulin resistance and hyperinsulinemia, oxidative stress, altered mitochondrial function and elevation of inflammatory cytokines[4] all of which are considered to be possible mechanisms to link diabetes and cancer. Antidiabetic therapy influences many of these processes, therefore, in absence of complete understanding of mechanisms linking diabetes and cancer, it is very logical to suspect whether the antidiabetic drugs can affect the risk of developing cancer in diabetic patients. T2D has been shown to be associated with risk of cancers of liver,[5] pancreas,[6] colorectum,[7] breast,[8] kidney,[9] uterus,[10] urinary bladder,[11] and hematologic malignancies like non-Hodgkin's lymphoma (NHL).[12]

DIABETES TREATMENT THERAPY AND CANCER RISK

The clear relationship between T2D and cancer makes it important to assess the potential role of any antidiabetic therapy in the cancer risk. Recent meta-analysis and studies, both comparative and cohort, have evaluated the risk of developing cancer in diabetic patients receiving treatment for it versus those who are not taking antidiabetic drugs. Well-established antidiabetic drugs include sulfonylureas (SUs), metformin, thiazolidinediones (TZDs), α-glucosidase inhibitors (acarbose only) along with exogenous insulin and insulin analogs like insulin glargine. The more new drug classes are dipeptidyl peptidase-4 (DPP-4) inhibitors, glucagon-like peptide-1 (GLP-1) receptor agonists or incretin mimetics, sodium-glucose cotransport 2 (SGLT2) inhibitors, D2-dopamine agonists (bromocriptine). Table 1[13] summarizes the cancer risk for both established and newer drugs, and outlines types of studies for their association with cancer risk.

The majority of studies have indicated protective role of metformin and provided conflicting data on other antidiabetic agents, mainly insulin and incretin-based therapies. Different mechanisms of action of these drugs may be responsible for such varying effects. However, possibly because of time-related biases[14] and some other limitations these studies differ from each other in the approach. The accuracy of studies depends on how precisely a drug exposure is measured but this important factor has not been given attention in detail yet and therefore the impact of antidiabetic drugs on cancer risk still remains a matter of controversy.[15]

TABLE 1: Risk of cancer from approved drugs for type 2 diabetes mellitus.[13]

Drugs	Cancer risk	Types of studies	Comments
Oral agents			
(A) Insulin sensitizers:			
Metformin	Lower	Case-control cohort retrospective database	Decreased risk of cancer-related death
Thiazolidinediones	Higher risk of bladder cancer; lower risk of breast and lung cancer	Case-control cohort	Slight dose-dependent increase in bladder cancer risk in cohort studies; no increased risk in randomized control trials
(B) Insulin secretagogues			
Sulfonylureas	Higher	Case-control cohort	Increased risk of cancer-related death compared with insulin sensitizers
Meglitinide	Higher	Case-control	Neutral to increased association of cancer risk (fewer available data compared with sulfonylurea)
(C) Other oral agents:			
Alpha-glucosidase inhibitors	Neutral	Case-control retrospective database	
Dipeptidyl peptidase-4 inhibitors	Possibly higher risk of pancreatic cancer	Expert opinion	Sitagliptin shows increased risk of acute pancreatitis, raising concerns about pancreatic cancer; to date, there is no evidence of increased risk of pancreatic cancer in humans
Sodium-glucose-linked cotransporter 2 inhibitors	Neutral	Randomized controlled clinical trials	
Injectable agents			
Glucagon-like peptide-1 receptor agonists	Higher risk of thyroid and Pancreatic cancer	• Adverse events reports • Expert opinion • Rodent studies	Medullary thyroid cancer and pancreatic cancer risk increased in rodents; potentially increased pancreatic cancer risk from adverse serious events reported for exenatide twice daily.
Insulin glargine	Neutral	Case-control randomized controlled	Median dose 0.4 U/kg/day at 6 years in the ORIGIN trial[16]
Insulin analogs	Higher	Case-control cohort retrospective database	

Insulin and Insulin Analogs: Conflicting Evidence

Insulin increases the risk of malignancy by its direct and indirect impact on cancer growth. It is a potent growth stimulating hormone which increases hepatic expression of insulin-like growth factor 1 (IGF-1) and acts through mitogenic type A insulin receptor, whose activation directly enhances cancer growth.[17]

In 2009, Hemkens et al. by a retrospective study, linked the long-acting insulin analog glargine to risk of cancer[18] leading to a situation of controversy and concern among the medical community and patients.

In an analysis published in the same year, an association between insulin glargine use and cancer incidence could not be established after evaluating 31 randomized clinical trials in a drug manufacturer's database.[19]

More recently, the Outcome Reduction with an Initial Glargine Intervention (ORIGIN) trial which involved 12,537 participants from 573 sites in 40 countries, did not reveal increased cancer risk among insulin users.[20] The results can be explained by relatively short duration of the studies, frequent use of metformin along with insulin, and relatively low doses of insulin used in the ORIGIN trial. It was also found that the risk of malignancy associated with insulin use does not depend neither on the insulin treatment regimen (basal, basal/bolus or premixed)[21] nor on the type of insulin (human or analog).[22]

As per specific malignancies, glargine use was linked with a lower risk of colon cancer and an increased risk of breast and prostate cancers when compared with human insulin use.

The dose of glargine could not be related to diagnosis.[23] Thus, there is no clear evidences correlating analog insulin with increased cancer risk so insulin initiation should not be delayed specially in uncontrolled diabetes. Further long-term prospective studies on insulin use and cancer are warranted.

Metformin: The Drug of Choice

Approved by the Food and Drug Association (FDA) in 1995 despite been in clinical use since 1950s, metformin is the drug of choice unless there are contraindications for its use. Metformin acts primarily by improving peripheral insulin sensitivity and inhibiting hepatic glucose production (gluconeogenesis). Its other beneficial effects include increase in glucagon-like peptide-1 (GLP-1) levels and induction of islet incretin-receptor gene expression,[24] lowering of cancer risk and increased survival of those with cancer among the diabetic population.

Libby et al. in an observational cohort study that compared 4,000 subjects with diabetes who had received metformin with 4,000 diabetic subjects who had not taken it,[25] found that 7.3% of metformin users had cancer compared with 11.6% among those who did not received metformin.

Li et al. in their study showed that diabetic patients receiving metformin had a significantly lower risk for pancreatic cancer compared with non-metformin users [95% confidence interval (CI), 0.22–0.69; P = 0.001]. Those who took metformin had a 62% reduction in the risk for developing pancreatic cancer.[26]

Wright et al. also concluded that use of metformin reduced the risk of prostate cancer by 44%.[27]

Most of the studies suggested adenosine monophosphate activated protein kinase (AMPK) for anti-cancer properties of metformin to be the key molecule. It phosphorylates proteins leading to cellular inhibition and tumor reduction. Thus, based on present literature metformin use and cancer appears to have a negative relationship and further prospective studies need to be conducted for better assessment.

Thiazolidinediones

Thiazolidinediones, such as pioglitazone, act by binding to peroxisome proliferator-activated gamma (PPAR-γ) receptors in the cell nucleus and increase insulin sensitivity along with reduction of hepatic gluconeogenesis. Various cohort studies have found a statistically significant increase in risk of urinary bladder cancer with the use of pioglitazone.[28] On the other hand TZDs use has been associated with a reduced risk of cancer of lung, colon and breast.[29]

In June 2011, the United States FDA (USFDA) announced pioglitazone use of >1 year may be associated with increased risk of bladder cancer. This was based on a nested case control study in diabetic patients and a 10-year observational study as well including 193,099 patients, aged >40 years, of Kaiser Permanente Northern California (KPNC) health plan.[30] Other various randomized controlled trials did not showed any significant increase in risk of bladder cancer with pioglitazone exposure.[30] Another cohort study suggested an increased risk of melanoma and NHL with the ever use of pioglitazone.[31]

Chronic irritation of bladder due to crystal formation was supposed to be the possible mechanism for the risk of bladder cancer with pioglitazone use.[32]

Rosiglitazone was not found to be associated with increased cancer risk even with cumulative dosage and increased duration of exposure.[32]

Meglitinides: Limited Evidence

Meglitinides increase insulin release by inhibiting potassium channels in the pancreas on a site different from SU. Only one retrospective study by Chang et al. showed that use of a meglitinide had a significantly increased risk for developing cancer, mainly liver cancer[33] possibly due to increase in insulin levels. Due to limited data a correlation between meglitinide use and cancer risk cannot be established.

Sulfonylureas: Evidence of Higher Risk

Sulfonylureas act by inhibition of potassium channels in the pancreatic cells leading to stimulation of endogenous insulin secretion. Limited studies done on cancer risk associated with SU indicate that there may be a increased incidence of cancer among those who receive them.

The nested case-control study done by Monami et al. demonstrated overall neutral effect on cancer risk associated with SU use. However, all SU derivatives were not equal as glibenclamide use was associated with increased risk, while gliclazide showed a reduced risk of malignancy. The study also positively correlated a greater length of exposure to a SU with increased risk of cancer compared with the control group of diabetic patients.[34]

Currie et al.[35] showed that SU monotherapy was associated with a 36% higher risk of cancer than metformin monotherapy while combined treatment with SU + metformin was associated with a neutral effect on cancer incidence.

Chang et al.[33] carried out a retrospective study in China in which out of 108,920 subjects included in the study, 8,194 developed cancer. Significant association was detected for increased risk of liver and pancreatic cancers with the use of first- and second-generation SU, but not with third-generation SU.

Another study by Yang et al. showed a decreased cancer risk among patients taking gliclazide and glibenclamide.[36]

The higher risk of cancer seen with SU remain a matter of concern like other antidiabetic drugs, they have only been evaluated in a retrospective manner, leading to invalidated conclusions.

Alpha-Glucosidase Inhibitors (Acarbose)

Glucosidase inhibitors act by inhibiting α-glucosidase enzymes in small intestines leading to delayed absorption of complex carbohydrates from alimentary tract thus reducing the glucose load of body. The limited data available does not appear to show that glucosidase inhibitors increase the cancer risk.

Incretin Mimetics

GLP-1 Receptor Agonists and DPP-4 Inhibitors

Glucagon-like peptide-1 is an incretin hormone secreted by L-type cells in distal ileum in response to food ingestion. GLP-1 agonists like exenatide and liraglutide promote glucose dependent insulin secretion and restore β–cell sensitivity along with increase in β-cell mass.

Glucagon-like peptide-1 is normally degraded by an enzyme DPP-4. Drugs that inhibit DPP-4 are vildagliptin, sitagliptin, linagliptin, teneligliptin, and recently added gemigliptin.

As pancreatitis is a known complication of incretin mimetics there is concern that long term use of these drugs increases pancreatic cancer risk and that of medullary thyroid carcinoma also because of C-cell hyperplasia leading to rise in serum calcitonin particularly with liraglutide[37] as evident from studies in rodents.

In 2011 Elashoff et al. found a 2.9 times higher incidence of pancreatic cancer and a 4-fold increase in thyroid cancer incidence in patients receiving exenatide as compared to other therapies.[38]

In the same year Koehler et al. showed that activation of GLP-1 receptor increases apoptosis leading to lysis of colon cancer cells while another study also found to have a protective effect of GLP-1 agonists on breast cancer.[39,40]

Alves et al.[41] meta-analyzed 25 studies and found that neither exenatide (no cases reported) nor liraglutide was associated with increased thyroid cancer risk.

Therefore, at this time there is no clear data to prove an increased cancer risk with incretin therapy and long-term prospective studies are needed to analyze specific outcomes.

Sodium-Glucose Linked Cotransporter 2 Inhibitors

Sodium glucose linked cotransporter 2 inhibitors are the newest class of drugs which lower blood glucose by inhibiting SGLT2 protein in the proximal renal tubules thus promoting glycosuria. Among this class, in those treated with dapagliflozin, higher incidence of bladder and breast cancer was noted as compared to the control group although it was not statistically significant. Canagliflozin was not found to have a positive relationship with increased cancer risk.[42]

As diabetes itself has been linked to carcinoma bladder, thus creating a chicken or egg scenario, further studies on long-term data are warranted to establish any association with increased cancer risk.

Bromocriptine Mesylate

Bromocriptine, an ergot derivative, has been proposed to reverse metabolic alterations of insulin resistance and obesity by changes in hypothalamic circadian system of monoamine neuronal activities. It was approved by FDA in 2009 for use in T2D in adults. In 2000, an Italy-based study showed that low-dose bromocriptine acutely

TABLE 2: Classification of studies by representation of dose, duration and continuity of exposure to drug of interest.[44]

	Drugs of interest	Dose (Y/N)	Duration (Y/N)	Continuity (Y/N)
Currie et al.[35]	Metformin, sulfonylureas	N	Y	N
Govindarajan et al.[45]	Any thiazolidinedione	N	N	N
Ramos-Nino et al.[46]	Pioglitazone, or rosiglitazone	N	N	N
Monami et al.[47]	Sulfonylureas	N	Y	N
Ferrara et al.[31]	Pioglitazone	Y	Y	Y
Libby et al.[25]	Metformin	Y	Y	N
Landman et al.[48]	Metformin	Y	N	N
Yang et al.[36]	Glibenclamide, gliclazide, glipizide	Y	N	N
Baur et al.[49]	Glucose-lowering drugs	N	N	N

(N: no; Y: yes.)

normalizes prolactin in patients with prostate cancer and in those with metastatic breast carcinoma[43] but it is still unclear whether bromocriptine affects cancer risk in diabetic patients.

DISCUSSION

Most of the data linking the use of antidiabetic drugs to cancer development is retrospective and still non-conclusive and only suggest an association rather than direct cause. The available data suggests a higher risk of cancer incidence with insulin, pioglitazone, and insulin secretagogues while metformin seems to have a protective effect against some cancers in diabetic patients. This nonconclusive nature of the available data has raised several epidemiological challenges for carrying out investigations of the association between antidiabetic drugs and risk of cancer.

Possible limitations of various studies may be as follows:

- Most of the patients are treated with many drugs making it difficult to identify the effect of one drug on cancer risk
- Large numbers of studies tend to combine all cancers for analysis, masking the risks for different cancer sites
- Most studies lack sufficient power to detect small associations
- Time-related biases are always present.

Table 2[44] depicts that only one study has taken into account the effects of drug exposure- i.e continuity of exposure.

The future studies therefore, need to have accurate representation of timing of exposure, dose and duration of drug use, and representation of continuity in order to obtain a fruitful data establishing a relationship between use of antidiabetic drugs and development of cancer.

CONCLUSION

In the absence of clear associations between antidiabetic drugs and cancer development risk, healthcare providers must weigh the benefits and the risks of agents for optimization of glycemic control and other metabolic factors in every patient.

Cancer screening in this high-risk population, education regarding lifestyle modifications which ameliorates many adverse metabolic states coexisting in diabetes and cancer and customization of therapy to individual patients with respect to personal and family history of cancer are the utmost weapons which physicians need to have in their armamentarium. Finally, health care providers need to be more thoughtful in selection of antidiabetic therapy by utilizing the available data in the best possible way.

REFERENCES

1. Whiting DR, Guariguata L, Weil C, et al. IDF diabetes atlas: global estimates of the prevalence of diabetes for 2011 and 2030. Res Clin Pract. 2011;94:311-21.
2. Cannata D, Fierz Y, Vijayakumar A, et al. Type 2 diabetes and cancer: what is the connection? Mt Sinai J Med. 2010;77:197-213.
3. Centers for Disease Control and Prevention. Diabetes public health resource (2014). National diabetes statistics report, 2014. Estimates of diabetes and its burden in the United States [online] Available from www.cdc.gov/diabetes/ pubs/estimates14.htm. [Accessed October, 2018].
4. Vigneri P, Frasca F, Sciacca L, et al. Diabetes and cancer. Endocr Relat Cancer. 2009;16:1103-123.

5. El-Serag HB, Hampel H, Javadi F. The association between diabetes and hepatocellular carcinoma: a systematic review of epidemiologic evidence. Clin Gastroenterol Hepatol. 2006;4:369-80.
6. Huxley R, Ansary-Moghaddam A, Berrington de González A, et al. Type-II diabetes and pancreatic cancer: a meta-analysis of 36 studies. Br J Cancer. 2005;92:2076-2083.
7. Larsson SC, Orsini N, Wolk A. Diabetes mellitus and risk of colorectal cancer: a meta-analysis. J Natl Cancer Inst. 2005;97:1679-87.
8. Larsson SC, Mantzoros CS, Wolk A. Diabetes mellitus and risk of breast cancer: a meta-analysis. Int J Cancer. 2007;121:856-62.
9. Washio M, Mori M, Khan M, et al. Diabetes mellitus and kidney cancer risk: the results of Japan Collaborative Cohort Study for Evaluation of Cancer Risk (JACC Study). Int J Urol. 2007;14:393-7.
10. Friberg E, Orsini N, Mantzoros CS, et al. Diabetes mellitus and risk of endometrial cancer: a meta-analysis. Diabetologia. 2007;50:1365-74.
11. Larsson SC, Orsini N, Brismar K, et al. Diabetes mellitus and risk of bladder cancer: a meta-analysis. Diabetologia. 2006;49:2819-23.
12. Mitri J, Castillo J, Pittas AG. Diabetes and risk of non-Hodgkin's lymphoma: a meta-analysis of observational studies. Diabetes Care. 2008;31:2391-7.
13. Ching Sun GE, Kashyap SR, Nasr C, et al. Diabetes therapy and cancer risk: Where do we stand when treating patients? Cleveland Clin J Med. 2014;81(10):620-8.
14. Suissa S, Azoulay L. Metformin and the risk of cancer: Time-related biases in observational studies. Diabetes Care. 2012;35(12):2665-73.
15. Seshasai SR, Kaptoge S, Thompson A, et al. Diabetes mellitus, fasting glucose, and risk of cause-specific death. N Engl J Med. 2011;364:829-41.
16. Colhoun HM. Use of insulin glargine and cancer incidence in Scotland: a study from the Scottish Diabetes Research Network Epidemiology Group. Diabetologia. 2009;52:1755-65.
17. Gallagher EJ, LeRoith D. Diabetes, antihyperglycemic medications and cancer risk: smoke or fire? Curr Opin Endocrinol Diabetes Obes. 2013;20(5):485-94.
18. Hemkens LG, Grouven U, Bender R, et al. Risk of malignancies in patients with diabetes treated with human insulin or insulin analogues: a cohort study. Diabetologia. 2009;52:1732-44.
19. Home PD, Lagarenne P. Combined randomised controlled trial experience of malignancies in studies using insulin glargine. Diabetologia. 2009;52:2499-506.
20. Gerstein HC, Bosch J, Dagenais GR, et al. ORIGIN Trial Investigators. Basal insulin and cardiovascular and other outcomes in dysglycemia. N Engl J Med. 2012;367(4):319-28.
21. Holden SE, Jenkins-Jones S, Morgan CL, et al. Glucose-lowering with exogenous insulin monotherapy in type 2 diabetes: dose association with all-cause mortality, cardiovascular events and cancer. Diabetes Obes Metab. 2015;17(4):350-62.
22. Evans JMM, Donnelly LA, Emslie-Smith AM, et al. Metformin and reduced risk of cancer in diabetic patients. BMJ. 2005;330(7503):1304-305.
23. Ruiter R, Visser LE, van Herk-Sukel MP, et al. Risk of cancer in patients on insulin glargine and other insulin analogues in comparison with those on human insulin: results from a large population-based follow-up study. Diabetologia. 2012;55:51-62.
24. Maida A, Lamont BJ, Cao X, et al. Metformin regulates the incretin receptor axis via a pathway dependent on peroxisome proliferator-activated receptor- in mice. Diabetologia. 2011;54:339-49.
25. Libby G, Donnelly LA, Donnan PT, et al. New users of metformin are at low risk of incident cancer: a cohort study among people with type 2 diabetes. Diabetes Care. 2009;32:1620-5.
26. Li D, Yeung SC, Hassan MM, et al. Antidiabetic therapies affect risk of pancreatic cancer. Gastroenterol. 2009;137:482-8.
27. Wright JL, Stanford JL. Metformin use and prostate cancer in Caucasian men: results from a population-based case-control study. Cancer Causes Control. 2009;20:1617-22.
28. Yki-Järvinen H. Thiazolidinediones. N Engl J Med. 2004;351:1106-118.
29. Colmers IN, Bowker SL, Johnson JA. Thiazolidinedione use and cancer incidence in type 2 diabetes: a systematic review and meta-analysis. Diabetes Metab. 2012;38:475-84.
30. US Food and Drug Administration (2011). FDA Drug Safety Communication: update to ongoing safety review of Actos (pioglitazone) and increased risk of bladder cancer [online] Available from www.fda.gov/Drugs/Drugsafety/ucm259150.htm. [Accessed October, 2018].
31. Ferrara A, Lewis JD, Quesenberry CP Jr, et al. Cohort study of pioglitazone and cancer incidence in patients with diabetes. Diabetes Care. 2011;34:923-9.
32. Azoulay L, Yin H, Filion KB, et al. The use of pioglitazone and the risk of bladder cancer in people with type 2 diabetes: nested case-control study. BMJ. 2012;344:e3645.
33. Chang C, Lin J, Wu L, et al. Oral insulin secretagogues, insulin, and cancer risk in type 2diabetes mellitus. J Clin Endocrin Metab. 2012;97(7):E1170-5.
34. Monami M, Colombi C, Balzi D, et al. Metformin and cancer occurrence in insulin-treated type 2 diabetic patients. Diabetes Care. 2011;34:129-31.
35. Currie CJ, Poole CD, Gale EA. The influence of glucose-lowering therapies on cancer risk in type 2 diabetes. Diabetologia. 2009;52:1766-77.
36. Yang X, So WY, Ma RC, et al. Use of sulphonylurea and cancer in type 2 diabetes –The Hong Kong Diabetes Registry. Diabetes Res Clin Pract. 2010;90:343-51.
37. Bjerre Knudsen L, Madsen LW, Andersen S, et al. Glucagon-like peptide-1 receptor agonists activate rodent thyroid C-cells causing calcitonin release and C-cell proliferation. Endocrinol. 2010;151:1473-86.
38. Elashoff M, Matveyenko AV, Gier B, et al. Pancreatitis, pancreatic, and thyroid cancer with glucagon-like peptide-1-based therapies. Gastroenterol. 2011;141:150-6.
39. Koehler JA, Kain T, Drucker DJ. Glucagon-like peptide-1 receptor activation inhibits growth and augments apoptosis in murine CT26 colon cancer cells. Endocrinol. 2011;152:3362-72.
40. Ligumsky H, Wolf I, Israeli S, et al. The peptide-hormone glucagon-like peptide-1 activates cAMP and inhibits growth of breast cancer cells. Breast Cancer Res Treat. 2012;132:449-61.
41. Alves C, Batel-Marques F, Macedo AF. A meta-analysis of serious adverse events reported with exenatide and liraglutide: acute pancreatitis and cancer. Diabetes Res Clin Pract. 2012;98:271-84.
42. Kim Y, Babu AR. Clinical potential of sodium-glucose co-transporter 2 inhibitors in the management of type 2 diabetes. Diabetes Metab Syndr Obes. 2012;5:313-527.
43. Iyer P, Molitch M. Positive prolactin response to bromocriptine in 2 patients with cabergoline-resistant prolactinomas. Endocr Pract. 2011;17:e55-8.
44. Walker JJ, Johnson JA, Wild SH. Diabetes treatments and cancer risk: the importance of considering aspects of drug exposure, Lancet Diabetes Endocrinol. 2013;1:132-9.
45. Govindarajan R, Ratnasinghe L, Simmons DL, et al. Thiazolidinediones and the risk of lung, prostate and colon cancer in patients with diabetes. J Clin Oncol. 2007;25:1476-81.
46. Ramos-Nino ME, MacLean CD, Littenberg B. Association between cancer prevalence and use of thiazolidinediones: results from the Vermont Diabetes Information System. BMC Med. 2007;5:17.
47. Monami M, Lamanna C, Marchionni N, et al. Rosiglitazone and risk of cancer: a meta-analysis of randomized clinical trials. Diabetes Care. 2008;31:1455-60.
48. Landman GWD, Kleefstra N, van Hateren KJJ, et al. Metformin associated with lower cancer mortality in type 2 diabetes: ZODIAC-16. Diabetes Care. 2010;33:322-6.
49. Baur DM, Klotsche J, Hamnvik OP, et al. Type 2 diabetes mellitus and medications for type 2 diabetes mellitus are associated with risk for and mortality from cancer in a German primary care cohort. Metabolism. 2011;60:1363-71.

Chapter 27

Cardiovascular Outcome Trials with Dipeptidyl Peptidase-4 Inhibitors

Rajesh Rajput

The primary objective of treatment of hyperglycemia is to prevent the various short-term and long-term complications of the same. It has been established that cardiovascular (CV) events are the most common causes for morbidity and mortality in type 2 diabetes mellitus (T2DM) patients. The CV benefit of a standard glucose lowering strategy was established in the landmark the United Kingdom Prospective Diabetes Study (UKPDS), where each 1% reduction in HbA1c led to a significant 14% reduction of all-cause mortality, a 14% reduction in myocardial infarction (MI), 12% reduction in stroke and 16% reduction in the events of heart failure (HF).[1] Subsequent studies conducted in patients of T2DM with established CV risk/cardiovascular disease (CVD) failed to show any superiority of intensive glucose control over standard control in terms of prevention of CV events.[2-4] One must, however, not forget that the UKPDS was conducted in newly diagnosed T2DM patients with no CV risk in contrast to ADVANCE (the Action in Diabetes and Vascular Disease: Preterax and Diamicron MR Controlled Evaluation), ACCORD (the Action to Control Cardiovascular Risk in Type 2 Diabetes) and VADT (the Veterans Affairs Diabetes Trial)[5] trial where patients with long-standing T2DM (8 years, 10 years and 11.5 years, respectively) and established CVD were recruited. In addition, another important difference between these trials was duration of follow-up; patients were followed up for a much longer duration in UKPDS than in the other three landmark CV outcome studies. Based on the lessons learned from these trials, one must achieve glycemic targets as early as possible in natural history of T2DM with drugs that are CV safe.

While there is an established positive correlation between glycemic lowering and the reduction of CV events, paradoxically, some of the glucose lowering agents were found to be associated with increased risk of future CV events. Meta-analysis of studies conducted with rosiglitazone, a popular oral antidiabetic of the thiazolidinedione class suggested a significant increase in overall CV events (21%), HF (27%) and MI (17%).[6] Therefore, it became clear that while glycemic lowering as a strategy could benefit the heart, all the drugs are not equally CV safe. This paradox was one of the key reasons for the drug regulators to create a directive to establish CV safety of the newer antidiabetic agents. The fundamental rationale of the CV safety outcome studies is to answer the question; if one ignores the "glucose lowering", will the new antidiabetic agents still be safe to be used in T2DM patients with a history of CV disease or at high risk of CV disease. The strategy to "ignore glucose lowering" was of course to compare the effect of the new drug with standard antidiabetic regimens in a manner that the glucose lowering is similar in both the arms of the study (glycemic equipoise). In July 2008, the United States Food and Drug Administration (US-FDA) provided a guidance on risk assessment to establish the safety of a new antihyperglycemic medications.[7]

It is important to understand the difference between CV Safety Outcome Trials (CVSOTs) and the glycemic efficacy trials (and their meta-analyses). The glycemic efficacy trials are primarily focused on the glucose lowering efficacy of the drug being studied; they are usually smaller in terms of drug exposure (subject number, usually in hundreds and duration of the study, usually in months) and mostly include low-risk patients. To draw any conclusion of CV safety, even from many such studies analyzed together may therefore be fallacious, especially because the studies individually examine primarily, glycemic control in the study arm, all other factors being similar. On the other hand, dedicated CVSOTs are much broader in scope, especially because they include a much larger number of patients at much higher risk of CV events and followed over a longer duration (at least 2 years). Most importantly their primary objective is to examine the CV safety of the study drug, all other parameters, including glucose control being like the comparator arm.

The dipeptidyl peptidase-4 (DPP-4) inhibitors or "gliptins" is a relatively new class of oral antidiabetics that were launched 2007 onward in all the major markets and soon thereafter became part of the standard of care for T2DM management. Sitagliptin, the first gliptin approved, demonstrated a glycemic efficacy profile comparable to all the other existing oral agents and was not associated with some of the well-recognized and largely accepted hazards of some of the older agents like hypoglycemia and weight gain [especially, with the sulfonylureas (SUs)]. Meta-analysis, Real World Studies and retrospective database analyses also consistently suggested that the gliptins were also safer than the SUs in terms of leading to CV events.[8-11]

Since the CVSOTs are extremely resource intensive and are conducted mostly because of the US-FDA mandate, antidiabetic medications not marketed in the USA are not put through this exercise. Apart from sitagliptin, which was marketed prior to the US-FDA mandate, the other gliptins which either underwent or are undergoing CVSOTs are the ones which are currently marketed in USA, i.e. alogliptin (EXAMINE), saxagliptin (SAVOR-TIMI 53) and linagliptin (CAROLINA and CARMELINA). At this point of time, there is no information about any planned CVSOTs with the other gliptins available elsewhere, namely, vildagliptin, teneligliptin, gemigliptin and trelagliptin. The once weekly omarigliptin which is marketed in Japan and was planned for an US launch also had a CVSOT underway that got terminated (although an interim analysis of data was published) once the sponsor decided not to launch the molecule in the USA.[12] Of the four gliptins marketed in the USA, we therefore have full results of CVSOTs conducted with three gliptins and topline result of CVSOT conducted with the remainder.

Of the three completed, presented and published CVSOTs with the gliptins, SAVOR-TIMI 53 and EXAMINE was aligned with the US-FDA guidance and analyzed a composite of CV death, nonfatal MI and nonfatal stroke as the primary outcome (a 3P-MACE, or three-point major adverse CV events), while sitagliptin, as was designed prior to the mandate also included hospitalization for unstable angina along with the other three, therefore had a 4P-MACE as the primary end-point.[13-15] The TECOS (Trial Evaluating Cardiovascular Outcomes With Sitagliptin) also analyzed a 3P-MACE as the secondary end-point.[16] There are in fact major differences among the five CVSOTs conducted with the 4 gliptins. SAVOR-TIMI 53 was conducted in a population at high risk of CV events (and not necessarily in patients with past CV event).[13] The EXAMINE was conducted in patients with recent onset acute coronary syndromes that included acute MI and unstable angina requiring hospitalization.[14] The TECOS was conducted in patients with established CV Disease.[15] There are, in fact, not one but two CVSOTs conducted with linagliptin. In CAROLINA, linagliptin is compared with glimepiride[16] while, CARMELINA was conducted in patients with an evidence of chronic kidney disease with or without CV disease.[17] In CARMELINA although the primary end-point was 3P-MACE, the secondary end-point primarily considered the renal events.

The primary endpoints for SAVOR-TIMI 53 [3P-MACE hazard ratio (HR): 1.00; confidence interval (CI): 0.89–1.12, $p < 0.001$], EXAMINE (3P-MACE HR: 0.96; CI ≤1.16, $p < 0.001$) and TECOS [4P-MACE HR: 0.98, CI: 0.88–1.09, $p < 0.001$; 3P-MACE (HR: 0.99, CI: 0.89–1.11, $p < 0.001$)] all suggested that the gliptins were just as safe as the existing standard of care in terms of CV safety in patients at high risk of CV events or in patients with history of CV events. None of the agents increased (or decreased) the occurrence of any of the individual components of the end-points, namely, CV death, nonfatal MI or nonfatal stroke. An imbalance was however noticed in the events of HF (recorded as hospitalization for heart failure, HHF) with saxagliptin (HR: 1.27, CI: 1.07–1.51, $p < 0.007$), a finding that was consistent across the patient subtypes and various subset analyses of the SAVOR-TIMI 53 study.[13] The HR for HHF was increased only numerically in EXAMINE (HR: 1.07, CI: 0.79–1.46, p = NS)[18] and was not increased in TECOS (HR: 1.00, CI: 0.83–1.20, $p > 0.1$).[15] Most importantly, the subsequent analysis of the TECOS data confirmed the safety of sitagliptin in terms of occurrence of HHF across patient subtypes including patients with or without any history of HF.[19]

As previously mentioned, it is often difficult to assess the specific CV hazard of a glucose lowering therapy, because the CV benefit of the glycemic lowering may mask the CV hazard. This is where the glycemic equipoise plays a big role. Glycemic equipoise was targeted and largely maintained in most but not all the CVSOTs conducted in the recent years. The between group difference of HbA1c at the end of the study period was 0.29% in TECOS (baseline HbA1c of 7.2%), 0.2% in SAVOR-TIMI 53 (baseline 8.0%) and 0.36% in EXAMINE (baseline 8.0%).[13-15]

In August 2017, the US-FDA updated the label of all the gliptins available in USA to include the observation of an association between DPP-4 inhibitor treatment and HF in CVOTs specifically for two members of the class (i.e. saxagliptin and alogliptin). Accordingly, clinicians were advised to consider the risks and benefits of gliptins prior to initiating treatment in patients at risk for HF, such as those with a prior history of HF and a history of renal impairment, and observe these patients for signs and symptoms of HF during therapy as well as to evaluate and manage and even consider discontinuation of therapy if HF develops.[20]

The CVSOTs with gliptins also confirmed and nullified a lot of other effects of the gliptin class. The gliptins, which are known as a reasonably well-tolerated class, were also well-tolerated in the CVSOTs. Events of interest like pancreatitis, pancreatic cancer, neoplasms, gastrointestinal disorders, musculoskeletal or connective tissue disorders, respiratory or renal disorders were not increased in these large studies conducted over reasonably long duration. These large studies are a gold mine for understanding how this class affects the diabetic patients and the many subsequent subset analyses are constantly adding to what we know about these drugs.

Summarizing, the CVSOTs with the gliptins, especially TECOS, proves that the gliptins could be a rational choice of therapy in a broad range of T2DM patients with preexisting CVD or at high risk of CV events, because they are just as effective as the usual standard of care in terms of glucose lowering and does not increase the risk of CV events compared to the same, at the same time being better tolerated than many of the older therapies which may be associated with therapeutic side effects like hypoglycemia and weight gain.

REFERENCES

1. Stratton IM, Adler AI, Neil HA, et al. Association of glycaemia with macrovascular and microvascular complications of type 2 diabetes (UKPDS 35): prospective observational study. BMJ. 2000;321:405-12.
2. Patel A, MacMahon S, Chalmers J, et al. Intensive Blood Glucose Control and Vascular Outcomes in Patients with Type 2 Diabetes. N Engl J Med. 2008;358:2560-72.
3. Gerstein HC, Miller ME, Byington RP, et al. Effects of intensive glucose lowering in type 2 diabetes. N Engl J Med. 2008;358:2545-59.
4. Ismail-Beigi F, Craven T, Banerji MA, et al. Effect of intensive treatment of hyperglycaemia on microvascular outcomes in type 2 diabetes: an analysis of the ACCORD randomised trial. Lancet. 2010;376:419-30.
5. Duckworth W, Abraira C, Moritz T, et al. Glucose control and vascular complications in veterans with type 2 diabetes. N Engl J Med. 2009;360:129-39.
6. Nissen SE, Wolski K. Effect of Rosiglitazone on the Risk of Myocardial Infarction and Death from Cardiovascular Causes. N Engl J Med. 2007;356:2457-71.
7. US-FDA. (2018). Guidance for Industry Diabetes Mellitus: Evaluating Cardiovascular Risk in New Antidiabetic Therapies to Treat T2 Diabetes. [online] Available from https://www.fda.gov/downloads/Drugs/Guidances/ucm071627.pdf [accessed October, 2018].
8. Zhang Y, Hong J, Chi J, et al. Head-to-head comparison of dipeptidyl peptidase-IV inhibitors and sulphonylureas—a meta-analysis from randomized clinical trials. Diabetes Metab Res Rev. 2014;30(3):241-56.
9. Engel SS, Golm GT, Shapiro D, et al. Cardiovascular safety of sitagliptin in patients with type 2 diabetes mellitus: a pooled analysis. Cardiovasc Diabetol. 2013;12:3.
10. Gamble JM, Thomas JM, Twells LK, et al. Comparative effectiveness of incretin-based therapies and the risk of death and cardiovascular events in 38,233 metformin monotherapy users. Medicine (Baltimore). 2016;95(26):e3995.
11. Gooßen K, Gräber S. Longer term safety of dipeptidyl peptidase-4 inhibitors in patients with type 2 diabetes mellitus: systematic review and meta-analysis. Diabetes Obes Metab. 2012;14(12):1061-72.
12. Gantz I, Chen M, Suryawanshi S, et al. A randomized, placebo-controlled study of the cardiovascular safety of the once-weekly DPP-4 inhibitor omarigliptin in patients with type 2 diabetes mellitus. Cardiovasc Diabetol. 2017;16(1):112.
13. Scirica BM, Bhatt DL, Braunwald E, et al. Saxagliptin and cardiovascular outcomes in patients with type 2 diabetes mellitus. N Engl J Med. 2013;369(14):1317-26.
14. White WB, Cannon CP, Heller SR, et al. Alogliptin after acute coronary syndrome in patients with type 2 diabetes. N Engl J Med. 2013;369(14):1327-35.
15. Green JB, Bethel MA, Armstrong PW, et al. Effect of Sitagliptin on Cardiovascular Outcomes in Type 2 Diabetes. N Engl J Med. 2015;373(3):232-42.
16. Biessels GJ, Janssen J, van den Berg E, et al. Rationale and design of the CAROLINA®—cognition substudy: a randomised controlled trial on cognitive outcomes of linagliptin versus glimepiride in patients with type 2 diabetes mellitus. BMC Neurol. 2018;18(1):7.
17. Rosenstock J, Perkovic V, Alexander JH, et al. Rationale, design, and baseline characteristics of the CArdiovascular safety and Renal Microvascular outcomE study with LINAgliptin (CARMELINA®): a randomized, double-blind, placebo-controlled clinical trial in patients with type 2 diabetes and high cardio-renal risk. Cardiovasc Diabetol. 2018;17(1):39.
18. Zannad F, Cannon CP, Cushman WC, et al. Heart failure and mortality outcomes in patients with type 2 diabetes taking alogliptin versus placebo in EXAMINE: a multicentre, randomised, double-blind trial. Lancet. 2015;385(9982):2067-76.
19. McGuire DK, Van de Werf F, Armstrong PW, et al. Association between Sitagliptin Use and Heart Failure Hospitalization and Related Outcomes in Type 2 Diabetes Mellitus: Secondary Analysis of a Randomized Clinical Trial. JAMA Cardiol. 2016;1(2):126-35.
20. US-FDA. (2017). Drug Safety Labeling Changes (SLC)—Sitagliptin Phosphate, (SUPPL-40). [online] Available from https://www.accessdata.fda.gov/scripts/cder/safetylabelingchanges/index.cfm?event=searchdetail.page&DrugNameID=799. [accessed October, 2018].

Chapter 28

Weekend Therapies in Diabetes Management

Sujeet Jha, Swati Waghdhare

Every year, hundreds of millions of dollars are spent in pursuit of diabetes therapies that are more evolved. This pursuit is modified by informed decision from payers, administrators, patients, physicians and caregivers. An ideal diabetes therapy is one that helps achieve glycemic control without unwarranted side effects of hypoglycemia or weight gain and at the same time be convenient and not taxing on lifestyle besides reducing suffering in terms of micro- and macrovascular complications including death. This broad level agreement has heterogeneity, when broken down into individual preferences, as each concerned person has a variety of preferences regarding the specific characteristics of progressively more favorable diabetes therapies (Table 1).[1]

In this chapter, we wanted to attempt how ease of use coupled with effectiveness and safety addresses some of the expectations that these various stakeholders have and especially so with once weekly therapy options.

A maximally effective drug would address the underlying cause of diabetes. This, in a type 1 diabetes context, should stop the autoimmune process and regenerate β-cells or mimic the physiological insulin secretion function of the pancreas without too much patient hassle or efforts. In a type 2 diabetes (T2D) context, would mean that the drug addresses both insulin resistance and progressive decline in β-cell function. Additional properties of providing robust glycemic control, with cardio and renal protection with weight loss if possible are additional parameters. Ease of use can be broadly defined by the amount of inconvenience associated with taking a drug, how much pain its dosing entails, the flexibility of its dosing, and its duration of action. From this perspective, an ideal therapy would have few steps involved in its administration, could be oral preferably and if injectable should have the flexibility of administration any time of the day without any correlation to meals and should have once daily or preferably once weekly administration.

In this regard, once weekly therapies are a reality in T2D management and specifically so with incretin options (Box 1).

Omarigliptin [Marizev (Japan)] is a small molecule dipeptidyl peptidase-4 (DPP-4) inhibitor developed by Merck for the oral treatment of T2D. Unlike the majority

TABLE 1: Multiple perspectives.[1]

Patient's perspectives	Physician's perspectives	Payer's perspectives
• Effective • Easy to use • Safe and tolerable • Affordable	• Improve patients' health and outcomes • Possess strong efficacy and speak to patients' desires that a drug retain its efficacy overtime • Provide robust glucose control as well as nonglycemic benefits, and address the underlying cause of disease • Safe, meaning that it would not increase the risk for cardiovascular events, cancer, or hypoglycemia	• Best outcomes at the lowest cost • Drug's ability to provide novel or added benefit • Decrease both short- and long-term treatment costs

Box 1: Once weekly/weekend therapies in diabetes.[2]

Dipeptidyl peptidase-4 inhibitors
- Omarigliptin#*: 25 mg weekly dose
- Trelagliptin#*: 100 mg weekly dose

Glucagon-like peptide-1 receptor agonists
- Exenatide once weekly
- Dulaglutide
- Semaglutide*
- Albiglutide*

*not approved in India.
#only approved in Japan.

of other approved agents of its class, which are usually administered once daily, omarigliptin is administered once weekly. Once weekly omarigliptin has received its first global approval in this indication in Japan, for use in adults.[3]

Trelagliptin (Zafatek) is an orally active DPP-4 inhibitor developed by Takeda and approved in Japan for the treatment of type 2 diabetes mellitus (T2DM). Unlike other approved agents of its class, which are usually administered once daily, trelagliptin can be administered once weekly. Phase II development of trelagliptin was discontinued in the USA and EU, as Takeda considered that the costs associated with obtaining approval in these markets were prohibitive.[4]

Once weekly, glucagon-like peptide-1 receptor-agonist (GLP-1RA) dulaglutide has been studied extensively in 6,700 patients in various AWARD [Assessment of Weekly Administration of LY2189265 (dulaglutide) in Diabetes] trials.[5] The efficacy of exenatide once weekly has been examined in six 24–30 weeks randomized trials—the DURATION (Diabetes Therapy Utilization: Researching Changes in A1C, Weight and Other Factors Through Intervention With Exenatide Once Weekly) trials.[6-11]

Once weekly therapies have the advantages of lower pill/injection burden enhanced convenience and adherence, with minimal requirement of self-monitoring of blood glucose. Because it is once weekly administration, there is a possibility of directly observed therapy (DOTs) administration in selected cases, where such schedule is warranted.[12]

The limitations of once weekly therapies are in terms of adverse events. Following administration, these drugs cannot be taken out of the body, rendering the side effects to persist for the extended half-life of the drug in some cases. Hence, a close review of the adverse events of members of this class is warranted.

In my clinical practice experience I have seen benefits, when we have used it as a second-line therapy after metformin. I have a large number of patients on once weekly GLP-1RA. One of the greatest beneficiaries are those who were on basal bolus regime, more so with large insulin requirement, in due course of time, they were shifted to one a week GLP-1RA, they do not require the rapid acting bolus insulin and the requirement of basal insulin also reduces significantly. Weight loss benefits have been significant and much more than what clinical trials have shown. Initially the patient tends to get gastrointestinal side effects on day 2 and 3 of initiation, but with 4th–6th dose of GLP-1RA the side effects subside. So the patient education is very important when introducing these once a week therapy. At our center we have done a retrospective study to analyze 25 obese patients [abstract submitted to the Research Society for the Study of Diabetes in India (RSSDI)] we have seen a significant reduction ($p < 0.001$) in body mass index (BMI), it was also evident from baseline with an mean reduction of 2.31 kg/m^2 [95% confidence interval (CI): 1.49–3.14]. The treatment was well tolerated, with a majority of patients (76%) experiencing no adverse events. Nausea was the most common adverse event reported in 12% of patients.

In conclusion, once weekly therapies might specifically benefit that subgroup of patients who have poor glycemic control, patients who are reluctant on initiating insulin due to the fear of daily multiple pricks, not compliant on multiple daily medications or find it difficult to accommodate daily administration of drugs in to their busy life schedule. Patient education on the effects and side effects of the therapy is very important. However, a close review of the efficacy and adverse events profile is required before embarking on any of these therapies.

REFERENCES

1. Rotenstein LS, Kozak BM, Shivers JP, et al. The Ideal Diabetes Therapy: What Will It Look Like? How Close Are We? Clinical Diabetes. 2012;30(2):44-53.
2. Kalra S, Gupta Y. Weekend therapy in diabetes. Prim Care Diabetes. 2016;66(5):627-8.
3. Burness CB. Omarigliptin: first global approval. Drugs. 2015;75(16):1947-52.
4. McKeage K. Trelagliptin: First Global Approval. Drugs. 2015;75(10):1161-4.
5. file:///C:/Users/c189272/Downloads/Priloha_Medical%20SPECIAL_AWARD%20Trials%20Compendium.pdf
6. Bergenstal RM, Wysham C, Macconell L, et al. Efficacy and safety of exenatide once weekly versus sitagliptin or pioglitazone as an adjunct to metformin for treatment of type 2 diabetes (DURATION-2): a randomised trial. Lancet. 2010;376(9739):431-9.

7. Blevins T, Pullman J, Malloy J, et al. DURATION-5: exenatide once weekly resulted in greater improvements in glycemic control compared with exenatide twice daily in patients with type 2 diabetes. J Clin Endocrinol Metab. 2011;96:1301-310.
8. Buse JB, Nauck M, Forst T, et al. Exenatide once weekly versus liraglutide once daily in patients with type 2 diabetes (DURATION-6): a randomised, open-label study. Lancet. 2013;381:117-24.
9. Diamant M, Van Gaal L, Stranks S, et al. Once weekly exenatide compared with insulin glargine titrated to target in patients with type 2 diabetes (DURATION-3): an openlabel randomised trial. Lancet. 2010;375:2234-43.
10. Drucker DJ, Buse JB, Taylor K, et al. Exenatide once weekly versus twice daily for the treatment of type 2 diabetes: a randomised, open-label, non-inferiority study. Lancet. 2008;372:1240-50.
11. Russell-Jones D, Cuddihy RM, Hanefeld M, et al. Efficacy and safety of exenatide once weekly versus metformin, pioglitazone, and sitagliptin used as monotherapy in drug-naive patients with type 2 diabetes (DURATION-4): a 26-week double-blind study. Diabetes Care. 2012;35: 252-8.
12. Kalra S, GuptaY. DOT (directly observed therapy) in diabetes: Current thought, future reality. Aust J Rural Health. 2014;22:206.

Chapter 29

Sodium-glucose Transporter 2 Inhibitors and Kidney

Manisha Sahay, Rakesh Sahay

INTRODUCTION

Diabetic kidney disease (DKD) is the leading cause of end-stage renal disease (ESRD) in India.[1] Our country has a population of 1.2 billion out of which 72 million are diabetics. About 30–40% of all diabetics progress to ESRD. Patients with ESRD need renal replacement therapy in the form of dialysis or transplantation both of which are available in India widely. However, the cost of these therapies is high. Dialysis costs around 30,000 INR per month while the cost of transplantation varies from 5 to 7 lakhs. Both these therapies are available free of cost in many states including our state, i.e. Telangana, but it imposes a huge economic burden on the government. Each dialysis requires about 120 L of water and generates a huge amount of biohazardous waste. Transplantation needs lifelong immunosuppression and increases the risk of infections and malignancies in the long-term. Thus, the best option is prevention of development of chronic kidney disease (CKD) in a diabetic patient.

The important measures to prevent development of DKD are glycemic control, control of hypertension, use of angiotensin-converting enzyme (ACE) inhibitors and angiotensin II receptor blockers (ARBs), control of dyslipidemia, avoidance of acute insults to the kidney, i.e. avoidance of nephrotoxic drugs, e.g. nonsteroidal anti-inflammatory drugs (NSAIDs), antibiotics like aminoglycosides, vancomycin, avoidance of high molecular weight contrast studies, e.g. CT contrast, etc., prompt treatment of infections, correction of volume depletion, removal of any obstruction in the urinary tract, low protein diet and restriction of salt to half tea spoon per day.[2]

A significant advancement in prevention of progression of CKD in a diabetic patient has been the development of hypoglycemic agents which in addition to control of glycemia cause renoprotection. These include liraglutide and sodium-glucose transporter 2 (SGLT2) inhibitors.

MECHANISM OF ACTION OF SODIUM-GLUCOSE TRANSPORTER 2 INHIBITORS

In normoglycemia the glomerular filtration rate (GFR) is about 180 L/day and blood glucose concentration is 90–100 mg/dL. Approximately 162–180 g of glucose passes from Bowman's capsule into the tubular lumen. The entire glucose load is reabsorbed by SGLT2 transporters. Tubular glucose reabsorption increases linearly with increasing blood glucose levels, until the glucose transport system becomes saturated. Transport maximum for the glucose (TmG) tubular transport system in adults is about 375 mg/min. TmG corresponds with a blood glucose level of approximately 300 mg/dL, which is referred to as the renal threshold for glucose.

Sodium-glucose transporter receptors are present on the luminal side of proximal convoluted tubules and transport glucose from luminal to intracellular space against the concentration gradient. There are two types of SGLT receptors in the tubule of which SGLT2 is responsible for 90% of glucose absorption (Fig. 1 and Table 1).[3] SGLT2 inhibitors decrease glucose reabsorption in the tubules and increase urine glucose excretion. Various SGLT2 inhibitors are available (Table 2).

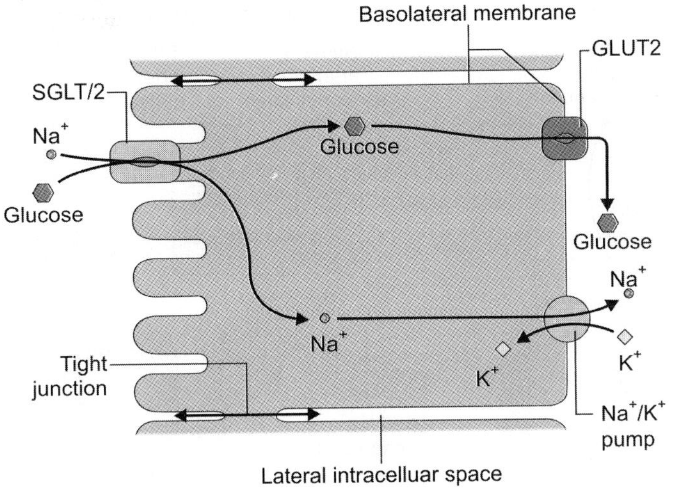

Figure 1 Sodium-glucose transporter 2 inhibitors (SGLT2) inhibitors in proximal tubule cells.

TABLE 1: SGLT1 and SGLT2 inhibitors.

Characteristics	SGLT1	SGLT2
Location	Small intestine; later part of PCT (segment 3) in kidney	Early PCT (segment 1, 2)
Capacity	Low	High
Affinity	High	Low
% glucose reabsorption	10%	90%
Disease if mutation	Glucose-galactose malabsorption	Familial renal glycosuria
Disease symptoms and signs	Diarrhea at few days age	None
Course	Fatal without glucose free/ galactose free diet	Benign
Inhibitors	Phlorizin	Currently available SGLT2 inhibitor

(PCT: proximal convoluted tubule; SGLT: sodium-glucose transporter.)

EFFECT ON RENAL HEMODYNAMICS

Inhibition of tubuloglomerular feedback: Brenner[4] demonstrated that glomerular hyperfiltration accompanied by glomerular capillary hypertension is a pathophysiological mechanism for initiation and progression of renal disease, regardless of the nature of the initial injury.

The two most important pathophysiological mechanisms leading to renal hyperfiltration are efferent arteriole constriction and/or afferent arteriole dilatation which are both affected in diabetes.

Changes in efferent arteriolar tone occur due to neurohormonal activation mostly due to renin-angiotensin-aldosterone system (RAAS) activation.

Afferent arteriolar dilation is controlled by tubular feedback. The tubular hypothesis states that hyperglycemia causes an increase in proximal tubule glucose filtered load in diabetes. This results in overactivity of SGLT2 and SGLT1 with increased tubular reabsorption of glucose and sodium.[5-8] This increased proximal sodium reabsorption leads to decreased sodium delivery to distal tubule and macula densa, with consequent reduction in adenosine triphosphate (ATP) breakdown and adenosine production. Adenosine is a strong vasoconstrictor, and its reduction causes vasodilatation of the afferent arteriole and thus hyperfiltration (Fig. 2). Abnormalities

TABLE 2: SGLT2 inhibitors.

Canagliflozin	Yes	100–300	Dose limited to 100 mg once daily in patients with eGFR >45 <60 mL/min/1.73 m^2 Stopped in patients with eGFR <45 mL/min/1.73 m^2
Empagliflozin	Yes	10-25	Dose adjustment in patients with creatinine clearance <60 mL/min Contraindicated in patients with creatinine clearance <45 mL/min No adjustment in hepatic failure
Dapagliflozin	Yes	5–10	Should not be initiated in patients with eGFR <60 mL/min/1.73 m^2 No dose adjustment in patients with eGFR >60 mL/min/1.73 m^2
Ipragliflozin	No	100–300	Dose limited to 100 mg once daily in patients with eGFR >45 <60 mL/min/1.73 m^2 Not recommended in patients with eGFR <45 mL/min/1.73 m^2
Luseogliflozin	No	–	–
Tofogliflozin	No	–	–

(eGFR: estimated glomerular filtration rate; SGLT2: sodium-glucose transporter 2.)

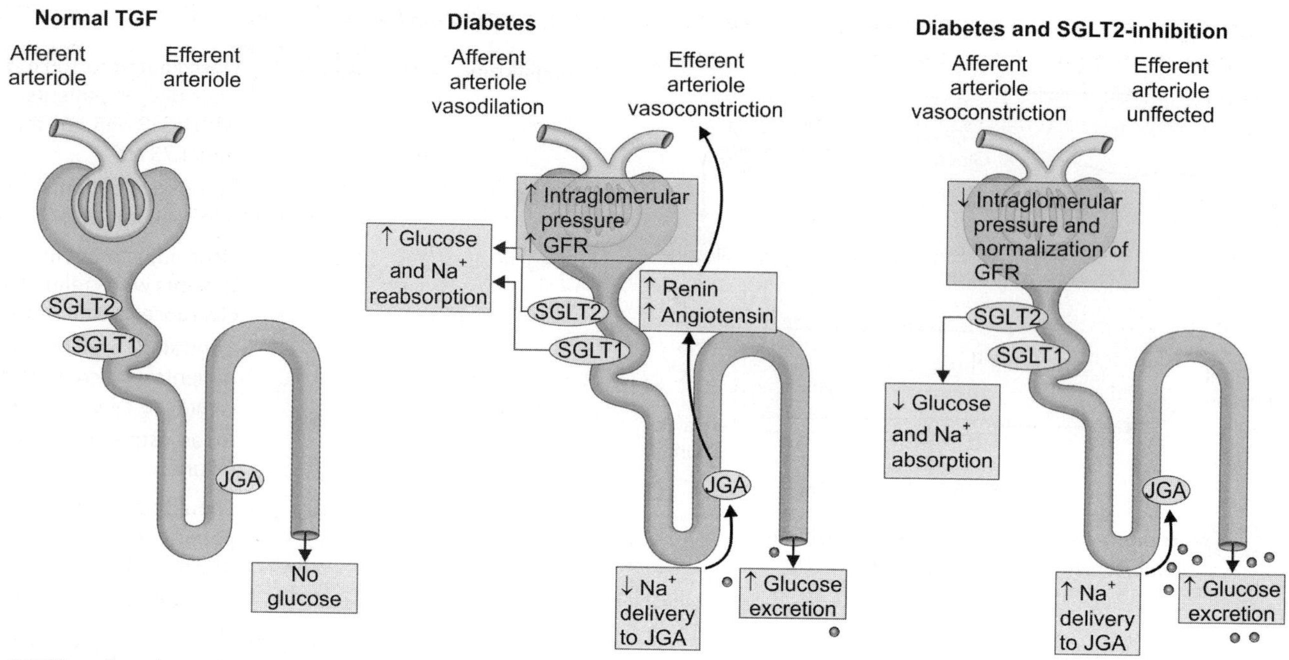

(SGLT1: sodium-glucose transporter 1; JGA: juxtaglomerular apparatus; GFR: glomerular filtration rate; Na: sodium; K: potassium.)

Figure 2 Mechanism of action of sodium-glucose transporter 2 (SGLT2) inhibitors.

in the tubuloglomerular feedback system and increased proximal tubular sodium reabsorption, with consequent reduction in distal delivery, have also been demonstrated in patients with type 1 or type 2 diabetes (T2D). SGLT 2 inhibitor cause afferent arteriolar constriction by tubuloglomerular feedback and hence decrease intraglomerular hypertension (Fig. 2).[5] Thus, the actions of ACE inhibitor and SGLT2 inhibitor are additive, ACE inhibitor act on the efferent arteriole and SGLT2 inhibitor act on the afferent arteriole.

GLYCEMIC EFFECTS

Sodium-glucose transporter 2 inhibitors are weak glucose-lowering agents, with mean reductions in HbA1c between 0.4 and 1.1% depending on baseline hyperglycemia. They can be used as monotherapy or in combination with Metformin, Sulfonylureas, Glitazones, Gliptins and Insulin. SGLT2 inhibitors approved in India are Dapagliflozin, Canagliflozin and Empagliflozin. Reduction in blood glucose is noninsulin-mediated. SGLT2 inhibitors have both basal and postprandial antihyperglycemic effects. Total insulin use can be decreased. However, SGLT2 inhibitors are not approved for type 1 diabetes mellitus (T1DM) as SGLT2 inhibitors are associated with euglycemic ketoacidosis especially in T1DM. SGLT2 inhibitors increase hepatic gluconeogenesis and decrease renal gluconeogenesis and increase pancreatic β-cell mass.[5,8,9]

EFFECT ON BLOOD PRESSURE

Sodium-glucose transporter 2 inhibitors consistently lower systolic blood pressure (BP) by ≈5 mm Hg and diastolic BP by ≈2 mm Hg in patients with type 2 diabetes mellitus (T2DM) and restore normal nocturnal BP dipping. Greater BP-lowering effect is observed with the combination of an SGLT2 inhibitor with a RAAS-blocker versus either agent alone.

Sodium-glucose transporter 2 inhibitors reduce BP by multiple mechanisms:

- These cause natriuresis. Even though natriuresis and plasma volume contraction are attenuated in CKD, there is a heightened sensitivity to even small changes in plasma volume, leading to persistent BP-lowering
- SGLT2 inhibition modulates renal lipid metabolism and inflammation via inhibition of CD68+ macrophage accumulation and expression of p65, toll-like receptor 4, monocyte chemoattractant protein-1, and osteopontin which decrease systolic BP
- SGLT2 inhibitor reduce arterial stiffness
- SGLT2 inhibitors act on ACE2-(angiotensin 1–7) pathways. Other neurohormones and RAAS are not affected. CKD patients have higher BPs and SGLT2

inhibition may lead to greater antihypertensive effects in those with higher BP at baseline.[10-14]

Weight reduction occurs due to natriuresis and diuretic effects and also due to loss of glucose in urine.

URIC ACID LOWERING EFFECT

Plasma uric acid levels have been associated with hypertension, cardiovascular disease (CVD) and renal disease. SGLT2 inhibitors are associated with a 10–15% reduction in plasma uric acid levels as a result of increased glycosuria, leading to secretion of uric acid in exchange for glucose reabsorption via the GLUT-9 transporter.[15]

LIPID-LOWERING EFFECTS

Sodium-glucose transporter 2 inhibitors reduce the levels of triglycerides and may increase high-density lipoprotein (HDL).[16]

CARDIOVASCULAR EFFECTS

Sodium-glucose transporter 2 inhibitors were found to be cardiovascular (CV) protective.[17] In two trials [Canagliflozin Cardiovascular Assessment Study (CANVAS) and CANVAS-R (renal)][18,19] to assess the effects of canagliflozin on CV and renal outcomes in patients with T2D and high CV risk, 10,142 patients (mean A1c 8.2%) were randomly assigned to canagliflozin or placebo. After a mean follow-up 3.6 years, the primary outcome, a composite of death from CV causes, nonfatal myocardial infarction or nonfatal stroke, occurred in fewer patients in the canagliflozin group. Similarly, EMPA-REG trial found empagliflozin to be cardioprotective.[20]

EFFECTS ON KIDNEYS

The SGLT2 inhibitors are renoprotective.[21,22] Dapagliflozin was shown to reduce albuminuria.[23] Several landmark trials confirmed the renoprotective effects of SGLT2 inhibitors (Table 2).

Canagliflozin Treatment and Trial Analysis versus Sulfonylurea (CANATA-SU) study included 1,450 type 2 diabetics with baseline estimated glomerular filtration rate (eGFR) >55 mL/min/1.73 m^2. All participants were treated with metformin, 60% were treated renin-angiotensin system (RAS) blocker. Each participant was randomly assigned to add-on therapy with one of two doses of canagliflozin or with glimepiride, used as an active control. Secondary analysis showed that over 2 years follow-up, decline in eGFR was significantly slower with either canagliflozin dose compared with glimepiride. Canagliflozin also reduced albuminuria, compared with glimepiride. These differences occurred with little difference in HbA1c between treatment groups, suggesting effects are not mediated by blood glucose.[24]

The EMPA-REG (Empagliflozin Cardiovascular Outcome Event Trial) conducted over 3 years in 7,020 patients was designed specifically to evaluate CV morbidity and mortality in patients with T2DM and established CVD (99.5%), mean GFR 83, 26% had GFR <60 microvascular disease was a prespecified secondary outcome. The composite microvascular endpoint (the initiation of retinal photocoagulation, vitreous hemorrhage, diabetes-related blindness or incident or worsening nephropathy) occurred in fewer patients in the empagliflozin group (14% vs. 20.5%).[25]

The CREDENCE (Canagliflozin and Renal Events in Diabetes with Established Nephropathy Clinical Evaluation) study is testing the effects of canagliflozin versus placebo on the occurrence of ESRD, doubling of serum creatinine and renal or CV death. CREDENCE was terminated early as there was a strong signal for favorable renal outcomes.

Data from CANVAS[18] and CANVAS-R trials[19] reported that the therapy was associated with a reduced risk of sustained kidney function lost, decline in eFGR and reduction in albuminuria versus placebo. The VERTIS trial for ertugliflozin, DECLARE and DAPA-CKD for dapagliflozin are all underway.

Cherney et al.[26] pooled data from 2,286 patients with T2D in five randomized, placebo-controlled, phase III clinical trials lasting 24 weeks and observed that there was a disconnect effect of empagliflozin on glycated hemoglobin (HbA1c) lowering and its effect on weight and BP reductions in renal impairment. HbA1c reductions and weight reduction with empagliflozin waned at lower levels of eGFR, whereas BP reductions were maintained.[26]

ADVERSE EFFECTS

Increased risk of genitourinary fungal infections and increased risk of urinary tract infection (UTI) due to glycosuria are seen.[27]

Euglycemic diabetic ketoacidosis (eu-DKA) is one of the most life-threatening complications of SGLT2 inhibitors. The following are the proposed mechanisms for eu-DKA:

- Glycosuria by SGLT2 lowers blood glucose which results in reduced secretion of insulin from pancreatic β-cells. This increases the secretion of glucagon from the pancreatic α-cells. Also, SGLT2 inhibitors are α-cell secretagogues and increase glucagon directly. Lack of insulin and elevation of glucagon causes increased glycogenolysis and gluconeogenesis in the liver. High glucose spills over into the urine and causes osmotic diuresis, polyuria, dehydration and polydipsia. Reduced insulin and increased glucagon levels initiate lipolysis in adipose tissues and β-oxidation of fatty acids, leading to the formation of ketone bodies in the liver and thus eu-DKA

- Sodium-glucose transporter 2 inhibitors may decrease excretion of ketone bodies synthesized in the body by reducing GFR.

In hyperglycemic DKA high blood sugar prompts testing for urine or blood ketones, leading to early diagnosis and management of DKA. Unfortunately, hyperglycemia is absent in type 1 diabetics taking SGLT2 inhibitors and eu-DKA ensues. In addition, as the blood sugar is not high, insulin dose is not increased and even may be reduced, thus worsening the acidosis. Significant delay in diagnosis and treatment occurs. The eu-DKA is one of the life-threatening side effects of SGLT2 inhibitor.

Risk factors for DKA include infection, dehydration, low-carbohydrate diet or reduced caloric intake, alcohol use, steroid use, reduced dose or discontinuation of insulin or oral insulin secretagogue therapy or change in insulin dose.

Sodium-glucose transporter 2 inhibitors are not Food and Drug Administration (FDA)-approved for use in people with type-1 diabetes and off label use should be avoided.

In people with T2D, there is no clear risk to suggest DKA with SGLT2 inhibitor. Case reports are however noted in the literature. In the EMPA-REG OUTCOME study the frequency of DKA in those exposed to dapagliflozin was <0.1%.

Sodium-glucose transporter 2 inhibitors should be interrupted during prolonged fasting, illness or surgery, low-carbohydrate diet, volume depletion, stress or changes in insulin or insulin-secretagogue doses.

ACUTE KIDNEY INJURY

Canagliflozin was licensed for use in March 2013 by the FDA. Subsequently FDA issued a warning in 2015 about the risk of DKA associated with SGLT2 inhibitor. The FDA has added this warning to the labels of all SGLT2 inhibitor. It is possible that SGLT2i inhibitor may predispose to acute kidney injury (AKI) by volume depletion because of their natriuretic properties, effects on tubuloglomerular feedback and various other mechanisms. In addition, the volume and intrarenal hemodynamic effects of SGLT2 inhibitors are synergistic when combined with RAAS antagonists and diuretics in T2DM. However, empagliflozin was not associated with increased risk of AKI in EMPA-REG OUTCOMES. Bone fractures are also reported to occur with SGLT2 inhibitor. There was an increase in the risk of lower limb amputations and fractures in canagliflozin-treated patients.

There were some reports of dapagliflozin and empagliflozin and bladder and breast cancer. However, this needs further study.

CONCLUSION

Sodium-glucose transporter 2 inhibitors are a second-line or later therapy option for the management of T2D. Unlike the glucose-lowering effects of SGLT2 inhibitor, the spill-over of sodium and glucose beyond the proximal nephron following SGLT2 inhibition triggers dynamic and reversible realignment of energy metabolism, renal filtration and plasma volume without relying on losses into the urine. In addition, these processes are observed in the absence the resetting of energy/salt/water physiology following SGLT2 inhibition has an impact, not only on adiposity, renal function and BP control, but also on the health and survival of patients with T2D. Patients should be educated about the risks of DKA.

Precautions before starting Sodium-glucose transporter 2

Prior to starting an SGLT2 inhibitor, volume status and renal function (serum creatinine with eGFR) should be assessed. Hypovolemia should be corrected prior to initiating an SGLT2 inhibitor. Liver function should be assessed prior to initiation of canagliflozin or dapagliflozin. Patients at risk for falls and fracture may benefit from assessment of bone density. If SGLT2 inhibitors are prescribed, then it should be used with extreme caution. Adequate patient counseling and close monitoring for sign and symptoms of ketosis is advisable in such cases. Urine or blood ketones should be regularly checked in patients taking SGLT2 inhibitor.

REFERENCES

1. Rajapurkar MM, John GT, Kirpalani AL, et al. What do we know about chronic kidney disease in India: first report of the Indian CKD Registry. BMC Nephrol. 2012;13:10.
2. Umanath K, Lewis JB. Update on Diabetic Nephropathy: Core Curriculum. Am J Kidney Dis. 2018;71(6):884-95.
3. Wright E, Loo D, Hirayama B. Biology of human sodium glucose transporters. Physiol Rev. 2011;91:733-94.
4. Brenner B, Hostetter T, Olson J, et al. The role of glomerular hyperfiltration in the initiation and progression of diabetic nephropathy. Acta Endocrinol Suppl (Copenh). 1981;242:7-10.
5. DeFronzo RA, Norton L, Abdul-Ghani M. Renal, metabolic and cardiovascular considerations of SGLT2 inhibition. Nat Rev Nephrol. 2017; 13:11-26.
6. Cherney DZ, Perkins BA, Soleymanlou N, et al. Renal hemodynamic effect of sodium-glucose cotransporter 2 inhibition in patients with type 1 diabetes mellitus. Circulation. 2014;129:587-97.
7. Tang SC, Lai KN. The pathogenic role of the renal proximal tubular cell in diabetic nephropathy. Nephrol Dial Transplant. 2012;27:3049-56.
8. Abdul-Ghani M, DeFronzo R. Inhibition of renal glucose reabsorption: a novel strategy for achieving glucose control in type 2 diabetes mellitus. Endocr Pract. 2008;14:782-90.
9. Vasilakou D, Karagiannis T, Athanasiadou E, et al. Sodium-glucose cotransporter 2 inhibitors for type 2 diabetes: a systematic review and meta-analysis. Ann Intern Med. 2013;159:262-74.
10. Lovshin JA, Gilbert RE. Are SGLT2-inhibitors reasonable antihypertensive drugs and renoprotective? Curr Hypertens Rep. 2015;17:551.
11. Novikov A, Vallon V. Sodium glucose cotransporter 2 inhibition in the diabetic kidney: an update. Curr Opin Nephrol Hypertens. 2015;24:1-9.
12. Cherney DZ, Perkins BA, Soleymanlou N, et al. The effect of empagliflozin on arterial stiffness and heart rate variability in subjects with uncomplicated type 1 diabetes mellitus. Cardiovasc Diabetol. 2014;13:28.
13. Kohan DE, Fioretto P, Tang W, et al. Long-term study of patients with type 2 diabetes and moderate renal impairment shows that dapagliflozin reduces weight and blood pressure but does not improve glycemic control. Kidney Int. 2014;85:962-71.
14. Mazidi M, Rezaie P, Gao HK, et al. Effect of sodium-glucose cotransport-2 inhibitors on blood pressure in people with type 2 diabetes mellitus: A systematic review and meta-analysis of 43 randomized control trials with 22,528 patients. J Am Heart Assoc. 20176(6). pii: e004007.
15. Lytvyn Y, et al. Glycosuria-mediated urinary uric acid excretion in patients with uncomplicated type 1 diabetes mellitus. Am J Physiol Renal Physiol. 2015;308(2):F77-83.
16. Stenlof K, Cefalu W, Kim K, et al. Efficacy and safety of canagliflozin monotherapy in subjects with type 2 diabetes mellitus inadequately controlled with diet and exercise. Diabetes Obes Metab. 2013;15:372-82.
17. Heerspink HJ, Perkins BA, Fitchett DH, et al. Sodium glucose cotransporter 2 inhibitors in the treatment of diabetes mellitus: Cardiovascular and kidney effects, potential mechanisms, and clinical applications. Circulation. 2016;134(10):752-72.
18. Neal B, Perkovic V, de Zeeuw D, et al. Rationale, design, and baseline characteristics of the Canagliflozin Cardiovascular Assessment Study (CANVAS)–a randomized placebo-controlled trial. Am Heart J. 2013;166: 217-23.
19. Neal B, Perkovic V, Matthews DR, et al. Rationale, design and baseline characteristics of the CANagliflozincardio Vascular Assessment Study-Renal (CANVAS-R): a randomized, placebo-controlled trial. Diabetes Obes Metab. 2017;19:387-93.
20. Zinman B, Wanner C, Lachin JM, et al. Empagliflozin, Cardiovascular Outcomes, and Mortality in Type 2 Diabetes. N Engl J Med. 2015;373: 2117-28.
21. Gilbert RE. Sodium-glucose linked transporter-2 inhibitors: potential for renoprotection beyond blood glucose lowering? Kidney Int. 2014;86: 693-700.
22. De Nicola L, Gabbai FB, Liberti ME, et al. Sodium/glucose co-transporter 2 inhibitors and prevention of diabetic nephropathy: targeting the renal tubule in diabetes. Am J Kidney Dis. 2014;64:16-24.
23. Fioretto P, Stefansson BV, Johnsson EKA, et al. Dapagliflozin reduces albuminuria over 2 years in diabetic patients with renal impairment (Abstract). J Am Soc Nephrol. 2015;26:1A.
24. Cefalu WT, Leiter LA, Yoon KH, et al. Efficacy and safety of canagliflozin versus glimepiride in patients with type 2 diabetes inadequately controlled with metformin (CANTATA-SU): 52 week results from a randomised, double-blind, phase 3 non-inferiority trial. Lancet. 2013;382:941-50.
25. Barnett AH, Mithal A, Manassie J, et al. EMPA-REG RENAL trial investigators. Efficacy and safety of empagliflozin added to existing antidiabetes treatment in patients with type 2 diabetes and chronic kidney disease: a randomised, double-blind, placebo-controlled trial. Lancet Diabetes Endocrinol. 2014;2:369-84.
26. Cherney DZI, Cooper ME, Tikkanen I, et al. Pooled analysis of Phase III trials indicate contrasting influences of renal function on blood pressure, body weight, and HbA1c reductions with empagliflozin. Kidney Int. 2018;93:231-44.
27. Filippas-Ntekouan S, Filippatos TD, Elisaf MS. SGLT2i: are they safe? Postgraduate Med. 2018;130(1):72-82.

Chapter 30

Intensive Glycemic Control Improves Survival (Against the Motion)

Vinod Mittal

INTRODUCTION

Type 2 diabetes mellitus (T2DM) is a strong risk factor for the cardiovascular (CV) outcome and the incidence of bad CV outcomes increases with the increase in degree of hyperglycemia.[1] In the past, the blood glucose levels up to 220 mg/dL was considered and only excessive hyperglycemia exceeding this value was considered for the treatment.[2] However, after the demonstrated mortality benefit in a subgroup of overweight patients receiving metformin in the UK Prospective Diabetes Study (UKPDS), attention has been focused on intensive glycemic control for prevention of CV events.[3] However, other large randomized controlled trials have yielded mixed findings with respect to the favorable effects of intensive glucose lowering.

In 2009, Veterans Affairs Diabetes Trial (VADT) compared the effects of intensive and standard glucose control on CV events. The study reported that the intensive glucose control had minimal effects on microvascular complications (severe renal changes, decreased glomerular filtration rate, laser treatment, cataract extraction, vitrectomy, and new neuropathy) during a period of 5–6 years (Fig. 1).[4]

A. Shows time until the first occurrence of a major CV event (the primary outcome), which was a composite of myocardial infarction (MI), stroke, death from CV causes, congestive heart failure (HF), surgery for vascular disease, inoperable coronary disease, and amputation for ischemic gangrene, in the standard-therapy group and the intensive-therapy group, with a hazard ratio (HR) in the intensive-therapy group of 0.88 [95% confidence interval (CI), 0.74–1.05]
B. Shows the time until death from a CV cause (a component of the primary outcome), with a HR of 1.32 (95% CI, 0.81–2.14)
C. Shows time until death from any cause (a secondary outcome), with a HR of 1.07 (95% CI, 0.81–1.42). Adapted from: Duckworth W et al.

However in 2012, ACCORD (Action to Control Cardiovascular Risk in Diabetes) was specifically designed to determine the effects of intensive treatment of blood glucose on atherosclerotic CV disease outcomes in patients with T2DM who were at high risk. The study demonstrated an increased risk of total mortality (HR, 1.22) and CVD death (HR, 1.35) with lack of benefit in either the primary CVD outcome or primary microvascular outcome (Fig. 2).[5]

Further, the Action in Diabetes and Vascular Disease: Preterax and Diamicron Modified Release Controlled Evaluation (ADVANCE) trial also reported no significant decrease in CV events with intensive glucose control.

Moreover, the ACCORDION trial, which included 8,601 T2DM subjects followed for mean duration of a median 8.8-year reported that intensive glucose lowering for a mean of 3.7 years had a neutral long-term effect on the first occurrence of composite CV outcome, defined as nonfatal MI, nonfatal stroke, or CV death; however, increased risk of CV death reported during ACCORD (1.49; 95% CI 1.19, 1.87; $p < 0.0001$) was still evident during long-term follow-up (1.20, 95% CI 1.03–1.40, $p = 0.02$).[6] This follow-on study do not demonstrate beneficial legacy

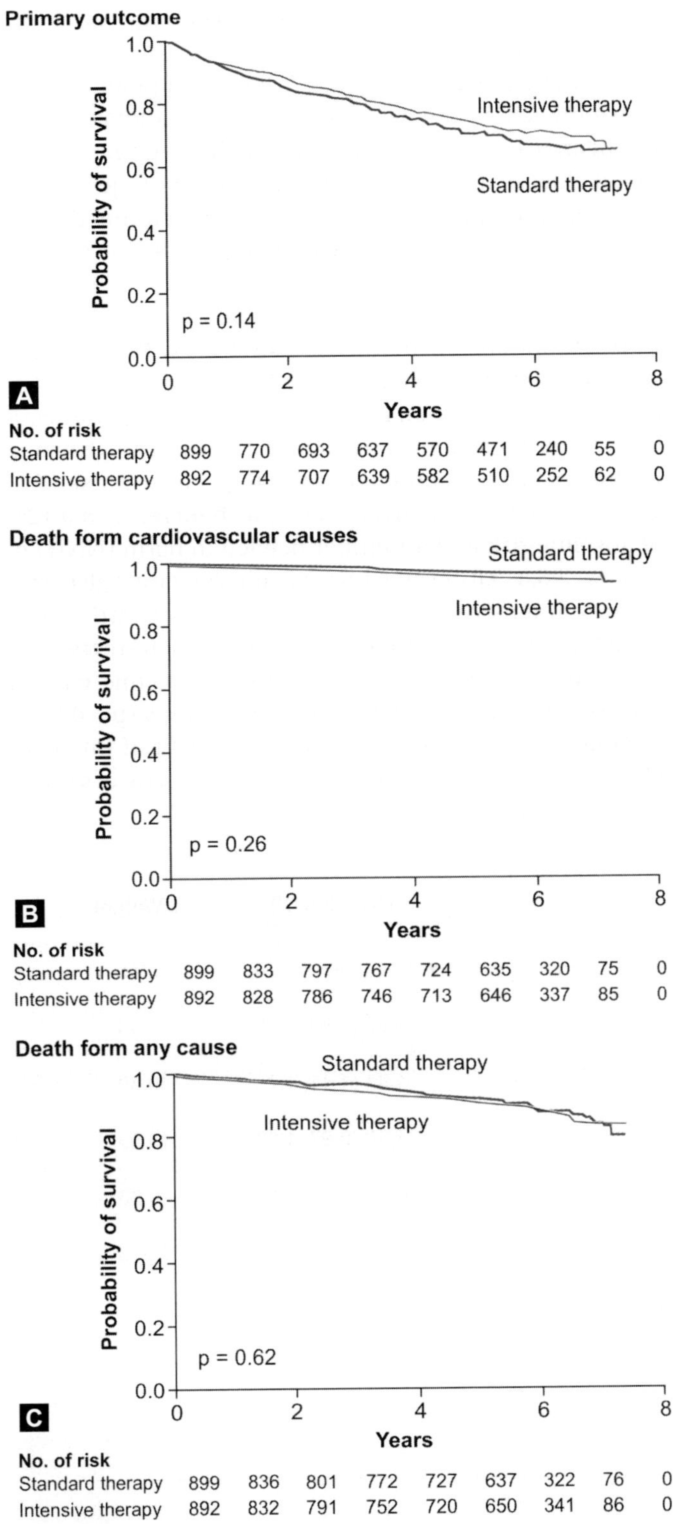

Figure 1 Kaplan–Meier curves for the time til the first occurrence of a primary or secondary outcome.

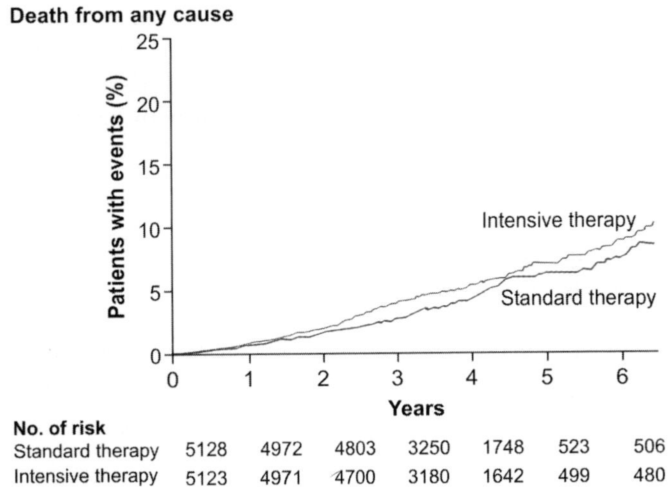

Figure 2 Kaplan–Meier curves for death from any cause after 3.4-year median duration follow-up.

of 3.7 years of intensive glucose lowering therapy on CV events and 20% higher risk of CV death in ACCORDIAN study can be attributed to absolute risk difference of 1.3% over years. Thus, pointing towards the absence of any clinical benefits from the intensive lowering over a median follow-up of 8.8 years in patients with T2DM and high CV risk.

In addition, in 2009, normoglycemia in intensive care evaluation-survival using glucose algorithm regulation (NICE-SUGAR) trial involved 6,104 adult participants admitted to the ICUs (intensive care units). Hyperglycemia is common in acutely ill patients, including those treated in ICUs and it has been associated with increased morbidity and mortality in such group of patients. The results of the NICE-SUGAR trial showed increased 90-day mortality in the intensive glucose control to target 81–108 mg/dL when compared to conventional glucose control to target ≤180 mg/dL (Fig. 3). Additionally, the risk of severe hypoglycemia was significantly higher in the intensive control group. Based on the findings of this study, intensive glucose control was not recommended for patients in the ICU.[7]

Another meta-analysis of randomized controlled trials comparing strategies of more versus less intensive glucose-lowering in patients with HF. As we know poor glycemic control has been associated with an increased risk of HF, it is unknown whether improved glycemic control reduces this risk. This study included 37,229 HF patients (from eight randomized trials). Meta-analytic pooling demonstrated that intensive glucose control did not influence the overall occurrence of HF and has been associated with a 20% increase of HF risk (Fig. 4), when compared with conventional treatment leading to a conclusion that in patients with T2DM, tight glycemic control does not reduce the risk of HF.[8]

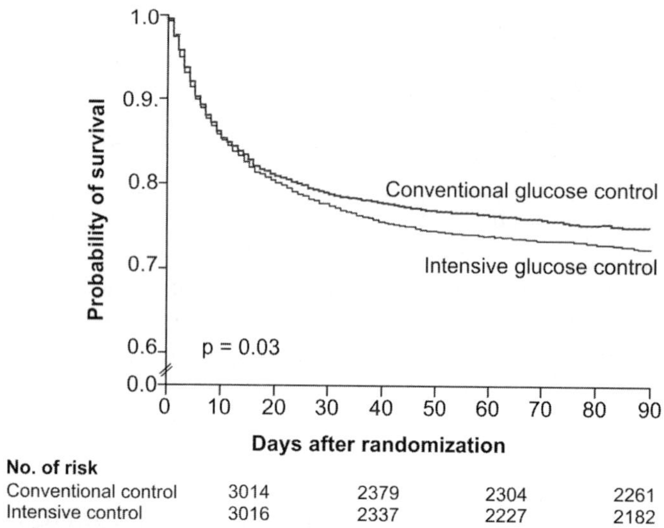

Figure 3 Kaplan–Meier estimates for the probability of survival, which at 90 days was greater in the conventional control group than in the intensive-control group (hazard ratio, 1.11; 95% confidence interval, 1.01–1.23; p = 0.03).

Further, the 2009 ACC/AHA focused update on ST-elevation acute MI gave a weak recommendation for the use of an insulin-based regimen to achieve and maintain blood glucose less than 180 mg/dL and Chatterjee S et al. decided to assess the validity of this recommendation. As, number of early trials comparing intensive glucose control in T2DM with an MI reported a decrease in mortality over a short period of follow up leading to a presumption of improved survival with intensive glucose control; however, shortly data disproved this hypothesis. A meta-analysis carried out by Chatterjee S et al. reported significantly higher rates of hypoglycemia in the intensive glucose control group [relative risk (RR) 13.40, 95% CI 3.69–48.61; p <0.01], with increase in a 12% of absolute risk and a number needed to harm (NNH) of 9 (95% CI 6.8–9.8)-even without achieving target glycemic control. Intensive control failed to improve cardiac HF, arrhythmias and reinfarction rates. Meta-regression revealed that mortality with intensive glycemic control was worse with increased duration of therapy (p = 0.001). Overall, this study recorded limited benefit of intensive glycemic control in T2DM with a significant risk of serious hypoglycemia.[9]

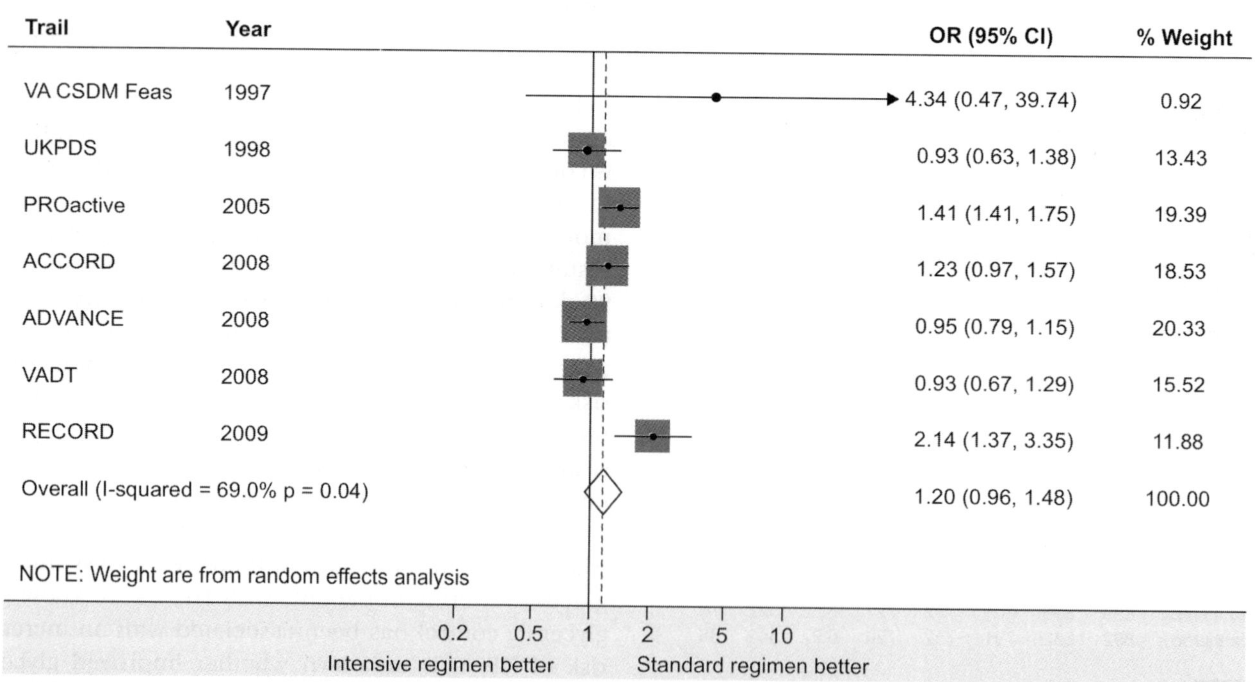

Figure 4 Probability of heart failure-related events with intensive glucose-lowering versus standard treatment. The size of the markers (squares) is approximately proportional to the statistical weight of each trial.

Despite the largely negative results in the individual trials described above, a recent systematic review that combined the results from several studies concluded that intensive management does not seem to reduce all-cause mortality in patients with T2D. In a meta-analysis performed by Hemmingsen et al. which included data from the UKPDS, ACCORD, ADVANCE, VADT and VA CSDM (Veterans Affairs Cooperative Study in Type 2 Diabetes Mellitus) studies etc, intensive glycemic control did not significantly affect the RRs of all-cause (1.02, 95% CI 0.91–1.13; 28,359 participants, 12 trials, Fig. 5) or CV mortality (1.11,0.92–1.35; 28,359 participants, 12 trials, Fig. 6).

Further, the trial reported that the risk severe hypoglycemia was significantly increased when intensive glycemic control was targeted (RR 2.39, 1.71–3.34; 27,844 participants, 9 trials, Fig. 7).

This meta-analysis provided sufficient evidence for:

- An absence of a 10% RR reduction in all-cause mortality
- Increased risk of severe hypoglycemia by 30% with intensive glycemic control versus conventional glycemic control in patients with T2DM.[10]

These observations showed that patients with T2DM often have comorbid conditions and tight glucose control is probably not always beneficial as an intensive glycemic control did not have any favorable effect on CV risk reduction and other risk parameters but the price of intensive glycemic control may be an increased risk of hypoglycemia. Therefore, it is important to set the glycemic targets based on each patient's unique risk profile and appreciation for the complex pathophysiology of vascular outcomes in T2DM.

CONCLUSION

Patients with type 2 diabetes are at increased risk of macrovascular and microvascular disease. Uncertainty exists as to whether intensive glycemic control reduces the risk of death, macrovascular disease, or microvascular disease. Only a few meta-analyses with a high risk of bias have estimated the effect of intensive glycemic control on microvascular complications. There is sufficient evidence that intensive glycemic control does not reduce all-cause mortality, cardiovascular mortality or non-fatal myocardial infarction. There is insufficient evidence to

Study	No. of events/total: Intensive control	Conventional control	Risk ratio (Mantel-Haenszel, random) (95% CI)	Weight (%)	Risk ratio (Mantel-Haenszel, random) (95% CI)
UGDP 1978	52/204	52/210		8.6	1.03 (0.74–1.44)
Service 1983	0/10	0/10		0.0	Not estimable
VA CSDM 1995	5/75	5/78		0.8	1.04 (0.31–3.45)
Jaber 1996	0/23	0/22		0.0	Not estimable
UKPDS 1998	539/3,071	213/1,138		25.9	0.94 (0.81–1.08)
Kumamoto 2000	3/55	6/55		0.6	0.50 (0.13–1.90)
Bagg 2001	0/21	0/22		0.0	Not estimable
ACCORD 2008	257/5,128	203/5,123		20.4	1.26 (1.06–1.51)
ADVANCE 2008	498/5,571	533/5,569		30.7	0.93 (0.83–1.05)
REMBO 2008	4/41	4/40		0.7	0.98 (0.26–3.64)
IDA 2009	0/51	0/51		0.0	Not estimable
VADT 2009	102/892	95/899		12.3	1.08 (0.83–1.41)
Total (95% CI)	1,460/15,142	1,111/13,217		100.0	1.02 (0.91–1.13)

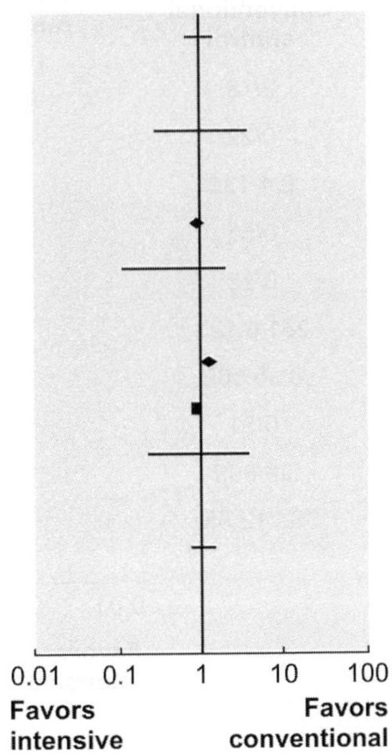

Test for heterogeneity: $\tau^2 = 0.01$, $\chi^2 = 10.07$, df = 7, p = 0.18, $I^2 = 30\%$

Test for overall effect: z = 0.33, p = 0.74

(CI: confidence interval.)

Figure 5 Forest plot for all-cause mortality.

Study	No. of events/total: Intensive control	No. of events/total: Conventional control	Weight (%)	Risk ratio (Mantel-Haenszel, random) (95% CI)
UGDP 1978	31/204	32/210	11.8	1.00 (0.63–1.57)
Service 1983	0/10	0/10	0.0	Not estimable
VA CSDM 1995	3/75	3/78	1.4	1.04 (0.22–4.99)
Jaber 1996	0/23	0/22	0.0	Not estimable
UKPDS 1998	301/3,071	91/1,138	23.9	1.23 (0.98–1.53)
Kumamoto 2000	1/55	1/55	0.5	1.00 (0.06–15.59)
Bagg 2001	0/21	0/22	0.0	Not estimable
ACCORD 2008	135/5,128	94/5,123	21.5	1.43 (1.11–1.86)
ADVANCE 2008	253/5,571	289/5,560	28.2	0.88 (0.74–1.03)
REMBO 2008	1/41	2/40	0.6	0.49 (0.05–5.17)
IDA 2009	0/51	0/51	0.0	Not estimable
VADT 2009	40/892	33/899	11.9	1.22 (0.78–1.92)
Total (95% CI)	765/15,142	545/13,217	100.0	1.11 (0.92–1.35)

Test for heterogeneity: $\tau^2 = 0.03$, $\chi^2 = 12.86$, df = 7, p = 0.08, $I^2 = 46\%$

Test for overall effect: z = 1.11, p = 0.27

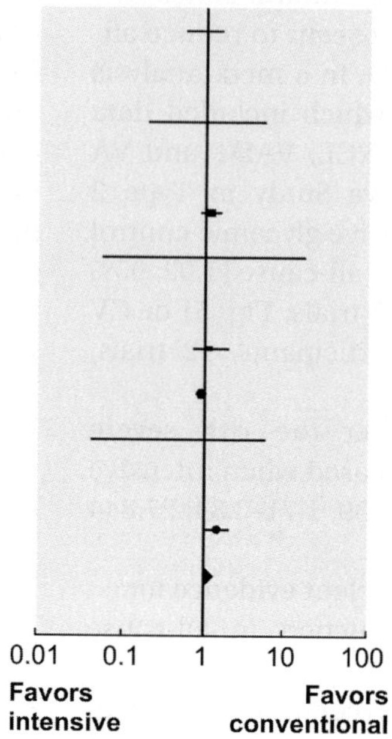

(CI: confidence interval.)

Figure 6 Forest plot for cardiovascular mortality.

Study	No. of events/total: Intensive control	No. of events/total: Conventional control	Weight (%)	Risk ratio (Mantel-Haenszel, random) (95% CI)
VA CSDM 1995	5/75	2/78	3.8	2.60 (0.52–12.99)
Jaber 1996	0/23	0/22	0.0	Not estimable
UKPDS 1998	33/3,071	8/1,138	12.3	1.53 (0.71–3.30)
Kumamoto 2000	0/55	0/55	0.0	Not estimable
Bagg 2001	0/21	0/22	0.0	Not estimable
ACCORD 2008	830/5,128	261/5,123	33.0	3.18 (2.78–3.63)
ADVANCE 2008	155/5,571	81/5,569	28.5	1.85 (1.42–2.42)
IDA 2009	0/51	0/51	0.0	Not estimable
VADT 2009	76/892	28/899	22.4	2.74 (1.79–4.18)
Total (95% CI)	1094/14,887	380/12,957	100.0	2.39 (1.71–3.34)

Test for heterogeneity: $\tau^2 = 0.08$, $\chi^2 = 15.01$, df = 4, p = 0.005, $I^2 = 73\%$

Test for overall effect: z = 5.10, p <0.001

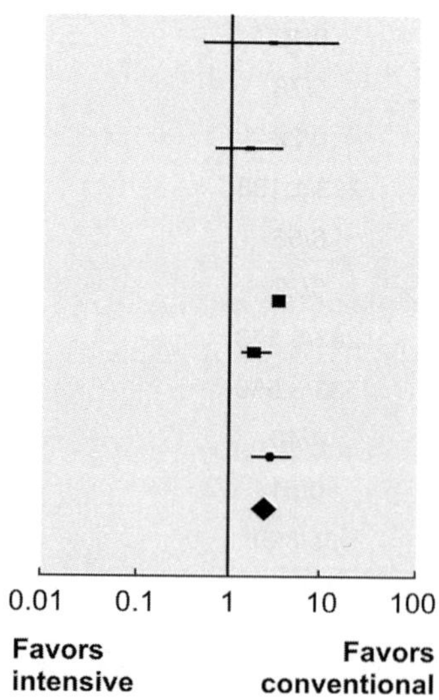

(CI: confidence interval.)

Figure 7 Forest plot for severe hypoglycemia.

support the conclusions that intensive glycemic control prevents the occurrence of microvascular disease assessed as a composite outcome, retinopathy, or nephropathy. There is also sufficient evidence exists that intensive glycemic control increases the risk of severe hypoglycemia by 30% compared with conventional glycemic control, which in fact may be associated with increase mortality.

REFERENCES

1. Gerstein HC, et al. Nine-Year Effects of 3.7 Years of Intensive Glycemic Control on Cardiovascular Outcomes. Diabetes Care. 2016 May;39(5): 701-708.
2. Vanhorebeek I, Langouche L, Van den Berghe G et al. Tight blood glucose control: What is the evidence? Crit Care Med. 2007;35(9 Suppl):S496-502.
3. Sardar P, Udell JA, Chatterjee S, et al. Effect of Intensive Versus Standard Blood Glucose Control in Patients With Type 2 Diabetes Mellitus in Different Regions of the World: Systematic Review and Meta-analysis of Randomized Controlled Trials. J Am Heart Assoc. 2015 May 5;4(5). pii: e001577.
4. Duckworth W Abraira C, Moritz T, et al. Glucose Control and Vascular Complications in Veterans with Type 2 Diabetes. N Engl J Med. 2009 Jan 8;360(2):129-39.
5. Genuth S, Ismail-Beigi F. et al. Clinical Implications of the ACCORD Trial. J Clin Endocrinol Metab. 2012 Jan;97(1):41-8.
6. ACCORDION: 9-Year Effects of 3.7 Years of Intensive Glycemic Control on Cardiovascular Outcomes The ACCORD Study Group Writing Committee Diabetes Care 2016.
7. Finfer S, Chittock DR, Su SY, et al. Intensive versus conventional glucose control in critically ill patients. N Engl J Med. 2009 Mar 26;360(13):1283-97.
8. Castagno D, Baird-Gunning J, Jhund PS, et al. Intensive glycemic control has no impact on the risk of heart failure in type 2 diabetic patients: Evidence from a 37,229 patient meta-analysis. Am Heart J. 2011 Nov;162(5):938-48.e2
9. Chatterjee S, Sharma A, Lichstein E, Mukherjee D. Intensive glucose control in diabetics with an acute myocardial infarction does not improve mortality and increases risk of hypoglycemia-a meta-regression analysis. Curr Vasc Pharmacol. 2013 Jan;11(1):100-104.
10. Hemmingsen B1, Lund SS, Gluud C, et al. et al. Intensive glycaemic control for patients with type 2 diabetes: systematic review with meta-analysis and trial sequential analysis of randomised clinical trials. BMJ. 2011 Nov 24;343:d6898.

Chapter 31

Triple or Quadruple Combination Therapy in Type 2 Diabetes—How Rational?

Vijay Panikar, Nikhil Nasikkar, Sanhita Walawalkar

INTRODUCTION

Type 2 diabetes mellitus (T2DM) and its complications have contributed tremendously to the burden of mortality and disability worldwide. Globally, the number of people with diabetes mellitus (DM) has quadrupled in the past three decades, and DM is the ninth major cause of death. About 1 in 11 adults worldwide now have DM, 90% of whom have T2DM. Asia is a major area of the rapidly emerging T2DM global epidemic (Fig. 1).[1]

India leads the world and stands at the second position after China, with 69 million persons affected by diabetes, posing a daunting challenge to the sustainable development of the nation, as almost every tenth adult (9.3%) in India is estimated to be affected by diabetes.[2]

CHALLENGES IN THE MANAGEMENT OF TYPE 2 DIABETES MELLITUS

Diabetes continues to present a significant clinical and economic burden. Maintaining glycemic control, as measured by glycated hemoglobin (HbA1c) levels, in patients with T2DM is crucial for reducing the serious clinical complications and subsequent economic costs associated with this chronic disease.[3]

However, managing the complex T2DM patient still presents a number of challenges to clinicians.

Over the years, understanding the pathophysiology of diabetes and its complications has changed the approach to the management of diabetes. It has highlighted the importance of lipid and blood pressure management. Newer oral antidiabetic drugs having different and synergistic actions have now made the treatment of diabetes easier and more effective. New treatment algorithms have helped in improving glycemic control.

Ominous Octet of Hyperglycemia

The pathogenesis of hyperglycemia has been very aptly described by Dr Ralph DeFronzo. The initial triumvirate was – (1) beta-cell failure (decreased insulin secretion), (2) increased hepatic glucose production and (3) insulin resistance in muscle and liver. The later additions were (4) increased lipolysis due to insulin resistance, (5) incretin deficiency, (6) α-cells hyperglucagonemia, (7) kidney (increased glucose reabsorption) and (8) brain (insulin resistance and neurotransmitter dysregulation). Collectively, these eight players comprise the "ominous octet" (Fig. 2)[4] and play important roles in the development of glucose intolerance in T2DM individuals.

Hepatic Glucose Production

DeFronzo in course of his Banting lecture at the American Diabetes Association conference (2009) stated – "Effective treatment of type 2 diabetes requires multiple drugs used in combination to correct the multiple pathophysiological defects. Treatment should be based on known pathogenic abnormalities and not simply on reduction of HbA1c. Therapy must be started early in the natural history of T2DM to prevent progressive β-cell failure."[4]

Insulin Resistance

Insulin resistance is a major defect in individuals with type 2 diabetes; there is a reduced biological response

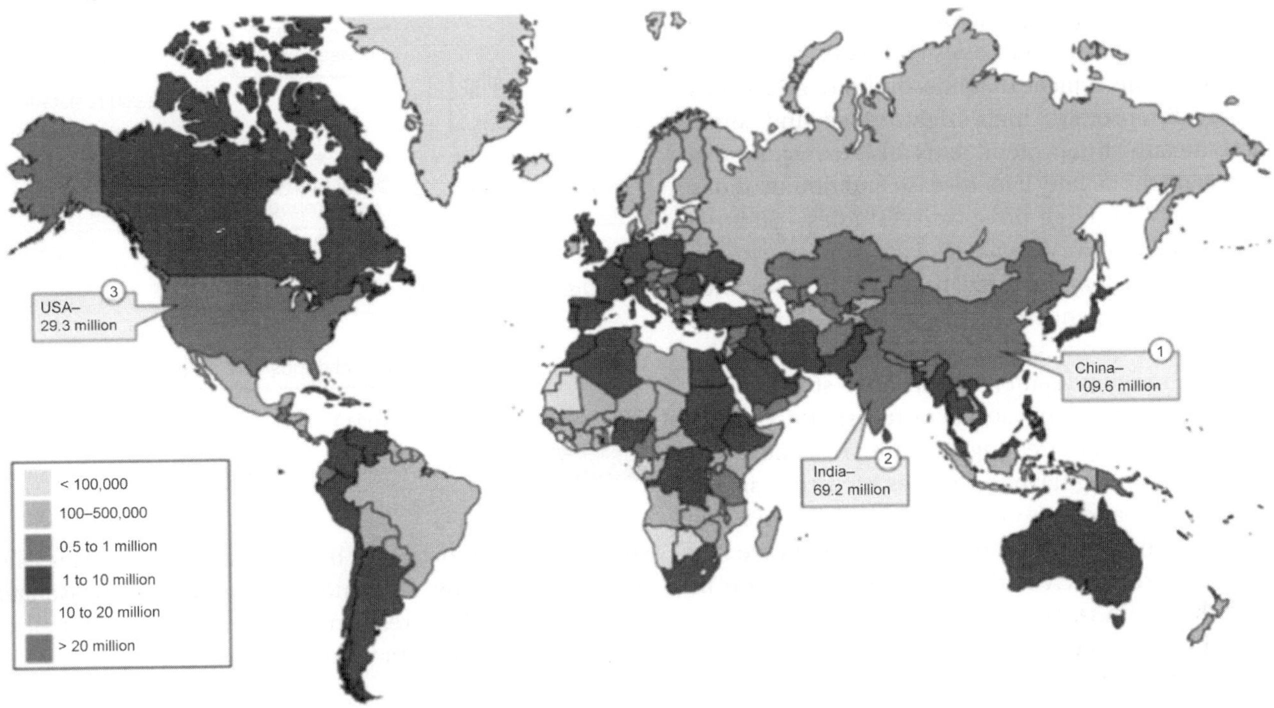

Figure 1 Estimated total number of adults (20–79 years) living with diabetes mellitus. ***(For color version, see Plate 1)***

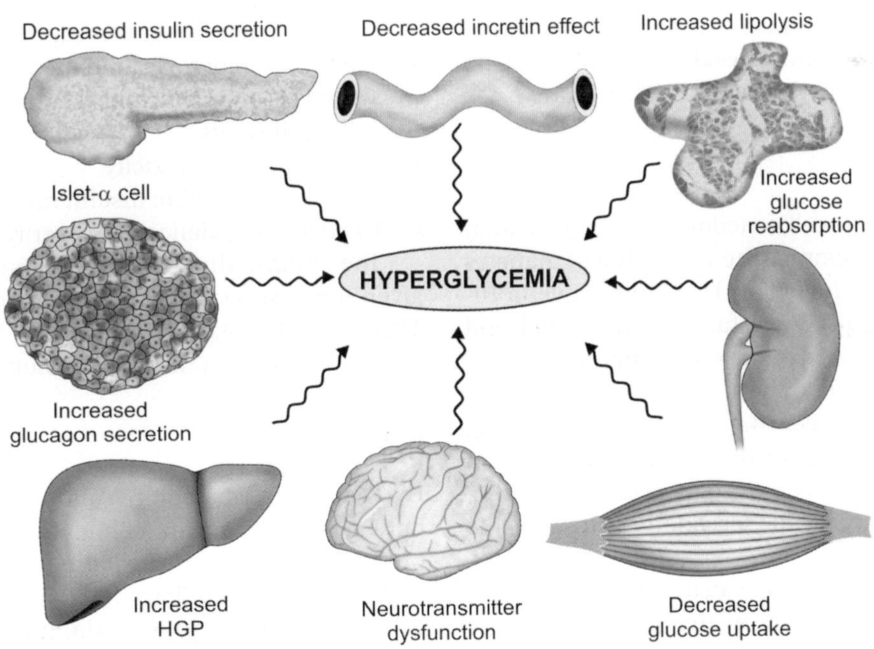

(HGP: hepatic glucose production.)

Figure 2 The ominous octet.

to insulin and is a strong predictor of type 2 diabetes. It is also closely associated with obesity. Insulin resistance is the cause of the typical diabetic dyslipidemia - low high-density lipoprotein, high triglycerides and small dense low-density lipoprotein. It is also considered a cause of nonalcoholic fatty liver disease and nonalcoholic steatohepatitis. Two large prospective studies—*Helsinki Policemen Study*[5] and *Verona Diabetes Complications Study*,[6] have each demonstrated that insulin resistance is a very strong independent predictor of cardiovascular (CV) disease, myocardial infarction (MI) and stroke. The recent insulin resistance intervention after stroke study "pioglitazone after ischemic stroke or transient ischemic attack"[7] showed that treating insulin resistance in nondiabetics with pioglitazone reduces recurrent stroke by 24%, MI by 24% and new onset of diabetes by 52%. For the first time, a therapy directed at insulin resistance has been shown to prevent CV and cerebrovascular events in patients with insulin resistance. Insulin resistance is the highest in Asian Indians, followed by white Caucasians and then by Afro-Caribbeans.[8]

Treatment options for insulin resistance: Nonpharmacological—These are diet, exercise and weight reduction. Pharmacological—Pioglitazone is the only drug available with a strong effect on insulin resistance, although metformin also has some effect in improving peripheral insulin sensitivity. In contrast, treatment with either sitagliptin or exenatide once weekly had no effect on insulin resistance as shown in 'DURATION 4' study.[9]

Beta Cell

The steady decline in β-cell function leading to insulin deficiency is the sole factor for the worsening of diabetes control over the years. The Belfast Diet Study[10] over a 10-year period showed that β-cell function worsened and insulin resistance remained relatively constant.

Multiple factors (Flowchart 1) may drive the progressive decline of β-cell function; the main being lipotoxicity, glucotoxicity, insulin resistance, insulin processing dysfunction, i.e., insulin-proinsulin ratio, amyloid deposition, protein glycation and possible decline in progenitor cells.

Peroxisome proliferator-activated receptor (PPAR) γ expression is suppressed by higher concentration of free fatty acid (FFA; not glucose). FFA also produces deleterious effect on β-cells by inhibiting glucose-stimulated insulin release by 80% as well as reduces islet insulin content by 75% and reduces insulin messenger ribonucleic acid expression. Pioglitazone prevents all of the damaging effects in vitro.[11]

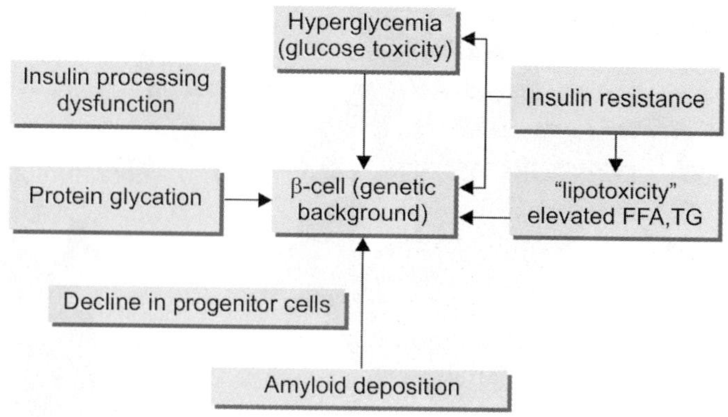

(FFA: free fatty acid; TG: triglyceride.)

Flowchart 1 Factors leading to decline of β-cell function.

PIOGLITAZONE AND PRESERVATION OF β-CELL FUNCTION

- Direct effect on the β-cell (PPAR γ)
- Amelioration of insulin resistance
- Reduction in plasma FFA (lipotoxicity)
- Mobilization of toxic lipid metabolites (fatty-acyl-CoA synthase, diacylglycerol, ceramides) out of the beta cell (lipotoxicity)
- Reversal of glucotoxicity
- Improve proinsulin: insulin ratio
- Decrease prevalence and severity of amyloid in β-cells.

The thiazolidinediones (TZDs) have consistently given the best results in diabetes prevention studies like TRIPOD, DREAM, PIPOD and ACT NOW, and have also shown durability in the ADOPT study.

Hypoglycemia

Hypoglycemia as a complication of treatment is commonly seen with insulin, sulfonylureas (SU) and glinides. Metformin, TZD, α-glucosidase inhibitors (AGIs), dipeptidyl peptidase-4 inhibitor (DPP4i), glucagon-like peptide 1 agonist (GLP1a) and sodium-glucose cotransporter 2 inhibitors (SGLT2i) have a very low incidence of hypoglycemia when used as a monotherapy.

Weight Gain

Weight gain is commonly seen with insulin, SU and TZD. Metformin and DPP4i are weight neutral. GLP1a and SGLT2i can reduce weight.

Potential Renal Benefits

DPP4i,[12] SGLT2i,[13] and pioglitazone[14] have shown clinically significant reduction of microalbuminuria when added to standard therapy.

Vascular Risk Reduction and Safety

Sulfonylureas other than gliclazide may be considered less cardiac friendly. The United States Food and Drug Administration has advised a heart failure warning label change for all available gliptins in the United States, namely, sitagliptin, linagliptin, saxagliptin and alogliptin. Other gliptins, such as vildagliptin, gemigliptin, or teneligliptin, have no CV outcome data till date. Drugs and studies which have shown benefits when considering the outcomes of combined endpoints of CV mortality, nonfatal MI, and stroke are - (1) Pioglitazone - PROactive study (2) Empagliflozin - EMPA-REG (3) Liraglutide - Leader (4) Semaglutide - SUSTAIN-6.[15]

CLINICAL CONSIDERATION FOR THE USE OF COMBINATION THERAPY

The review of pathophysiology and challenges in the management of T2DM demonstrate an effective treatment of T2DM will require multiple drugs in combination. Ample evidence is available to prove that aggressive glycemic control in T2DM leads not only to an improvement in symptoms and short-term health, but also in delaying/minimizing/reducing long-term complications.[16]

Combination treatment in T2DM should be individualized based on efficacy, risk-benefit profile, patient preference, and cost.

NEED OF TRIPLE AND QUADRUPLE COMBINATION THERAPIES

As understanding of the pathophysiology of T2DM grows, it is becoming apparent that early use of targeted combination therapy has the potential to slow disease progression, potentially through the correction of known pathologies and the preservation of β-cell function.[17] Given this finding, why not hit hard from the start and use several drugs together to nullify many of the known defects of T2DM and preserve β-cell function early.

In patients with more recent disease, triple oral therapy with metformin, SU and a DPP4i may help to address key disease aspects, including decreased insulin secretion and increased hepatic glucose production. In patients with inadequate glycemic control despite metformin and SU dual therapy, the addition of a DPP4i, or a SGLT2i, or a TZD has been shown to improve glycemic control.[17]

The results of the review conducted by Downes et al. have demonstrated that the addition of a third pharmaceutical class to metformin + SU therapy is statistically and clinically more effective at reducing HbA1c than dual therapy with metformin + SU.[18] Abdul-Ghani et al.[19] evaluated initial triple combination therapy of metformin/pioglitazone/exenatide, which targets known pathophysiologic defects in new-onset T2DM patients, produces greater and more durable HbA1c reduction (5.95% p <0.001), less hypoglycemia and weight loss versus weight gain in drug-naïve subjects with recently diagnosed T2DM. The results of this study demonstrate that combination therapy with metformin/pioglitazone/exenatide in newly diagnosed T2DM patients produces greater and more reduction in HbA1c than sequential add-on therapy with metformin, SU and basal insulin after a mean follow-up 6 years.

If HbA1c target is not achieved after about 3 months on triple therapy, the guidelines recommend combination injectable therapy. However, there may be situations where insulin and other injectables are not an option. A quadruple therapy regimen is a possible approach in these patients.[20] Chien et al. conducted the study to examine the effectiveness and tolerability of add-on sitagliptin in elderly T2DM patients inadequately controlled with SU + metformin + AGI combination. The addition of sitagliptin 100 mg to existing combination regimens significantly reduced HbA1c (–1.3%), fasting plasma glucose (-38.3 mg/dL) and 2-hour postprandial plasma glucose (-60.0 mg/dL) (all p <0.0001) at 24 weeks compared with baseline value but no significant reductions in these parameters were found in the control group.

Possible Pathophysiological Cocktails

Fixed drug combinations:
- Metformin/Pioglitazone + Gliptin/SGLT2i (two pills)
- Metformin + Gliptin/SGLT2i (two pills)
- Metformin + Pioglitazone + SGLT2i.

Such combinations could address most of the pathophysiological targets in treating T2DM with the advantage of – (1) long durable glycemic control by preserving the β-cells; (2) treating insulin resistance and its associated complications; (3) very less chances of hypoglycemia; (4) no weight gain or even cause weight loss; and (5) CV benefits.

Thus, a treatment paradigm shift is recommended in which multiple drug combination should be initiated, based not only on the drug's glucose-lowering efficacy/durability but also on its effect on weight, blood pressure, lipids, CV protection and side effect profile.

CONCLUSION

Type 2 DM is a significant health problem with an increasing worldwide prevalence. The management of T2DM is relatively challenging. If health care professionals are to have any chance of controlling the burden of T2DM, then interventions to limit or reduce its associated pathophysiologic defects ("ominous octet") and complications are vital. However, treatment with a single or dual glucose-lowering agent can only address limited targets and does not provide adequate glycemic control in many cases.

If you treat the underlying defects responsible for type 2 diabetes, you can be assured of durable glycemic control and inevitably fewer diabetes complications. This can be achieved by using multiple drug therapy with synergistic actions (2, 3, or 4 agents) as a first-line therapy in the treatment of T2DM.

REFERENCES

1. Zheng Y, Ley SH, Hu FB. Global aetiology and epidemiology of type 2 diabetes mellitus and its complications. Nat Rev Endocrinol. 2018;14(2):88-98.
2. Akhtar SN, Dhillon P. Prevalence of diagnosed diabetes and associated risk factors: evidence from the large-scale surveys in India. J Soc Health Diabetes. 2017;5(1):28.
3. Morgan, L. Challenges and opportunities in managing type 2 diabetes. Am Health Drug Benefits. 2017;10(4):197-200.
4. DeFronzo RA, Eldor R, Abdul-Ghani M. Pathophysiologic approach to therapy in patients with newly diagnosed type 2 diabetes. Diabetes Care. 2013;36(Suppl 2):S127-38.
5. Pyörälä M, Miettinen H, Halonen P, et al. Insulin resistance syndrome predicts the risk of coronary heart disease and stroke in healthy middle-aged men: the 22-year follow-up results of the Helsinki Policemen Study. Arterioscler Thromb Vasc Biol. 2000;20:538-44.
6. Bonora E, Formentini G, Calcaterra F, et al. HOMA-estimated insulin resistance is an independent predictor of cardiovascular disease in type 2 diabetic subjects: prospective data from the Verona Diabetes Complications Study. Diabetes Care. 2002;25:1135-41.
7. Kernan WN, Viscoli CM, Furie KL, et al. Pioglitazone after ischemic stroke or transient ischemic attack. N Engl J Med. 2016;374:1321-31.
8. The UK prospective diabetes study 16. Overview of 6 years' therapy of type II diabetes: a progressive disease. U.K. Prospective Diabetes Study Group. Diabetes. 1995;44:1249-58.
9. Russell-Jones D, Cuddihy RM, Hanefeld M, et al. Efficacy and safety of exenatide once weekly versus metformin, pioglitazone, and sitagliptin used as monotherapy in drug-naive patients with type 2 diabetes (DURATION-4): a 26-week double-blind study. Diabetes Care. 2012;35:252-8.
10. Levy J, Atkinson AB, Bell PM, et al. Beta-cell deterioration determines the onset and rate of progression of secondary dietary failure in type 2 diabetes mellitus: the 10-year follow-up of the Belfast Diet Study. Diabet Med. 1998;15(4):290-6.
11. Lupi R, Del Guerra S, Marselli L, et al. Rosiglitazone prevents the impairment of human islet function induced by fatty acids: evidence for a role of PPARgamma2 in the modulation of insulin secretion. Am J Physiol Endocrinol Metab. 2004;286(4):E560-6.
12. Groop PH, Cooper M, Perkovic V, et al. Linagliptin lowers albuminuria on top of recommended standard treatment for diabetic nephropathy. Diabetes. 2012;61(Suppl 1):A243.
13. Yale JF, Bakris G, Cariou B, et al. Efficacy and safety of canagliflozin in subjects with type 2 diabetes and chronic kidney disease. Diabetes Obes Metab. 2013;15(5):463-73.
14. Hanefeld M, Brunetti P, Schernthaner GH, et al. One-year glycemic control with a sulfonylurea plus pioglitazone versus a sulfonylurea plus metformin in patients with type 2 diabetes. Diabetes Care. 2004;28:141-7.
15. Schemthaner G, Sattar N. Lessons from SAVOR and EXAMINE: Some important answers, but many open questions. J Diabet Complications. 2014;28(4):430-3.
16. Cahn A, Cefalu WT. Clinical considerations for use of initial combination therapy in type 2 diabetes. Diabetes Care. 2016;39(Suppl 2):S137-45.
17. Levin PA. Practical combination therapy based on pathophysiology of type 2 diabetes. Diabetes Metab Syndr Obes. 2016;9:355-69.
18. Downes MJ, Bettington EK, Gunton JE, et al. Triple therapy in type 2 diabetes; a systematic review and network meta-analysis. Peer J. 2015;3:e1461.
19. Abdul-Ghani M, Puckett CL Jr, Triplitt CL, et al. Durable HbA1c Reduction with Initial Combination Therapy with Metformin/Pioglitazone/Exenatide in Subjects with New-Onset Diabetes—Six-Year Follow-Up of the EDICT Study. Diabetes. 2018;67(Supplement 1):123.
20. Chien MN, Lee CC, Chen WC, et al. Effect of sitagliptin as add-on therapy in elderly type 2 diabetes patients with inadequate glycemic control in Taiwan. Int J Gerontol. 2011;5(2):103-6.

Chapter 32

Gut Microbiota and Diabetes Mellitus—The Link

Ranjit Mohan Anjana

INTRODUCTION

The global prevalence of type 2 diabetes mellitus (T2DM) has dramatically increased over the last three decades,[1,2] and this increase has been accompanied by decreased life expectancy and quality of life among affected populations.[3] As of 2017, >425 million adults have diabetes mellitus (DM) and this number is estimated to increase to 629 million by 2045.[1] More than 95% of all adults with DM have T2DM. The rise in numbers will be highest in low- and middle-income countries, where 75% of the population and more than 80% of all people with undiagnosed diabetes live. India is one of the epicenters of the global DM epidemic and has the second highest number of people with the disease in the world.[4] The recent National study (ICMR-INDIAB) also showed that the corresponding projections for India would be 62.4 million people with diabetes and 77.2 million people with prediabetes.[4] Despite the availability of clinically effective therapies for diabetes, achieving good glycemic control in patients with diabetes is a tough task and the consequences of poor glycemic control are reflected in progression to microvascular complications (diabetic neuropathy, retinopathy and nephropathy) and macroangiopathy (ischemic heart disease, stroke and peripheral vascular disease).[5] T2DM, which leads to a series of vascular co-morbidities as well as premature mortality, is therefore becoming a major public health menace worldwide.

Type 2 diabetes mellitus is characterized by impaired glucose homeostasis resulting from a combination of β-cell dysfunction and insulin resistance.[5] In addition to well-established risk factors for T2DM, including genetic predisposition, poor physical activity, fetal programming and obesity,[6] an altered configuration of the microbial community in gut-the microbiota-has emerged as a new candidate that may be linked to T2DM.[7,8] Recent studies on T2DM have identified the gastrointestinal tract or gut as one of the main players in the pathogenesis of the disease (part of the "ominous octet").[9] One of the ways in which the gut is postulated to influence the development of metabolic disease is through the actions of the myriad microorganisms contained therein, otherwise called the gut microbiota. In this context, the evidence base is growing to suggest that the gut microbiota are significant environmental factors and key players in the onset and development of diabetes and therefore, there is an imperative need to study the link between gut microbiota and T2DM in all possible ways in order to target therapeutics. This chapter is an attempt to give a glimpse of current happenings in this field with a focus on future perspectives.

ROLE OF GUT MICROBIOTA AND HUMAN METABOLISM

The gut microbiota is an integral part of a complex network coordinating the physical and chemical elements of the intestinal barrier with almost all organ systems of the human body.[10] The human gut hosts an enormous number and variety of micro-organisms, including bacteria (i.e. 100 trillions) belonging to over 1,000 species.[11,12] The gut microbiome which exerts several trophic, metabolic and protective functions on the hosts exceeds the size of the human genome by two orders of magnitude. It is made up of more than 200 prevalent bacterial species and up to 1000 less common species, the gut microbiome functions like a virtual organ system.[11-14] Dominated by three major groups of bacteria namely Firmicutes, Bacteroidetes and Actinobacteria that represent >95% of the total microbiota, the composition of the gut microbiota is often affected by diet, host genetics and the immune status.[10,11] The important message is that the gut microbiota of all human beings fulfill core functions but differ in specialized functions. As a consequence some communities are linked to human diseases and obesity more than others.[15]

THE LINK BETWEEN GUT MICROBIOTA AND TYPE 2 DIABETES

As the understanding grows, it is being realized that the gut is not only associated with digestion and excretion but also that gut hormones may have an important therapeutic potential. This is increasingly drawing the attention and interest of medical researchers. The 'gut connection' to T2DM received even more attention in recent years because of the fact that there is an intricate relationship between intestinal microbiota and development of metabolic diseases with special reference to diabetes. The potential of the human microbiome as an early detection biomarker for diagnostic and prognostic purposes for metabolic disorders in general and diabetes in particular is a very active area of research.

In 2004, the first evidence was published from studies on germ-free mice, suggesting that the gut microbiota might contribute to alterations in glucose metabolism.[16] Subsequently, several studies have investigated the role of the human gut microbiota in T2DM. The most comprehensive studies to date used metagenomic sequencing in Chinese[7] and Swedish[8] individuals and both studies established that human T2DM was characterized by dysbiotic gut microbiota. Despite discrepancies between the two studies - which may partly reflect differences in ethnicity, diet and intake of medication - both studies reported that patients with T2DM had less butyrate-producing bacteria (*Roseburia* species and *Faecalibacterium prausnitzii*). Earlier studies in humans as well as in mice reported that obesity and impaired glucose metabolism were associated with an altered ratio between the two major *phyla* in the human gut, Firmicutes and Bacteroidetes.[17,18] However, neither the Swedish nor the Chinese study confirmed these findings. Wu et al.[19] reported a reduced abundance of *bifidobacteria* in T2DM by qPCR as well as in sequencing results as a possible characteristic of diabetes. When obese and lean individuals with/without T2DM were evaluated for the presence of *Faecalibacterium prausnitzii*—a prominent member of the human gut microbiota belonging to the Firmicutes group[20] it was observed that there was a reduction in the levels of *Faecalibacterium prausnitzii* in patients with T2DM. The reduction correlated with increased levels of inflammatory markers indicating that an increase in the number of *Faecalibacterium prausnitzii* may alleviate inflammation and insulin resistance. Differences in the abundance and diversity of microbiota in T2DM and obesity were also reported in a small study in Austria.[21]

The landmark Chinese study[7] showed the involvement of intestinal flora with T2DM. Approximately 60,000 microbial genes were found to be differentially abundant in patients with T2D who were also characterized by a moderate degree of gut microbial dysbiosis, a decrease in the abundance of some universal butyrate-producing bacteria and an increase in various opportunistic pathogens. Another study by Zhang et al.[22] has also reported distinct gut microbiota changes in subjects with impaired glucose tolerance (IGT) and patients with T2DM compared to subjects with normal glucose tolerance (NGT). Interestingly in this study also, butyrate-producing bacteria were more abundant in the NGT group than others. In addition, Verrucomicrobiae was speculated as a potential marker of T2DM.

Karlsson et al.[8] have used shotgun sequencing to characterize the fecal metagenome of 145 European women with NGT, IGT or T2DM. Observing compositional and functional alterations in the metagenomes of women with T2DM, they have developed a mathematical model based on metagenomic profiles (defined as 'metagenomic clusters' or MGCs) that identified T2DM with high accuracy. They classified women with IGT into subgroups with T2DM- or NGT-like metabolism on the basis of their fecal microbiome and this classification appears to offer a potentially new approach to identify individuals at high risk of developing T2DM. Recent studies by Zupancic et al.[23] have identified a subset of bacterial taxa (26 bacterial species) that are linked to metabolic syndrome traits including glucose intolerance.

Studies from India have reported that the distinctive feature of Indian gut microbiota is the predominance of genus *Prevotella* and *Megasphaera*.[24] These studies also observed that *Escherichia* counts were elevated in T2DM with HbA1c of 6.5–8.5% suggesting that lipopolysaccharides present in the cell wall of gram-negative bacteria may be responsible for low-grade inflammation as evidenced by elevated levels of inflammatory markers in T2DM with the same HbA1c levels. Bhute et al.[25] showed depletion of the butyrate producing family Ruminococcaceae among patients with T2DM in India. Another recent study on Finnish individuals with prediabetes has also indicated a decreased abundance of the family Ruminococcaceae.[26] Interestingly, the Data from the Epidemiological Study on the Insulin Resistance Syndrome (DESIR) study has recently reported that blood microbiota dysbiosis is also associated with the onset of cardiovascular events.[27]

Very little information has so far been provided in any of the published studies on effects of antidiabetic medication on gut microbiota. In the Swedish study, diabetic patients treated with metformin had increased levels of Enterobacteriaceae and decreased levels of *Clostridium* and *Eubacterium*[8], yet the significance of these observations was not clear. By taking advantage of the large metagenomic datasets from the Swedish and Chinese studies[7,8] respectively, it was in fact possible, based on just a few metagenomic markers subjected to receiver operator curve analysis, to discriminate between patients with and without T2DM with an accuracy of above 80%. It remains, however, to be established whether this discriminative power represents discrimination between individuals with T2DM and normal glucose tolerance or discrimination between individuals receiving or not receiving metformin treatment. Metformin, the first-line drug of choice for the treatment of T2DM, increases the levels of *Akkermansia* species in high-fat diet-fed mice in parallel to its beneficial effects on glucose metabolism.[28] Supplying mice with *A. muciniphila* orally has been reported to result in improvements of glucose tolerance and metabolic dysfunctions such as metabolic endotoxemia and adipose tissue inflammation.[28,29] These promising results not only suggest novel glucose-lowering mechanisms of metformin, but also provide future potential targets for altering glucose regulation by means of bacterio-therapy.

GUT MICROBIOTA AND TYPE 1 DIABETES

Type 1 diabetes (T1DM) results from autoimmune destruction of pancreatic β-cells in genetically predisposed individuals.[30] The β-cell destruction involves innate and adaptive immune responses and when around 80% of the β-cells are affected, the first signs of diabetes become manifested.[31] The mechanisms associating gut microbiota and T1DM development are yet to be fully understood. Studies in humans tend to suggest this possibility; however, these results have not yet proven a direct relationship between changes in intestinal microbiota and the development of autoimmune diseases. Increased intestinal permeability may facilitate the absorption of antigens which can injure pancreatic β-cells.[32] Individuals susceptible to T1DM and other autoimmune diseases present inadequately functioning intestinal barrier,[33] allowing greater exposure of antigens to the immune system. However, the mechanisms resulting in this condition–leaky gut–before T1DM has developed are not yet been fully understood.

While analyzing the metabolic profiles of T1DM patients, Orešic et al.[34] observed that certain metabolites correlated with the disease. These differences were observed even before the onset of the first autoantibodies and thus are potential biomarkers of the disease. Since many of these metabolites were produced by the gut microbiota it is postulated that alterations in these could promote the development of T1DM. In fact the study by Giongo et al.[35] has identified alterations in gut microbiota associating with progression towards T1DM. Mining 16S rRNA data from T1DM patients showed an association of gut microbiota alterations with development of autoimmunity.[36] Significant differences have been reported in the gut microbiota of children with T1DM as compared to that of healthy children.[37]

This emphasize that more studies are needed to explore the role of the gut in T1DM development. Despite numerous studies showing health benefits of probiotics, the enthusiasm for their application as well as other means to alter the intestinal microbial ecosystem in the prevention of T1DM needs to be tempered due to the current lack of knowledge of the normal developing intestinal microbiota, in addition to questions as to how it affects the developing immune system. Future studies using newly developed techniques to evaluate intestinal microbiota, coupled with the rapidly emerging fields of proteomics and metabolomics, are certainly needed.

GUT MICROBIOTA AND HOST METABOLISM

Gut microbiota is under control of host genetics as documented in knock-out studies in mice.[38] Likely, the reported associations to blood groups in humans also mirror this regulatory mechanism. Microbiota on its side impact on gene regulation in its host and one of the mechanisms appears to be mediated through microbial circulating non-coding RNA.[39] Also gut microbiota is known to affect the innate immune response of the host, e.g. through intestinal uptake of bacterial LPS, resulting in a metabolic endotoxaemia, i.e. a systemic low-grade inflammation and insulin resistance.[40] Similarly, bacterial metabolites including SCFAs (short chain fatty acids), TMAO (Trimethylamine-N-Oxide) and hippurate have biological activities that regulate host functions. For instance, SCFAs (majorly acetate, propionate and butyrate), which are produced by bacterial fermentation of dietary fibers not only act as local nutrient sources but also trigger the release of anorectic hormones like GLP-1 and PYY.[41]

Bacterial lipopolysaccharides (LPS), derived from the outer membranes of gram-negative bacteria have been intensively studied and are known to induce metabolic endotoxemia by promoting secretion of pro-inflammatory cytokines.[42] Studies in both animal models and humans have shown that a high-fat diet can modulate the gut microbiota and increase circulating levels of LPSs, probably by uptake of LPSs in chylomicrons secreted from intestinal epithelial cells or through increased intestinal permeability.[42-44] It is likely that the gut microbiota may exert effects on glucose and lipid metabolism through several complementary mechanisms, but, for many of these signaling pathways, a common feature is an altered intestinal integrity of the gut epithelial wall. While there is very little information available on these aspects, it is important to know whether these microbial components and metabolites serve as systemic biomarkers in relation to changes in gut microbiota in metabolic disorders.

Since elevated circulatory levels of LPS combined with other metabolic abnormalities may pose a potent risk for the genesis of diabetes itself and also for the later development of micro and macrovascular complications, measurement of LPS activity thus appears as a new biomarker tool to estimate the metabolic risk profile in humans.[45] In this context, we recently reported for the first-time a clinically relevant study in India which demonstrated the association of increased LPS levels and LPS activity in patients with T2DM.[46] Increased circulatory levels of LPS and Zonulin (a marker of gut permeability) in patients with T2DM appear to expand our understanding of the emerging role of gut and gut microbiota in the pathogenesis of diabetes. The biomarker potential of LPS is also inferred by several other studies. An increase in plasma LPS occurs in healthy individuals after a high-fat meal,[47] whereas a chronic state of low-grade endotoxemia as measured by plasma LPS[48] or LPS-binding protein[49] is evident in patients with obesity and insulin resistance. Once elevated in circulation, LPS can target various tissues (macrophages, adipose, skeletal muscle and liver) where they can interact with specific receptors (toll like receptors, pattern-recognition receptors), induce the secretion of inflammatory cytokines and negatively regulate insulin signaling. Interestingly, LPS-producing *Enterobacter cloacae* isolated from a morbidly obese patient was shown to trigger obesity and insulin resistance in germ-free mice[50].

CONCLUSION

Collectively, present evidence suggests that changes in the gut microbiota from a healthy to dysbiotic may result in a leaky gut epithelium with increased gut permeability causing absorption of macromolecules from the intestinal content triggering systemic immune alterations, altered signaling pathways affecting lipid and glucose metabolism and low-grade inflammation eventually leading to insulin resistance and possibly to T2DM. However, studies in humans have so far not been able to answer the question of whether the gut microbiota is a cause or consequence–or both–of T2DM.

The first step could be implementation of well-designed prospective studies, ideally with carefully phenotyped prediabetic individuals. If such longitudinal studies support a link between the gut microbiota and future development of T2DM, microbiota in those prediabetic individuals who develop T2DM and in those who do not develop T2DM should be further tested and characterized in mechanistic mice experiments. Finally, to establish causality, proper randomized clinical intervention trials are needed in which subjects are randomized to receive treatment with health-promoting bacteria or placebo. Future research should also focus on the complex hormonal, immunomodulatory and metabolic mechanisms that influence host-microbiota interactions and evaluated through well designed studies that measure specific endpoints.

REFERENCES

1. International Diabetes Federation Website. Accessed at www.idf.org/diabetesatlas on 08 Oct 2018.
2. Danaei G, Finucane MM, Lu Y, et al. National, regional, and global trends in fasting plasma glucose and diabetes prevalence since 1980: systematic analysis of health examination surveys and epidemiological studies with 370 country-years and 2·7 million participants. Lancet. 2011;378:31-40.
3. Abegunde DO, Mathers CD, Adam T, et al. The burden and costs of chronic diseases in low-income and middle-income countries. Lancet. 2007; 370: 1929-511.
4. Anjana RM, Pradeepa R, Deepa M, et al. ICMR–INDIAB Collaborative Study Group. Prevalence of diabetes and prediabetes (impaired fasting glucose and/or impaired glucose tolerance) in urban and rural India: phase I results of the Indian Council of Medical Research-INdia DIABetes (ICMR-INDIAB) study. Diabetologia. 2011;54:3022-7.
5. Defronzo, RA. Banting Lecture. From the triumvirate to the ominous octet: a new paradigm for the treatment of type 2 diabetes mellitus. Diabetes 2009;58:773-95.

6. Grarup N, Sandholt CH, Hansen T, Pedersen O. Genetic susceptibility to type 2 diabetes and obesity: from genome-wide association studies to rare variants and beyond. Diabetologia. 2014;57:1528-41.
7. Qin J, Li Y, Cai Z, et al. A metagenome-wide association study of gut microbiota in type 2 diabetes. Nature. 2012;490:55-60.
8. Karlsson FH, Tremaroli V, Nookaew I, et al. Gut metagenome in European women with normal, impaired and diabetic glucose control. Nature. 2013;498:99-103.
9. Defronzo RA. Banting Lecture. From the triumvirate to the ominous octet: a new paradigm for the treatment of type 2 diabetes mellitus. Diabetes. 2009;58:773-95.
10. Benson AK, Kelly SA, Legge R, et al. Individuality in gut microbiota composition is a complex polygenic trait shaped by multiple environmental and host genetic factors. Proc Natl Acad Sci. 2010;107:18933-8.
11. Turnbaugh PJ, Ridaura VK, Faith JJ, et al. The effect of diet on the human gut microbiome: a metagenomic analysis in humanized genotobiotic mice. Sci Transl Med 2009;1:6.
12. Qin J, Li R, Raes J, et al. Human gut microbial gene catalogue established by metagenomic sequencing. Nature 2010;464:59-65.
13. Ley RE, Hamady M, Lozupone C, et al. Evolution of mammals and their gut microbes. Science. 2008;320:1647-51.
14. Kurokawa K, Itoh T, Kuwahara T, et al. Comparative metagenomics revealed commonly enriched gene sets in human gut microbiomes. DNA Res. 2007;14:169-81.
15. Gerritsen JJ, Smidt HH, Rijkers GT, et al. Intestinal microbiota in human health and disease: the impact of probiotics. Genes Nutr. 2011;6:209-40.
16. Backhed F, Ding H, Wang T, et al. The gut microbiota as an environmental factor that regulates fat storage. PNAS 2004;101:5718-23.
17. Ley RE, Turnbaugh PJ, Klein S, et al. Microbial ecology: human gut microbes associated with obesity. Nature 2006;444:1022-1023.
18. Turnbaugh PJ, Ley RE, Mahowald MA, et al. An obesity- associated gut microbiome with increased capacity for energy harvest. Nature. 2006;444:1027-1031.
19. Wu X, Ma C, Han L, et al. Molecular characterisation of the faecal microbiota in patients with type II diabetes. Curr Microbiol. 2010;61:69-78.
20. Furet JP, Kong LC, Tap J, et al. Differential adaptation of human gut microbiota to bariatric surgery-induced weight loss: links with metabolic and low-grade inflammation markers. Diabetes. 2010;59:3049-57.
21. Remely M, Dworzak S, Hippe B, et al. Abundance and Diversity of Microbiota in Type 2 Diabetes and Obesity. J Diabetes Metab. 2013;4:253.
22. Zhang X, Shen D, Fang Z, et al. Human gut microbiota changes reveal the progression of glucose intolerance. PLoS One. 2013;8:e71108.
23. Zupancic ML, Cantarel BL, Liu Z, et al. Analysis of the gut microbiota in the old order Amish and its relation to the metabolic syndrome. PLoS One. 2012;7(8):e43052.
24. Pushpanathan P, Srikanth P, Seshadri KG, et al. Gut Microbiota in Type 2 Diabetes Individuals and Correlation with Monocyte Chemoattractant Protein1 and Interferon Gamma from Patients Attending a Tertiary Care Centre in Chennai, India. Indian J Endocrinol Metab. 2016;20(4):523-30.
25. Bhute S, Pande P, Shetty SA, et al. Molecular Characterization and Meta-Analysis of Gut Microbial Communities Illustrate Enrichment of Prevotella and Megasphaera in Indian Subjects. Front Microbiol. 2016 May 9;7:660.
26. Org E, Blum Y, Kasela S, et al. Relationships between gut microbiota, plasma metabolites, and metabolic syndrome traits in the METSIM cohort. Genome Biol. 2017;18(1):70.
27. Amar J, Lange C, Payros G, et al. D.E.S.I.R. Study Group. Blood microbiota dysbiosis is associated with the onset of cardiovascular events in a large general population: the D.E.S.I.R. study. PLoS One. 2013;8:e54461.
28. Shin NR, Lee JC, Lee HY, et al. An increase in the Akkermansia spp. population induced by metformin treatment improves glucose homeostasis in diet-induced obese mice. Gut. 2014;63:727-35.
29. Everard A, Belzer C, Geurts L, et al. Cross-talk between Akkermansia muciniphila and intestinal epithelium controls diet-induced obesity. PNAS. 2013;110:9066-71.
30. Bluestone JA, Herold K, Eisenbarth G. Genetics, pathogenesis and clinical interventions in type 1 diabetes. Nature. 2010;464:1293-1300.
31. Dabelea DRA, Bell RB, D'Agostino J, et al. Incidence of diabetes in youth in the United States. JAMA 2007;297:2716-24.
32. Vehik K, Dabelea D. The changing epidemiology of type 1 diabetes: why is it going through the roof? Diabetes Metab Res Rev 2011;27:3–13.
33. Neu J, Reverte CM, Mackey AD, et al. Changes in intestinal morphology and permeability in the biobreeding rat before the onset of type 1 diabetes. J Pediatr Gastroenterol Nutr. 2005;40:589-95.
34. Oresic M, Simell S, Sysi-Aho M, et al. Dysregulation of lipid and amino acid metabolism precedes islet autoimmunity in children who later progress to type 1 diabetes. J Exp Med. 2008;205:2975-84.
35. Giongo A, Gano KA, Crabb DB, et al. Toward defining the autoimmune microbiome for type 1 diabetes. ISME J. 2011;5:82–91.
36. Brown CT, Davis-Richardson AG, Giongo A, et al. Gut microbiome metagenomics analysis suggests a functional model for the development of autoimmunity for type 1 diabetes. PLoS One. 2011;6:e25792.
37. Murri M, Leiva I, Gomez-Zumaquero JM, et al. Gut microbiota in children with type 1 diabetes differs from that in healthy children: a case-control study. BMC Med. 2013;11:46.
38. Zhang C, Zhang M, Wang S, et al. Interactions between gut microbiota, host genetics and diet relevant to development of metabolic syndromes in mice. ISME J 2010;4:232-41.
39. Dalmasso G, Nguyen HT, Yan Y, et al. Microbiota modulates host gene expression via microRNAs. PLoS One. 2011;6:e19293.
40. De Bandt JP, Waligora-Dupriet AJ, Butel MJ. Intestinal microbiota in inflammation and insulin resistance: relevance to humans. Curr Opin Clin Nutr Metab Care. 2011;14:334-40.
41. Zhou J, Martin RJ, Tulley RT, et al. Dietary resistant starch up regulates total GLP-1 and PYY in a sustained day-long manner through fermentation in rodents. Am J Physiol Endocrinol Metab. 2008;295:E1160-66.
42. Cani PD, Amar J, Iglesias MA, et al. Metabolic endotoxemia initiates obesity and insulin resistance. Diabetes. 2007;56:1761-72.
43. Erridge C, Attina T, Spickett CM, et al. A high-fat meal induces low-grade endotoxemia: evidence of a novel mechanism of postprandial inflammation. American Journal of Clinical Nutrition. 2007;86:1286-92.
44. Harte AL, Varma MC, Tripathi G, et al. High fat intake leads to acute postprandial exposure to circulating endotoxin in type 2 diabetic subjects. Diabetes Care. 2012;35:375-82.
45. Creely SJ, McTernan PG, Kusminski CM, et al. Lipopolysaccharide activates an innate immune system response in human adipose tissue in obesity and type 2 diabetes. Am J Physiol Endocrinol Metab. 2007;292:E740-7.
46. Jayashree B, Bibin YS, Prabhu D, et al. Increased circulatory levels of lipopolysaccharide (LPS) and zonulin signify novel biomarkers of proinflammation in patients with type 2 diabetes. Mol Cell Biochem. 2014 Mar;388(1–2):203-10.
47. Erridge C, Attina T, Spickett CM, et al. A high-fat meal induces low-grade endotoxemia: evidence of a novel mechanism of postprandial inflammation. Am J Clin Nutr. 2007;86:1286-92.
48. Cani PD, Amar J, Iglesias MA, et al. Metabolic endotoxemia initiates obesity and insulin resistance. Diabetes. 2007;56:1761-72.
49. Sun L, Yu Z, Ye X, et al. A marker of endotoxemia is associated with obesity and related metabolic disorders in apparently healthy Chinese. Diabetes Care. 2010;33:1925-32
50. Fei N, Zhao L. An opportunistic pathogen isolated from the gut of an obese human causes obesity in germfree mice. ISME J. 2013;7:880-4.

Chapter 33

Glucagon—Missing Piece in Type 2 Diabetes Mellitus Management

Sanjay Kalra

INTRODUCTION

Glucagon, a 29 amino acid long peptide, secreted by the α-cells of the islets of Langerhans, has always been overshadowed by its more flamboyant cousin, the β-cells insulin. In recent decades, however, our understanding of glucagon's role, and its importance in the metabolic homeostasis, has grown. Glucagon has also been utilized as a diagnostic and therapeutic tool, as well as a target for therapy. Conceptually, glucagon levels can be used to assist in personalized choice of glucose-lowering therapy.

Though glucagon was identified and named in 1923, it was recognized to be a distinct hormone, originating from the α-cells, in the 1950s.[1] The bihormonal hypothesis of Unger and Orci (1975) postulated the need to control glucagon secretion so as to treat diabetes properly.[2] Recently, Kalra and Gupta proposed a metabolic fulcrum, which balances two hormones, insulin and glucagon, with opposing actions.[3] It is suggested that the islets of Langerhans be considered as one endocrine organ, instead of approaching the α-and β-cells as two different glands.

Pharmaceutical advances have kept pace with improvements in pathophysiological understanding of glucagon's role. The development of a prefilled glucagon injection and nasal glucagon.[4–6] designed to manage hypoglycemia, and addition of glucagon to advanced insulin pump systems are examples of such advances. Even more relevant to management of hyperglycemia is the development of drugs which specifically focus on glucagon as a target for glycemic lowering.

PHYSIOLOGICAL BASIS

Glucagon secretion is stimulated by hypoglycemia, most amino acids/acids, stress, and exposure to cold. On the other hand, it is inhibited by intake of glucose/carbohydrate meal, isoleucine, nonesterified fatty acids, and ketones. The glucagon insulin ratio determines the energy homeostasis of body. A high insulin glucagon ratio promotes protein biosynthesis, inhibits glucose production, and reduces lipolysis. A low insulin glucagon ratio increases hepatic gluconeogenesis and lipolysis, allowing the body to utilize nutrients scored in the liver and adipose tissue.

PHARMACOLOGICAL RELEVANCE

The insulin glucagon ratio can therefore be used as a marker of metabolic status. A high insulin glucagon ratio represents what we call "maladaptive anabolism", while a low ratio implies predominant catabolism. This demarcation can be used to choose appropriate glucose lowering therapy. A person with type 2 diabetes with high insulin glucagon ratio would benefit from insulin sparing drugs like glucagon-like peptide-1 receptor agonist (GLP-1RA) and sodium-glucose co-transporter 2 (SGLT2) inhibitor, while one with low insulin glucagon ratio may respond better to insulin secretagogues or insulin.[7] This concept can be considered as "Endometabolic Precision Medicine", as opposed to pharmacogenomics based precision medicine.

CHALLENGES

However, this is easier said than done. It is difficult to measure glucagon, and there is significant variation in sensitivity and specificity of various assays. Portal and systemic circulations of glucagon differ, and individual variations in porto-systemic gradient of glucagon prevent extrapolation of data obtained from venous sampling to a comprehensive understanding of glycemic homeostasis.[8]

INCRETIN-BASED THERAPY

The incretin hormones, glucagon-like peptide-1 (GLP-1) and gastric inhibitory polypeptide, are able to improve α-cell sensitivity. They do so by inhibiting glucagon secretion during hyperglycemia, and increasing it during hypoglycemia. Thus, glucagon acts as a therapeutic target which mediates not only correction of hyperglycemia, but the prevention of hypoglycemia as well. This improvement in α-cell sensitivity also helps reduce the burden on the β-cell, which is able to reduce its insulin secretion. This effect is evident in the insulin-sparing effect of GLP-1RA therapy.[9,10]

In toto, GLP-1RA acts as an islet cell de-stressor, by reducing the burden on both α-and β-cell, reducing both insulin and glucagon concentrations, and normalizing the insulin glucagon ratio. In fact, one-third of the glucose suppressive effect of GLP-1RA is thought to be due to glucagon suppression.[11]

We propose "The Hypothesis of Endocrine Parsimony" to explain the beneficial cardio metabolic effects noted with GLP-1RA. The word "parsimony" means effective use of limited available resources.[12] Islet distress leads to reduction of both insulin and glucagon, this optimizes the insulin glucagon metabolic fulcrum, and saves the energy spent by the body in maintaining a high stress conflict zone in the islets of Langerhans. This create a virtuous cascade throughout the body, facilitating distress of the cardiovascular endothelium, and promoting cardiovascular health.

SGLT2 INHIBITOR THERAPY

The SGLT2 inhibitors also act to destress the β-cell, but their use is associated with an increase in glucagon secretion.[13] Combinations of incretin-based therapy with SGLT2 inhibitors have therefore been studied, and found to have good results in glucose lowering.

GLUCAGON AS A THERAPEUTIC TARGET

Glucagon receptor antagonists are a new class of drugs under development. However, early clinical studies have shown side effects such as transaminitis, liver fat deposition, increase in body weight, systolic blood pressure, low density lipoprotein cholesterol, and α-cell hyperplasia. This has limited the utility of their beneficial effects on glycemia. Glucagon receptor/GLP-1 receptor co-agonism has also emerged as a therapeutic strategy for diabesity. Molecules in preclinical development act to stimulate both glucagon and GLP-1 receptors, to reduce appetite and weight. Neither of these therapeutic classes has reached clinical use, however.[11]

GLUCAGON AS A THERAPY

Glucagon is utilized as a treatment for major or severe hypoglycemia of varied etiology. Available as an injectable, it can be administered by intravenous, subcutaneous or intramuscular route. Children <25 kg in weight need a 0.5 mg dose (or 20–30 μg/kg) while in those above 25 kg, and adults, 1 mg is indicated. If weight is unknown, the age of 6 years can be taken as a threshold for administering 1 mg. Glucagon should be avoided concomitantly with anticholinergic drugs and indomethacin. It is also contraindicated for use in pheochromocytoma, insulinoma, glucagonoma and prolonged fasting or starvation. Nausea, vomiting and tachycardia are the commonest side effects.[14]

Nasal glucagon has also been developed, and is currently awaiting approval by regulatory authorities. A 3 mg dose has been found effective and convenient in correcting hypoglycemic events in type 1 diabetes.[4]

CONCLUSION

Glucagon is an essential part of the homeostasis of glucose, and contributes substantially to the pathophysiology of diabetes. It has found use in multiple

Box 1: Use of glucagon in endocrinology

Diagnostic
- Growth hormone deficiency
- Secondary adrenal insufficiency
- Etiology of hypoglycemia in liver metastasis
- Pheochromocytoma
- Earlier diagnosis of pancreatic cancer
- To facilitate barium enema
- To facilitate endoscopic retrograde cholangiopancreatography

Therapeutic target
- Incretin-based therapy
- Pramlintide (amylin mimetic)
- Glucagon receptor antagonists
- Glucagon receptor/glucagon-like peptide-1 receptor co-agonists

Therapeutic tool
- Hypoglycemia
- Bihormonal pumps

situations, as a diagnostic and therapeutic tool (Box 1), and as a target for therapy. However, optimal utilization of this important peptide still remains the missing link in diabetes management.

REFERENCES

1. Ahrén B. Glucagon early breakthroughs and recent discoveries. Peptides. 2015;67:74-81.
2. Unger R, Orci L. The essential role of glucagon in the pathogenesis of diabetes mellitus. The Lancet. 1975;305(7897):14-6.
3. Kalra S, Gupta Y. Choice of Glucose-lowering Therapy— A Metabolic Fulcrum-based Approach. US Endocrinology, 2015;11(2):79-80
4. Pontiroli AE, Ceriani V. Intranasal glucagon for hypoglycaemia in diabetic patients. An old dream is becoming reality? Diabetes, Obesity and Metabolism. 2018 Apr 13. Available at: https://doi.org/10.1111/dom.13317
5. Wilson LM, Castle JR. Stable Liquid Glucagon: Beyond Emergency Hypoglycemia Rescue. J Diabetes Sci and Technol. 2018 Feb 1: 1932296818757795.
6. El-Khatib FH, Balliro C, Hillard MA, et al. Home use of a bihormonal bionic pancreas versus insulin pump therapy in adults with type 1 diabetes: a multicentre randomised crossover trial. The Lancet. 2017; 389(10067):369-80.
7. Kalra S, Gupta Y. The insulin: glucagon ratio and the choice of glucose-lowering drugs. Diabetes Therapy. 20161;7(1):1-9.
8. Kalra S, Gupta Y. Letter to the Editor: Comment on "The Impact of Chronic Liraglutide Therapy on Glucagon Secretion in Type 2 Diabetes: Insight from the LIBRA Trial" by Kramer CK, et al. J Clin Endocrinology & Metabolism. 2015;100(11):L116-7.
9. Kalra S. Choosing appropriate glucagon-like peptide 1 receptor agonists: A patient-centered approach. Diabetes Therapy. 2014;5(1):333-40.
10. Prasad-Reddy L, Isaacs D. A clinical review of GLP-1 receptor agonists: efficacy and safety in diabetes and beyond. Drugs in Context. 2015;4:212283.
11. Hædersdal S, Lund A, Knop FK, Vilsbøll T. The role of glucagon in the pathophysiology and treatment of type 2 diabetes. InMayo Clinic Proceedings 2018 Jan 5. Elsevier.
12. Kalra S, Gupta Y, Sahay R. The law of therapeutic parsimony. Indian journal of endocrinology and metabolism. 2016;20(3).
13. Kalra S, Jacob JJ, Gupta Y. Newer antidiabetic drugs and calorie restriction mimicry. Indian Journal of Endocrinology and Metabolism. 2016;20(1):142.
14. Briscoe VJ, Davis SN. Hypoglycemia in type 1 and type 2 diabetes: physiology, pathophysiology, and management. Clinical Diabetes. 2006; 24(3):115-21.

Chapter 34

Algorithm for Management of Type 2 Diabetes—India Specific

Rajeev Chawla, Shalini Jaggi

INTRODUCTION

India today has the dubious distinction of being the "diabetic capital of the world" with 69.2 million known diabetics in 2015 and a projected number of more than 123.5 million by 2040 as per the International Diabetes Federation (IDF) estimates (IDF Diabetes Atlas, 7th edition, 2015. Diabetes has globally assumed epidemic proportions with its monumental load of microvascular as well as macrovascular complications and comorbidities resulting in a huge social as well as economic burden of the disease. This load can be minimized by early screening as well as optimal management of diabetes and even prediabetes and most of the life-changing complications can be prevented with an early and aggressive intervention to control hyperglycemia.

An ideal diabetes management strategy aims at not only treating the acute symptoms of hyperglycemia but also maintaining euglycemia with minimal glycemic excursions so as to prevent/delay the development of various diabetic complications and restoring the quality of life of patients. Treatment should also work to preserve beta-cell function and prevent or slow the rate of apoptosis to delay the natural progression of the disease characterized by an inevitable decline in insulin secretion. Lifestyle management, weight loss in overweight/obese patients, regular exercise with increase in physical activity and a healthy diet through medical nutrition therapy form the backbone of any diabetes treatment strategy. Pharmacotherapy using oral or injectable agents may be used in addition to lifestyle modification therapies to achieve a target glycosylated hemoglobin (HbA1c) target of less than 7% for all diabetic patients as far as possible to prevent complications.

A better understanding of the multiple pathophysiologies of type 2 diabetes along with introduction of new drugs with evolving times has led to an era of pathophysiology-based pharmacotherapeutic approach to the management of hyperglycemia. Several guidelines all across the world provide different treatment algorithms on ways in which these glucose-lowering agents can be used either alone or in combination. This review is based on consensus developed by the Research Society for the Study of Diabetes (RSSDI) in India adapted from the IDF Guidelines 2014 that was subsequently published in Oct 2015 in IJJDC Oct 2015[1] and revised second version got published in IJJDC Jan-Mar 2018.[2]

PHARMACOTHERAPEUTIC APPROACH TO THE MANAGEMENT OF HYPERGLYCEMIA

Glucose-lowering medications may be started when lifestyle interventions alone are unable to maintain blood glucose control at target levels. It is necessary to continue lifestyle measures all along the management algorithm along with medical nutrition therapy alongside pharmacotherapy. The choice of medication should be based on individual needs of the patient with adequate consideration given to the cost-benefit ratio of each agent along with its efficacy and pharmacological action. Each initiation or dose increment may be monitored for response in 2–3 months and ineffective therapies may accordingly be discontinued if needed. Therapy decision should also take into consideration hypoglycemia, effect on weight as well as the adverse event profile of the agent besides the pathophysiology it addresses.

First-line Oral Therapy

- Begin therapy with metformin unless there is evidence of renal impairment or any other contraindication
- Titrate the dose over early weeks to minimize discontinuation due to gastrointestinal (GI) intolerance
- Monitor renal function and use metformin with caution if estimated glomerular filtration rate (eGFR) <45 mL/min/1.73 m^2
- Other options include initiating with a sulfonylurea (SU) (or glinide) for rapid response where glucose levels are high, or a (DPP-4) inhibitor or alpha-glucosidase inhibitor (AGI)—these agents can also be used initially in place of metformin where it is not tolerated or is contraindicated
- In some circumstances dual therapy may be indicated right for initiation where a single agent alone is unlikely to achieve glucose targets, underlining the need for an early aggressive approach to intensify glycemic control to prevent the "legacy effect" and ensuing complications of prolonged hyperglycemia.

Second-line Therapy

- When glucose control targets are not being achieved, add a SU
- Other options include adding metformin if not used first-line, AGI, a DPP-4 inhibitor or a thiazolidinedione based on the individual profile of the patient
- A non-SU insulin secretagogue (glinides) is an alternative option to SU especially if there is predominantly post prandial hyperglycemia
- Sodium-glucose cotransporter-2 (SGLT2) inhibitors can also be considered as second line agents when weight and hypoglycemia are major concerns as well as their proven cardiovascular (CV) safety in type 2 diabetic patients with CV disease
- Glucagon-like peptide-1 (GLP-1) analogs are also a good choice due to their efficacy as well as multiple pleiotropic benefits of weight loss properties, less hypoglycemia, reduced appetite and cardioprotection, but due to their high cost, GI intolerance and mode of administration (injectable), they are prescribed as second line agents to a very niche set of patients in India.

Third-line Therapy

- When glucose control targets are no longer being achieved with two agents, it is recommended to either start insulin or add a third agent
- If starting insulin, add basal insulin or use premix insulin
- If adding a third oral agent options include an AΓI, a DPP-4 inhibitor, an SGLT2 inhibitor or a thiazolidinedione
- Another option is to add a GLP-1 analog
- Since 2014 DCGI has approved hydroxychloroquine as an adjuvant to diet and exercise to aid in glycemic control in type 2 diabetes patients in addition to metformin and SU dual therapy.

Fourth-line Therapy

- Begin insulin therapy in combination with a sensitizing agent (metformin or glitazone) when optimized oral blood glucose lowering medications (and/or GLP-1 analogs) and lifestyle interventions are unable to maintain target glucose control
- Intensify insulin therapy in patients already using insulin.

CONSIDERATIONS

The decision on choice of oral antidiabetic therapy in type 2 diabetes mellitus (T2DM) patients should be based on the cost and efficacy factors in Indian context besides their efficacy and other actions.

RATIONALE AND EVIDENCE

Antidiabetic Agents

Biguanide

Metformin remains the first-line type 2 diabetes drug due to its efficacy as well as properties such as weight neutrality and low cost and no major adverse effects such as hypoglycemia etc. It works by reducing hepatic glucose output thus working as an excellent insulin sensitizer.[3,4] Metformin is associated with initial GI side effects, and caution also needs to be taken to avoid its use in patients at an increased risk for lactic acidosis (e.g. those with advanced renal insufficiency, alcoholism, hypoxemic states etc.). Antiproliferative as well as CV benefits of this drug have also been reported though robust clinical trial data is still awaited.

Sulfonylurea

It is the oldest oral hypoglycemic agent class available and is characterized as an insulin secretagogue. SU agents cause closure of adenosine triphosphate-sensitive potassium channels in beta-cells thus stimulating insulin release.[5] Although they are effective in controlling glucose levels, their use is associated with modest weight gain and increased risk of hypoglycemia. The modern SUs particularly gliclazide modified release and glimepiride have a lower risk of hypoglycemia than the older generation agents such as glibenclamide and are recommended as preferred SUs to be used. Glibenclamide should be used only in case of nonavailability of these agents. Studies have demonstrated increased chances of secondary failure with these agents probably due to an exacerbation of islet dysfunction over time.[6] Shorter-acting secretagogues, the meglitinides (commonly called glinides), also stimulate insulin release through similar mechanisms (acting at a different site away from the SU site) but are associated with comparatively less hypoglycemia,[7] though they require more frequent dosing.

Thiazolidinediones

Thiazolidinediones (TZDs) or glitazones are peroxisome proliferator activated receptor-γ activators[7] that improve insulin sensitivity in skeletal muscle and reduce hepatic glucose production.[3,4] The risk of hypoglycemia is negligible with these agents and they are more durable than SUs and metformin in their effects.[6] Pioglitazone demonstrated pleiotropic effects on CV events as a secondary outcome in one large trial involving patients with overt macro vascular disease.[8,9] Recently, pioglitazone was controversially linked with a possible increased risk of bladder cancer[10] though it was not substantiated. Data from a retrospective study in India involving 2,222 T2DM patients including patients with age >60 years, duration of diabetes >10 years and uncontrolled diabetes (1,111 pioglitazone users and 1,111 pioglitazone nonusers) found no evidence of bladder cancer in any group.[11] The commonly recognized side effects of TZDs include weight gain, increased risk of bone fractures, fluid retention leading to edema and/or increased incidence of heart failure in predisposed individuals.[6,9]

Incretin-based Therapies

The injectable GLP-1 receptor agonists (incretin mimetics) mimic the effects of endogenous GLP-1, thereby stimulating pancreatic insulin secretion in a glucose dependent fashion. They also suppress pancreatic glucagon output, slow gastric emptying and reduce appetite. Their main advantage is weight loss, which ranges from modest to significant in most patients. A limiting side effect is nausea and vomiting, particularly early in the course of treatment. There have been concerns regarding an increased risk of pancreatitis, but recently published ELIXA study and LEADER study did not show any increased risk of pancreatitis, pancreatic cancer or thyroid cancer with lixisenatide[12] or liraglutide.[13]

The DPP-4 inhibitors or incretin enhancer therapies enhance circulating concentrations of active GLP-1 and glucose-dependent insulinotropic polypeptide by preventing their immediate degradation by the DPP-4 enzyme.[14,15] Their major effect appears to be in the regulation of insulin and glucagon secretion; besides being oral agents, they are weight neutral. Recent CV studies with DPP-4 inhibitors have shown that these agents do not increase CV risk.[16-18] Typically, none of the incretin-based classes cause hypoglycemia by themselves.

Sodium–glucose Cotransporter 2 Inhibitors

The SGLT2 inhibitors provide insulin-independent glucose lowering by blocking SGLT2 receptors thus inhibiting increased glucose reabsorption in the proximal renal tubule. These agents also provide modest weight loss and blood pressure reduction. Although there are three FDA approved agents for use in patients with type 2 diabetes, there is insufficient data to recommend clinical use in type 1 diabetes at this time.[19] SGLT2 inhibitors have the potential to reduce CV risk in patients with T2DM not only through optimization of glycemic control, but also via beneficial effects on body weight, blood pressure, lipids and serum uric acid.[20,21]

Other Agents

Two agents that are used infrequently in management of type 2 diabetes are AGIs, which retard gut carbohydrate absorption,[22] and colesevelam, a bile acid sequestrant whose mechanism of glucose-lowering action remains poorly understood with its major additional benefit of low-density lipoprotein cholesterol reduction.[23] Both have GI effects, mainly flatulence with AGIs and constipation with colesevelam. The dopamine agonist bromocriptine (quick release formulation) is also available as an antihyperglycemic agent that supposedly acts by mimicking the morning surge of dopamine.[24] Its mechanism of action and precise role are unclear. Another agent, the amylin agonist, pramlintide (not available in India), is typically reserved for patients treated with intensive insulin therapy, usually in type 1 diabetes mellitus; it decreases postprandial glucose excursions by inhibiting glucagon secretion and slowing gastric emptying.[25]

The glucose-lowering effectiveness of non-insulin pharmacological agents is said to be high with metformin, SUs, TZDs and GLP-1 agonists (expected HbA1c reduction ~1.0–1.5%),[26-28] and comparatively lower for meglitinides, DPP-4 inhibitors, SGLT2 inhibitors, AGIs, colesevelam and bromocriptine (~0.5–1.0%). However, older drugs have typically been tested in clinical trial participants with higher baseline HbA1c, which is associated with greater treatment emergent glycemic reductions, irrespective of therapy type. In head-to-head trials, any differential effects on glucose control are small. So agent- and patient-specific properties, such as ease of administration, dosing frequency, side-effect profiles, cost and other benefits often help in their selection.

INDIVIDUALIZING THERAPY

ABCDEFGH approach for diabetes management as proposed in" RSSDI Therapeutic Wheel"[1]

Choice of any antidiabetic agent should take into account the patient's general health status and associated medical disorders. This patient centric approach may be referred to as the ABCDEFGH approach for diabetes management. As shown in the Figure 1, for any T2DM patient first line of therapy should be metformin unless not tolerated or contraindicated.

Individualized Treatment

- For an individual who has been diagnosed with diabetes, consider a combination of metformin and one of these treatment options based on the following parameters—**A**ge, **B**MI, **CKD**, **D**uration of Diabetes, **E**stablished CVD, **F**inancial condition, **G**lycemic status and **H**ypoglycemia concern
- Drug choice should be based on patient preferences as well as presence of various comorbidities and complications, and drug characteristics, with the goal of reducing blood glucose levels while minimizing side effects, especially hypoglycemia and weight gain
- A comparative effectiveness meta-analysis[1] suggests that overall each new class of noninsulin agents added to initial therapy lowers HbA1c around 0.9–1.1%.[28]

Age

- Estimated glomerular filtration rate adjusted doses of gliptins may be a suitable addition to metformin for elderly patients in whom one will like to avoid hypoglycemia and weight gain[29]
- Agents belonging to AGI could also be important choice in elderly patient. These agents have moderate efficacy but minimal side effects
- In elderly males, glitazones may be a safer alternative in patients with preserved cardiac function. However, postmenopausal females must be spared for its use because of high predisposition to osteoporosis.
- While SU's, GLP-1 receptor agonist (GLP-1 RA), SGLT2 inhibitors or glinides should emerge as last choice since there are adverse effects as well as premium price associated with these agents. Risk benefits ratio must be properly evaluated before using them.

Body Mass Index

- Glucagon-like peptide-1 receptor agonist seem to be the best add on therapy for those having high body mass index (BMI). This group of medications have highest weight reducing property in addition to the excellent efficacy
- The SGLT 2 inhibitors also have a weight reduction property albeit less than that of GLP-1 RA. The medicines in this group has an additional advantage of excellent tolerance and can be given orally as compared to GLP-1 RA. However, their glycemic efficacy seems to be less than that of GLP-1 RA. The experience with this group of agents is less than that with GLP-1 RA[30]
- The AGIs and gliptins are weight neutral and so can be used as third line of agents
- The last option for such kind of patients should be SU's, insulin or glitazones since they are having weight gain properties.

Chronic Kidney Disease

- In the same manner if we focus on complications (renal impairment) preference of therapy would be

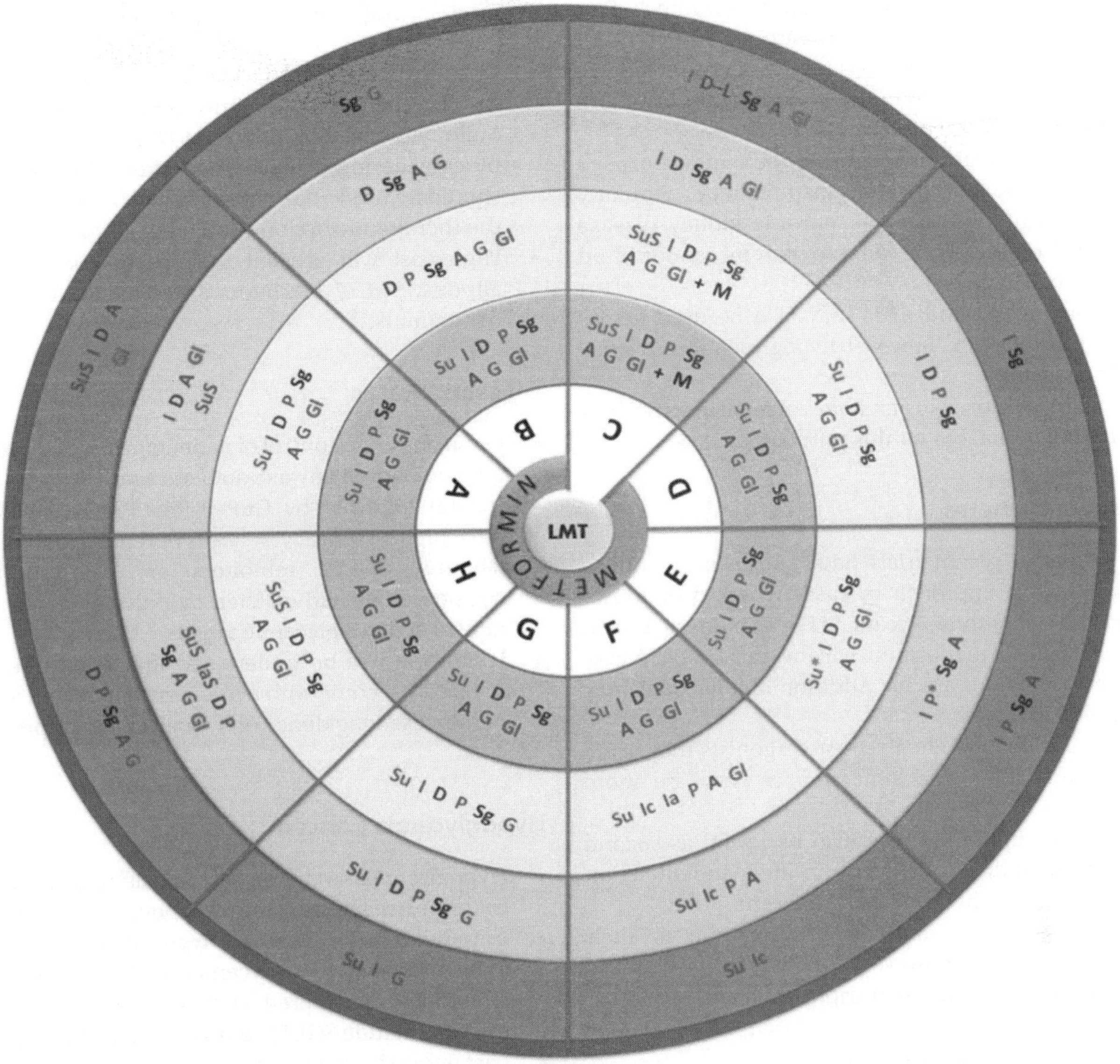

Su	– Sulfonylurea	Ia	– Insulin analogs	P*	– Pioglitazone if EF >40%
Su*	– Preferably glimiperide or gliclazide	IaS	– Short-acting insulin analogs	Sg	– SGLT2 inhibitors
SuS	– Short-acting sulfonylureas	D	– DPP-4 inhibitors	A	– Alphaglucosidase inhibitors
I	– Insulin	D-L	– Linagliptin	G	– GLP analogs
Ic	– Conventional insulins	P	– Pioglitazone	Gl	– Glinides

From innermost to outermost: A: Age = Advancing Age; B: BMI = Increasing BMI; C: CKD = Advancing CKD; D: Duration of diabetes = Increasing duration; E: Established CVD = Low CVD risk to Established CVD risk; F: Finance = Adequate-to-limited; G: Glycemic status = Worsening glycemic control; H: Hypoglycemia = Hypoglycemia concern.

Lesser options available   Wider options available

(BMI: body mass index; CKD: chronic kidney disease; CVD: cardiovascular disease; DPP-4: dipeptidyl peptidase-4; EF: ejection fraction; GLP: glucagon-like peptide; SGLT2: sodium-glucose cotransporter 2.)

Figure 1 RSSDI diabetes therapeutic wheel. ***(For color version, see Plate 2)***

gliptins as add on therapy with metformin.[31] Few of the gliptins need dose adjustment as per eGFR while vildagliptin needs dose adjustment in hepatic insufficiency. Linagliptin does not require any dose adjustment in renal disease

- Repaglinide is another agent which may be used across all stages of renal insufficiency. Similarly glitazones may be used in chronic kidney disease (CKD), however, one has to careful about fluid retention
- Short acting SU and AGIs may also be used across renal insufficiency, however hypoglycemia is a huge limiting factor
- Insulin may be used in any stages of renal insufficiency and is the best agent for this purpose.

Duration of Diabetes

- As results of recent trials have suggested to utilize an aggressive approach in cases where duration of diabetes is less than 5 years, SU or glinide, as an add on therapy to metformin, will be the best choices, being very potent agents. Addition of glitazones may be useful at this stage[32]
- Glucagon-like peptide-1 receptor agonists may score over gliptins for this indication as they are more efficacious than gliptins
- The SGLT2 inhibitors may also be useful as second add on agent due to their insulin-independent action which is patho physiologically different
- Gliptins and AGIs are last choices due to their moderate efficacy, however, they may be used as add on agents at any stage after triple drug fails.

Established Cardiovascular Disease

- In patients with established cardiovascular disease (CVD), DPP4 inhibitors may be preferred agents after pioglitazone, SGLT inhibitors and AGIs because of low risk of hypoglycemia. GLP-1 analogs may be a suitable alternative for patients who are overweight or obese. AGIs may be preferred in patients with postprandial hyperglycemia
- Pioglitazone has also been shown in different studies to reduce CVD risk
- Recent data from EMPA-REG study has shown that SGLT inhibitors reduce CV risk and CV mortality, and may be preferred.

Financial Condition

- Cost of therapy also plays an essential role considering the treatment remains continued lifelong
- Sulfonylureas should be first choice with metformin by considering its cost. Then after AGIs or glitazone should be used at next therapy level,[33] in the next level the therapeutic option should be glinides or insulin
- High cost will prevent the use of insulin analogs, gliptins, SGLT2 inhibitors and GLP-1 RA in most of the patients.[34]

Glycemic Status

- Good glycemic control of patients is directly correlated with efficacy of any antidiabetic agent
- Insulin followed by GLP-1 RA, SUs and glitazones have highest efficacy in terms of reducing HbA1c[35]
- Gliptins, SGLT2 inhibitors or AGIs should be considered as add on therapy if these agents are not able to achieve glycemic targets
- It is always to be understood that good efficacy, in most cases, come with a price written on it in the form of increased incidence of hypoglycemia or prohibitive cost.

Hypoglycemia Concern

- Hypoglycemia is the biggest hurdle that any medical fraternity is facing during treatment course of diabetes
- In patients with history of hypoglycemia or for those at high risk of hypoglycemia, GLP-1 RA or gliptins should be considered as first choice with.[36] Other options include SGLT2 inhibitors, glitazones and AGIs
- Last option for such patients should be either glinides, SU's or insulin since there are high chances of hypoglycemia with these agents
- Group of patients where one will require avoiding hypoglycemia include:
    - Those with established CVD
    - Elderly patients
    - Those suffering from retinopathy and cannot perform self-monitoring blood glucose without help of others
    - Those who stay alone, especially in remote areas
    - Those who are having poor longevity
    - Those who are having documented hypoglycemia unawareness

 - Those who met with severe symptomatic hypoglycemia requiring hospitalization.

CONCLUSION

How to use the RSSDI Diabetic Therapeutic Wheel?

- The RSSDI therapeutic wheel is designed to be a simple user friendly approach to decide the appropriate antidiabetic agent to be used in T2DM
- When you see a patient in your clinic:
  - Prescribe lifestyle intervention to all and metformin to most patients as mentioned in the inner core of the wheel (white and light blue rings)
  - Then identify the 2/3 most important concerns/factors (from ABCDEFGH) that you feel should influence your choice of antidiabetic agent, e.g. age/CKD/finance etc.
  - Identify the best choices available to you from the outer rings of the wheel (orange and red)
  - Further fine tune your choices if more concerns exist in a given patient and reach a rational final choice in an "individualized approach".

REFERENCES

1. Madhu SV, Saboo B, Chawla R, et al. RSSDI Clinical Practice Recommendations for Management of Type-2 Diabetes Mellitus 2015. Int J Diabetes Dev Ctries. 2015;(Suppl1):S1-71.
2. Bajaj S, Saboo B, Chawla R, et al. RSSDI Clinical Practice Recommendations for Management of Type-2 Diabetes Mellitus 2018 ; Int J Diabetes Dev Ctries. 2018;38(Suppl1).
3. Bailey CJ, Turner RC. Metformin. N Engl J Med. 1996;334(9):574-9.
4. Lamanna C, Monami M, Marchionni N, et al. Effect of metformin on cardiovascular events and mortality: a meta analysis of randomized clinical trials. Diabetes Obes Metab. 2011;13(3):221-8.
5. Bryan J, Crane A, Vila-Carriles WH, et al. Insulin secretagogues, sulfonylurea receptors and K(ATP) channels. Curr Pharm Des. 2005;11(21):2699-716.
6. Kahn SE, Haffner SM, Heise MA, et al. Glycemic durability of rosiglitazone, metformin, or glyburide monotherapy. N Engl J Med. 2006;355:2427-43.
7. Gerich J, Raskin P, Jean-Louis L, et al. PRESERVE-β: two-year efficacy and safety of initial combination therapy with nateglinide or glyburide plus metformin. Diabetes Care. 2005;28:2093-9.
8. Yki-Jarvinen H. Thiazolidinediones. N Engl J Med. 2004;351(11):1106-18.
9. Dormandy JA, Charbonnel B, Eckland DJ, et al. Secondary prevention of macrovascular events in patients with type 2 diabetes in the PROactive study (PROspectivepioglitAzone Clinical Trial InmacroVascular Events): a randomised controlled trial. Lancet. 2005;366(9493):1279-89.
10. Lewis JD, Ferrara A, Peng T, et al. Risk of bladder cancer among diabetic patients treated with pioglitazone: interim report of a longitudinal cohort study. Diabetes Care. 2011;34(4):916-22.
11. Gupta S, Gupta K, Ravi R, et al. Pioglitazone and the risk of bladder cancer: An Indian retrospective cohort study. IJEM. 2015;19(5):639-43.
12. Bentley-Lewis R, Aguilar D, Riddle MC, et al. Rationale, design, and baseline characteristics in Evaluation of LIXisenatide in Acute Coronary Syndrome, a long-term cardiovascular end point trial of lixisenatide versus placebo. Am Heart J. 2015;169(5):631-8.e7.
13. Marso SP, Daniel GH, Brown-Frandsen K, et al. Liraglutide and cardiovascular outcomes in type 2 diabetes; N Engl J Med. 2016;375:311-22.
14. Deacon CF. Dipeptidyl peptidase-4 inhibitors in the treatment of type 2 diabetes: a comparative review. Diabetes Obes Metab. 2011;13(1):7-18.
15. Chawla S, Kaushik N, Singh NP, et al. Effect of addition of either sitagliptin or pioglitazone in patients with uncontrolled type 2 diabetes mellitus on metformin: A randomized controlled trial. J Pharmacol Pharmacother. 2013;4(1):27-32.
16. Scirica BM, Bhatt DL, Braunwald E, et al. Saxagliptin and cardiovascular outcomes in patients with type 2 diabetes mellitus. N Engl J Med. 2013;369(14):1317-26.
17. White WB, Cannon CP, Heller SR, et al. Alogliptin after acute coronary syndrome in patients with type 2 diabetes. N Engl J Med. 2013;369(14):1327-35.
18. TECOS: Sitagliptin Cardiovascular Outcome Study. ClinicalTrials.gov identifier: NCT00790205.
19. Chiang JL, KirkmanMS, Laffel LM, et al. Type 1 Diabetes Sourcebook Authors. Type 1 diabetes through the life span: a position statement of the American Diabetes Association. Diabetes Care. 2014;37(7):2034-54.
20. Basile JN. The potential of sodium glucose cotransporter 2 (SGLT2) inhibitors to reduce cardiovascular risk in patients with type 2 diabetes (T2DM). J Diabetes Complications. 2013;27(3):280-6.
21. Baker WL, Smyth LR, Riche DM, et al. Effects of sodium-glucose cotransporter 2 inhibitors on blood pressure: a systematic review and meta-analysis. J Am SocHypertens. 2014;8(4):262-75.e9.
22. Van de Laar FA, Lucassen PL, Akkermans RP, et al. Alpha-glucosidase inhibitors for people with impaired glucose tolerance or impaired fasting blood glucose. Cochrane Database Syst Rev. 2006;(4):CD005061.
23. Fonseca VA, Handelsman Y, Staels B. Colesevelam lowers glucose and lipid levels in type 2 diabetes: the clinical evidence. Diabetes Obes Metab. 2010;12(5):384-92.
24. Defronzo RA. Bromocriptine: a sympatholytic, D2- dopamine agonist for the treatment of type 2 diabetes. Diabetes Care. 2011;34(4):789-94.
25. Singh-Franco D, Robles G, Gazze D. Pramlintide acetate injection for the treatment of type 1 and type 2 diabetes mellitus. ClinTher. 2007;29(4):535-62.
26. Bolen S, Feldman L, Vassy J Wilson L, et al. Systematic review: comparative effectiveness and safety of oral medications for type 2 diabetes mellitus. Ann Intern Med. 2007;147(6):386-99.
27. Peters A. Incretin-based therapies: review of current clinical trial data. Am J Med. 2010;123:S28-37.
28. Bennett WL, Maruthur NM, Singh S, et al. Comparative effectiveness and safety of medications for type 2 diabetes: an update including new drugs and 2-drug combinations. Ann Intern Med. 2011;154(9):602-13.
29. Type 2 diabetes - newer agents (partial update); NICE Clinical Guideline. 2009 Available at: patient.info/doctor/antihyperglycaemic-agents-used-for-type-2-diabetes [Last accessed on 27 Aug 2015].
30. Cauthon K, Yendapally R. A Review of GLP-1 Receptor Agonists and SGLT2 inhibitors for Type 2 Diabetes.
31. S Ghoshal-BMJ Blogs: Gliptins – where are we now? 30Jan 2013
32. Hanefeld M. Pioglitazone and sulfonylureas: effectively treating type 2 diabetes. Int J ClinPract Suppl. 2007;(153):20-7.
33. Kalra S, Chadha M, Sharma SK, et al. Untapped diamonds for untamed diabetes: The α-glucosidase inhibitors. Indian J EndocrinolMetab. 2014;18(2):138–41.
34. Second- and Third-Line Pharmacotherapy for Type 2 Diabetes: Update. Ottawa (ON): Canadian Agency for Drugs and Technologies in Health; 2013.
35. Gallwitz B. The Future of Combination Therapies of Insulin with a Glucagon-like Peptide-1 Receptor Agonists in Type 2 Diabetes – Is it Advantageous? Eur Endocrinol. 2014;10(2):98-9.
36. McCulloch DK, Nathan DM, Mulder JE. Management of persistent hyperglycemia in type 2 diabetes mellitus. 2015.

Chapter 35

Novel Markers for Screening Diabetes Complications

Sudha Vidyasagar

INTRODUCTION

Type 2 diabetes is associated with microvascular and macrovascular complications, involving various organ systems. These lead to increased mortality and morbidity, which is 2–4-fold higher than in the general population.[1] Since these complications are due to long-term glycemia, the early detection of these complications is important in making a difference to the quality of life to these patients. The traditional markers of glycemia such as glycated hemoglobin have been used to predict the occurrence of these. However, there have been problems in the accuracy of such predictions.

Hence, novel biomarkers, which constitute inflammatory molecules growth factors and cytokines, have been explored to understand the subgroup of patients who are susceptible to these complications and would constitute a high-risk group. In this article, we will explore the various complications of diabetes and their predictability using biomarkers.

DIABETIC NEPHROPATHY

This is an important microvascular complication of diabetes, most commonly present in type 1 diabetes, after 5–10 years and also in type 2 diabetes, though at a lesser rate. Traditionally, the presence of microalbuminuria with albumin excretion rate of more than or 200 μg/min has been observed as a warning signal for the onset of diabetic kidney disease. However, the accuracy of this investigation to predict progression to end-stage renal disease has been doubted. For example, 30% of diabetics with renal dysfunction have normoalbuminuria.

Various other factors such as blood pressure, plasma lipid profile, glomerular filtration rate (GFR) measurements, and presence of diabetic retinopathy (DR) have also been used to identify those who will progress to chronic kidney disease. However, the pathology of diabetic kidney disease is complex and involves structural remodeling of the kidney with activation of several signaling pathways. For example, the role of renin–angiotensin–aldosterone system (RAAS) as proinflammatory, involving cytokines such as tumor necrosis factor alpha (TNF-α) and interleukin-1 (IL-1) beta has been noted. The role of protein kinase C (PKC) as a mediator of mesangial hypotrophy and renal fibrosis by way of upregulation of vascular endothelial growth factor (VEGF) has been discovered.[2] Several other cytokines also play a role in the renal inflammation such as IL-1, IL-6, and IL-18.

Biomarkers in renal disease have been classified as glomerular, tubular, and other proteins (Table 1). Glomerular biomarkers include transferrin, type IV collagen, glycosaminoglycans (GAGs) and ceruloplasmin. The role of micro-RNAs (miRNAs), which are short noncoding mRNAs that regulate urine proteomics, highlights their epigenetic role in development of diabetic nephropathy (DN). Urinary transferrin is also a better marker of glomerular injury. In fact, it predicts the development of microalbuminuria in type 2 diabetes mellitus (T2DM) patients who have no albumin in patients.[3] However, this lacks specificity as it can be present in several other systemic diseases. Type IV collagen is a more specific biomarker in type 1 diabetes mellitus (T1DM) as an early predictor of nephropathy.[4] Urinary fibronectin is also being explored in comparison to albuminuria.

TABLE 1: Classification of the novel biomarkers.

Glomerular biomarkers	Tubular biomarkers	Biomarkers of oxidative stress	Biomarkers of inflammation	Miscellaneous biomarkers
• Transferrin • Albumin • IgG • Ceruloplasmin • Type IV collagen • Laminin • GAGs • Fibronectin • L-PGDS	• NGAL • KIM-I • NAG • Cystatin C • L-FABP • Alpha-1-microglobulin	• 8oHdG	• TNF-α‡ • IL-Iβ‡ • IL-8‡ • IL-18‡ • IP-10‡ • MCP-1‡ • G-CSF‡ • Eotaxin‡ • Orosomucoid • RANTES‡	• VEGF‡ • Podocalyxin‡ • Nephrin‡ • H-FABP# • Retinol-binding protein# • AGEs

Notes: ‡Also regarded as glomerular biomarkers.

#Also regarded as tubular biomarkers.

(IgG: immunoglobulin G; GAGs: glycosaminoglycans; L-PGDS: lipocalin-type prostaglandin D synthase; NGAL: neutrophil gelatinase -associated lipocalin; KIM-I: kidney injury molecule I; NAG: N-acetyl-glucosamine; L-FABP: liver-type fatty acid-binding protein; 8oHdG: 8-oxo-7,8-dihydro-2 -deoxyguanosine; TNF-α: tumor necrosis factor α; IL: interleukin; IP-10: interferon gamma-induced protein: MCP-1: monocyte chemoattractant protein-I: G-CSF: granulocyte colony stimulating factor; RANTES: regulated on activation, normal T cell expressed and secreted; VEGF: vascular endothelial growth factor; H-FABP: heart fatty acid-binding protein; AGEs: advanced glycation end products.)

Tubular biomarkers include neutrophil gelatinase-associated lipocalin (NGAL) may be elevated before microalbuminuria in T2DM. Alpha-1 microglobulin is filtered and reabsorbed in the proximal tubule normally. In tubular dysfunction, it is excreted and may mark the onset of diabetic tubular disease. Cystatin C and NGAL and urinary liver type fatty acid binding protein are also markers of tubular dysfunction.

Further biomarkers of inflammation such as IL-8 and granulocyte colony-stimulating factor (G-CSF) have been found to be increased in the urine of patients with DN. Advanced glycation end product (AGE) levels in the urine have also been found to be high in patients with microalbuminuria, more than in patients with normoalbuminuria.[5]

In conclusion, all these biomarkers need to be followed up in long-term studies to assess the significance of these in prediction and progression of DN.

DIABETIC RETINOPATHY

Diabetic retinopathy is the leading cause of blindness all over the world in type 1 and type 2 DM patients. One of chief reasons for the progression to blindness is uncontrolled sugar as evidenced from data from Diabetes Control and Complications Trial (DCCT) and United Kingdom Prospective Diabetes Study (UKPDS). Retinopathy can begin even in the prediabetes stage.[6] Screening for DR by fundus examination by an ophthalmologist is advised, but in resource-poor countries, the logistics of this exercise is enormous, and near impossible. Hence, the search has been on for biomarkers, which can identify a high-risk group of patients, who may need prompt intervention.

The DR is classified into proliferative and nonproliferative retinopathy. Neovascularization is the hallmark of proliferative retinopathy, and is due to retinal ischemia, leading to increased amounts of vascular endothelial growth factor (VEGF). Macular edema also contributes to visual loss. The breaking of the blood-retinal barrier (BRB) is the beginning of retinopathy, and this is due to several proinflammatory markers, cytokines, and AGEs. An attempt has been made to detect these markers early in the course of the disease to prevent further progression of the disease.

Hyperglycemia-induced oxidative stress on the mitochondrial chain causes PKC activation and resulting in inflammation. Higher levels of C-reactive protein (CRP) have been shown in patients with DR.[7] This chronic inflammation is fueled by IL-1 and IL-6, in addition to TNF-α, leading to increased expression of adhesion molecules. The toll-like receptors are also activated by oxidative stress due to high sugars. There is thus damage to BRB and pericytes, causing leak into the retina, and DR.[8] Hyperglycemia also causes increased AGE, the most important of which is (carboxymethyl)lysine (CML).[9] In addition, increased levels of plasminogen activator inhibitor 1 has also been shown to correlate with the risk of progression of proliferative retinopathy.[10]

The VEGF causes angiogenesis and endothelial growth, causing neovascularization and increased vascular permeability. PKC is known to act in concert with this post-transcriptionally. In addition, the RAAS pathway involving angiotensin-II is upregulated in diabetes, and this increases secretion of VEGF resulting in uncontrolled angiogenesis (Fig. 1). There is a positive correlation between levels of VEGF and the incidence and severity of retinopathy.[11]

The theory that DR is probably due to alteration in neuroprotective factors is also gaining ground. There is increase in glutamate, which is the excitatory neurotransmitter, and decrease in pigment epithelium-derived factor (PEDF), and brain-derived neurotrophic factor (BDNF). The latter inhibits apoptosis of retinal cells, and its decrease contributes to loss of integrity of retina.[12]

Further, the role of miRNAs in the angiogenesis has been addressed by two trials, such as (1) Diabetic Retinopathy Candesartan Trial (DIRECT) and (2) PROTECT1. These have demonstrated that certain miRNAs are potential biomarkers for DR.[13]

BIOMARKERS IN DIABETIC NEUROPATHY

Diabetic neuropathy is painful often and can completely alter the quality of life for the diabetic patient. It has been found that those with painful neuropathy may have higher concentrations of inflammatory markers, which may account for the low-grade inflammation common in these patients.[14] There is also the role of anti-inflammatory cytokines, which may have a protective role, such as IL-1 receptor antagonist. The final impact of several glycemic markers, cytokines, and pro- and anti-inflammatory markers looks complex. The relative role of each of this and their impact is not very clear. The Flowchart 1 shows the complexity of their whole interaction.

CARDIOVASCULAR BIOMARKERS IN DIABETES

Cardiovascular (CV) morbidity and mortality are the leading causes of death in diabetes, all over the world. It is well known that this complication is risk stratified by factors beyond glycemia, and it is important to incorporate several comorbidities into this picture, which contribute to this important complication.

The CV morbidity seems to be a combination of pathophysiology such as low-grade chronic inflammation, endothelial dysfunction, insulin resistance, poor tissue repair, all culminating in accelerated atherosclerosis. All these lead to cardiac disease in the form of coronary artery disease leading to myocardial infarction, congestive cardiac failure due to cardiomyopathy, fatal arrhythmias, and thromboembolism. Identifying these early would go a long way in reducing CV events in these patients.

Low-grade inflammation in DM is characterized by increase in proinflammatory substances such as CRP. However, it was found that this marker did not have sufficient specificity and sensitivity to identify those

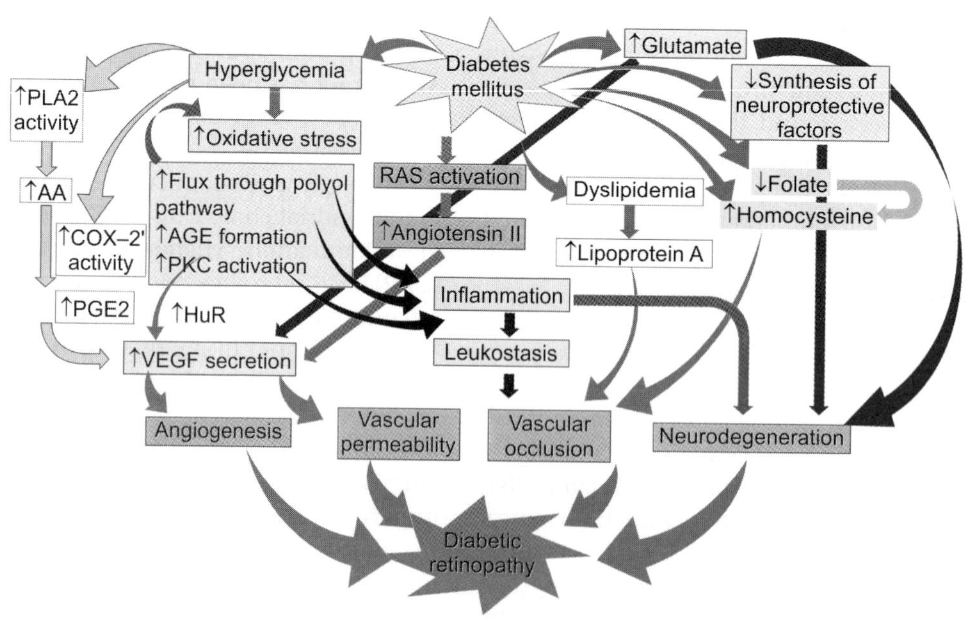

(PLA2: phospholipases A2; AA: arachidonic acid; COX2: cyclooxygenase-2; PGE2: postaglandin E2; AGE: advanced glycation end product; PKC: potein kinase C; VEGF: vascular endothelial growth factor; RAS: renin–angiotensin system.)

Figure 1 Simplified overview of the multiple interacting pathways leading to the pathogenesis of diabetic retinopathy.

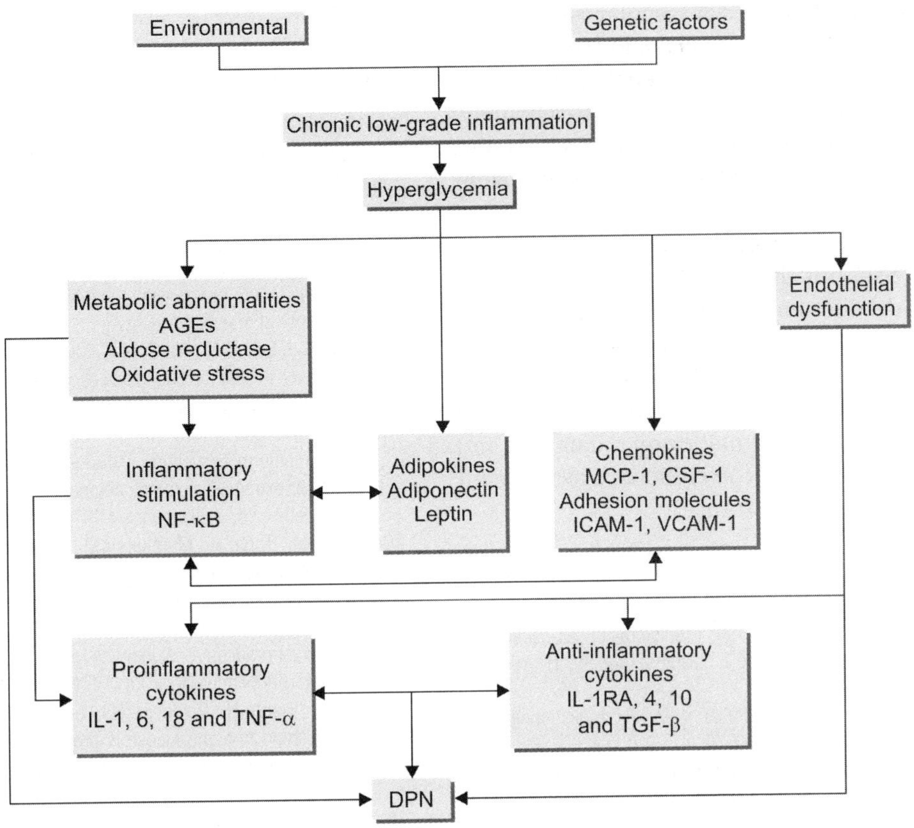

(CSF: colony-stimulating factor; DPN: diabetic peripheral neuropathy; IL: interleukin; ICAM: increased expression of adhesion molecules; MCP: monocyte chemoattractant protein; TGF: transforming growth factor; TNF: tumor necrosis factor; VCAM: vascular cell adhesion molecule.)

Flowchart 1 Complexity of whole interaction of biomarkers in diabetic neuropathy.

patients who may have higher CV risk. It is well known that cytokines such as IL-6, IL-1, IL-10, and IL-18, CRP and TNF-α are other candidates for this inflammatory state.[15] All these are known to affect plaque stability, endothelial remodeling, and accelerated atherosclerosis, thus making a huge impact on CV risk.[16,17] In addition, novel biomarkers have emerged such as galectin-3, which is involved in the modulation of proliferation of fibroblasts. Thus, it contributes to proliferation and inflammation of the vessel wall.[18] The plasma concentration of this biomarker correlates closely with CV risk.[19] However, its ability to predict mortality is probably similar to CRP and other markers such as natriuretic peptide.

Natriuretic peptide has emerged as an important biomarker due to role in the protective functions such as vasodilatation, lusitropy, increased insulin sensitivity, and diuresis. This has been found to be consistently lesser in patients with DM.[20] Conversely, the role of N-terminal pro-brain natriuretic peptide (NT-proBNP) in DM patients can be high possibly due to the already evidenced cardiac problems, and hence has no predictive value.

Endothelial-derived microparticles have major role in tissue repair, and these have been found to be lower in patients with DM. These have major role in the vasculogenesis and intercellular information, which modulate repair. An imbalance between proliferation, repair, and apoptosis, which is signaled by these miRNAs may contribute to CV risk.[21]

Matricellular proteins, which are involved in vascular remodeling such as osteopontin, osteonectin, etc. may be surrogate markers of vascular calcification and endothelial dysfunction. The exact role of these is yet to be defined.[22] Cardiac troponins are routinely used as markers of myocardial damage, but whether they can be used as predictive biomarkers in DM is not clear.

Growth defining factor 15 (GDF15) is secreted from macrophages, liver, and fat. These may have some role in expression on the cardiac myocytes, but their purpose is unclear as of now. In a population-based study, however, these were found to be predictive of CV mortality revising interest in them.[23] Elevated levels of fibroblast growth factor 23 has also been associated with heart failure and CV risk.[24]

The SUMMIT VIP Study looked at vascular assessments and biomarkers to predict the CV events in patients with T2DM.[25] They concluded that in patients with T2DM, markers of inflammation such as IL-6, high-sensitivity C-reactive protein (hsCRP), matrix metalloproteins, endothelial mitogens, etc. did reflect CV risk. But further studies are needed to confirm these findings.

In conclusion, there is a role for all these biomarkers in predicting CV risk, but the extent to which they can contribute to clinical decisions is still uncertain.

Thus biomarkers have emerged as having a singular role in the identification and prediction of risk of complications of diabetes. These may play a vital role in early intervention in patients likely to progress to major organ damage, and may form an important part of the clinician's assessment of patients with diabetes, in the future.

REFERENCES

1. Raffield LM, Hsu FC, Cox AJ, et al. Predictors of all-cause and cardiovascular disease mortality in type 2 diabetes: Diabetes Heart Study. Diabetol Metab Syndr. 2015;7(1):58.
2. Asaba K, Tojo A, Onozato ML, et al. Effects of NADPH oxidase inhibitor in diabetic nephropathy. Kidney Int. 2005;67(5):1890-8.
3. Kazumi T, Hozumi T, Ishida Y, et al. Increased urinary transferrin excretion predicts microalbuminuria in patients with type 2 diabetes. Diabetes Care. 1999;22(7):1176-80.
4. Kotajima N, Kimura T, Kanda T, et al. Type IV collagen as an early marker for diabetic nephropathy in non-insulin-dependent diabetes mellitus. J Diabetes Complications. 2000;14(1):13-7.
5. Turk N, Mornar A, Mrzljak V, et al. Urinary excretion of advanced glycation end products in patients with type 2 diabetes and various stages of proteinuria. Diabetes Metab. 2004;30(2):187-92.
6. Ford ES, Zhao G, Li C. Pre-diabetes and the risk for cardiovascular disease: a systematic review of the evidence. J Am Coll Cardiol. 2010;55(13):1310-7.
7. Van Hecke MV, Dekker JM, Nijpels G, et al. Inflammation and endothelial dysfunction are associated with retinopathy: the Hoorn Study. Diabetologia. 2005;48(7):1300-306.
8. Lupo G, Motta C, Giurdanella G, et al. Role of phospholipases A2 in diabetic retinopathy: in vitro and in vivo studies. Biochemical pharmacology. 2013;86(11):1603-613.
9. Li L, Han L, Fu Q, et al. Formation and inhibition of N -(carboxymethyl) lysine in saccharide-lysine model systems during microwave heating. Molecules. 2012;17(11):12758-70.
10. Rajab HA, Baker NL, Hunt KJ, et al. DCCT/EDIC Group of Investigators. The predictive role of markers of inflammation and endothelial dysfunction on the course of diabetic retinopathy in type 1 diabetes. J Diabetes Complications. 2015;29(1):108-114.
11. Ozturk BT, Bozkurt B, Kerimoglu H, et al. Effect of serum cytokines and VEGF levels on diabetic retinopathy and macular thickness. Mol Vis. 2009;15:1906.
12. Liu Y, Tao L, Fu X, et al. BDNF protects retinal neurons from hyperglycemia through the TrkB/ERK/MAPK pathway. Mol Med Rep. 2013;7(6):1773-8.
13. Zampetaki A, Willeit P, Burr S, et al. Angiogenic microRNAs linked to incidence and progression of diabetic retinopathy in type 1 diabetes. Diabetes. 2016;65(1):216-27.
14. Doupis J, Lyons TE, Wu S, et al. Microvascular reactivity and inflammatory cytokines in painful and painless peripheral diabetic neuropathy. J Clin Endocrinol Metab. 2009;94(6):2157-63.
15. Koya D, Jirousek MR, Lin YW, et al. Characterization of protein kinase C beta isoform activation on the gene expression of transforming growth factor-b, extracellular matrix components and prostanoids in the glomeruli of diabetic rats. J Clin Invest. 1997;100(1):115-26.
16. Taira M, Toba H, Murakami M, et al. Spironolactone exhibits direct renoprotective effects and inhibits renin-angiotensin-aldosterone system in diabetic rats. Eur J Pharmacol. 2008;589(1-3):264-71.
17. Guo C, Martinez-Vasquez D, Mendez GP, et al. Mineralocorticoid receptor antagonist reduces renal injury in rodent models of types 1 and 2 diabetes mellitus. Endocrinology. 2006;147(11):5363-73.
18. Xia L, Wang H, Goldberg HJ, et al. Mesangial cell NADPH oxidase upregulation in high glucose is protein kinase C dependent and required for collagen IV expression. Am J Physiol Renal Physiol. 2006;290(2): F345-56.
19. Moriwaki Y, Yamamoto T, Shbutani Y, et al. Elevated levels of interleukin-18 and tumor necrosis factor-alpha in serum of patients with type 2 diabetes mellitus: relationship with diabetic nephropathy. Metabolism. 2003;52(5):605-8.
20. Ruggenenti P, Remuzzi G. Time to abandon microalbuminuria? Kidney Int. 2006;70(7):1214-22.
21. Currie G, McKay G, Delles C. Biomarkers in diabetic nephropathy: present and future. World J Diabetes. 2014;5(6):763-76.
22. Lee SY, Choi ME. Urinary biomarkers for early diabetic nephropathy: beyond albuminuria. Pediatr Nephrol. 2015;30(7):1063-75.
23. Sthaneshwar P, Chan SP. Urinary type IV collagen levels in diabetes mellitus. Malays J Pathol. 2010;32(1):43-7.
24. Miyake H, Nagashima K, Yagi H, et al. Urinary laminin P1 as an index of glycemic control in children with insulin-dependent diabetes mellitus. Diabetes Res. 1992;23(3):131-8.
25. Shore AC, Colhoun HM, Natali A, et al. Use of Vascular Assessments and Novel Biomarkers to Predict Cardiovascular Events in Type 2 Diabetes: The SUMMIT VIP Study. Diabetes Care. 2018;41(10):2212-9.

Chapter 36

Diabetic Ketoacidosis in Type 1 Diabetes

Siddhant Trehan, Rajeev Chawla

INTRODUCTION

Diabetic ketoacidosis (DKA) is an acute, major, life-threatening complication of diabetes caused by insulin deficiency. It is characterized by hyperglycemia, hyperketonemia and metabolic acidosis. It occurs in patients with type 1 diabetes, but it is not uncommon in some patients with type 2 diabetes. Although the incidence of this complication has been reducing due to increased awareness among patients and physicians, this tends to cause serious effects in patients, resulting in significant mortality and morbidity. A recurring and central theme in the management of diabetes and related complications is the need for implementing preventive strategies, which include routine monitoring and patient education.

EPIDEMIOLOGICAL ASPECTS

Available data indicate the incidence of DKA at 1 per 2,000 patients. Results of the Rhode Island Hospital Study from Fishbein et al. showed an estimated DKA incidence of 4.6 per 1000 diabetic patients per year with a greater incidence in younger age groups and women. DKA occurs mostly in patients with type 1 diabetes but is not uncommon among patients with type 2 diabetes. The mortality rate is 5% in experienced centers.

Pathogenesis of Diabetic Ketoacidosis

Relative or absolute insulin deficiency in the presence of catabolic counter-regulatory hormones (glucagon, catecholamines, growth hormones and cortisol) is the basic underlying mechanism (Fig. 1). This leads to hepatic overproduction of glucose, release of free fatty acids into the circulation from adipose tissue (lipolysis) and to unrestrained hepatic fatty acid oxidation to ketone bodies [β-hydroxybutyrate (β-OHB) and acetoacetate], with resulting ketonemia and metabolic acidosis.[1] Hyperglycemia results in osmotic diuresis leading to dehydration and loss of electrolytes. Sodium depletion is worsened as insulin deficiency further diminishes renal sodium reabsorption. Metabolic acidosis leads to loss of intracellular potassium in exchange for hydrogen ions, and insulin deficiency also causes potassium loss from cells.[1] Thus, there is high circulating plasma potassium.

Precipitating Factors for Diabetic Ketoacidosis

The most common precipitating factor is intercurrent infection. The other common factors are listed in Box 1. The frequency of each factor varies according to the age and ethnicity. Many a times, no obvious cause could be determined. Recurrent DKA is particularly seen in young girls.

Presenting Features for Diabetic Ketoacidosis

The symptoms of DKA include increasing polyuria and thirst, weight loss, weakness, drowsiness and eventually coma (in about 10% of cases) (Box 2).

On physical examination, there is dehydration, hypotension, tachycardia and hypothermia. Acidosis stimulates the respiratory center resulting in deep and rapid (Kussmaul) respiration. In some patients, the smell of acetone may be obvious in patient's breath.

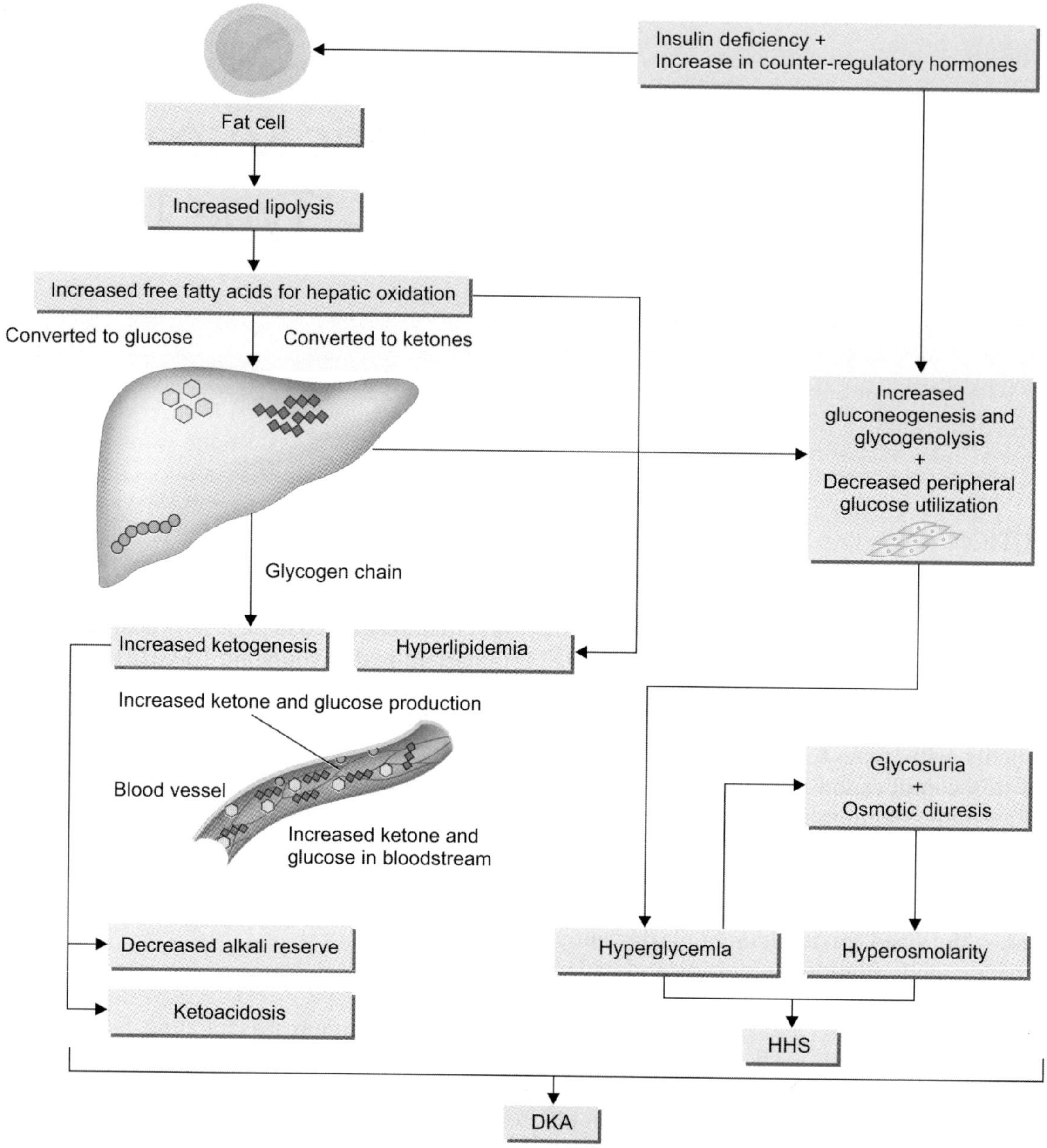

(DKA: diabetic ketoacidosis; HHS: hyperosmolar hyperglycemic state.)

Figure 1 Schematic representation of pathogenesis of diabetic ketoacidosis and hyperosmolar hyperglycemic state.[2]

Box 1: Precipitating factors for diabetic ketoacidosis.

- Infection
- Insulin error/omission
- Newly diagnosed cases
- Cardiovascular (myocardial infarction/stroke)
- Pancreatitis
- Pulmonary embolism
- Alcohol excess
- Steroid use

Box 2: Clinical features of diabetic ketoacidosis.

- Polyuria and nocturia
- Thirst
- Weight loss
- Weakness
- Blurred vision
- Acidotic (Kussmaul) respiration
- Abdominal pain, especially in children
- Leg cramps
- Nausea and vomiting
- Confusion and drowsiness
- Coma

Evaluation of a Patient for Diabetic Ketoacidosis

Diabetic ketoacidosis is a medical emergency. Therefore, a rapid history, physical examination and bedside tests should allow a provisional diagnosis in the emergency department and avoid treatment delays (Flowchart 1).[3]

- When DKA is suspected in a child or young person with known diabetes measure the blood ketones (beta-hydroxybutyrate), using a near-patient method if available.[4] If the level is elevated, immediately send them to a hospital with acute pediatric facilities. When DKA is suspected in a child or young person with known diabetes and it is not possible to measure the blood ketones (beta-hydroxybutyrate) using a near-patient method, immediately send them to a hospital with acute pediatric facilities. If DKA is suspected or confirmed in a child or young person, explain to them and to their family members or carers (as appropriate) that DKA is a serious matter that needs urgent hospital assessment
- When a child or young person with suspected or known DKA arrives at hospital,[4] measure their:
  - Capillary glucose levels
  - Capillary blood ketones (beta-hydroxybutyrate) if testing facility is available or urine ketones
  - Capillary or venous pH and bicarbonate.
- Diagnose DKA in children and young people with diabetes who have:
  - Acidosis (indicated by blood pH below 7.3 or plasma bicarbonate below 18 mmol/L) and ketonemia (indicated by blood beta-hydroxybutyrate above 3 mmol/L) or ketonuria (++ and above on the standard strip marking scale).[4]
- Diagnose severe DKA in children and young people with DKA who have a blood pH below 7.1
- Children and young people with DKA should be cared for in a facility that can provide the level of monitoring and care for DKA specified in these recommendations
- Children and young people with DKA should be cared for with one-to-one nursing either on a high-dependency unit (preferably a pediatric unit), or on a general pediatric ward, if: they are younger than 2 years or they have severe DKA (indicated by a blood pH below 7.1)[4]
- Think about inserting a nasogastric tube if a child or young person with DKA has a reduced level of consciousness and is vomiting, to reduce the risk of aspiration
- Seek urgent anesthetic review and discuss with a pediatric critical care specialist if a child or young person with DKA cannot protect their airway because they have a reduced level of consciousness

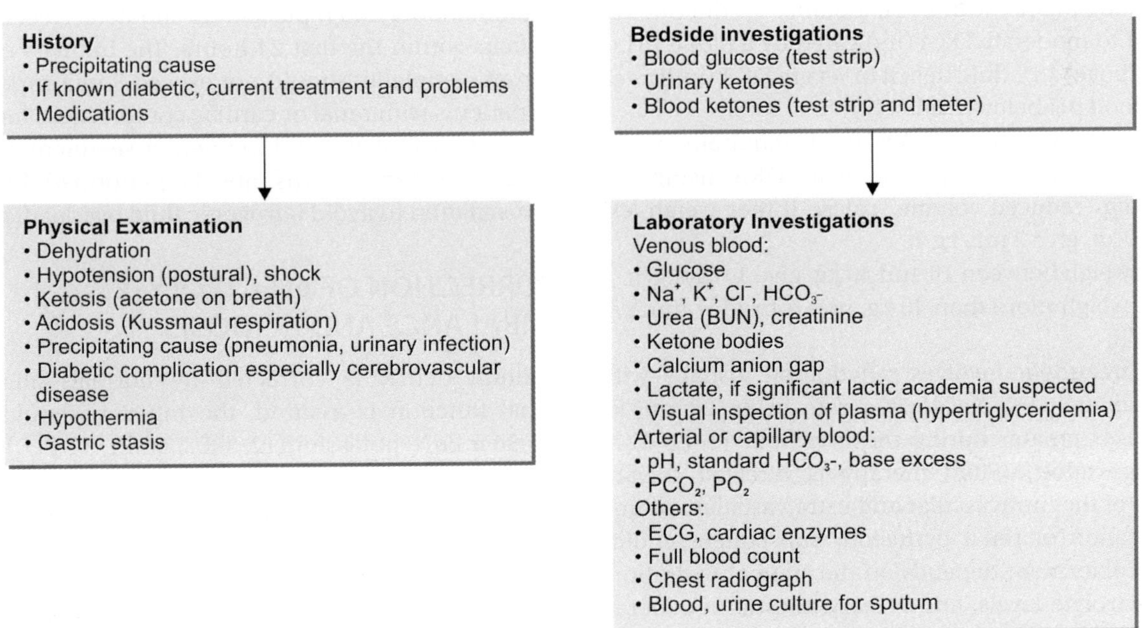

(BUN: blood urea nitrogen; ECG: electrocardiogram.)

Flowchart 1 Initial evaluation for diabetic ketoacidosis.

- Discuss the use of inotropes with a pediatric critical care specialist if a child or young person with DKA is in hypotensive shock. Think about sepsis in a child or young person with DKA who has any of the following:
    - Fever or hypothermia
    - Hypotension
    - Refractory acidosis
    - Lactic acidosis.

Diagnostic Criteria for Diabetic Ketoacidosis

Based on the biochemical and clinical characteristics, DKA can be arbitrarily divided into mild, moderate and severe (Table 1).

Table 1: Diagnostic criteria for diabetic ketoacidosis.

	DKA		
	Mild	Moderate	Severe
Plasma glucose (mg/dL)	>250	>250	>250
Arterial pH	7.25–7.30	7.00–7.24	<7.00
Serum bicarbonate (mEq/L)	15–18	0 <15	<10
Urine ketones*	Positive	Positive	Positive
Serum ketones*	Positive	Positive	Positive
Effective serum osmolality (mOsm/kg)†	Variable	Variable	Variable
Anion gap‡	>10	>12	>12
Alteration in sensoria or mental obtundation	Alert	Alert/ drowsy	Stupor/ coma

*Nitroprusside reaction method; †calculation: 2[measured Na (mEq/L)] + glucose (mg/dL)/18; ‡calculation: (Na^+) (Cl + HCO_3) (mEq/L).
(DKA: diabetic ketoacidosis.)

Treatment Goals for Diabetic Ketoacidosis

Successful treatment of DKA aims for correction of dehydration, hyperglycemia, and electrolyte imbalances and identification of comorbid precipitating events; and above all, frequent patient monitoring (Flowchart 2).

Fluid Correction in the Management of Diabetic Ketoacidosis[4]

The total body water and electrolyte deficit is shown in Table 2.

- When calculating the fluid requirement for children and young people with DKA, assume: 5% fluid deficit in mild to moderate DKA (indicated by a blood pH of 7.1 or above) 10% fluid deficit in severe DKA (indicated by a blood pH below 7.1)
- Calculate the maintenance fluid requirement for children and young people with DKA using the following "reduced volume" rules: If they weigh less than 10 kg, give 2 mL/kg/h
- If they weigh between 10 and 40 kg, give 1 mL/kg/h
- If they weigh more than 40 kg, give a fixed volume of 40 mL/h.

Initial treatment involves rehydration, usually with isotonic saline (0.9% NaCl) at a rate of 15-20 mL/kg body wt/h or greater during the first hour (1-1.5 L in the average adult). Fluid therapy is directed toward expansion of the intravascular and extra vascular volume and restoration of renal perfusion. Subsequent choice for fluid replacement depends on the state of hydration, serum electrolyte levels, and urinary output. In general, 0.45% NaCl infused at 4-14 mL/kg/h is appropriate if the corrected serum sodium is normal or elevated; 0.9% NaCl at a similar rate is appropriate if corrected serum sodium is low.

The success of fluid replacement is observed by hemodynamic monitoring (improvement in blood pressure), measurement of fluid input/output, and clinical examination. Fluid replacement should correct estimated deficits within the first 24 hours. The induced change in serum osmolality should not exceed 3 mOsm/kg H_2O/h. In patients with renal or cardiac compromise, monitoring of serum osmolality and frequent assessment of cardiac, renal, and mental status must be performed during fluid resuscitation to avoid iatrogenic fluid overload.

CORRECTION OF ELECTROLYTE IMBALANCE AND ACIDOSIS

Sodium deficit is corrected by normal saline. Once renal function is assured, the infusion should include 20–30 mEq/L potassium (2/3 KCl and 1/3 KPO_4) until the patient is stable and can tolerate oral supplementation. Although phosphate and magnesium depletion are also present, there is no evidence that routine replacement is beneficial. However, serum phosphate levels <0.35 mmol/L can cause muscle weakness and myocardial dysfunction and need correction. Similarly, serum magnesium levels <0.7 mmol/L should also be corrected.

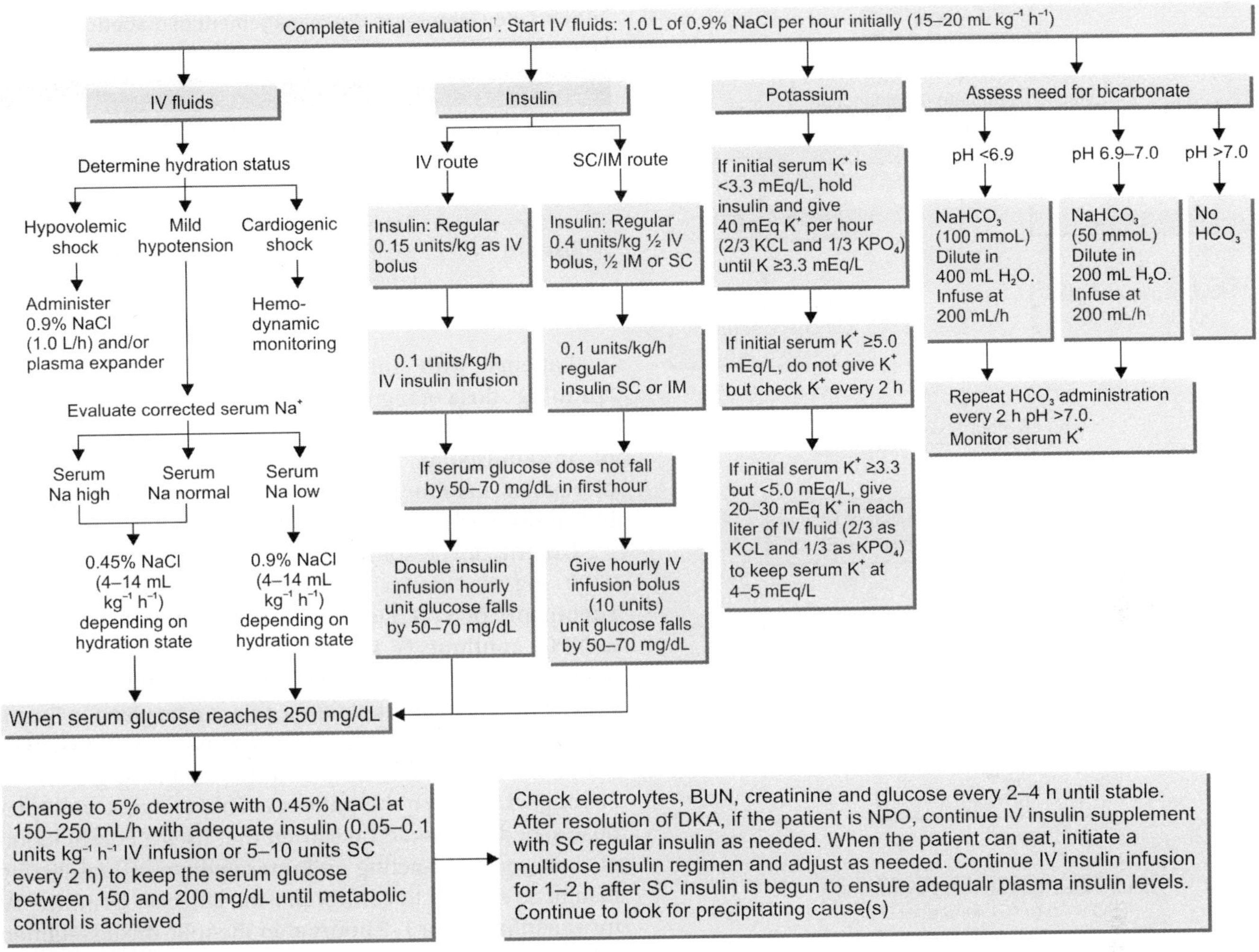

(BUN: blood urea nitrogen; DKA: diabetic ketoacidosis; IM: intramuscular; IV: intravenous; SC: subcutaneous.)

Flowchart 2 Initial evaluation for diabetic ketoacidosis.

TABLE 2: Typical total body deficits of water and electrolytes in diabetic ketoacidosis.

	DKA
Total water (L)	6
Water (mL/kg)	100
Na^+ (mEq/kg)	7–10
Cl (mEq/kg)	3–5
K^+ (mEq/kg)	3–5
PO_4 (mmol/kg)	5–7
Mg^{++} (mEq/kg)	1–2
Ca^{++} (mEq/kg)	1–2

(DKA: diabetic ketoacidosis.)

The role of intravenous (IV) bicarbonate is controversial. There is no proven benefit in patients with arterial pH ≥6.9. There are good theoretical reasons why IV bicarbonate should not be added and its use is associated with the development of cerebral edema. The American Diabetes Association (ADA) guidelines recommend 100 mmol diluted and given over 2 hours in patients with a pH <6.9 or in whom the acidosis is thought to be contributing to deteriorating clinical status (Flowchart 3 and 4).[5]

MANAGEMENT OF HYPERGLYCEMIA IN DIABETIC KETOACIDOSIS[6]

Unless the episode of DKA is mild, regular insulin by continuous IV infusion is the treatment of choice. In adult

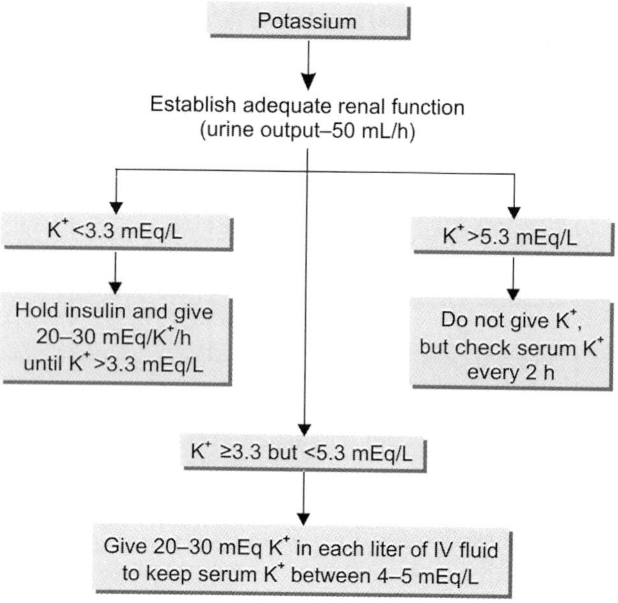

(IV: intravenous.)

Flowchart 3 Protocol for correcting electrolyte imbalance.

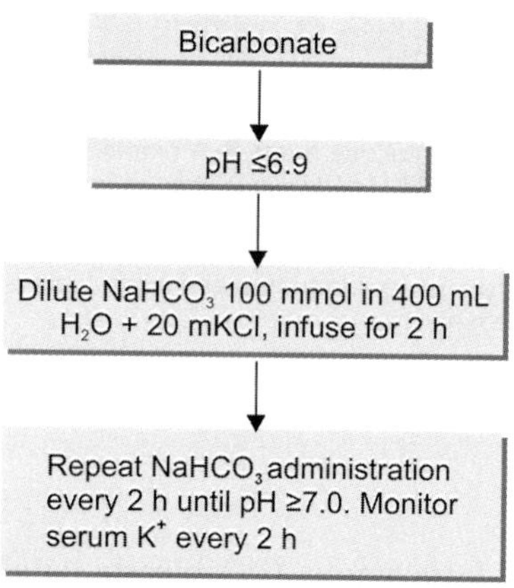

Flowchart 4 Management of acidosis.

patients, once hypokalemia (K^+ <3.3 mEq/L) is excluded, an IV bolus of regular insulin at 0.15 units/kg body weight, followed by a continuous infusion of regular insulin at a dose of 0.1 unit/kg/h (5–7 units/h in adults), should be administered (Table 3).

When the plasma glucose reaches 250 mg/dL, it may be possible to decrease the insulin infusion rate to 0.05–0.1 unit/kg/h (3–6 units/h), and dextrose (5–10%) may be added to the IV fluids. Thereafter, the rate of insulin administration or the concentration of dextrose may need to be adjusted to maintain the above glucose values until acidosis is resolved.

TABLE 3: Key features in the management of diabetic ketoacidosis.

	DKA
Insulin treatment	Immediate insulin therapy is extremely crucial for reversal of DKA and must be initiated at the earliest
Electrolyte imbalance	Potassium loss is lesser in DKA as compared to HHS; however, potassium replenishment is needed in patients with DKA

(DKA: diabetic ketoacidosis; HHS: hyperosmolar hyperglycemic state.)

Patients with mild DKA should first receive a "priming" dose of regular insulin of 0.4–0.6 units/kg body weight,[6] half as an IV bolus and half as a subcutaneous or intramuscular injection. Thereafter, 0.1 unit/kg/h of regular insulin should be given subcutaneously or intramuscularly.

Criteria for resolution of DKA includes a glucose <200 mg/dL, serum bicarbonate ≥18 mEq/L, and a venous pH of >7.3. Once DKA is resolved, if the patient is NPO, continue IV insulin and fluid replacement and supplement with subcutaneous regular insulin as needed every 4 hours. In adult patients, this can be given in 5-unit increments for every 50 mg/dL increase in blood glucose above 150 mg/dL for up to 20 units for blood glucose of 300 mg/dL. In case the patient is able to eat, a multiple-dose schedule should be started that uses a combination of short- or rapid-acting and intermediate-or long-acting insulin as needed to control plasma glucose. Continue IV insulin infusion for 1–2 hours after the split-mixed regimen is begun to ensure adequate plasma insulin levels.

Complications of Diabetic Ketoacidosis

The most common complications of DKA include:

- Hypoglycemia due to overzealous treatment with insulin
- Hypokalemia due to insulin administration and treatment of acidosis with bicarbonate
- Hyperglycemia secondary to interruption/discontinuance of IV insulin therapy after recovery without subsequent coverage with subcutaneous insulin
- Hyperchloremia caused by the use of excessive saline for fluid and electrolyte replacement and transient non-anion gap metabolic acidosis as chloride from IV fluids replaces ketoanions lost as sodium and potassium salts during osmotic diuresis.

Cerebral edema is a rare but frequently fatal complication of DKA, occurring in 0.7–1.0% of children with DKA. Hypoxemia and, rarely, noncardiogenic pulmonary edema may also complicate the treatment of DKA.

Preventive Measures for Diabetic Ketoacidosis

Better access to medical care, proper education, and effective communication with a healthcare provider during an intercurrent illness may be helpful in preventing many cases of DKA. Cessation of insulin therapy for economic reason is disturbing and needs to be addressed.

Better education of care givers as well as patients regarding signs and symptoms of new-onset diabetes; conditions, procedures and medications that worsen diabetes control; and the use of glucose monitoring could potentially decrease the incidence and severity of DKA

CONCLUSION

- Insulin deficiency with raised levels of counter regulatory hormones leads to DKA and hyperosmolar hyperglycemic state (HHS)
- DKA occurs mostly in type 1 diabetes, whereas HHS is more common in type 2 diabetes
- Increased lipolysis and increased supply of FFA for hepatic fatty acid oxidation lead to ketoacidosis
- The most common symptoms of DKA are polydipsia and polyuria. The most common symptom of HHS is altered sensorium
- Metabolic acidosis in DKA needs to be corrected by IV bicarbonate infusion, only if pH ≤6.9
- Glucose levels must be reduced with caution in children to avoid cerebral edema.

REFERENCES

1. Kitabchi AE, Umpierrez GE, Miles JM, Fisher JN. Hyperglycemic crises in adult patients with diabetes. Diabetes Care. 2009;32(7):1335-43.
2. Kitabchi A, Umpierrez GE, Murphy MB. Diabetic ketoacidosis and hyperglycemic hyperosmolar state. In: De-Fronzo R, Ferrannini E, Keen HPZ, (Eds). International Textbook of Diabetes Mellitus. 3rd edn. Chichester: John Wiley & Sons;2004:1101-19.
3. McNaughton CD, Self WH, Slovis C. Diabetes in the Emergency Department: Acute Care of Diabetes Patients. Clin Diabetes. 2011;20(2):51-9.
4. Diabetes in children and young people NICE 2018.
5. Standards of medical care in diabetes-2015 abridged for primary care providers. Clin Diabetes. 2015;33(2):97-111.
6. Inzucchi SE, Bergenstal RM, Buse JB, et al. Management of hyperglycemia in type 2 diabetes, 2015: a patient-centered approach: update to a position statement of the American Diabetes Association and the European Association for the Study of Diabetes. Diabetes Care. 2015 Jan;38(1):140-9.

Chapter 37

Updates in Diabetic Retinopathy Management in Last Decade

Deependra Vikram Singh

INTRODUCTION

Diabetes mellitus (DM) is a chronic disease that can lead to sight-threatening conditions like diabetic macular edema (DME), proliferative diabetic retinopathy (PDR), retinal vascular occlusions and retinal detachments.[1] Asia is now home to approximately 80% of the world's diabetic population, including >60 million Indians and the total number of diabetic persons is expected to increase to >100 million by 2030.[2,3] Alongside, this rapidly increasing disease incidence is an increase in the associated complications, including diabetic retinopathy (DR), which is estimated to affect >93 million worldwide.[4] Although the burden of DR is significant, early treatment is effective, and an estimated 90% of severe vision loss can be prevented.[5]

In this chapter, we will summarize the key advancements that have taken place in detection and management of DR over last one and a half decade.

OVERVIEW OF MANAGEMENT PROTOCOLS FOR DIABETIC RETINOPATHY BEFORE 2002

Screening frequency for DR as recommended by American academy of ophthalmology was annually for patients with no retinopathy changes and quarterly for patients with any DR changes.[6] Also, fundus photography (FP) was not considered as an effective screening method. Recommended method for screening was dilated slit lamp biomicroscopy and indirect ophthalmoscopy.

Management protocols for DR have been revolving around five pivotal studies; DR Study (DRS), early treatment for DRS (ETDRS), DR vitrectomy study (DRVS), diabetes control and complications trial (DCCT) and United Kingdom prospective DRS (UKPDS).

The DCCT demonstrated 35–76% reduction in microvascular complications after intensive therapy (INT) that lowered hemoglobin A1c (HbA1c) from a median of 9–7%.[7]

The UKPDS trials also highlighted that control of blood glucose, blood pressure and serum lipids reduce the incidence and severity of DR in patients with type 1 or 2 diabetes.[8] Based on both DCCT and UKPDS, it was recommended to have strict glycemic control along with control of hypertension and lipid levels to reduce the incidence and severity of DR.

Landmark studies, DRS and ETDRS evaluated role of laser photocoagulation for DR and found the laser photocoagulation reduces the risk of severe vision loss in PDR by 50% and reduces the risk of moderate vision loss in patients with macular edema by 50%. These studies also identified the stage of DR at which interventions including laser would be most beneficial and provided definitions of high risk characteristics (HRC) in patients with PDR and clinical significant macular edema (CSME) for DME. ETDRS not only laid down the guidelines for photography for screening and grading DR but also introduced the concept of sharing digital pictures for grading.

The DRVS explored the results of early vitrectomy and found it to be beneficial for type 1 diabetics and resulting in better chances of restoring good (> 6/12) vision.

So, a good metabolic control with regular screening for DR with institution of timely laser for PDR and DME along with institution of early vitrectomy for type 1 diabetics had been the cornerstone in the management of DR till 2002.

KEY ADVANCES

Increasing popularity of digital fundus images for DR screening and automated DR detection, addition of optical coherence tomography (OCT) as important imaging modality and anti-vascular endothelial growth factor (VEGF) injections have been the key advances in management of DR after 2002.

Digital Fundus Images and Automation

While FP has been proposed as an effective and alternative screening tool much earlier, it could not become popular till digital fundus images became available in 2002. Early studies in 2002 evaluating digital fundus imaging as screening tool reported sensitivities and specificities of around 90%.[9,10] Challenges associated with these systems were high capital cost, nonportable, required dilatation of all patients and trained personnel for capturing. So, next advancement was utilization of nonmydriatic (NM) FP for screening. Between 2000 and 2009, there are hundreds of studies which reported the usefulness of NM FP.[11,12] Next development was on combining NM FP with telescreening utilizing internet and cloud. To make it more accessible to target population, these NM cameras were installed at the community level; at primary healthcare clinics and optical clinics. All the major studies found this telescreening much more effective than hospital-based screening in detecting sight-threatening DR (STDR).

Once the affectivity of telescreening for DR was established, the next phase was introduction and popularity of low cost fundus cameras. This brought new challenge of "handling too many images" and who does the grading for these images and also how to reduce the "turn over time" for reporting. Researchers and healthcare planners have already realized that even if an adequate number of ophthalmologists are available, using ophthalmologists to screen every person with DM usually is not feasible and is likely to be an inefficient use of resources.[13] Few studies did explore the reliability and accuracy of digital NM FP-based screening for DR by family physicians, general ophthalmologists and optometrists.[14,15] The agreement between graders were found to be excellent. Study[14] also reported incidence of DR to be as high as 39% with STDR at 10% on screening diabetics at primary health care at Hong kong. The literature has been flooded with reports on affectivity of internet supported and NM FP-based screening for DR from all over the world. This is now accumulating enormous amount of retinal images and led the path to automated detection and grading of DR by artificial intelligence (AI).[16] DR with its characteristic and striking features on retinal images is most suited target for deep learning and automated detection and grading. There are already numerous reports claiming reliability and validating role of AI for DR screening. Information technology (IT) giants like IBM and GOOGLE have already reached an advanced stage in this development. In April 2018, the food and drug administration (FDA) granted marketing approval to IDx for the first medical device utilizing AI to detect referable DR from color FP after they reported results of their pivotal trial.[17] Although AI still has to be validated in field trials across different ethnic groups, its availability for DR screening would probably enhance the detection rates and is expected to reduced the incidence of diabetic blindness.

Optical Coherence Tomography

Optical coherence tomography, with its noninvasive visualization of retinal structures in unprecedented resolution, is the most powerful in vivo diagnostic tool in modern medicine. Spectral domain (SD)-OCT is widely available and represents the gold standard in diagnostic imaging in the management of the leading macular diseases including DME. A conventional three-dimensional (3D) OCT image is based on 20,000–52,000 A-scans per second offering a resolution of 5–7 μm. OCT is now regarded as the most sensitive method for detection and assessment of DME. The retinal map scan is useful in locating the area with retinal thickening; single line scans are useful in detailing the specific DME morphologic changes such as intraretinal cysts, subretinal fluid or detachment, and vitreoretinal traction. Availability of OCT has been most remarkable advancement for DR since 2002. The OCT scans not only help clinicians detect subclinical DME, it helps in quantifying, classifying DME (Fig. 1) but can also detect coexisting pathologies like traction or retinal thinning. These all attributes have immense prognostic significance. Digitalization also allows serial monitoring, patient education, sharing on cloud as well as automated detection. Excellent correlation of structural assessment of macula by OCT and visual function makes it a great tool for assessing the efficacy of different treatment algorithms for DME. Another big change facilitated by availability of OCT is attention of ophthalmologist and retinologists to DME and restoring near vision in patients with DME. There is a paradigm shift in treatment goals for DR, from preventing blindness and visual impairment to restoring good vision for maximum patients and thereby helping them stay independent and thus manage their DM better.

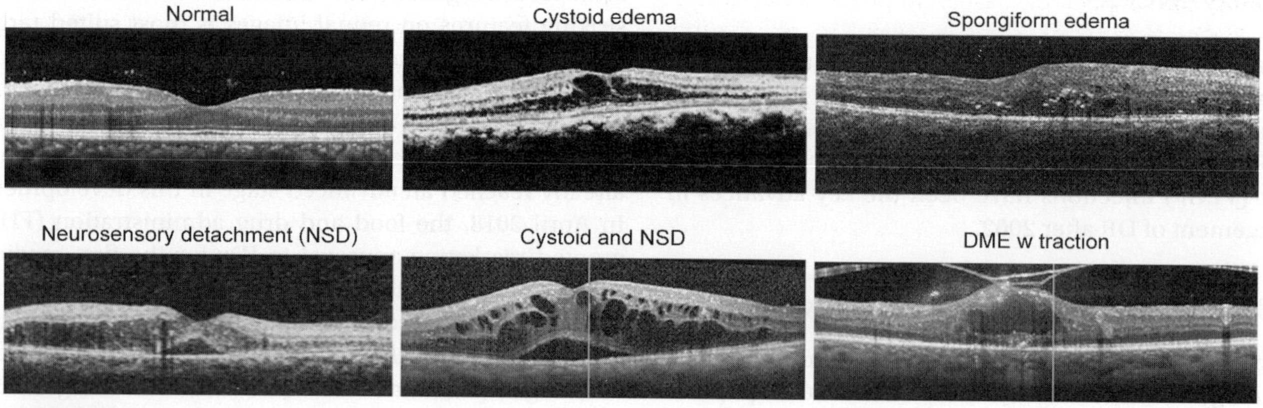

Figure 1 Morphological types of diabetic macular edema on optical coherence tomography.

Anti-vascular Endothelial Growth Factor Injections for Diabetic Macular Edema

Although the pathogenesis of DR is not completely understood, it seems that hyperglycemia is the primary insult because poor glycemic control is associated with progression of retinopathy. Hyperglycemia causes damage to retinal blood vessels, resulting in hemorrhages, microaneurysms and capillary closure. Capillary closure causes retinal hypoxia, which long has been known to be associated with retinal neovascularization,[18] but more recently has also been linked to DME. Hypoxic retina produces high levels of VEGF, which can stimulate retinal neovascularization, but also causes leakiness of retinal vessels when injected into the vitreous cavity of mice and causes macular edema when provided by sustained release in the vitreous of primates.[19] This provided the rationale for testing VEGF antagonists in patients with DME. In a pilot trial, it was found that five intraocular injections of 0.5 mg ranibizumab (RBZ) over the span of 7 months resulted in a mean reduction in excess foveal thickness of 85% and an average improvement in best-corrected visual acuity (BCVA) of 12 letters.[20] Initial success was followed by a large number of randomized controlled trials where role of intravitreal anti-VEGF injections for DME as an adjunctive treatment to laser was successfully established followed by confirmation of their efficacy (and eventually) superiority to laser as monotherapy for DME. Detailed discussion of these studies is beyond the scope of this update but at current moment, intravitreal anti-VEGF injections have become a first line treatment for DME involving center of macula (CIDME). Most studies including Diabetic Retinopathy Clinical Research Network (DRCR.net) have demonstrated the benefits of treating CIDME. Patients should be monitored almost monthly with OCT to consider the need for treatment. Typically, the number of injections is 6–8 in the first year, 2 or 3 during the second year, 1–2 during the third year, and 0–1 in the fourth and fifth years of treatment.

Intravitreal Steroid Implants

Inflammation has an important role in the pathogenesis of DME. The use of intravitreal corticosteroids for the treatment of DME has been extensively evaluated, due to their ability to inhibit proinflammatory cells and leukostasis,[21] inhibit the expression of prostaglandins, proinflammatory cytokines and VEGF, and to enhance the barrier function of vascular tight junctions. Steroid agents are also increasingly being used for the treatment of DME. Triamcinolone, fluocinolone and dexamethasone can be administered in the form of intravitreal injections or implants. Most effective and popular is dexamethasone implant that has favorable safety profile and efficacy lasting 3 months. They are best suited to patients who would need prolonged treatment.[22]

While anti-VEGF agents are considered as first-line therapy for DME, intraocular steroids have become a good alternative for patients with pseudophakia, persistent suboptimal response to anti-VEGF agents, or systemic vascular comorbidities that preclude the use of anti-VEGF agents.

Paradigm Shift from Preventing Vision Loss to Visual Improvement and Quality of Life

Together with availability of OCT and more effective treatment of DME with injections, lot of studies are evaluating the impact on visual improvement, unlike before 2002 when treatment goals were to reduce the loss of vision or visual improvement. Important outcome parameters that are evaluated now include reading acuity, night vision and driving abilities. There are more parameters being added to evaluate the mobility status of these patients and over all quality of life (QoL).

Anti-VEGF Injections for Proliferative DR and Reversal of Diabetic Retinopathy – Reductions in DRS Diabetic Retinopathy Severity Scales

Recently, a phase 3 trial with level 1 evidence challenged the laser photocoagulation as primary treatment for PDR and found that anti-VEGF injections cannot only halt progression of PDR but have potential for better outcomes at 2 years than laser. Popularly known as "protocol-s" from DRCR.net study, the results are being read with extreme caution at present. Worldwide, retinologists have still advocated laser as a primary treatment for PDR, especially in low resource setting like India, where compliance and adherence to follow-up is suboptimal. Laser photocoagulation is not only cost-effective but also is considered as a finite treatment for PDR.

Another interesting question that was pondering retinologists was whether we can reverse DR. This was supported by observation from long-term studies on anti-VEGF drugs for DME. The studies (RIDE and RISE trials) reported a greater proportion of RBZ-treated patients experiencing a 2-step or more or 3-step or more improvement in Diabetic Retinopathy Severity Scales score compared with sham-treated patients and a smaller proportion in whom PDR developed or who underwent Pan-Retinal Photocoagulation (PRP).[23] Although this improvement in DR severity scale was assessed by FP, same is being evaluated in fundus fluorescein angiography (FFA)-based studies.

Biomarkers in Retinal Imaging for Early Detection Prior to Microaneurysms

Another major update in DR is focus on early detection. There is an interval between the development of DM and the first clinical signs of DR; however, neural retinal damage and clinically invisible microvascular changes progress during the asymptomatic phase.[24] Last decade a lot of retinal structural and function and molecular biomarkers have been identified that can detect subclinical DR. Earlier reports focused on choroidal thickness as a biomarker but more recently investigators have found the retinal vessel caliber and enlargement of foveal avascular zone on OCT angiography as potential biomarkers for early DR. Besides them, contrast sensitivity, microperimetry and electroretinography have also been proposed as potential biomarkers. Studies have found significant increases in the levels of inflammatory cytokines, particularly interferon gamma, interleukin-1a, interleukin-3 and monocyte chemotactic protein-2 in diabetic patients with retinopathy compared to controls. They have also found increased level of VEGF-R2 receptors in retinal capillary endothelium. Clinical relevance of most of these biomarkers remains to be tested by future studies. The affordability of these diagnostic tests for the general population, their unknown accuracy without an established gold standard test at the no DR stage and the lack of longitudinal trials to define predictability prevent the use of these diagnostic modalities in routine clinical practice at present.

Surgical Advances

Last 16 years have also seen a tremendous advancement in the field on vitreoretinal surgeries. This has been made possible by wide angle viewing systems, high speed, and small gauge (25 and 27G) vitrectomy systems, more refined lasers and preoperative anti-VEGF injections that have made dissections less complex and safer. Pars plana vitrectomy for tractional retinal detachment (TRD) continues to be one of the most complex vitreoretinal procedures. Smaller gauge systems offer several advantages including the possibility of self-sealing sclerotomies, improved retinal stability and ease of tissue manipulation. Most recent studies of diabetic TRD repair report anatomical success in the range of 83–94% with vision loss in <25% of cases. A very recent study reports 92.6% of the cases achieving successful reattachment, 57.6% with Best-corrected visual acuity (BCVA) of 20/400 or greater, and vision loss in <20% of eyes.[25] Future trends are to operate these cases much earlier before neuronal damage from traction becomes irreversible.

CONCLUSION

Acceptance of digitalized fundus images as a valid screening method combined with technologies like cloud internet and deep learning and involvement of nonspecialist for screening has been a major update for DR detection. Revolutionary changes have been brought by OCT scans and intravitreal injections and together they are preventing vision loss in DR patients. It is also heartening to know that efforts are directed to restore vision and may be reverse changes in patients with DR thereby making them more ambulatory and thus improving their DM control and possibly QoL.

REFERENCES

1. Bali J, Bali RT. Pathological ocular angiogenesis in diabetes: a perspective of emerging paradigms and current evidence. J Clin Ophthalmol Res. 2013;1(1):3-10.
2. Anjana RM, Pradeepa R, Deepa M, et al. Prevalence of diabetes and prediabetes (impaired fasting glucose and/or impaired glucose tolerance) in urban and rural India: phase I results of the Indian Council of Medical Research-India DIABetes (ICMRINDIAB) study. Diabetologia. 2011;54:3022-7.
3. Hu FB. Globalization of diabetes: the role of diet, lifestyle, and genes. Diabetes Care. 2011;34:1249-57.
4. Yau JWY, Rogers SL, Kawasaki R, et al. Global prevalence and major risk factors of diabetic retinopathy. Diabetes Care. 2012;35:556-64.
5. Ferris FL III How effective are retinopathy treatments. JAMA. 1993;269: 1290-1.
6. American Academy of Ophthalmology (1993). Retinal Panel of the American Academy of Ophthalmology Quality of Care Committee. Preferred Practice Pattern: Diabetic retinopathy [online] Available from: https://www.aao.org/Assets/dba38b76-3095-4360.../diabetic-retinopathy-ppp-pdf. [Accessed October 2018].
7. The Diabetes Control and Complications Trial Research Group. The relationship of glycemic exposure (HbA1c) to the risk of development and progression of retinopathy in the diabetes control and complications trial. Diabetes. 1995;44:968-83.
8. UK Prospective Diabetes Study (UKPDS) Group. Intensive blood-glucose control with sulphonylureas or insulin compared with conventional treatment and risk of complications in patients with type 2 diabetes (UKPDS 33). Lancet. 1998;352:837-53.
9. Rudnisky CJ, Hinz BJ, Tennant MT, et al. High resolution stereoscopic digital fundus photography versus contact lens biomicroscopy for the detection of clinically significant macular edema. Ophthalmol. 2002;109:267-74.
10. Fransen SR, Leonard-Martin TC, Feur WJ, et al. Clinical evaluation of patients with diabetic retinopathy; accuracy of the Inoveon Diabetic retinopathy-3DT system. Ophthalmol. 2002;109:595-60.
11. Lin DY, Blumenkranz MS, Brothers RJ, et al. The sensitivity and specificity of single-field nonmydriatic monochromatic digital fundus photography with remote image interpretation for diabetic retinopathy screening: a comparison with ophthalmoscopy and standardized mydriatic color photography. Am J Ophthalmol. 2002;134(2):204-13.
12. Vujosevic S, Benetti E, Massignan F, et al. Screening for diabetic retinopathy: 1 and 3 nonmydriatic 45-degree digital fundus photographs vs 7 standard early treatment diabetic retinopathy study fields. Am J Ophthalmol. 2009;148(1):111-8.
13. Horton MB, Silva PS, Cavallerano JD, et al. Operational components of telemedicine programs for diabetic retinopathy. Curr Diabetes Rep. 2016;16(12):128.
14. Lian JX, Gangwani RA, McGhee SM, et al. Systematic screening for diabetic retinopathy (DR) in Hong Kong: prevalence of DR and visual impairment among diabetic population. Br J Ophthalmol. 2016;100(2):151-5.
15. Cunha LP, Figueiredo EA, Araújo HP, et al. Non-mydriatic fundus retinography in screening for diabetic retinopathy: agreement between family physicians, general ophthalmologists, and a retinal specialist. Front Endocrinol (Lausanne). 2018;9:251.
16. Gulshan V, Peng L, Coram M, et al. Development and validation of a deep learning algorithm for detection of diabetic retinopathy in retinal fundus photographs. JAMA. 2016;316:2402-10.
17. Abràmoff MD, Lavin PT, Birch M, et al. Pivotal trial of an autonomous AI-based diagnostic system for detection of diabetic retinopathy in primary care offices. NPJ Digi Med. 2018;1(1).
18. Shimizu K, Kobayashi Y, Muraoka K. Midperipheral fundus involvement in diabetic retinopathy. Ophthalmol. 1981;88:601-12.
19. Ozaki H, Hayashi H, Vinores SA, et al. Intravitreal sustained release of VEGF causes retinal neovascularization in rabbits and breakdown of the blood-retinal barrier in rabbits and primates. Exp Eye Res. 1997;64:505-17.
20. Nguyen QD, Tatlipinar S, Shah SM, et al. Vascular endothelial growth factor is a critical stimulus for diabetic macular edema. Am J Ophthalmol. 2006;142:961-9.
21. Tamura H, Miyamoto K, Kiryu J, et al. Intravitreal injection of corticosteroid attenuates leukostasis and vascular leakage in experimental diabetic retina. Invest Ophthalmol Vis Sci. 2005;46:1440-4.
22. Felinski EA, Antonetti DA. Glucocorticoid regulation of endothelial cell tight junction gene expression: Novel treatments for diabetic retinopathy. Curr Eye Res. 2005;30:949-57.
23. Ip MS, Domalpally A, Hopkins JJ, et al. Long-term effects of ranibizumab on diabetic retinopathy severity and progression. Arch Ophthalmol. 2012;130:1145e-52.
24. Safi H, Safi S, Hafezi-Moghadam A, et al. Early detection of diabetic retinopathy. Surv Ophthalmol. 2018;63(5):601-8.
25. Storey PP, Ter-Zakarian A, Philander SA, et al. Visual and anatomical outcomes after diabetic traction and traction-rhegmatogenous retinal detachment repair. Retina. 2018;38(10):1913-9.

Chapter 38

Alarming Signs of Diabetic Kidney Disease—Time to a Nephrologist

Arvind Gupta, Alok Jain, Rajeev Gupta

INTRODUCTION

Diabetic kidney disease (DKD) is a widespread public health problem with substantial morbidity and mortality. It occurs in 20–40% of all patients with type 2 diabetes mellitus (DM) and is the leading cause of end-stage renal disease (ESRD).[12]

In a study published in NHANES III USRDS 2013,[1] estimated glomerular filtration rate (eGFR) <60 mL/min/1.73 m^2 was present in 19.3% patients and albumin creatinine ratio (ACR) >30 mg/gm was present in 9.3% patient suffering from diabetes. This is important because, according to the Kidney International August 2017,[18] diabetes with early renal involvement may decrease life expectancy by 16 years. Early DKD had higher mortality across all eGFR levels as well as in all the levels of proteinuria.

Now with the help of microalbuminuria or macroalbuminuria, we are able to diagnose diabetic nephropathy within 5–10 years of type 1 DM.

Type 2 DM patients do not follow the same course as type 1 DM patients. These patients may even present with proteinuria or they can have diabetic nephropathy even before Type 2 diabetes is diagnosed.

Another important point to remember is that in patient of type 2 diabetes the macrovascular complications like cardiac disease or death due to cardiovascular disease can occur at any point of time, but in patients of type 1 diabetes, risk of cardiovascular disease is not seen till advance kidney disease.

EARLY REFERRAL TO NEPHROLOGIST

Chronic kidney disease (CKD) patients with DM are recommended for early referral to prevent the rapid progression of kidney disease and improve patient survival. Kessler et al. and Kinchen et al.[19-21] reported that the most prevalent referral time for DKD patients is between 4 and 12 months.

A more direct method of assessing primary care physician (PCP) recognition of DKD was used by Boulware et al.[3] using a national survey of family physicians, internists and nephrologists. In their study, 304 physicians were presented with a clinical and laboratory data including a progressively worsening creatinine (2.1–2.3 mg/dL) at the time of initial visit. They were not provided eGFR value, but were provided with all other for the calculation— physician and internist was given the task to diagnostic CKD stage and need for referral. Results of the study showed 59% and 78% of physicians and internists were able to categorize CKD and its staging as compare to 97% of nephrologist.

The Kidney Disease Outcomes Quality Initiative[13] (KDQOI) guidelines recommends referral to a nephrologist at stage 4; however, few physician recommended referral (76% family medicine and 81% internal medicine) compared with 99% of nephrologists. These studies suggest that there is decreased awareness of renal disease in primary care.

Boulware et al.[3] surveyed physician and nephrologist referring pattern and their acquaintance with KDOQI guidelines, time for ideal reference and information from reference. About 47% of the physicians and 31% of the internist reported to have difficulty in refereeing the patient to nephrologist as has little time and 52% and 29% had difficulty because of lack of local nephrologist. Less than 10% in both groups were of the opinion that nephrologist should take the complete care of the patient. Physicians who had <10 years of practice and are familiar with the CKD were the doctors who used to refer the patients to the nephrologist early.

In a study done by Martinez Ramirez et al.[25] regarding early and late reference to nephrologist by physician, at the end of 1 year the conclusion was that those patients who have been referred early to nephrologist have stable glomerular filtration rate (GFR), better blood pressure control, increase use of renin-angiotensin-aldosterone system blockers, and decrease use of nonsteroidal anti-inflammatory drugs, and this benefit was more in group having microalbuminuria.

Definitions of late referral vary among studies but generally imply a rapid initiation of renal replacement therapy (RRT) following referral (<1–4 months) without adequate time to counsel patients on options for ESRD care (including transplantation) or to obtain a fistula if possible, or otherwise a graft. The prevalence of late referrals varies by study and definition, but is commonly reported to be between 20 and 40% in the CKD[45,46] population. Early referral is >12 months prior to the start of dialysis. The benefits of early referral to nephrologists are well known, and early referral improves patient survival and quality of life and reduces hospitalization, length of hospital stay and medical costs.

Timing of referral of patients with CKD to a nephrology service affects their outcomes. The majority of patients with renal disease are referred close to the time of initiation of RRT, which contributes to poor patient outcomes on RRT.

In a review of referral patterns of European patients with type 2 DM who were starting RRT, 25–30% patients were referred to a nephrologist <1 month before initiation of dialysis. Data from the Australia and New Zealand Dialysis and Transplant Registry (ANZ-DATA)[26] show that of 2,300 patients starting RRT in 2002, 26% were referred <3 months prior to commencing dialysis. This timely referral has reported benefits like reduction in rate of GFR decline, increased use of RAAS blockers, and improved mortality. Potential harms of late referral include suboptimal management of mineral bone disorders and anemia, higher rates of dialysis catheter use versus fistulas when initiating RRT, and increased mortality both overall and in the first year of dialysis.

Consequences of late referral are:

- Increased mortality and morbidity
- Increased cost and duration of hospitalization
- More need of temporary vascular access in patient
- Increased need for urgent dialysis
- Suboptimal management for ESRD.
- Reduced access to renal transplantation services.

Important observation in this study[26] was that highly educated patients like graduates from University or uneducated patients were associated with the long referral time as compared to those patient who has elementary or middle school education.

National Institute for Clinical Excellence (NICE)[30] guidelines:

- People with stage 4 and 5 CKD (+ diabetes)
- Heavy proteinuria [ACR ≥70 mg/mmol, or protein creatinine ratio (PCR) ≥100 mg/mmol, or urinary protein excretion ≥1 g/24 h] unless diabetic and already treated
- Proteinuria (ACR ≥30 mg/mmol, or PCR ≥50 mg/mmol, or urinary protein excretion ≥0.5 g/24 h) with hematuria
- Rapidly declining eGFR (>5 mL/min/1.73 m^2 in 1 year, or >10 mL/min/1.73 m^2 within 5 years)
- Hypertension poorly controlled despite the use of at least four antihypertensive drugs at therapeutic doses
- People with, or suspected of having rare or genetic causes of CKD
- Suspected renal artery stenosis.

Summation of Guidelines as when to Refer to a Nephrologist

The recommendation for referring to the nephrologist is in the following situation:

- Stage 4 or 5 CKD of any cause having eGFR of <30 mL/min/1.73 m^2
- Having ACR >30 mg/mmol or urine protein excretion of >500 mg/day that is patient is having a persistent significant albuminuria
- A consistent decline in estimated glomerular filtration rate from a baseline of <60 mL/min/1.73 m^2 (a decline >5 mL/min/1.73 m^2 over a 6-month period which is confirmed on at least three separate readings) (1C).

We suggest referral to a specialist renal service or nephrologist in the following situations:

- Glomerular hematuria with macroalbuminuria (2C)
- Chronic kidney disease and hypertension difficult to control despite at least three antihypertensive agents (2C)
- We suggest discussing management issues with a specialist by letter, email or telephone in cases where it may not be necessary for the person with CKD to be seen by the specialist (2D)
- Once a referral has been made and a plan jointly agreed, routine follow-up could be done take physician's clinic and recommendation about criteria for future referral or re-referral should also be specified (1D).

Other criteria which is also required for referral to nephrologist are:

- Acute deterioration of renal function that is eGFR decline >25% in <1 month after exogenous factors being excluded
- Renal progression that is decline of eGFR of >5 mL/min/year
- Serum potassium >5.5 or <3.5 mEq/L
- If the patient is suffering from anemia that is Hb <10.5 g/dL with CKD and has a corrected transferrin saturation of >20% and serum ferritin >100 ng/mL.

A number of studies[2,7,8,11,16,17,24,34,37,40] have showed that if the patient is referred early in serious CKD then there is decrease rate of kidney failure decline, decrease duration and need for hospitalization, increase likelihood of use of permanent dialysis access, increase chances of kidney transplantation[4,5] and decrease in the morbidity and mortality rate.

In a series from Australia,[26] 30% of the patients who are suffering from CKD were referred "late" to nephrologist that is within 3 months of requiring renal replacement therapy. This patients has decreased survival rate on dialysis and also had less chances to receive a kidney transplant.

Several studies[6,17,23,39] have shown that early reference to nephrologist has good outcome but there is no high-level clinical evidence in support as well as there is no assessment on the economics of implementing such guidelines as well as there was complexities in making the decisions for referral of CKD patients like poor predictability of progression, multiple comorbid medical problems, loss of functional and cognitive impairment in making decisions.[14,27-29,32,35,36] Even the chances of cardiovascular morbidity and mortality were also high. PCPs were less aware of the guidelines[15,22,34] and the recommendation to the renal specialist when they were presented with a hypothetical clinical situation of CKD. Survey of 479 internal medicine residents in USA[1] was done to determine there decision to refer to a nephrologist in CKD management and the results showed reduction in (proteinuria (45%), uncontrolled hypertension (64%), hyperkalemia (26%), anemia (28%), CKD bone disorder (45%), GFR) <30 mL/min/1.73 m^2 (90%) and rapid decline in GFR (79%).[1]

BENEFITS OF EARLY REFERRAL

In general, the main potential benefits associated with timely, appropriate renal services referral includes:

- Optimizing patient planning and preparation for dialysis or renal transplantation (including of permanent dialysis access)
- Improved diagnosis and management of treatable kidney disease (e.g. glomerulonephritis) requiring renal biopsy or immunosuppression
- Slow CKD progression by improving control of CKD risk factors
- Improved management of complications, related to CKD such as renal anemia (hemoglobin <10 g/dL), chronic kidney disease-mineral and bone disorder (CKD-MBD) and refractory hypertension.

The potential disadvantages of referral to nephrologist are:

- Saturation of or decrease number of nephrologist manpower and resources, thereby limiting the access of high risk CKD patients who can be benefited from specialist renal care
- Inefficient utilization of health care
- May be unnecessary or costly health care investigation with less serious CKD which is easily manageable in primary health care.

There is no randomized controlled trial of the outcome in the population who is getting treatment in primary or institutional healthcare as far is nephrologist referral is concerned. In a nonrandomized controlled trial of 52 diabetic patients in whom CKD was detected in primary practice on the basis of an abnormal routine eGFR report and/or proteinuria, Martinez-Ramirez et al.[25] demonstrated that patients who were subsequently referred to a nephrologist exhibited better preservation of renal function than those who remained treated by only their family doctors. Albuminuria increased more in patients treated by family doctors and systolic blood pressure was not as well controlled. The nephrologist significantly increased ($p < 0.05$) the use of angiotensin-converting enzyme inhibitors (ACEI), angiotensin receptor blockers (ARBs), and statins and discontinued non-steroidal anti-inflammatory drugs more than family doctors (study, 42%, 43%, 39% and –11% versus control, 17%, 4%, –7% and 27%, respectively). Glycemic, lipid control and quitting of smoking were not attained by either the nephrologist or by family doctors. However, these results may have been limited by indication bias, since the decision to refer a diabetic CKD patient to a specialist renal service was non-random. Moreover, the sample size was too small to allow for adequate adjustment for demographic and clinical factors.

Black et al.[45] conducted a systematic analysis of the evidence of clinical effectiveness, cost-effectiveness and economic analysis of early referral strategies for management of people with markers of renal disease. Only seven studies (all nonrandomized) were identified as relevant to assessing the clinical effectiveness of early referral strategies for CKD. Five retrospective studies examining patients who had commenced renal replacement therapy found that early referral (>12 months prior to renal replacement therapy) was associated with reduced odds of mortality for up to 5 years after renal replacement therapy commencement.

Studies have shown that as far as long-term care is concerned both nephrologist and PCP wants that PCP should remain the primary care giver,[15,22] but the areas of clinical practice should be clearly demarcated in between all the care providers. There should be a multidisciplinary approach and intervention to give the care to CKD patients. Effective communication also plays a crucial role in treating the patients of CKD.

STRATEGIES TO MANAGE DKD

A model of DKD care should consist of at least the following elements:

- Clearly delineated areas of clinical practice agreed on between all providers in advance
- An effective outcomes measurement system and QI strategy
- Integration of multidisciplinary teams with multifactorial interventions
- Effective communication strategy using a shared EMR with access to a fully functional patient chart.

Every clinician has its role in treating the patients of DKD. The Table 1 gives us information regarding proper care of CKD patients in various subsets of presentation and complication.

Predialysis education and information can help the patient to choose his dialysis modality as well as increases the awareness about the various aspects of end-stage renal disease. It may also help the patient to think about transplant and has also shown that this predialysis education will decrease the cost at the start of the dialysis, need of urgent dialysis and days of hospitalization during first month of dialysis initiation.

ALARMING SIGNS OF DKD

The evidence-based pearls in this article will help PCPs understand these concepts and avoid common pitfalls in the recognition and treatment of such disorders and guide their decision to refer their patients to a specialist.

- A "normal" serum creatinine level may not be normal- Normal creatinine values may vary among different laboratories, and some patients with serum creatinine levels within the "normal" range may have substantial reduction in kidney function. For example, a 65-year-old man with a serum creatinine level of 1.4 mg/dL would have an eGFR of 52.4 mL/min/1.73 m^2 (CKD-EPI) corresponding to stage 3 CKD. The interpretation of serum creatinine level also depends on muscle mass, age, sex, height and limb amputation. A patient with an amputation and a high-normal creatinine level may actually have advanced CKD
- Know the medications that spuriously elevate the serum creatinine level- The antibiotic trimethoprim-sulfamethoxazole and the H2-blocker cimetidine are two commonly used drugs that decrease the secretion of creatinine. Other drugs are Famotidine, Ranitidine and cefoxitin
- Cause should be ascertained in patient with decrease gfr or proteinuria-Positive urine dipstick test result should be confirmed by spot urinary protein to urinary creatinine ratio or by 24 hour urinary protein ratio. Risk of CKD progression is higher if the urine

TABLE 1: **Management of chronic kidney disease in various subsets of presentation and complication.**

	CKD stage 3			CKD stage 4			CKD stage 5		
Clinical focus areas	Physician	Nephro-logist	Endo-crinologist	Physician	Nephrolog-ist	Endo-crinologist	Physician	Nephro-logist	Endo-crinologist
DM Mgt	+		+	+		+	+		
HTN Mgt	+				+			+	
Diet and lifestyle	+	+	+	+	+	+	+	+	+
MBD	+	+			+			+	
Anemia of CKD	+	+			+			+	

Note: Areas of focus for the physician, nephrologist and endocrinologist with progression of DKD following development of stage 3 CKD.
(CKD: chronic kidney disease; DM: diabetes mellitus; DKD: diabetic kidney disease; HTN: hypertension; MBD: mineral bone disorders; Mgt: management.)

protein to creatinine ratio is >1 and if the patient is having high proteinuria or active sediment or having deterioration in renal function then he should be referred to nephrologist to ascertain the cause, evaluation and for treatment

- Referral to nephrologist in early-stage ckd-If the patient is having stage 5 CKD, or having uncontrolled complications like uncontrolled blood pressure, secondary hyperparathyroidism, active urinary sediment or nephrotic range proteinuria, then these patient should be referred early to the nephrologist to slow the progression of CKD
- Anemia in ckd should be treated not overtreated-National kidney foundation dialysis outcome quality initiative KDOQI guidelines suggest that the hemoglobin level in patients of CKD should be between 11 and 12 and is to be treated by erythropoietin and iron till that level is reached and if the level is above 13 gm% then erythropoietin should be discontinued. There are high chances of cerebrovascular events, thrombosis and hypertension
- Caution in using bowl preparation containing phosphates-This can cause acute phosphate nephropathy so polyethylene glycol which is not causing volume shifts or abnormalities in electrolytes can be used
- Avoid oral preparation containing magnesium or aluminium-As it may cause aluminium toxicity or hypermagnesemia which can be hazardous. In CKD there can be an increased risk of aluminium accumulation which may lead to bone disease or neurotoxicity. Calcium or potassium citrate and even sodium citrate can increase aluminium absorption in gut
- Use ACEIs or arbs as they are wonder drugs-To prevent the progression of CKD with proteinuria these are the drugs of choice. When these drugs are started, there can be an increase of creatinine by 20–30% which is acceptable as well as patient can have a rise in serum potassium level up to 5.5 mEq/L. As long as patient is stable we should not discontinue this drug and only when it goes beyond the level stated above then these drugs should be discontinued temporarily and restarted with a titrated dose. To combat hyperkalemia by ACEIs or ARBs, frusemide or metolazone can be used in treatment of hypertension and hyperkalaemia in CKD
- Search for secondary causes of hypertension in patients of ckd-Resistant or severe or difficult to control hypertension or if there is sudden worsening of HT or associated other clinical findings then we should always think of an underlying cause of hypertension other than CKD. Secondary hypertension should always be ruled out in these scenarios. If there is deterioration of renal function or hypertension gets worsens with ACEIs or ARBs, it may suggest probability of renal artery stenosis
- Search for cause of recurrent nephrolithiasis-It is a commonly encountered problem in primary care by physicians which leads to significant morbidity. The chance of development of renal stone disease till age 70 years is around 15% and 10-year recurrence rate of calcium oxalate stones is 50% without treatment, so these patients should be evaluated for any metabolic cause. Those patients who are suffering from inflammatory bowel disease, recurrent UTI, having a family history of stones should be referred to nephrologist for further evaluation. Detailed evaluation which includes diet history, medications which can lead to formation of stone, urine analysis and detailed measurement of levels of serum calcium, phosphorus, electrolytes and uric acid along with detailed analysis of urine should be done in these patients to treat effectively.

CONCLUSION

Chronic kidney disease is the disease which is primarily being treated by physicians. However, they should be able to recognize early in the course of CKD, evaluate in details and give appropriate treatment or do timely referral to nephrologist, (Fig. 1) then there can be a substantial reduction in morbidity and mortality in patients of CKD.

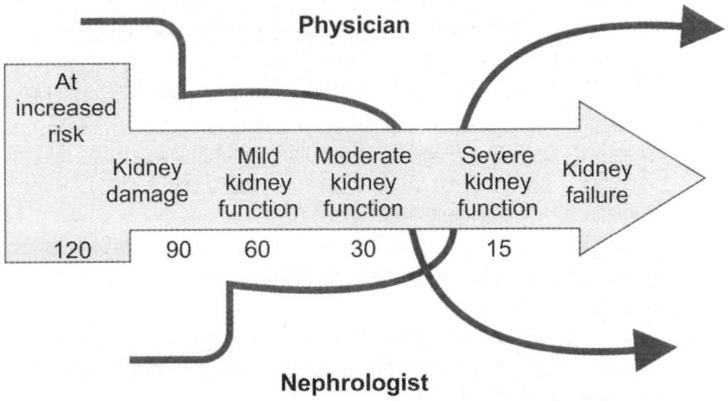

Figure 1 Co-management of chronic kidney disease.

REFERENCES

1. Agrawal V, Ghosh AK, Barnes MA, et al. Perception of indications for nephrology referral among internal medicine residents: a national online survey. Clinical Journal of The American Society of Nephrology: CJASN. 2009;4:323-8.
2. Binik YM, Devins GM, Barre PE, et al. Live and learn: patient education delays the need to initiate renal replacement therapy in end-stage renal disease. J Nerv Ment Dis. 1993;181:371-6.
3. Boulware LE, Troll MU, Jaar BG, et al. Identification and referral of patients with progressive CKD: a national study. AM J Kidney Dis. 2006;48:192-204.
4. Campbell KH, Dale W, Stankus N, et al. Older adults and chronic kidney disease decision making by primary care physicians: a scholarly review and research agenda. J Gen Intern Med. 2008;23:329-36.
5. Cass A, Cunningham J, Snelling P, et al. Late referral to a nephrologist reduces access to renal transplantation. Am J Kidney Dis. 2003;42:1043-9.
6. Chadban S, Snelling P, Harvie B, et al. Chronic Kidney Disease Management in General Practice. 2007, Kidney Health Australia.
7. Chan MR, Dall AT, Fletcher KE, et al. Outcomes in patients with chronic kidney disease referred late to nephrologists: a meta-analysis. Am J Med. 2007;120:1063-70.
8. Churchill DN. An evidence-based approach to earlier initiation of dialysis. American Journal of Kidney Diseases. Am J Kidney Dis. 1997;30:899-906.
9. Clement R, Chevalet P, Rodat O, et al. Withholding or withdrawing dialysis in the elderly: the perspective of a western region of France. Nephrology Dialysis Transplantation. 2005;20:2446-52.
10. Crowe E, Halpin D, Stevens P, et al. Early identification and management of chronic kidney disease: summary of NICE guidance. BMJ. 2008; 337:a1530.
11. Curtis BM, Ravani P, Malberti F, et al. The short- and long-term impact of muti-disciplinary clinics in addition to standard nephrology care on patient outcomes. Nephrol. Dial. Transplant. 2005;20:147-154.
12. Comanagement of Diabetic Kidney Disease by the Primary Care Provider and Nephrologist , Brendan T. Bowman, MD, Amanda Kleiner, MD, W. Kline Bolton, MD,Med Clin N Am 97 (2013) 157–173.
13. KDOQI clinical practice guidelines and clinical practice recommendations for diabetes and chronic kidney disease. Am J Kidney Dis 2007;49(2 Suppl 2): S12–154.
14. Forrest CB, Nutting PA, Starfield B, et al. Family physicians' referral decisions: results from the ASPN referral study. J Fam Pract. 2002;51:215-22.
15. Fox CH, Brooks A, Zayas LE, et al. Primary care physicians' knowledge and practice patterns in the treatment of chronic kidney disease: an Upstate New York Practice-based Research Network (UNYNET) study. J Am Board Fam Med. 2006;19:54-61.
16. Jungers P, Joly D, Nguyen-Khoa, T et al. [Continued late referral of patients with chronic kidney disease. Causes, consequences, and approaches to improvement]. Presse Medicale. 2006;35:17-22.
17. Jungers P, Zingraff J, Albouze G, et al. Late referral to maintenance dialysis: detrimental consequences. Nephrol Dial Transplant. 1993;8:1089-93.
18. Jungers P, Zingraff J, Page B, et al. Detrimental effects of late referral in patients with chronic renal failure: a case-control study. Kidney International - Supplement. 1993;41:S170-3.
19. Kinchen KS, Cooper LA, Levine D, et al. Referral of patients to specialists: factors affecting choice of specialist by primary care physicians. Ann Fam Med. 2004;2:245-52.
20. Kinchen KS, Cooper LA, Wang N-Y, et al. The impact of international medical graduate status on primary care physicians' choice of specialist. Med Care. 2004;42:747-55.
21. Kinchen KS, Sadler J, Fink N, et al. The timing of specialist evaluation in chronic kidney disease and mortality. Ann Intern Med. 2002;137:479-86.
22. Lea JP, McClellan WM, Melcher C, et al. CKD risk factors reported by primary care physicians: do guidelines make a difference? Am J Kidney Dis. 2006;47:72-7.
23. Levin A, Hemmelgarn B, Culleton B, et al. Guidelines for the management of chronic kidney disease. CMAJ. 2008;179(11):1154-62.
24. Levinsky NG. Specialist evaluation in chronic kidney disease: too little, too late. Ann Intern Med. 2002;137:542-3.
25. Martinez-Ramirez HR, Jalomo-Martinez B, Cortes-Sanabria L, et al. Renal function preservation in type 2 diabetes mellitus patients with early nephropathy: a comparative prospective cohort study between primary health care doctors and a nephrologist. Am J Kidney Dis. 2006;47:78-87.
26. McDonald SM, Excell L, and Livingston B, ANZDATA Registry Report 2008. 2008, Australian and New Zealand Dialysis and Transplant Registry.
27. McKenzie JK, Moss AH, Feest TG, et al. Dialysis decision making in Canada, the United Kingdom, and the United States. Am J Kidney Dis. 1998;31:12-8.
28. Mendelssohn DC, Kua BT, Singer PA. Referral for dialysis in Ontario. Arch. Int Med. 1995;155:2473-8.
29. Montgomery AJ, McGee HM, Shannon W, et al. Factors influencing general practitioner referral of patients developing end-stage renal failure: a standardized case-analysis study. BMC Health Serv Res. 2006;6:114.
30. National Collaborating Centre for Chronic Conditions, Chronic kidney disease: National clinical guideline for early identification and management in adults in primary and secondary care. Royal College of Physicians: London, 2008.
31. O'Neill L, Kuder J. Explaining variation in physician practice patterns and their propensities to recommend services. Med Care Res Rev. 2005;62:339-57.
32. Parry RG, Crowe A, Stevens JM, et al. Referral of elderly patients with severe renal failure: questionnaire survey of physicians. BMJ. 1996;313:466.
33. Piccoli GB, Grassi G, Mezza E, et al. Early referral of Type 2 diabetic patients: are we ready for the assault? Nephrol Dial Transplant. 2002;17:1241-7.
34. Ratcliffe PJ, Phillips RE, Oliver DO. Late referral for maintenance dialysis. Br Med J Clin Res Ed. 1984;288:441-3.
35. Sekkarie M, Cosma M, Mendelssohn D. Nonreferral and nonacceptance to dialysis by primary care physicians and nephrologists in Canada and the United States. Am J Kidney Dis. 2001;38:36-41.
36. Sekkarie MA, Moss AH. Withholding and withdrawing dialysis: the role of physician specialty and education and patient functional status. Am J Kidney Dis. 1998;31:464-72.
37. Sesso R, Belasco AG. Late diagnosis of chronic renal failure and mortality on maintenance dialysis. Nephrol Dial Transplant. 1996;11:2417-20.
38. Sigel P, Leiper R. GP views of their management and referral of psychological problems: a qualitative study. Psychol Psychother. 2004;77:279-95.
39. SIGN, Diagnosis and management of chronic kidney disease: A national clinical guideline. 2008, Scottish Intercollegiate Guidelines Network.
40. Smart NA, Titus TT. Outcomes of early versus late nephrology referral in chronic kidney disease: a systematic review. Am J Med. 2011;124:1073-80.e2.
41. Paige NM, Nagami GT. The top 10 things nephrologists wish every primary care physician knew. Mayo Clin Proc. 2011;124:1073-80.e2.
42. Umanath K, Lewis JB. Update on Diabetic Nephropathy: Core Curriculum 2018. Am J Kidney Dis. 2018;71(6):884-95.
43. Ritz E. Consequences of late referral in diabetic renal disease. Acta Diabetol 2002;39(Suppl 1):S3–8.
44. Arora P, Obrador GT, Ruthazer R, et al. Prevalence, predictors, and consequences of late nephrology referral at a tertiary care center. J Am Soc Nephrol 1999;10:1281–6.
45. Black C, Sharma P, Scotland G et al. Early referral strategies for management of people with markers of renal disease: a systematic review of the evidence of clinical effectiveness, cost-effectiveness and economic analysis. Health Technology Assessment (Winchester, England). 2010; 14:1-184.

Chapter 39

Novel Agents for Diabetic Neuropathy Management

Ashu Rastogi

INTRODUCTION

Diabetes mellitus is one of the most prevalent noncommunicable diseases that affect the mankind across all races and geographical locations. An increasing prevalence of diabetes in recent times has contributed to swelling number of patients with diabetic complications, including diabetic neuropathy (DN). One-half to two-thirds of patients with diabetes are affected by peripheral neuropathy depending upon the modality used for the diagnosis. However, DN is a diagnosis of exclusion after carefully considering chronic alcoholism, vitamin B12 deficiency, malnutrition and varied other common etiologies of peripheral neuropathy. The distal symmetrical polyneuropathy (DSPN) is by far the most common type of DN, which affects more than 90% of the subjects with DN. DSPN may have myriad presentation ranging from negative sensations such as abnormal feeling of the floor, walking on cotton, insensitivity to burns or thorn pricks without pain suggesting loss of temperature and touch perception. Otherwise, patients may report positive sensations like burning sensations, electric shock like sensations, stabbing pain, or insect crawling on foot, etc. Sometimes, the symptoms may even be debilitating like excruciating night pains in legs and foot, insulin neuritc pain or thigh pain associated with amyotrophy. Painful diabetic peripheral neuropathy (DPN) is thus another aspect of DN affecting 10–26% of diabetic patients presenting with predominant hyperalgesia or allodynia. DPN markedly affects the quality of life, influencing the ability to perform activities of daily living. Subjects affected with DPN usually refrain from social and recreational activities, and depressed mood plays a crucial role in this disability. More commonly, all the above-mentioned symptoms are present in the same patient because of affliction of both the large as well as small nerve fibers.

Diabetic neuropathy continues to embody a therapeutic challenge as the lurking pathophysiological processes for DN are not yet fully understood. The pharmacological treatments, with exception to those targeted to the glycemic control, are symptomatic, not focused on the pathophysiological mechanism, limited by side effects and by the development of tolerance. This review focuses on the novel agents targeted toward the symptoms of DN and also therapies aimed at reversing the process of DN.

NOVEL AGENTS FOR SYMPTOMATIC RELIEF IN DIABETIC PERIPHERAL NEUROPATHY

Although the pathophysiology of DPN is not fully understood, both central and peripheral mechanisms are likely involved in the genesis of pain, which complicates the management of patients with painful DPN. Duloxetine and pregabalin are considered as the first-line treatment options for pain related to DPN and are approved by the US Food and Drug Administration (FDA) for this indication. Generally, in clinical trials, treatment is considered successful, if patient would obtain at least 50% reduction in the pain level associated with some additional beneficial effects on sleep, fatigue, depression and quality of life. Various other agents that are in clinical use for symptomatic relief include antidepressants, namely, amitriptyline, nortriptyline; anticonvulsants like gabapentin, pregabalin, topiramate; opioids, namely, tramadol, oxycodone; and topical agents, namely, capsaicin, lidocaine patch, isosorbide nitrate sprays or a combination of all these classes of drugs.[1] These drugs, used alone or in combination, have been shown to reduce neuropathic pain compared with placebo in randomized controlled trials, still, pain relief remains inadequate for most patients. Hence, there is a dire need of newer therapeutic agents to address DPN, but unfortunately, no new agents are approved by FDA over the past 20 years.

Recent advances in the understanding of the pathophysiology, especially the implication of inflammatory molecules has led to the development of novel agents though still in preclinical phases that may see light of the day in future.

Most promising novel agents that are investigated and have gain acceptance for DPN are the opioid analgesics. Oxycodone, an opioid analgesic has been tried in DN with some favorable results, but a recent Cochrane review concluded that there is no convincing, unbiased evidence that oxycodone controlled-release (CR) is of value in treating patients who have painful DPN. Oxycodone CR is therefore best reserved as add-on for selecting patients only who are at little risk of opioid abuse and dependence.[2] Tapentadol extended-release (ER) is a new class of centrally acting analgesic combining two mechanisms of action: μ-opioid receptor (MOR) agonism and norepinephrine reuptake inhibitor (NRI). It has been shown to provide pain relief in doses of 100–250 mg, given twice a day up to 1 year of treatment.[3] In another larger study, patients who received tapentadol ER achieved clinically meaningful improvements in pain intensity and health status, based on responder rate analyses. In addition, significant differences in the Short Form-36 physical functioning, rolephysical, bodily pain, social functioning and role-emotional subscale scores, and the physical component summary score were observed with tapentadol compared to placebo. More than 50% of the patients who received tapentadol ER throughout the study achieved a clinically meaningful 30% improvement in pain intensity from the start of titration to the end of the maintenance period, and approximately 39% achieved a 50% improvement in pain intensity. A numerically greater difference was observed in the mean change in pain intensity amongst females and opioid naïve patients.[4] As compared to oxycodone CR, tapentadol ER treatment is associated with better gastrointestinal tolerability, thus, improving compliance with therapy and may be a better option for the long-term management of chronic pain. The NRI activity of tapentadol may contribute to an opioid-sparing effect, resulting in the improved gastrointestinal tolerability. Tapentadol ER received FDA approval in August 2012 for the management of neuropathic pain associated with DPN when a continuous, around-the-clock opioid analgesic is needed for an extended period of time.

Another class of drugs investigated for DPN is cannabinoid (CB) receptor agonists. Nabilone, a synthesized CB (CB1 predominant) receptor agonist, in doses of 1–4 mg/day effectively relieved DPN symptoms, improved disturbed sleep, quality of life and overall patient status. However, meta-analyses of studies with selective CBs suggested that pain scores did not demonstrate analgesic benefit (mean difference −0.72 points; 95% confidence interval −2.04 to 0.59 points; $p = 0.28$, $I^2 = 75\%$). The use of nabiximols and dronabinol, but not nabilone, conferred analgesic benefit among the various selective CBs. Selective CBs were associated with the improvements in the quality of life and sleep and enhanced patient satisfaction, but the impact on physical and psychological function was unclear. Serious adverse effects were rare with the doses of selective CBs used in these trials.[5] Palmitoylethanolamide (PEA), a fatty acid amide of the N-acylethanolamine family, is capable of exerting important analgesic, anti-inflammatory, and neuroprotective effects. PEA potentiates anandamide action at CB1 and CB2 receptors and/or transient receptor potential vanilloid 1 (TRPV1) channels, while having no appreciable affinity for these receptors. PEA-micronized treatment resulted in a significant reduction in the pain symptoms characteristic of DN.[6]

Tricyclic antidepressants and selective serotonin reuptake inhibitorsare in common use for DPN, but therapeutic effectiveness is limited. Therefore dual serotonin and NRI (SNRI), i.e. duloxetine and venlafaxine are used. Desvenlafaxine is the newer congener, most potent metabolite of the parent compound venlafaxine and has been recently evaluated in patients with painful DPN. In a Phase III multicenter, randomized placebo-controlled trial with more than 400 patients, desvenlafaxine in doses of 200 and 400 mg/day was found to be effective in relieving pain and improving activity.[7] Compounds that act at nicotinic acetylcholine receptors have antinociceptive activities. Among these compounds, tebanicline (a potent nicotinic acetylcholine receptor agonist) has demonstrated analgesic effects across a broad range of preclinical models of nociceptive and neuropathic pain. Another, nicotinic acetylcholine receptor agonist, A-366833 (at 1, 3 or 6 mg/kg) exerts antinociceptive activity and reduces mechanical hyperalgesia in diabetes-induced neuropathic rat models.[8] Minocycline, an inhibitor of microglial activation, inhibits the development of neuropathic pain by preventing the release of proinflammatory cytokines. Chronic administration of minocycline before peripheral nerve injury attenuates and delays the development of neuropathic pain.[9]

Therapeutic treatment with PKF275-055, a long-acting novel dipeptidyl peptidase-IV inhibitor, corrects the alterations in sodium-potassium adenosine triphosphatase (Na/K-ATPase) activity and nerve conduction velocity that are present in untreated diabetics. PKF275-055 treatment increases mechanical sensitivity thresholds by approximately 50% and progressively improves alterations in thermal responsiveness. PKF275-055 has an anabolic effect, improves oral glucose tolerance and counteracts the alterations in Na/K-ATPase activity, nerve conduction velocity, and nociceptive thresholds observed in diabetic rats.[10] TRPV1 channel in sensory neurons are involved in thermal hyperalgesia. Intrathecal administration of resiniferatoxin, a potent TRPV1 agonist, attenuates thermal hyperalgesia but not mechanical allodynia and also prevents increases in TRPV1-mediated neuropeptide release in spinal cord tissues.[11] MK801, an *N*-methyl-D-aspartate receptor antagonist in combination with electroacupuncture, prolongs antihyperalgesia, increases p35 expression, and decreases the cleavage of p35 to p25 during diabetic neuropathic pain.[12]

In a Phase III multicenter, randomized placebo-controlled trial (n = 412), graduated doses of 200 and 400 mg/day desvenlafaxine were found to be effective in relieving pain and improving activity.

Tanezumab is a fully humanized anti–nerve growth factor immunoglobulin G type-2 monoclonal antibody, which has high selectivity and specificity for nerve growth factor (NGF) that prevent interaction between NGF and its receptors by tightly binding NGF, thereby disrupting ongoing pain signaling. Tanezumab in doses of 20 mg subcutaneous administered on day 1 and week 8 showed a reduction in DPN pain but no improvement in patients' global assessment of pain.[13]

Inflammation is considered as the perpetuator of nociceptive stimulus and initiation of DPN. Clinical trials of a novel p38 mitogen-activated protein kinases inhibitor produce rapid relief of neuropathic pain and decreased systemic inflammation acutely but not on extended treatment.[14] Chemokine ligand type 12 (CXCL12)/chemokine receptor type 4 (CXCR4) signaling is necessary for the development of mechanical allodynia, a pain hypersensitivity behavior common in painful DN, and therapies targeting CXCL12/CXCR4 signaling may be novel agents, being tested in preclinical studies.[15] Mesenchymal stem cells that have anti-inflammatory properties have also been tested in diabetic mice, and an improvement in radiant heat assays and mechanical stimuli tests with lower serum levels of many proinflammatory cytokines was demonstrated.[16] Type 2 diabetes is associated with substantial downregulation of miR-146a. Systemic administration of miR-146a mimics to diabetic mice elevates miR-146a levels in plasma and sciatic nerve tissue and significantly increased motor and sensory nerve conduction velocities by 29% and 11%, respectively, and regional blood flow by 50% in sciatic nerve tissue. All the novel pharmaceutical agents for symptomatic relief in DPN are summarized in Table 1.

In addition to pharmacological agents, certain interventional therapies have been considered in select patients with refractory neuropathic pain, including spinal cord stimulation, electrical stimulation therapy through stocking electrodes, pulsed magnetic field therapy, transcutaneous nerve stimulation, acupuncture, laser therapy and monochromatic infrared light therapy (MIRE).

A small study of 19 patients with low-level laser therapy irradiated through scanning mode with dosage of 3.1 J/cm^2 on the plantar and dorsum of the foot and 3.4 J/cm^2 with contact method for 10 days showed a significant reduction in neuropathic pain using visual analog scale (VAS) and Michigan Neuropathy Screening Instrument (MNSI).[17] Experience with MIRE therapy is mixed with initial few studies showing improvement in pain intensity measured by 10 cm VAS, sensation assessed with 10 g monofilament, and balance. Our experience suggested no significant change in primary outcome of distal leg intraepidermal nerve fiber density or vibration perception threshold (VPT), DN symptoms, neuropathy disability scores and MNSI questionnaire in the MIRE cohort when compared with sham therapy. However, we observed a statistically significant improvement in the VAS and Norfolk Quality of Life scores post-therapy with MIRE therapy. However, other authors have refuted the effect of MIRE therapy based on their results of no improvement in quality of life, the MNSI, VPT, Semmes-Weinstein monofilaments, or nerve conduction velocities.[18] Presently, none of the above-mentioned interventional therapies are approved by FDA for symptomatic DPN.

NOVEL AGENTS TARGETED AT THE PATHOPHYSIOLOGY OF DIABETIC NEUROPATHY

No specific treatment has been approved by most regulatory agencies to modify the course of DSPN, although

TABLE 1: Novel therapeutic agents for symptomatic benefits in diabetic neuropathy.

Drug	Drug class	Side effects	Doses
Resiniferatoxin	TRPV1 agonist	Musculoskeletal hyperalgesia	2 µg/kg intrathecal
Tebanicline	Nicotinic acetylcholine receptor agonist	Hypothermia and seizures	0.05–1.6 mol/kg, SC
A-366833	Nicotinic acetylcholine receptor agonist	Nausea, dizziness, vomiting and asthenia	1, 3 and 6 mg/kg
Minocycline	Microglial activation inhibitor	Lightheadedness, nausea and vomiting	2-week treatment: 40 or 80 mg/kg (IP) Single dose: 30 or 100 mg/kg (IP)
PKF275-055	DPP-IV inhibitor	Hypoglycemia, dizziness and dysrhythmia	3 mg/kg
Nabilone	Synthetic CB1 predominant receptor	Drowsiness, dizziness, euphoria and dry mouth	1–4 mg/day
MK-801	NMDA receptor antagonist	Hyperactivity and truncal ataxia	0.5 mg/kg SC
Oxycodone	Opioids	Constipation, nausea, pruritus and fatigue	100–250 mg twice a day
Tapentadol	MOR-NRI	Nausea, headache, dizziness and somnolence	50–100 mg 4–6 times a day
PEA	N-acylethanolamine		300 or 600 mg daily
Desvenlafaxine	Serotonin-norepinephrine reuptake inhibitor	Nausea, dry mouth, hyperhidrosis and insomnia	200 and 400 mg/day
Tanezumab	Humanized monoclonal IgG2 antibody	Peripheral edema and paresthesia	20 mg SC

(CB: cannabinoid; DPP-IV: dipeptidyl peptidase-IV; IgG2: immunoglobulin G2; IP: interphalangeal; MOR: µ-opioid receptor; NMDA: N-methyl-D-aspartate; NRI: norepinephrine reuptake inhibitor; PEA: palmitoylethanolamide; SC: subcutaneous; TRPV1: transient receptor potential vanilloid 1.)

an aldose reductase inhibitor is approved for use in DSPN in Japan. Drugs aimed at the underlying pathogenesis of DSPN have failed in Phase III clinical trials, despite some promising results in Phase II studies. Interventions that have failed include aldose reductase inhibitors (tolrestat, zopolrestat, zenarestat and ranirestat), NGF, acetyl-L-carnitine, ruboxistaurin, α-lipoic acid, C-peptide, vitamins and vasodilators.

CONCLUSION

Diabetic neuropathy remains the most debilitating complication of diabetes affecting the quality of life of patients afflicted with diabetes. Inspite of various pharmaceutical agents tested for the symptomatic relief of neuropathy, no new agents have been approved lately, despite the established agents efficacy far from being perfect. Amongst novel agents, tapentadol, a MOR agonist and NRI and CBs receptor agonists have shown promise for neuropathic pain and are the light at the end of the tunnel.

REFERENCES

1. Pop-Busui R, Boulton AJM, Feldman EL, et al. Diabetic neuropathy: a position statement by American Diabetic Association. Diabetes Care. 2017;40:136-54.
2. Gaskell H, Moore RA, Derry S, et al. Oxycodone for neuropathic pain and fibromyalgia in adults (review). Cochrane Database Syst Rev.2014;6:CD010692.
3. Afilalo M, Morlion B. Efficacy of tapentadol ER for managing moderate to severe chronic pain. Pain Physician. 2013;16:27-40.
4. Schwartz S, Etropolski MS, Shapiro DY, et al. A pooled analysis evaluating the efficacy and tolerability of tapentadol extended release for chronic, painful diabetic peripheral neuropathy. Clin Drug Investig. 2015;35:95-108.
5. Meng H, Johnston B, Englesakis M, et al. Selective cannabinoids for chronic neuropathic pain: a systematic review and meta analysis. Anesth Analg. 2017;125:1638-52.
6. Schifilliti C, Cucinotta L, Fedele V, et al. Micronized palmitoylethanolamide reduces the symptoms of neuropathic pain in diabetic patients. Pain Res Treat. 2014;2014:849623.
7. Allen R, Sharma U, Barlas S. Clinical experience with desvenlafaxine in treatment of pain associated with diabetic peripheral neuropathy. J Pain Res. 2014;7:339-51.
8. Nirogi R, Jabaris SL, Jayarajan P, et al. Antinociceptive activity of 4 2* neuronal nicotinic receptor agonist A-366833 in experimental models of neuropathic and inflammatory pain. Eur J Pharmacol.2011;668(1-2):155-62.

9. Padi SS, Kulkarni SK. Minocycline prevents the development of neuropathic pain, but not acute pain: possible anti-inflammatory and antioxidant mechanisms. Eur J Pharmacol. 2008;601(1-3):79-87.
10. Bianchi R, Cervellini I, Porretta-Serapiglia C, et al. Beneficial effects of PKF275-055, a novel, selective, orally bioavailable, long-acting dipeptidyl peptidase IV inhibitor in streptozotocin-induced diabetic peripheral neuropathy. J Pharmacol Exp Ther. 2012;340(1):64-72.
11. Bishnoi M, Bosgraaf CA, Abooj M, et al. Streptozotocin-induced early thermal hyperalgesia is independent of glycemic state of rats: role of transient receptor potential vanilloid 1(TRPV1) and inflammatory mediators. Mol Pain. 2011;7:52.
12. Hwang HS, Yang EJ, Lee SM, et al. Antiallodynic effects of electro acupuncture combined with MK-801 treatment through the regulation of p35/p25 in experimental diabetic neuropathy. Exp Neurobiol. 2011;20:144-52.
13. Bramson C, Herrmann DN, Carey W, et al. Exploring the role of tanezumab as a novel treatment for the relief of neuropathic pain. Pain Med. 2015;16:1163-76.
14. Genovese MC, Cohen SB, Wofsy D, et al. A 24-week, randomized, double-blind, placebo-controlled, parallel group study of the efficacy of oral SCIO-469, a p38 mitogen-activated protein kinase inhibitor, in patients with active rheumatoid arthritis. J Rheumatol. 2011;38(5):846-54.
15. Jayaraj ND, Bhattacharyya BJ, Belmadani AA, et al. Reducing CXCR4-mediated nociceptor hyperexcitability reverses painful diabetic neuropathy. J Clin Invest. 2018;128(6):2205-25.
16. Waterman RS, Morgenweck J, Nossaman BD, et al. Anti-inflammatory mesenchymal stem cells (MSC2) attenuate symptoms of painful diabetic peripheral neuropathy. Stem Cells Transl Med. 2012;1(7):557-65.
17. CGSK, Maiya AG, Hande HM, et al. Efficacy of low level laser therapy on painful diabetic peripheral neuropathy. Laser Ther. 2015;24(3):195-200.
18. Lavery LA, Murdoch DP, Williams J, et al. Does anodyne light therapy improve peripheral neuropathy in diabetes? A double-blind, sham-controlled, randomized trial to evaluate monochromatic infrared photoenergy. Diabetes Care. 2008;31:316-21.

Chapter 40

Genetics and the Quest for Novel Therapies in Painful Diabetic Neuropathy

SK Singh, Rujul Jain

INTRODUCTION

Diabetes mellitus is a menacing global health problem assuming epidemic proportion worldwide. Peripheral neuropathy is the most common microvascular complication of diabetes, affecting approximately 50% of the patients.[1] Peripheral neuropathy is the forerunner of recurrent foot ulcerations and nontraumatic foot amputations in diabetic patients, leading to significant morbidity. Distal symmetrical polyneuropathy is the most common form of neuropathy, which causes stocking—glove (distal to proximal) pattern of nerve damage.[1] Early in the course of the disease, patients feel symmetrical burning pain and tingling sensation, typically worse at night. Later, patients develop distal weakness.[2]

Apart from the complex biochemical pathways involved in the pathogenesis of diabetic peripheral neuropathy (DPN), recent studies have also given insight into the various genetic factors which lead to increased susceptibility to neuropathy. Understanding these genetic factors will help in prognosticating response to various treatment modalities as well as pave the way for other novel therapies.

PATHWAYS IMPLICATED IN DIABETIC NEUROPATHY

A complex myriad of biochemical pathways ultimately culminate in mitochondrial dysfunction leading to oxidative stress. Polyol pathway is the most studied pathway implicated in the pathogenesis. Conversion of excess glucose to sorbitol via the enzyme aldose reductase (ALR) leads to the depletion of intracellular myoinositol and nicotinamide adenine dinucleotide phosphate hydrogen, predisposing cells to oxidative stress.[3] Shunting of glycolytic intermediates due to excess glucose into the hexosamine pathway leads to inflammation and cellular damage in peripheral nerves.[4] Similarly, accumulation of diacylglycerol leads to activation of neuronal protein kinase C which produces vasoconstriction and neuronal hypoxia.[5]

Binding of advanced glycation end products (AGEs) to receptor AGE (RAGE) activates a cascade of events which leads to altered vascular permeability and increased procoagulant activity in the neurons.[6] Latest emerging concept is that diabetic neuropathy is a disorder of defective energy transfer in the oxidative phosphorylation pathway. This results in decreased adenosine triphosphate production and increased reactive oxygen species production leading to neuronal dysfunction.[7]

PATHOGENESIS OF PAINFUL DIABETIC NEUROPATHY

Neuronal hyperexcitability of the sensory neurons leads to increased sensitivity to the thermal and mechanical stimuli in patients with painful diabetic neuropathy.

Dysfunction of the voltage-gated sodium channels (VGSCs), which are important for the generation of the action potential in dorsal root sensory neurons has been implicated in the pathogenesis of pain in diabetic neuropathy. Voltage-gated sodium (Nav) 1.7, 1.8, and 1.9 are the most abundant α subunits of VGSCs of which Nav 1.8 has been shown to be the major contributor to the generation of action potential.[8] Recently, TRPA1 (transient receptor potential ankyrin 1)[9] and voltage-gated calcium (Cav) 3.2 T-type Ca^{2+} channels[10] have also shown to be important in the pathogenesis of pain-related hypersensitivity in diabetic neuropathy. Methylglyoxal, a highly reactive metabolite, is increased in diabetes and causes posttranslational modification of ion channels. This leads to nociceptor hyperexcitability.[10]

INTERPLAY OF GENETIC FACTORS

It is intriguing as to why some patients with diabetes develop neuropathy, while some do not. A study showed a heritable component to diabetic neuropathy as 56% of the patients had a family history of neuropathy.[11] In the past few decades, genome-wide profiling based on microarrays has provided an insight into the transcriptome changes in human peripheral nerves affected by diabetes. Over 500 genes with differential expression have been identified based on profiling of transcriptome of sural nerve biopsies.[12]

Specific polymorphisms within the *ACE, APOE, AKR1B1, NOS3, NF-κB, TLR2, TLR4*, and *SREBP-1* genes are associated with diabetic neuropathy. Basically the genes implicated are important in immune response, lipid metabolism, adipokine signaling and adipogenesis which suggest that an interaction between glucotoxicity and dyslipidemia might lead to the onset and progression of diabetic neuropathy.[13]

Angiotensin-converting enzyme (ACE) encoded by *ACE* gene converts angiotensin I to angiotensin II which has been implicated in endothelial dysfunction and oxidative stress. ACE I/D (insertion/deletion) polymorphism of a 287-base pair Alu sequence in intron 16 of the *ACE* gene has been associated with diabetic neuropathy.[14] D allele has been shown to be a risk factor for diabetic neuropathy, while I/I genotype is protective. Variation in the ACE I/D can also affect the therapeutic efficacy to ACE inhibitors and angiotensin receptor blockers used to treat diabetic complications.[14]

In a study done in North Indian population, ALR nucleotide C(-106)T polymorphism was shown to be associated with a higher-risk of peripheral neuropathy in type 2 diabetes.[15] This variant can lead to more rapid and severe neuropathological deterioration in the sural nerve.

Polymorphism in apolipoprotein E (Apo E) which has an important role in lipid metabolism has been implicated in diabetic neuropathy. Apo E4 allele may be associated with an increased risk, while APO E2 allele may be protective.[16] Two genes, namely *SCN9A* (sodium channel gene) and *OPRM1* (opioid receptor gene), have been reported to be associated with increased risk of painful diabetic neuropathy.[17]

TREATMENT OF PAINFUL DIABETIC NEUROPATHY

Painful diabetic neuropathy places a significant economic burden on patients due to poor quality of life. The pain can be distressing and discomforting to the patient. Optimal glycemic control is of paramount importance in the management of any diabetic microvascular complication. This can ameliorate the progression of neuropathy.

Various drugs such as antidepressants (amitriptyline, desipramine, duloxetine, and venlafaxine), anticonvulsants (pregabalin, sodium valproate) and Capsaicin cream have been used in the past for the treatment of painful diabetic neuropathy. Lidocaine patch, α-lipoic acid, isosorbide dinitrate topical spray, acetyl-L-carnitine and nonsteroidal anti-inflammatory drugs are some of the other treatment modalities that have been tried with uncertain results. Transcutaneous electric nerve stimulation and even spinal cord stimulation using implantable electrodes to stimulate dorsal columns of the spinal cord have been used to ameliorate the pain associated with neuropathy in refractory cases. Sometimes there may be spontaneous resolution of pain in patients with painful diabetic neuropathy.[18]

NOVEL THERAPIES FOR PAINFUL DIABETIC NEUROPATHY

The limitation of the conventional therapies used for the treatment of painful diabetic neuropathy is that none of the treatment options is disease-modifying. However, recent advances in genome-wide profiling could lead to a more individualized treatment approach, based on the genotype of the patient.

Selective blockers of VGSCs (Na_v 1.7, 1.8, and 1.9) are in research phase for their possible use in painful diabetic neuropathy. These drugs offer an exciting prospect in their ability to be disease-modifying agents as dysfunction of these ion channels leads to axonal degeneration.[19] If these drugs could lead to sural nerve regeneration during the course of the disease, it would be a game changer in the treatment of neuropathy. Further experimental research is needed to validate the hypothesis.

Similarly, plausible mechanism in the pathogenesis of DPN could be a target of intervention. ALR overexpression in individuals due to gene and gene environment interactions might render them more prone to develop DPN. If such an alteration is identifiable, it may be an option for therapeutic target to diminish the level of ALR production. With the help of proteomics, patients with risk of having DPN could be identified, and personalized medicine would be possible for them.

Another ray of hope is from transient receptor potential channels A (TRPA1) antagonists that was shown to reduce pain-related hypersensitivity in rat models. Trials are currently underway for their applicability in humans.[20]

We hope that genomics and proteomics will be the future of treating disease, which is currently having ineffective treatment options, as is the challenge for DPN.

CONCLUSION

The pathogenesis of diabetic neuropathy has undergone a paradigm shift from being focused on single biochemical pathways to a more genetic centric approach. An individualized treatment approach based on the patient's phenotype and genotype could be a reality in future. Development of disease-modifying drugs, which could prevent axonal degeneration, could be a revolutionary step in the management of painful diabetic neuropathy. The idea that axonal regeneration can occur in the course of diabetic neuropathy can soon become a reality.

REFERENCES

1. Tesfaye S, Boulton AJ, Dyck PJ, et al. Diabetic neuropathies: update on definitions, diagnostic criteria, estimation of severity, and treatments. Diabetes Care. 2010;33(10):2285-93.
2. Finnerup NB, Attal N, Haroutounian S, et al. Pharmacotherapy for neuropathic pain in adults: a systematic review and meta-analysis. Lancet Neurol. 2015;14(2):162-73.
3. Oates PJ. Aldose reductase, still a compelling target for diabetic neuropathy. Curr Drug Targets. 2008;9:14.
4. Brownlee M. Biochemistry & molecular cell biology of diabetic complications. Nature. 2001;414:813.
5. Das Evcimen N, King GL. The role of protein kinase C activation and the vascular complications of diabetes. Pharmacol Res. 2007;55:498.
6. Thornally PJ. Glycation in diabetic neuropathy: characteristics, consequences, causes, and therapeutic options. Int Rev Neurobiol. 2002; 50:37.
7. Vincent AM, Callaghan BC, Smith AL, et al. Diabetic neuropathy: cellular mechanisms as therapeutic targets. Nat Rev Neurol. 2011;7:573-83.
8. Blair NT, Bean BP. Roles of tetrodotoxin (TTX)-sensitive Na^+ current, TTX-resistant Na^+ current, and Ca^{2+} current in the action potentials of nociceptive sensory neurons. J Neurosci. 2002;22:10277-90.
9. Andersson DA, Gentry C, Moss S, et al. Transient receptor potential A1 is a sensory receptor for multiple products of oxidative stress. J Neurosci. 2008;28:2485-94.
10. Messinger RB, Naik AK, Jagodic MM, et al. In vivo silencing of the Ca(V)3.2 T-type calcium channels in sensory neurons alleviates hyperalgesia in rats with streptozocin-induced diabetic neuropathy. Pain. 2009;145:184-95.
11. Galer BS, Gianas A, Jensen MP. Painful diabetic polyneuropathy: epidemiology, pain description, and quality of life. Diabetes Res Clin Pract. 2000;47:123-8.
12. Hur J, Sullivan KA, Pande M, et al. The identification of gene expression profiles associated with progression of human diabetic neuropathy. Brain. 2011;134:3222-35.
13. Witzel II, Jelinek HF, Khalaf K, et al. Identifying common genetic risk factors of diabetic neuropathies. Front Endocrinol. 2015;6:88.
14. Li Y, Tong N. Angiotensin-converting enzyme I/D polymorphism and diabetic peripheral neuropathy in type 2 diabetes mellitus: a meta-analysis. J Renin Angiotensin Aldosterone Syst. 2015;16(4):787-92.
15. Gupta B, Singh SK. Association of aldose reductase gene polymorphism (C-106T) in susceptibility of diabetic peripheral neuropathy among north Indian population. J Diabetes Complications. 2017;31(7):1085-9.
16. Monastiriotis C, Papanas N, Veletza S, et al. APOE gene polymorphisms and diabetic peripheral neuropathy. Arch Med Sci. 2012;8(4):583-8.
17. Li QS, Cheng P, Favis R, et al. SCN9A variants may be implicated in neuropathic pain associated with diabetic peripheral neuropathy and pain severity. Clin J Pain. 2015;31:976-82.
18. Griebeler ML, Morey-Vargas OL, Brito JP, et al. Pharmacologic interventions for painful diabetic neuropathy: an umbrella systematic review & comparative effectiveness network meta-analysis. Ann Intern Med. 2014;161:639.
19. Han C, Huang J, Waxman SG. Sodium channel Nav1.8: emerging links to human disease. Neurology. 2016;86:473-83.
20. O'Brien PD, Sakowski SA, Feldman EL. Mouse models of diabetic neuropathy. ILAR J. 2014;54:259-72.

Chapter 41

Silent Coronary Artery Disease in Diabetes Mellitus: How Far to Investigate?

Ashok K Taneja, Harpreet Pasricha

INTRODUCTION

Cardiovascular disease (CVD) in type 2 diabetes mellitus (T2DM) is the leading cause of morbidity and mortality and accounts for large fraction of death index. T2DM is recognized as a stronger risk factor for silent ischemia and infarction. Among patients of T2DM the 7 years risk of developing a first myocardial infarction (MI) is 10-folds and akin to recurrent MI in normal persons who had a previous MI.[1] The prevalence of coronary artery disease (CAD), especially the multivessel CAD is 10 times greater amongst diabetics than age-sex matched nondiabetic persons. The reason, thereof, is the fact that T2DM is considered as an accelerated atherosclerosis state and poses a considerable risk for development of cardiovascular (CV) metabolic disease. Large studies confirmed that a glycemic control with hemoglobin A1c (HbA1c) of 7% resulted in approximately 50% reduction in incidence of CVD.[2] With further tight control, the risk reduction may further be expected. Hence, a comprehensive approach that recognizes and controls multiple risk factors is the most effective management strategy in diabetics.

Many associations, the world over, suggested that a risk factor guided screening protocol be developed to identify such diabetic persons who are having asymptomatic CAD. Because delayed identification of CAD in such patients unquestionably worsens their prognoses. Thus, there should be a clear need to identify T2DM patients who are at risk for CV events before the onset of symptoms. Unfortunately, the protocols used for screening patients with T2DM for asymptomatic coronary atherosclerosis remains debatable.

Prevalence of silent ischemia or significant CV event varies widely due to different parameters used by different investigators. Framingham study, initiated in 1948, also calculated the CV risk in asymptomatic diabetic individuals and found that at least 25% of diabetic individuals (followed for 30 years) had MIs, previously having normal electrocardiogram (ECG). Hence, the various protocols used have serious limitations. American Diabetes Association (ADA) (2008) and American Endocrine Society (2010) proposed a screening module based on age, gender, hypertension and dyslipidemia for early detection of CAD in T2DM patients.[3] However, subsequent studies have shown that the traditional risk factors do not accurately predict the risk for CV events in T2DM patients.[3] This led to the developing a rationale module for an aggressive screening approach for CAD in asymptomatic patients with T2DM, independent of other risk factors. Nevertheless, there is no uniform policy regarding CAD screening in patients with T2DM, reflecting the statistical challenges of screening patients at low risk and the decisions to be made per se.

In November 2013, the American College of Cardiology (ACC) and American Heart Association (AHA) released new guidelines on assessment of CV risk based on a new tool, the race- and sex-specific pooled cohort equations. These are comprehensive multivariable, multiethnic population (age 40–70 years) based risk analysis equations to predict 10-year CV risk. In these calculations, 10-year risk is defined as the risk of developing a first atherosclerotic CVD event (nonfatal or fatal MI and nonfatal or fatal stroke) over a 10-year period amongst people not having any previous CVD.[4,5] Indian guidelines are also not evaluated or updated any protocol. Individuals, however one can develop his/her own protocol. Suggested guidelines are discussed here in this chapter.

PROPOSED METHODOLOGY

Many protocols are in vogue, but the most useful and practical is the one which is easy to implement, easy to analyze and cost-effective. Following are the various parameters being used:

Clinical Evaluation

A detailed history and complete general physical examination (including weight, height and waist circumference) will be performed for each subject following which they will be investigated for routine investigations (hemoglobin, total and differential leucocyte count, erythrocyte sedimentation rate, fasting and postprandial blood sugar, fasting serum lipid profile, blood urea, serum creatinine, serum bilirubin and serum liver enzymes, urine routine and microscopy and ECG).

Risk Factor Assessment

- *Age:* 40–79 years; but in India, we should consider 35–75 years of age
- *Gender:* Higher male preponderance. After menopause male: female ratio is equal
- Smoking/tobacco/alcohol/other addictions
- *Body mass index:* Obesity as indicated by body mass index (BMI) >27 kg/m^2
- *Waist circumference:* Central obesity as indicated by waist circumference (WC) >90 cm in males and >80 cm in females
- *Blood pressure:* Routine check and 24 hours ambulatory blood pressure monitoring (ABPM). Hypertension evidenced by blood pressure (BP) ≥140/90 mm Hg. Intense lowering of BP to <130 mm may not be required. As per ACCORD Trial (Action to Control Cardiovascular Risk in Diabetes) trial, the reduction of systolic BP to 120 mm Hg instead of 140 mm Hg, did not yield any further benefit in CV outcome. The ADVANCE Trial (Action in Diabetes and Vascular Disease: Preterax and Diamicron MR Controlled Evaluation) trial also indicated that intense lowering of glycemia with adequate control of BP reduced the risk of CV events[6]
- *Fasting serum lipid profile:* Hypercholesterolemia ≥200 mg/dL, hypertriglyceridemia ≥150 mg/dL, high low-density lipoprotein (LDL) cholesterol ≥100 mg/dL and low high-density lipoprotein (HDL) cholesterol <40 mg/dL in males and <50 mg/dL in females. In the lipid arm of the ACCORD trial, the control of dyslipidemia along with HbA1c to <7.0 was associated with reduction in CV events. Hence, it is very important to measure the lipid levels and control it by lifestyle change and medication[7]
- *Electrocardiogram:* Abnormalities of ischemia/infarction/left ventricular hypertrophy. Also look for pathological Q waves, left bundle block (in men), trifascicular block or deep T inversion. Framingham study evidenced very clearly that over a follow-up period of 30 years, with the baseline ECG normal, the chances of getting CV events is reduced to almost 25%, by controlling lipids and glycemic parameters[1]
- *Echocardiography:* Evidence of regional wall motion abnormality (in all 16 segments), diastolic dysfunction, or low ejection fraction. Routine calculation of left atrial (LA) volumes [suggestive of diastolic dysfunction (DDF)] and Tei index should be encouraged among the investigators. Strain rate imaging is very useful echo mode to evaluate myocardial functioning. The high sensitivity of both tissue Doppler imaging (TDI)-derived and two dimensional (2D) speckle tracking derived strain and strain rate are good for the early detection of myocardial dysfunction[8]
- *Stress testing-treadmill test (TMT):* ST segment variation, heart rate (HR) and BP response to exercise and origin of ventricular arrhythmias (Grade III and above)
- *Stress/Dobutamine echocardiography:* Look for evidence of stress induced hyperkinesia (assess all 16 segments); newer regurgitation in mitral or aortic valve or area of dyskinesia. Calculate E:A ratio or LA volumes (s/o diastolic dysfunction) in pre-exercise and postexercise phase. It is a good marker of ischemia if DDF appears afresh or increases in postexercise phase[9]
- *Serum homocysteine levels:* Suggest the high likelihood prevalence of CV events in future. Exact usefulness unclear
- High-sensitivity cardiac troponin T (hs-cTnT) and amino-terminal probrain natriuretic peptide (NT-proBNP) are useful in indicating to detect cardiac injury or failure. But the sensitivity and specificity of these tests to detect silent myocardial ischemia in T2DM is unknown at present
- *Carotid intima-media thickness (CIMT):* The CIMT test is a measure used to diagnose the extent of carotid

atherosclerotic vascular disease. The test measures the thickness of the inner two layers of the carotid artery the intima and media when patients are still asymptomatic. Early detection may indicate the need for a more aggressive approach for managing the risk factors associated with heart disease and stroke[8,9]

- *Calcium scoring on cardiac computed tomography:* Since the calcium is a marker of CAD, the amount of calcium detected on a cardiac computed tomography (CT) scan is a helpful diagnostic and prognostic tool. The findings on cardiac CT are expressed as a calcium score as it calculates the amount of calcium in atherosclerotic plaque which gives a clue to the extent of atherosclerosis in coronaries in asymptomatic individual[7,8]
- *Gadolinium enhanced cardiac magnetic resonance imaging:* Cardiac magnetic resonance (CMR) study with images on LV long and short axis should be performed wherever possible. Gadolinium enhanced circumferential resection margin (CRM) yields better results. Analyzing endocardial and epicardial contours drawn on longitudinal and short axis of all chambers, peak global longitudinal strain, systolic strain rate and early and late diastolic strain rates provide useful information on the presence of silent myocardial ischemia[10]
- Prevalence of metabolic syndrome as determined by the National Cholesterol Education Program Expert Panel (NCEP) Adult Treatment Panel III (ATP III) criteria (with South Asian cut-offs)
- Atherosclerotic cardiovascular disease (ASCVD) risk score (American College of Cardiology) charts.

CONCLUSION

The prevalence of silent MI is found to be 17% on detailed evaluation in diabetics. Earlier the detection, earlier the management and better the good results in reducing CV events. We should adopt an approach which should be clinical (clinical evaluation) and investigational. Combining the two with an economical protocol (India) shall yield good results. Practically clinical examination, ECG, echocardiography, stress testing and CIMT should give us a clear picture. For more clarity one can add calcium scoring strain imaging (echo) and NT-proBNP.

REFERENCES

1. Kannel WB, Abbott RD. Incidence and prognosis of unrecognized myocardial infarction. An update on the Framingham study. N Eng J Med. 1984;311:1144-7.
2. Prevalence of unrecognized silent myocardial ischemia and its association with atherosclerotic risk factors in noninsulin-dependent diabetes mellitus Milan Study on Atherosclerosis and Diabetes (MiSAD) Group. Am J Cardiol. 1997;79:134-9.
3. Wackers FJ, Young LH, Inzucchi SE, et al. Detection of silent myocardial ischemia in asymptomatic diabetic subjects: the DIAD study. Diabetes Care. 2004;27:1954-61.
4. Faerman I, Faccio E, Milei J, et al. Autonomic neuropathy and painless myocardial infarction in diabetic patients. Histologic evidence of their relationship. Diabetes. 1977;26:1147-58.
5. Ambepityia G, Kopelman PG, Ingram D, et al. Exertional myocardial ischemia in diabetes: a quantitative analysis of anginal perceptual threshold and the influence of autonomic function. J Am Coll Cardiol. 1990;15:72-7.
6. Langer A, Freeman MR, Josse RG, et al. Metaiodobenzylguanidine imaging in diabetes mellitus: assessment of cardiac sympathetic denervation and its relation to autonomic dysfunction and silent myocardial ischemia. J Am Coll Cardiol. 1995;25:610-8.
7. Gottlieb SO, Gottlieb SH, Achuff SC, et al. Silent Ischemia on Holter monitoring predicts mortality in high-risk postinfarction patients. JAMA. 1988;259(7):1030-5.
8. Young LH, Wackers FJ, Chyun DA, et al. Cardiac outcomes after screening for asymptomatic coronary artery disease in patients with type 2 diabetes: the DIAD study: a randomized controlled trial. JAMA. 2009;301(15):1547-55.
9. Frye RL, August P, Brooks MM, et al. A randomized trial of therapies for type 2 diabetes and coronary artery disease. N Eng J Med. 2009;360:2503-15.
10. American Diabetes Association. Standards of medical care in diabetes—2011. Diabetes Care. 2011;34(Suppl 1):S11-61.

Chapter 42

Etiopathogenesis and Management of Diabetic Heart Failure

Dheeraj Kapoor, Ranjana Bhatt

INTRODUCTION

Diabetes and heart failure (HF) are among the most frequently seen diseases in practice today. The risk ratio of HF in a progressive disease like diabetes is twice more in contrast to the nondiabetic population.[1,2] HF is subdivided into two major categories, one with preserved ejection fraction (EF) and the other with reduced EF, where both the subdivisions are seen in the diabetic population. However, the morbidity and mortality in cases of diabetic HF is far more than HF in nondiabetic population. It has been observed that contribution to the occurrence of congestive HF is partially seen as a direct effect from diabetes and the rest from the various comorbidities seen onboard with hyperglycemia, which are considered as individual risk factors for HF like hypertension, lipid disorders, kidney disease, overweight/obesity, sleep disorder, aging and coexisting cardiovascular diseases. Considering the bidirectional relationship predisposition to a state of insulin resistance in the cases of HF is supported by the CHARM program in the United States adult subgroup (Candesartan Heart Failure Assessment of Reduction in Mortality and Morbidity Program),[3] where the presence of newly diagnosed cases of diabetes was significant in the follow-up years. The DIAMOND (Danish Investigations of Arrhythmia and Mortality on Dofetilide) study, Survival and Ventricular Enlargement trial and Valsartan in Acute Myocardial Infarction Trial—all showed significant increase in mortality in the case of HF in diabetic population as compared to the nondiabetic subgroup.[4,5] Considering the two diseases, diabetes and HF separately, HF is a much more serious condition management of which among diabetic population is all the more challenging and difficult, resulting in poor outcomes and mortality. Thus the early identification of signs and symptoms, followed by a quick prioritized multidisciplinary approach, is required in the cases of congestive HF for stabilization.

ETIOPATHOGENESIS

Numerous alteration in the structure and function of cardiac musculature contributed by the defective metabolism of energy substrates is one of the prime mechanisms resulting in myocardial dysfunction. Excess of cardiac glucose in the setting of decreased insulin or insulin resistance shifts the metabolism of glucose to oxidation of free fatty acid (FFA), which results in the accumulation of various by-products of lipid. It is believed that these lipid fragments activate protein kinase C and NF-κB that further hampers the signaling of insulin molecule.[6] Raised fatty acid levels suppress the various glucose metabolism pathways like uptake of glucose, glycolysis and pyruvate oxidation in mitochondria via inhibition of various glucose transporters (GLUT 1 and GLUT 4). The adenosine triphosphate is a basic source of energy for functioning myocardium, which is generated ineffectively by FFA oxidation. High levels of fatty acids and glucose stimulate the tricarboxylic acid (TCA) cycle to provide electrons as power donor to the respiratory chain; however, inadequate need of such high energy creates a supersaturated state where these electrons leak out and under extreme oxidative stress form reactive oxygen species, which are the culprit molecules for cardiac fibrosis and all the diabetic complications.[7,8] The activation of sympathetic nervous system and accumulation of advance glycosylated end products further compromise the cardiac functioning.[9]

Role of other associated comorbidities with their pathophysiology:

- *Coronary heart disease (CHD)*: Mortality from CHD is commonly seen in diabetic population. Atherosclerosis progression to diffuse, multivessel disease with marked ischemia and calcification is the underlying pathology
- *Diabetic cardiomyopathy*: Defective signaling of calcium-associated proteins leads to decrease availability of calcium in the sarcolemma with progressive myocardial thickening, fibrosis and microvascular changes contributing to dysfunction in systolic motion of the heart[10]
- *Hypertension*: Activation of the renin–angiotensin system causes cardiac remodeling and hence, adequate suppression of renin–angiotensin–aldosterone system and blood pressure control is a priority in HF management[11]
- *Chronic kidney disease (CKD)*: Nephropathy and microalbuminuria act as a strong marker for HF and progression to cardiorenal syndrome[12]
- *Anemia*: Anemia can be seen as a part of CKD profile due to decreased red blood cell lifespan, deficiency of erythropoietin or iron deficiency, more frequently seen in a diabetic renal disease than other renal diseases.[13] Adverse impact of anemia is seen as multiple target organ damage due to deficient oxygenation and associated compensatory tachycardia, ventricular hypertrophy and volume overload state contributing either to worsening of previously compromised cardiac function as in cases of cardiomyopathy or manifest as new onset congestive cardiac failure[14]
- *Obesity*: Higher the body mass index higher is the risk. Deposition of excess fat in viscera alters the mobilization of fats and through the release of various cytokines with proinflammatory action and activation of neural pathways causes ventricular remodeling and cardiac dysfunction[15]
- *Oral diabetic drugs*: The thiazolidinediones group causes retention of fluid with enhanced absorption of sodium[16] and is hence contraindicated in patients of NYHA class III/IV.[17] Dipeptidyl peptidase-4 inhibitors except sitagliptin also aggravate the pumping inability of myocardium and so are another group of drugs to be cautiously used in cases with left ventricular (LV) dysfunction.[18] Increased possibility of hypoglycemic episodes with sulfonylurea has its own detrimental effect in HF patients and thus should be used under careful monitoring.

MANAGEMENT

Basic approach involves a two-step process with immediate management of HF in the diabetic subgroup, followed by standardized glycemic control in such patients using agents that are helpful in maintaining the cardiovascular safety profile.

- Heart failure treatment in diabetic subgroup includes three major groups of drugs—β-blockers, angiotensin-converting enzyme (ACE) inhibitors and mineralocorticoid receptor antagonists in various combinations
  - *Beta-blockers:* It has been observed that the use of selective β-blockers with nonvasodilation properties results in the resistance of insulin by alteration in perfusion of the skeletal muscle. However, the nonselective, vasodilating drugs like carvedilol, due to their insulin-sensitizing effect improve glycemic control, lipid derangement and risk of albuminuria.[19] β-blockers show significant results when used with diuretics and in patients with systolic HF
  - *Angiotensin-converting enzyme inhibitors and angiotensin receptor blockers (ARBs):* Significant increase of survival in HF patients with diabetes is seen with the use of ACE inhibitors and ARBs, as explained by some animal trials possibly due to the enhancement in insulin sensitivity as the blood flow to the peripheral tissues is restored in lieu of decreased angiotensin II levels and raised bradykinin.[20,21]
  - *Aldosterone receptor antagonists:* Spironolactone is a nonselective, while eplerenone is a selective aldosterone receptor antagonist used in cases where nonsignificant improvement occurs after β-blockers and ACE/ARBs.[22] In view of coexisting nephropathy being commonly associated in cases of diabetes and HF, careful monitoring of serum potassium levels is a must
  - *Cardiac resynchronization therapy (CRT):* Patients nonresponding to the abovementioned medical treatment, who have poor ventricular functioning along with prolonged quick response system duration, should be managed with CRT
- *Diabetes management in HF*: The target glycemic control should be 7% HbA1c and more lenient in critical cases as strict control of 6–6.5% HbA1c is associated with adverse outcomes as seen in ACCORD, ADVANCE, UKPDS and VADT trials
  - *Lifestyle modification*: Optimal dietary control, acceptable levels of exercise and regular blood

sugar monitoring are the cornerstone measures in the management of diabetes

- *Biguanides*: Metformin being the first-line drug is used as an insulin-sensitizing agent in combination with other oral hypoglycemic agents or along with insulin, except in cases of acute decompensated HF and renal insufficiency, to avoid risk of lactic acidosis
- *Insulin*: Insulin as infusion, premixed, or basal bolus regimen in the form of monotherapy or in combination with oral antidiabetic drugs is widely accepted and preferred therapy for glycemic control
- *Sodium-glucose cotransporter-2 inhibitors*: Drugs of this group play a significant role in diabetic cases with reduced EF in offloading excess of fluid and sugar through urine with optimal glycemic control, as seen in the EMPA-REG OUTCOME Trial where the drug empagliflozin was used[23]
- *Sulfonylureas*: It can be used in stable cases of HF with special caution to avoid episodes of hypoglycemia
- *Dipeptidyl peptidase-4 inhibitors*: Stabilized patients can be managed with sitagliptin Trial Evaluating Cardiovascular Outcomes with Sitagliptin trial; however, safety of other drugs of this group in patients with poor LV function is not yet achieved.

CONCLUSION

All diabetic patients should be screened regularly for their cardiac functional status, and adequate optimization in the management of diabetes should be done accordingly as once established the prognosis of HF is much poorer in diabetics than the nondiabetic population.

REFERENCES

1. Kannel WB, Hjortland M, Castelli WP. Role of diabetes in congestive heart failure: the Framingham study. Am J Cardiol. 1974;34(1):29-34.
2. Dei Cas A, Khan SS, Butler J, et al. Impact of diabetes on epidemiology, treatment, and outcomes of patients with heart failure. JACC Heart Fail. 2015;3(2):136-45.
3. Preiss D, Zetterstrand S, McMurray JJ, et al. Predictors of development of diabetes in patients with chronic heart failure in the Candesartan in Heart Failure Assessment of Reduction in Mortality and Morbidity (CHARM) program. Diabetes Care. 2009;32:915-20.
4. Gustafsson I, Brendorp B, Seibaek M, et al. Influence of diabetes and diabetes-gender interaction on the risk of death in patients hospitalized with congestive heart failure. Danish Investigation of Arrhythmia and Mortality on Dofetilde StudyGroup. J Am Coll Cardiol. 2004;43(5):771-7.
5. Aguilar D, Solomon SD, Køber L, et al. Newly diagnosed and previously known diabetes mellitus and 1-year outcomes of acute myocardial infarction: the VALsartan In Acute myocardial iNfarcTion (VALIANT) trial. Circulation. 2004;110(12):1572-8. Epub 2004 Sep 13.
6. Fink BD, Bai F, Yu L, et al. Impaired utilization of membrane potential by complex II-energized mitochondria of obese, diabetic mice assessed using ADP recycling methodology. Am J Physiol Regul Integr Comp Physiol. 2016;311(4):R756-63.
7. Giacco M. Brownlee oxidative stress and diabetic complications. Circ Res. 2010;107:1058-70.
8. Sverdlov AL, Elezaby A, Qin F, et al. Mitochondrial reactive oxygen species mediate cardiac structural, functional, and mitochondrial consequences of diet-induced metabolic heart disease. J Am Heart Assoc. 2016; 5(1): pii: e002555.
9. Doehner W, Frenneaux M, Anker SD. Metabolic impairment in heart failure: the myocardial and systemic perspective. J Am Coll Cardiol. 2014;64: 1388-400.
10. Bugger H, Abel ED. Molecular mechanisms of diabetic cardiomyopathy. Diabetologia. 2014;57(4):660-71.
11. Mandavia CH, Aroor AR, Demarco VG, et al. Molecular and metabolic mechanisms of cardiac dysfunction in diabetes. Life Sci. 2013;92(11): 601-8.
12. Emdin CA, Rahimi K, Neal B, et al. Blood pressure lowering in type 2 diabetes: a systematic review and meta-analysis. JAMA. 2015;313(6): 603-15.
13. Hockensmith ML, Estacio RO, Mehler P, et al. Albuminuria as a predictor of heart failure hospitalizations in patients with type 2 diabetes. J Card Fail. 2004;10(2):126-31.
14. Bosman DR, Winkler AS, Marsden JT, et al. Anemia with erythropoietin deficiency occurs early in diabetic nephropathy. Diabetes Care. 2001;24(3): 495-9.
15. Anand I, McMurray JJ, Whitmore J, et al. Anemia and its relationship to clinical outcome in heart failure. Circulation. 2004;110(2):149-54.
16. Guan Y, Hao C, Cha DR, et al. Thiazolidinediones expand body fluid volume through PPARgamma stimulation of ENaC-mediated renal salt absorption. Nat Med. 2005;11:861-6.
17. Kaul S, Bolger AF, Herrington D, et al. Thiazolidinedione drugs and cardiovascular risks: a science advisory from the American Heart Association and American College of Cardiology Foundation. J Am Coll Cardiol. 2010;55:1885-94.
18. Green JB, Bethel MA, Armstrong PW, et al. Effect of sitagliptin on cardiovascular outcomes in type 2 diabetes. N Engl J Med. 2015;373(3):232-42.
19. Haas SJ, Vos T, Gilbert RE, et al. Are beta-blockers as efficacious in patients with diabetes mellitus as in patients without diabetes mellitus who have chronic heart failure? A meta-analysis of large-scale clinical trials. Am Heart J. 2003;146:848-53.
20. Aguilar D, Solomon SD. ACE inhibitors and angiotensin receptor antagonists and the incidence of new-onset diabetes mellitus: an emerging theme. Drugs. 2006;66:1169-77.
21. Henriksen EJ, Jacob S, Kinnick TR, et al. ACE inhibition and glucose transport in insulin resistant muscle: roles of bradykinin and nitric oxide. Am J Physiol. 1999; 277(1 Pt 2):R332-6.
22. Pitt B, Remme W, Zannad F, et al. Eplerenone, a selective aldosterone blocker, in patients with left ventricular dysfunction after myocardial infarction. N Engl J Med. 2003;348:1309-21.
23. Zinman B, Wanner C, Lachin JM, et al. Empagliflozin, cardiovascular outcomes, and mortality in type 2 diabetes. N Engl J Med. 2015;373: 2117-28.

Chapter 43

Diabetes and Stroke

Prakash Keswani, Shrikant Sharma

INTRODUCTION

Diabetes has been a major cause of human suffering since ancient times. Its prevalence has been increasing exponentially for last two decades. It is considered a multisystem disease, and with increasing duration, diabetic patients are predisposed to develop a number of complications like dyslipidemia, hypertension, coronary artery disease, and cerebrovascular disease (stroke).

Diabetes per se is an important cause of stroke worldwide, but associated conditions further increase the risk and worsens the outcome.[1] Hypertension, dyslipidemia, and smoking are the chief modifiable risk factors for stroke, which is the cause of highest mortality in diabetics especially in women.[2]

EPIDEMIOLOGY

Diabetes mellitus has been found to increase the rate of development of stroke by two to four times, particularly in women. The different studies including UKPDS have documented the prevalence of diabetes in acute stroke patients in the range of 8 to 24%.[3,4] The Drug Information Association study from Italy conducted on unselected type 2 diabetes mellitus population, found that the age standardized incidence of stroke (per 1,000 person-years) was 5.5 in men and 6.3 in women with no previous history of cardiovascular disease. In persons with cardiovascular disease, this was as high as 13.7 in men and 10.8 in women. It is further seen that HbA1c, microvascular complications, low high-density lipoprotein (HDL) cholesterol, therapy for diabetes either insulin or oral hypoglycemic agents are associated with stroke occurrence and contribute to the rise in the prevalence.[5]

What is the Connection Between Diabetes and Stroke?

The interaction between diabetes and stroke is bidirectional. These are indeed two common diseases, arising together and having a close relationship. Both have some common risk factors, and lifestyle modifications are beneficial in the prevention of both. Diabetes leads to an increase in incidence of stroke and is also associated with poorer outcome of patients in stroke. This underlines the need of multifactorial treatment, so as to decrease incidence of these two diseases.

A systematic review and meta-analysis of 64 cohorts to assess diabetes as a risk factor in men and women found that the pooled maximum adjusted relative risk of stroke associated with diabetes was 2.28 [95% confidence interval (CI), 1.93–2.69] in women and 1.83 (1.60–2.08) in men. This was found to be independent of sex differences in other important cardiovascular risk factors. The Greater Cincinnati/Northern Kentucky Stroke Study states diabetes as the most important risk factor for ischemic stroke, especially in subjects less than 65 years.[6] Another study by Arvanitakis et al. observed that diabetes was associated with cerebral infarction but not Alzheimer's disease in older individuals.[7] A meta-analysis of records of diabetes, fasting blood glucose in people with no initial vascular disease was done by Sarwar et al. from 102 prospective studies.[8] It suggested a two fold excess risk for coronary artery disease, stroke and deaths attributed to vascular diseases in patients with type 2 diabetes mellitus. The hazard ratio for ischemic stroke was 2.27 and for hemorrhagic stroke was 1.56. Janghorbani et al. showed that both type 1 and type 2 diabetes are associated with increased risk of stroke in women. In 116,316 women studied, they found that women with type 1 disease showed a four-fold higher risk [relative risk 4.7 (95% CI, 3.3–6.6)] than women with type 2 disease [1.8 (1.7–2.0)] where risk was increased by two-fold. A stronger association was seen with type 1 diabetes mellitus due to young age, long duration, prolonged and increased insulin deficiency, and complications like hypertension, diabetic nephropathy, coagulation disorders, increased platelet aggregation and frequent episodes of hypoglycemia.[9]

Increased susceptibility for development of coronary, femoral, and cerebral artery atherosclerosis is seen in diabetics.[10] The Honolulu Heart Program Study observed the diabetes, to be associated with thromboembolic but not hemorrhagic stroke.[11] Studies on the recurrence after stroke implicate hypertension, diabetes mellitus and abnormal admission computed tomogram to increase the risk of stroke.[12] Stroke also causes alterations in metabolism of glucose, thus affecting recovery.

Epidemiology of Stroke and Diabetes in India

The crude prevalence rate of stroke in India is 471.58 per 100,000 subjects. In men, it was 495.91 per 100,000 and, in females, it was 444.43 per 100,000 (95% CI, 414.99–533.83).[13] In a study conducted by Das et al., the annual incidence of first stroke was 123.15 per 100,000 persons per year. In males, it was calculated to be 99.54/100,000, while in females it was 149.49/100,000 (95% CI, 102.46–232.50).[13] A community-based study to compare prevalence of neurological diseases in urban and rural population found annual incidence rate of stroke to be 148/100,000 persons per year (95% CI, 120–170).[14] The observations suggest that annual incidence rate in India is greater than that of Europe and North America.[15-19]

The prevalence of diabetes in Indian adults ranges from 10 to 15% and is on rising trend. Therefore complications arising because of diabetes are also likely to increase in Indian population. The stroke which is quite common a disease among Indians is expected to occur more frequently in Indian diabetic population.

PATHOPHYSIOLOGY

Diabetes increases both macrovascular and microvascular disease by causing vascular endothelial dysfunction, thereby leading to early onset stiffening of arteries, thickening of basement membrane of capillaries, and inflammation. These seem to be the chief mechanisms leading to stroke. Various mechanisms have been proposed in the pathogenesis of stroke in diabetes mellitus population. Multiple factors interplay in the pathogenesis of stroke in diabetes (Flowchart 1).

Hyperglycemia is associated with an increase in oxidative stress leading to vascular complications. There is an increased production of reactive oxygen species (ROS),due to the free radicals causing breakage of DNA strand, which in turn activates the DNA repair enzyme poly ADP-ribose polymerase, thereby inhibiting glycolysis by affecting the enzyme glyceraldehyde 3-phosphate

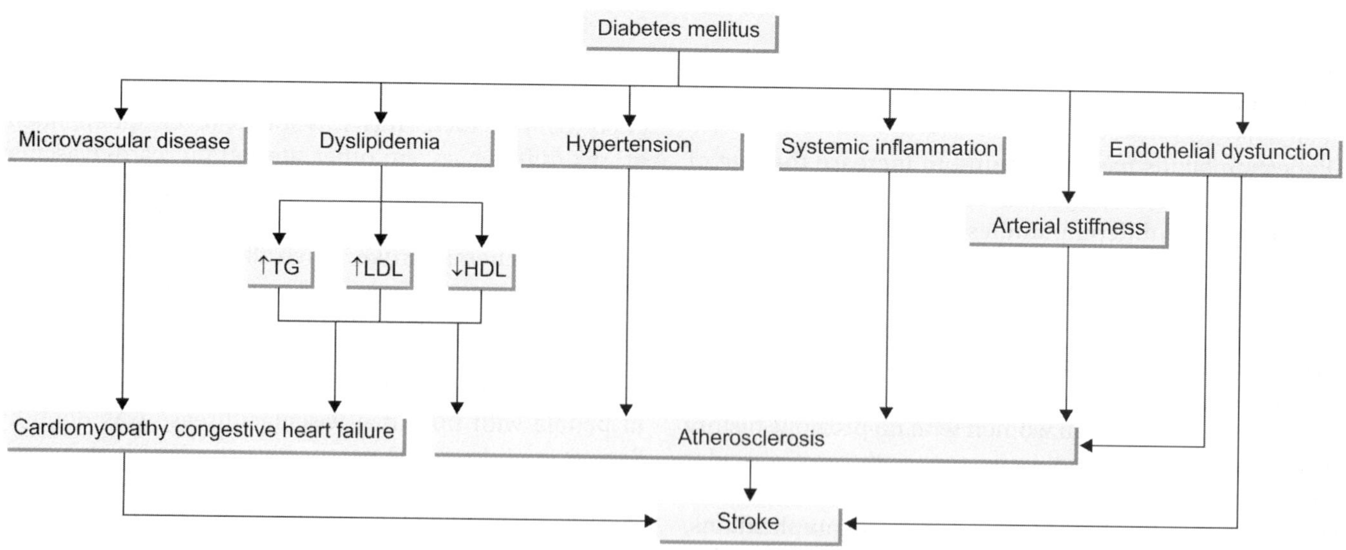

(LDL: low-density lipoprotein; HDL: high-density lipoprotein; TG: triglyceride.)

Flowchart 1 Pathogenesis of stroke in diabetes.

dehydrogenase. Thus intermediates in the glycolysis pathway are increased, which causes many chemical reactions contributing to endothelial dysfunction and diabetes-related microvascular disease. These include increased formation of advanced glycation end products (AGEs) along with increased expression of their receptors. Advanced glycation end products after binding to their receptors promote low-density lipoprotein uptake and oxidation thus increasing foam cell production. Glucose is diverted to aldose reductase pathway, and isozymes of protein kinase C are activated.[20-23] Polyol pathway flux, activation of protein kinase C isoforms, and excessive activation of hexosamine pathway take place leading to microvascular damage.

Diabetics have impairments in the nitric oxide (NO)–mediated vasodilation due to increased inactivation of NO. The response of smooth muscle to NO is also impaired. The tight junctions are weakened, and the expression of adhesion molecules is altered. Increased inflammation evidenced by markers like C-reactive protein, cytokines and adiponectin is common in diabetics. Due to all these factors, a procoagulant state develops. In addition, the platelets in diabetic patients are also prothrombotic, with increased aggregation. These along with basement membrane thickening cause atherosclerosis. Diabetes mellitus is also associated with increased intima-medial thickness, which is an early sign of atherosclerosis. These all changes along with basement membrane thickening cause atherosclerosis.

ROLE OF HYPERGLYCEMIA IN ACUTE STROKE

Hyperglycemia is seen in 30–40% of stroke patients with or without a previous history of diabetes. Possibly this occurs because of the release of stress hormones like cortisol and epinephrine, and stimulation of autonomic nervous system. Hyperglycemia is implicated in increasing the infarct size and worsening of damage. This may be due to disorders in coagulation and fibrinolytic pathways mediated by hyperglycemia, resulting in altered recanalization and decreased reperfusion.[24,25] Even short-term hyperglycemic spikes show an impact on endothelial dysfunction independent of long-term glycemic control.[26] Capes et al. found that the relative risk of mortality after an ischemic stroke in hyperglycemic subjects without prior diabetes at admission was 3.3 as compared to normoglycemics.[27] It was also observed that hyperglycemia leads to poorer outcome in thrombo-embolic stroke as compared to lacunar stroke. A study from Glasgow, United Kingdom, observed a higher plasma glucose in stroke had poorer prognosis, even after correcting for age, stroke subtype and severity.[28,29]

DIABETES MELLITUS AND ACUTE STROKE

The metabolic changes during acute stroke can be studied by magnetic resonance spectroscopy. High-energy phosphate metabolism and acidosis are implicated in neurological dysfunction and infarction. Due to disturbances in pH-dependent membrane transfer mechanisms, there is a deterioration of energy status in brain.[30,31] This stimulates the anaerobic glycolysis and accumulation of lactic acid leading to tissue acidosis.[32,33]

Blood and brain glucose levels affect the tissue acidosis. When brain receives uninterrupted glucose either due to reperfusion or incomplete ischemia, glycolysis is stimulated and metabolic acidosis is increased. Low glucose level decreases ischemic brain acidosis, thereby reducing infarction while hyperglycemia increases acidosis, which adversely affects recovery after neuronal ischemia. Pulsinelli also observed that neurologic outcome was poorer in diabetics as compared to nondiabetics.[34,35] The complications of diabetes are considered to have a causative role in poor outcome. In diabetics a proper collateral blood flow is not established, because of proliferative angiopathy of small cerebral blood vessels along with arteriosclerosis. In addition to this, the procoagulant state of diabetics, increased blood viscosity, impaired autoregulation of cerebral blood flow contribute to the worsening of infarct.

ROLE OF INSULIN RESISTANCE

Insulin resistance is an important factor for developing metabolic syndrome and atherosclerosis. Kernan et al. in their studies have implicated insulin resistance as a risk factor for stroke.[36] Insulin resistance in diabetics affects plasminogen activator inhibitor type 1, von Willebrand factor and fibrinogen. Insulin fails to suppress lipolysis activity causing excessive free fatty acid mobilization which enters various cells in the body. There is overproduction of ROS, along with dyslipidemia, which causes platelet aggregation.

ROLE OF DYSLIPIDEMIA

Dyslipidemia is twice as common in diabetics as in general population and is a major risk factor for cerebrovascular disease. Hyperinsulinemia affects apoprotein production by the liver and regulates lipoprotein lipase and cholesteryl ester transfer protein and causes lipid abnormalities. Diabetic dyslipidemia is characterized by low levels of HDL cholesterol, hypertriglyceridemia and postprandial rise in the levels of lipids. These accelerate the damage at the macrovascular level. In a study conducted in Japan, it was found that atherothrombotic occlusion of the internal carotid and basilar arteries were commoner in diabetics.[37] A multidisciplinary approach is needed for the correction of dyslipidemia in diabetics to prevent stroke. On the contrary, the UKPD Study did not find association of dyslipidemia and obesity with stroke in diabetics.[4]

ROLE OF HYPERTENSION

Diabetes and hypertension are independent risk factors to develop stroke. Hypertension leads to the development of both macro- and microvascular disease leading to stroke. A meta-analysis by Bangalore S reported a decrease in the risk of stroke by lowering blood pressure (BP) in patients with type 2 diabetes, impaired glucose tolerance, or impaired fasting glucose.[38] Presence of hypertension and diabetes have been found to be associated with rapid progression and poorer prognosis of patients with stroke.[39] There was a 17% reduction in stroke and 10% reduction in mortality due to all causes by lowering the BP intensively. The use of angiotensin-converting enzyme inhibitors decreases the risk of cardiovascular events in high-risk diabetics as evidenced by the Heart Outcomes Prevention Evaluation study.[40] Physicians should aim at a target systolic BP of 130–135 mm Hg.

METABOLIC SYNDROME AND STROKE

Metabolic syndrome comprises of hyperglycemia, hypertension, obesity and dyslipidemia, which are the risk factors of cardio and cerebrovascular disease. The Northern Manhattan Study found a statistically significant association between metabolic syndrome and ischemic stroke.[41] A prospective cohort study by Koren-Morag et al. found 2.29-fold increased odds of developing stroke in frank diabetes when seen in metabolic syndrome.[42] Metabolic syndrome is thought to be a proinflammatory condition showing increased levels of interleukin 6, C-reactive protein, and plasminogen activator and thus can lead to the development of stoke.

ATRIAL FIBRILLATION, HEART FAILURE AND STROKE

Patients with atrial fibrillation show an increased risk of developing ischemic stroke. The clinical predictive risk score, the CHA2DS2-VASc (congestive heart failure-1, hypertension-1, age >75 years-2, diabetes-1, stroke/TIA/thromboembolism-2, vascular disease-1, age 65–74 years-1, sex—female-1) score shows that diabetes is a risk factor to develop persistent atrial fibrillation and stroke.[43,44] A meta-analysis of case-control and cohort studies by Huxley RR studying the risk of atrial fibrillation in diabetes concluded that 25% of diabetes patients develop atrial fibrillation.[45] Another study to ascertain the effect of duration of diabetes on the risk of developing stroke in patients of the ATRIA cohort (Anticoagulation and Risk factors in Atrial Fibrillation) suggested that the risk increases with longer duration of diabetes.[46] The newer oral anticoagulants like rivaroxaban and apixaban have been helpful in preventing stroke in atrial fibrillation in both diabetic and nondiabetic population.[47]

Patients with heart failure and diabetes without atrial fibrillation showed a 27% increase in the relative risk of developing ischemic stroke. The CHA_2DS_2-VASc score was studied in subjects with heart failure without atrial fibrillation, and it was found that the risk of thromboembolic complications was higher in this group with heart failure.[48]

How Stroke is Different in Diabetes?

Uncontrolled diabetes shows an increase in the occurrence of both hemorrhagic and ischemic stroke, however, more so in ischemic stroke. Diabetes contributes to systemic and intracranial atherosclerosis and inflammation of the vessels leading to stroke. In diabetics, small vessel disease is more common than large vessel disease. A large multicentric study on diabetic European subjects observed that the frequency of intracerebral hemorrhage was lower, the rate of lacunar stroke was higher, the recovery of handicap was worse though mortality was not increased in diabetics.[49] Another study also showed that diabetics had lower relative prevalence of intracerebral hemorrhage and higher prevalence of subcortical infarction.[50] Lacunar strokes, characterized by noncortical infarcts of a single penetrating branch of a large cerebral artery, are the most common type of stroke in diabetics. Hypertension has been regarded as the most important risk factor for lacunar stroke; however, the association of diabetes mellitus with lacunar stroke is independent of hypertension. Diabetes mellitus patients with foot ulceration also have a worse cerebrovascular risk profile. Patients with diabetes have poorer prognosis and higher risk of death from stroke,[51] and diabetes is considered as a risk factor for death in stroke.

GLYCEMIC CONTROL DURING THE ACUTE PHASE OF STROKE

Hyperglycemia is a common clinical finding in stroke, irrespective of prior diabetes. Acute hyperglycemia leads to poorer outcome by increasing the size of the infarct, thereby increasing morbidity, prolonged hospitalization, delayed and poor functional recovery and mortality. Hyperglycemia by itself increases the risk of death at 90 days, 1 year and 6 years after stroke.

The American Heart Association/American Stroke Association guidelines for managing hyperglycemia in acute stroke are aimed at achieving a serum glucose concentration between 140 and 180 mg/dL in the first 24 hours.[52] European stroke initiative guidelines recommend insulin administration, if blood glucose level exceeds 180 mg/dL.[53] Subcutaneous insulin according to the sliding scale or intravenous glucose-insulin-potassium infusion is used commonly.[54] Several studies have observed an increased survival rate in patients, whose blood glucose was normalized gradually but within 48 hours.[55] The THIS (National Institute of Neurological Disorders funded Treatment of Hyperglycemia in Ischaemic Stroke) trial[56] and the GRASP (Glucose Regulation in Acute Stroke Patients) trial[57] label insulin therapy as a safe and effective treatment. However, the United Kingdom Glucose Insulin in Stroke Trial[54] did not observe significant difference in outcome with insulin therapy in stroke with mild-to-moderate hyperglycemia, rather the episodes of hypoglycemia were observed in 41% patients. The occurrence of hypoglycemia has been found to be associated with poorer outcome. The importance of glycemic management with oral therapy is less clear. Insulin during this period has not shown to improve results. Thus, gradual reduction of blood glucose levels with regular monitoring and keeping blood glucose levels to 140–180 mg% is advisable in acute phase of stroke.

LONG-TERM GLYCEMIC CONTROL

In type 1 and type 2 diabetes, good glycemic control over longer periods leads to decrease in microvascular complications. The DCCT/EDIC (Diabetes Control and Complications Trial, Epidemiology of Diabetes Interventions and Complications) study shows the reduction in cardiovascular complications and overall mortality risk and a small absolute risk reduction (1/1,000 patient years) in newly diagnosed type 1 diabetics.[58] A 10-year follow-up of intensive glucose control in type 2 diabetes mellitus by Holman et al. showed a reduction in microvascular complications (15%, $p = 0.01$), and overall mortality due to various causes (13%, $p = 0.007$) without showing any effect on stroke incidence.[59]

The ADVANCE (Action in Diabetes and Vascular Disease) and ACCORD (Action to Control Cardiovascular Risk in Diabetes) trials showed no benefit of prolonged glycemic control in stroke patients.[60,61] Moreover, the ACCORD trial was terminated due to increase in mortality rates in intensively treated patients.

Therefore, it can be inferred that strict glucose and HbA1c control should not be the sole aim in long-term treatment of stroke in diabetics. The role of HbA1c control in reduction of stroke is more in type 1 diabetes than type 2 diabetes. As shown in Box 1, individualized targets should be there for patients, according to their life expectancy, duration of disease and hyperglycemic status to maintain a balance between desired benefits and adverse effects.

Insulin therapy is still the mainstay of managing diabetes in patients with acute stroke. An advance in insulin delivery mechanisms and glucose monitoring reduces the risk of stroke in type 1 disease. The IRIS (Insulin Resistance Intervention after Stroke) trial showed that pioglitazone decreases incidence of stroke as compared to controls in insulin-resistant patients.[36] The management of hyperglycemia in stroke can be shifted from the traditional insulin infusion to metformin and

Box 1: American Diabetes Association guidelines for target HbA1c in various groups

HbA1c <6.5%
- Short duration
- Long life expectancy
- Diabetes controlled with lifestyle modification and metformin
- Absence of significant vascular or cardiovascular disease

HbA1c <8.0%
- History of severe hypoglycemia
- Long duration of diabetes
- Less life expectancy
- Presence of microvascular and macrovascular complications
- Presence of comorbidities

pioglitazone which are especially efficacious in insulin-resistant population. Glucagon-like peptide-1 analogs have been found to improve cardiovascular outcomes and cause weight and BP reduction (Liraglutide and Cardiovascular Outcomes in Type 2 diabetes trial).[62]

STROKE PREVENTION

Primary stroke prevention in diabetics involves control of blood glucose levels between 70 and 120 mg/dL before meals, and not >180 mg/dL after meals (intensive diabetes therapy—DCCT).[58] More stringent goals are applied to relatively young patients with no underlying complications, whereas less intensive goals should be set for elderly patients with long-standing diabetes, who may have established macrovascular disease and in whom the risks associated with hypoglycemia could be significant. Lifestyle modifications will decrease the risk of stroke by correcting dyslipidemia, hyperglycemia and decreasing BP. Weight control, decreased fat intake, increasing fiber in diet, and physical exercise are important measures to be taken care of. An intensified multifactorial intervention is necessary as can be seen in Box 2. In the Steno-2 study, subjects from the intensive therapy showed beneficial results in respect to the development of cardiovascular disease and deaths resulting from them as compared to the conventional treatment group. Intensive therapy targets in this included HbA1c at <6.5, serum total cholesterol level < 175mg/dL, serum triglyceride <150 mg/dL, and BP <130/80 mm Hg.[63] BP control in diabetics is an important factor as that in nondiabetics. The UKPD study showed decreased risk of stroke when BP was controlled around 140/80 mm Hg.[64] The ACCORD study suggested to maintain a target systolic BP <120 mm Hg to reduce the risk of stroke.[65]

CONCLUSION

Ischemic stroke is an important cause of morbidity, mortality, and disability worldwide, and its incidence is rising day by day. A higher prevalence of stroke is seen in diabetes mellitus patients. Risk factors like hyperglycemia, hypertension and dyslipidemia, contribute to the development of stroke in diabetes. All these lead to the formation of an atherogenic milieu, and both micro- and macrovascular disease lead to stroke. Diabetes is commonly associated with ischemic stroke which manifests as lacunar infarcts. Hyperglycemia during acute stroke needs proper management as it is associated with poorer outcomes. A good glycemic control is essential in the initial management of stroke but hypoglycemia must be avoided. Long-term tight glycemic control is desired in all patients but has to be recommended after considering the whole clinical profile and life expectancy of patients as uncontrolled diabetes is an intense procoagulant state.[66] Treatment of other associated risk factors like hypertension, dyslipidemia and obesity along with lifestyle modification would greatly benefit diabetic individuals and prevent vascular complications. This is very essential in the present time when the prevalence of diabetes is rising alarmingly. Health policy makers need to address this to reduce the physical, psychological and economic burden caused by the duo of diabetes and stroke.

Box 2: Principles to prevent stroke in diabetes

- Good glycemic control
- Good control of hypertension
- Weight reduction
- Dietary modifications
- Regular exercises
- Correction of dyslipidemia
- Cessation of smoking

KEY POINTS

- Incidence of diabetes is increasing worldwide
- Diabetics have a two- to four-time increased risk of developing stroke and greater sequelae
- Hypertension, dyslipidemia and insulin resistance contribute in the development of stroke
- Systemic complications of diabetes lead to poor outcome in stroke
- Glycemic control during acute stroke is crucial in management
- Maintaining blood glucose around normal limits in patients at risk of developing stroke can help in prevention
- Lifestyle modification and treatment of associated factors is also warranted.

REFERENCES

1. Shou J, Zhou L, Zhu S, et al. Diabetes is an independent risk factor for stroke recurrence in stroke patients: a meta-analysis. J Stroke Cerebrovasc Dis. 2015;24:1961-8.
2. Dutton GR, Lewis CE. The Look AHEAD trial: implications of life style interventions in type 2 diabetes mellitus. Prog Cardiovasc Dis. 2015;58:69-75.
3. Dalal PM, Parab PV.Cerebrovascular disease in type 2 diabetes mellitus. Neurol India. 2002; 50:380-5.

4. Davis TM, Millins H, Statton IM, et al. Risk factors for stroke in type 2 diabetes mellitus. United Kingdom Prospective Diabetes Study (UKPDS29). Arch Intern Med. 1999;159:1097-103.
5. Giorda CB, Avogaro A, Maggini M, et al.Incidence and risk factors for stroke in type 2 diabetic patients: the DAI study. Stroke. 2007;38:1154-60.
6. Kissela BM, Khoury J, Kleindorfer D, et al. Epidemiology of ischemic stroke in patients with diabetes: the greater Cincinnati/Northern Kentucky Stroke Study. Diabetes Care. 2005;28:355-9.
7. Arvanitakis Z, Schneider JA, Wilson RS, et al. Diabetes is related to cerebral infarction but not to Alzheimer disease pathology in older persons. Neurology. 2006;67(11):1960.
8. Sarwar N, Gao P, Seshasai SR, et al. Diabetes mellitus, fasting blood sugar concentration, and risk of vascular disease: a collaborative meta-analysis of 102 prospective studies. Lancet. 2010;375(9733):2215.
9. Janghorbani M, Hu FB, Willett WC, et al. Prospective study of type 1 and type 2 diabetes and risk of stroke subtypes: The Nurses' Health Study. Diabetes Care. 2007;30(7):1730.
10. Davis ND, Hachinski V. Epidemiology of cerebrovascular disease. In: Anderson D, (ed). Neuroepidemiology. A tribute to Bruce Schoenberg. Boca Raton, FL: CRC Press; 1991.pp. 27-53.
11. Sacco RL, Wolf PA, Kennel WB, et al. Survival and recurrence: the Framingham Study. Stroke. 1982;13:290-5.
12. Hier DB, Foulkes MA, Swiontoniowski M, et al. Stroke recurrence within two years after ischaemic infarction. Stroke. 1991;22:156-61.
13. Das SK, Banerjee TK, Biswas K, et al. A prospective community-based study of stroke in Kolkata, India. Stroke. 2007;38:906-10.
14. Gourie-Devi M, Gururaj G, Satishchandra P, et al. Prevalence of neurological disorders in Bangalore, India. A community-based study with comparison between urban and rural areas. Neuroepidemiology. 2004;23:261-8.
15. Ahmad OB, Boschi-Pinto C, Lopez AD, et al. Age standardization of rates: a new WHO standard. Geneva, Switzerland: World Health Organization. GPE discussion paper series no. 31, EIP/GPE/EBD.
16. Dalal PM, Bhattacharya M. Stroke epidemic in India: hypertension-stroke control programme is urgently needed. J Assoc Physicians India. 2007;55:689-91.
17. Brown RD, Whisnant JP, Sicks JD, et al. Stroke incidence, prevalence, and survival: secular trends in Rochester, Minnesota, through 1989.Stroke. 1996:27:373-80.
18. Thrift AG, Dewey HM, MacDonnell RA, et al. Incidence of major stroke subtypes: initial findings from the North East Melbourne Stroke Incidence Study (NEMESIS). Stroke. 2001;32:1732-8.
19. Jiang B, Wang WZ, Chen H, et al. Incidence and trends of stroke and its subtypes in China: results from three large cities. Stroke. 2006;37:63-8.
20. Baynes JW, Thorpe SR. Role of oxidative stress in diabetic complications: a new perspective of an old paradigm. Diabetes. 1999;48:1-9.
21. Schmidt AM, Yan SD, Wautier JL, et al. Activation of receptor for advanced glycation end products: a mechanism for chronic vascular dysfunction in diabetic vasculopathy and atherosclerosis. Circ Res. 1999;84:489-97.
22. Idris I, Gray S, Donnelly R. Protein kinase C activation: isoenzyme specific effects on metabolism and cardiovascular complications in diabetes. Diabetologia. 2001;44:659-73.
23. Strano A, Hoppensteadt D, Walenga JM, et al. Plasma levels of the molecular markers of coagulation and fibrinolysis in patients with peripheral arterial disease. Semin Thromb Hemost. 1996;22Suppl 1:35-40.
24. Crepaldi G, Fellin R, Calabro A, et al. Double blind multicentre trial on a new medium molecular weight glycosaminoglycan. Current therapeutic effects and perspectives for clinical use. Atherosclerosis. 1990; 81:233-43.
25. Vaidyula VR, Rao AK, Mozzoli M, et al. Effects if hyperglycemia and hyperinsulinemia on circulating tissue factor procoagulant activity and platelet CD40 ligand. Diabetes. 2006;55:202-8.
26. Tun NN, Arunagirinathan G, Munshi SK, et al. Diabetes mellitus and stroke: a clinical update. World J Diabetes. 2017;8(6):235-48.
27. Capes SE, Hunt D, Malmberg K, et al. Stress hyperglycemia and prognosis of stroke in non-diabetic and diabetic patients: a systematic overview. Stroke. 2001;32:2426-32.
28. Uyttenboogaart M, Koch MW, Stewart RE, et al. Moderate hyperglycemia is associated with favourable outcome in acute lacunar stroke. Brain. 2007;130:1626-30.
29. Bruno A, Biller J, Adams HPJr, et al. Acute blood glucose level and outcome from ischemic stroke. Trial of ORG 10172 in Acute Stroke Treatment (TOAST) Investigators. Neurology. 1999;52:280-4.
30. Asplund K, Hagg E, Helmers C, et al. The natural history of stroke in patients. Acta Med Scand. 1980;207:417-24.
31. Myers RE, Yamaguchi S. Nervous system effects of cardiac arrest in monkeys. Preservation of vision. Arch Neurol. 1977;34:65-74.
32. McMillan DE, Utterback NG, La Puma J. Reduced erythrocyte deformability in diabetes. Diabetes. 1978;27:895-901.
33. Wautier JL, Paton RC, Wautier MP, et al. Increased adhesion of erythrocytes to endothelial cells in diabetes mellitus and its relation to vascular complications. N Engl J Med. 1981;305:237-42.
34. Pulsinelli W, Waldman S, Sigsbee B, et al. Experimental hyperglycemia and diabetes mellitus worsen stroke outcome. Trans Am Nuerol Assoc. 1980;105:21-4.
35. Pulsinelli WA, Levy DE, Sigsbee B, et al. Increased damage after ischemic stroke in patients with hyperglycemia with or without established diabetes mellitus. Am J Med. 1977;34:65-74.
36. Kernan WN, Viscoli CM, Furie KL, et al. Pioglitazone after ischaemic stroke or transient ischaemic attack. N Engl J Med. 2016;374:1321-31.
37. Toshitaka U, Takahiko K, Nigishi H. Pathogenesis and neuroimaging of cerebral large and small vessel disease in type 2 diabetes: a possible link between cerebral and retinal microvascular abnormalities. J Diabetes Investig. 2017;8(2):134-48.
38. Bangalore S, Kumar S, Lobach I, et al. Blood pressure targets in subjects with type 2 diabetes mellitus/impaired fasting glucose: observations from traditional and Bayesian random-effects meta-analysis of randomized trials. Circulation. 2011;123:2799-810.
39. Jørgensen HS, Nakayama MD,Raaschou HO, et al. Effect of blood pressure and diabetes on stroke in progression. Lancet. 1994;344(8916):156-9.
40. Yusuf S, Sleight P, Pogue J, et al. Effects of an angiotensin-converting enzyme inhibitor, ramipril, on cardiovascular events in high risk patients. N Engl J Med. 2000;342:145-53.
41. Boden-Albala B,Sacco RL, Lee HS, et al. Metabolic syndrome and ischaemic stroke risk: northern Manhattan Study. Stroke. 2008;39:30-5.
42. Koren-Morag N, Goldbourt U, Tanne D. Relation between the metabolic syndrome and ischaemic stroke or transient ischaemic attack: a prospective cohort study in patients with atherosclerotic cardiovascular disease. Stroke. 2005;36:1366-71.
43. January CT, Wann LS, Alpert JS, et al. AHA/ACC/HRS guideline for the management of patients with atrial fibrillation: a report of the American college of Cardiology /AHA task force on Practice Guidelines and the Heart Rhythm Society. J Am Coll Cardiol. 2014;64:el76.
44. Lip GY, Nieuwlaat R, Pisters R,et al. Refining clinical risk stratification for predicting stroke and thromboembolism in atrial fibrillation using a novel risk-factor based approach: the Euro Heart Survey on atrial fibrillation. Chest. 2010;137:263-72.
45. Huxley RR, Filion KB, Konety S, et al. Meta-analysis of cohort and case control studies of studies of type 2 diabetes mellitus and risk of atrial fibrillation. Am J Cardiol. 2011;108:56-62.
46. Go AS, Hylek EM, Borowsky LH, et al. Warfarin use among ambulatory patients with non-valvular atrial fibrillation: the anti-coagulation and risk factors (ATRIA) study. Ann Intern Med. 1999;131:927-34.

47. Sadlon AH, Tsakiris DA. Direct anticoagulants in the elderly, systematic review and meta-analysis of evidence, current and future directions. Swiss Med Wkly. 2016;146:w14356.
48. Melgaard L, Gorst-Rasmussen A, Lane DA, et al. Assessment of the CHA2DS2–VASc Score in predicting ischaemic score, thromboembolism and death in patients with heart failure with and without atrial fibrillation. JAMA. 2015;314:1030-8.
49. Megherbi SE, Milan C, Minier D, et al. European BIOMED study of stroke care group. Association between diabetes and stroke subtype on survival and functional outcome 3 months after stroke: data from the European BIOMED study project. Stroke. 2003;34:688-94.
50. Karapanayiotides T, Piechowski-Jozwiak B, van Melle G, et al. Stroke patterns, etiology and prognosis in patients with Diabetes Mellitus. Neurology. 2004;62:1558-62.
51. Tuomilehto J, Rastenyte D, et al. Diabetes mellitus as a risk factor for death from stroke. Prospective study of the middle-aged Finnish population. Stroke. 1996;27:210-5.
52. Jauch EC, Saver JL, Adams HP, et al. Guidelines for the early management of patients with acute ischaemic stroke—a guideline for healthcare professionals fromAmerican Heart Association/AmericanStroke Association. Stroke. 2013;44:870-947.
53. Oslen TS, Langhorne P, Diener HC, et al. European stroke initiative recommendations for stroke management—update 2003. Cerebrovasc Dis. 2003;16:311-37.
54. Gray CS, Hildreth AJ, Sandercock PA, et al. Glucose–potassium–insulin infusion in management of post stroke hyperglycemia. The UK Glucose Insulin in stroke Trial (GIST-UK). Lancet Neurol. 2007;6:397-406.
55. Chen R, Bruce O, Wuwei F. Diabetes and stroke: epidemiology, pathophysiology, pharmaceuticals and outcomes. Am J Med Sci. 2016;351(4):380-6.
56. Bruno A, Kent TA, Coull BM, et al. Treatment of hyperglycemia in ischaemic stroke (THIS): a randomized pilot trial. Stoke. 2008;40:384-9.
57. Johnston KC, Hall CE, Kissela BM, et al. Glucose regulation in acute stroke patients (GRASP) trial: a randomized pilot trial. Stroke. 2009;40:3804-9.
58. Nathan DM, Cleary PA, Blacklund JY,et al. Intensive diabetes treatment and cardiovascular disease in patients with type 1 diabetes. N Engl J Med. 2005;353:2643–53.
59. Holman RR, Paul SK, Bethel MA, et al. 10 Year follow up of intensive glucose control in type 2 diabetes. N Engl J Med. 2008;359:1577-89.
60. Gerstein HC, Miller ME, Byington RP, et al. Effects of intensive glucose lowering in type 2 diabetes. N Engl J Med. 2008;358:2545-59.
61. Patel A, MacMohan S, Chalmers J, et al. Intensive blood glucose control and vascular outcomes in patients with type 2 diabetes. N Engl J Med. 2008;358:2560-72.
62. Marso SP, Daniels GH, Brown-Frandsen K, et al. Liraglutide and cardiovascular outcomes in type 2 diabetes. N Engl J Med. 2016; 375:311-22.
63. Gaede P, Lund-Anderson H, Parving HH, et al. Effects of a multifactorial intervention on mortality in type 2 diabetes. New Engl J Med. 2008;358: 580-91.
64. UK Prospective Diabetes Study Group. Tight blood pressure control and risk of macrovascular and microvascular complications in type 2 diabetes: UKPDS 38. UK Prospective Diabetes Study Group. Br Med J. 1998;317:703-13.
65. Cushman WC, Evans GW, Byington RP, et al. Effects of intensive blood pressure control in type 2 mellitus. New Engl J Med. 2010;362:1575-85.
66. Gentile NT, Vaidyula VR, Kanamalla U, et al. Factor VIIa and tissue factor procoagulant activity in diabetes mellitus after acute ischaemic stroke: impact of hyperglycemia. Thromb Haemost. 2007;98:1007-13.

Chapter 44

Cellular Mechanism of Atherosclerosis in Diabetes Mellitus

Mayur Agrawal, Subhash Yadav

INTRODUCTION

Atherosclerosis usually causes focal occlusion of vessel but may also lead to diffuse nonocclusive disease. Depending on the vessel involves, it has varied presentation. Coronary artery involvement leads to angina and myocardial infarction; central nervous system (CNS) artery atherosclerosis leads to transient ischemic attack (TIA) and stroke; peripheral artery atherosclerosis causes claudication and gangrene; whereas, mesentery artery involvement causes mesenteric ischemia.

Atherosclerosis usually involves the bifurcation of artery as there is altered hemodynamics at these sites. It is a slow process, develops usually over years. There is usually prolonged silent period followed by clinical manifestation. It can begin as early as childhood, with initial lesion as fatty streak.[1]

It is well documented in the literature that both type 1 and type 2 diabetes are powerful and independent factor factor for the coronary artery disease, cerebrovascular stroke and the peripheral disease. More than 75% of all the hospitalization for the diabetes complication are attributable to the cardiovascular disease. Long exposure to the hyperglycemia is now very well-known factor as a primary cause for the pathogenesis of the diabetes complications.[2] Hyperglycemia in the diabetes lead to the number of the alteration in the vascular tissue and that potentially promote accelerated atherosclerosis. Currently, there are the three major mechanisms which can lead to the pathogenic changes in the vascular tissue in diabetes: (1) nonenzymatic glycosylation of proteins and lipids, (2) protein kinase C (PKC) activation and (3) oxidative stress. More important fact regarding these factors is that they are dependent upon each other to cause the pathogenic changes.[3]

HISTOLOGY

Fatty streaks are the initial lesion occurring as thickening of the intima with deposition of foam cells with extracellular matrix. Foam cells are lipid-laden macrophages. There is also proliferation of the smooth muscle cells, which may arise from the hematopoietic stem cells. Foam cells are the hallmark of atheroma. As the lesion progresses, smooth muscle cells within the fatty streaks undergo apoptosis, thus further increasing macrophage accumulation. This fatty streak then develops into plaques. These plaques further undergo modification, develops fibrous cap which is relatively acellular, made up of dense collagen. Within the fibrous cap lies the lipid core. As the time passes, atherosclerotic plaque expands and develop its vascular supply; these thin-walled vessel (vasa vasorum) are prone to rupture and lead to hemorrhage within the plaque. Atheroma is also associated with remodeling, both negative and positive remodeling. In positive remodeling, it is compensatory mechanism; there is expansion of external elastic membrane and vessel size, thus preventing luminal narrowing and vascular compromise.[4]

PATHOGENESIS

The abnormal metabolic state that accompanies diabetes causes arterial dysfunction. Many factors work in synergy for atherosclerosis. Main contributors include endothelial dysfunction, dyslipidemia, diabetes, hypertension, smoking and other inflammatory and immunologic

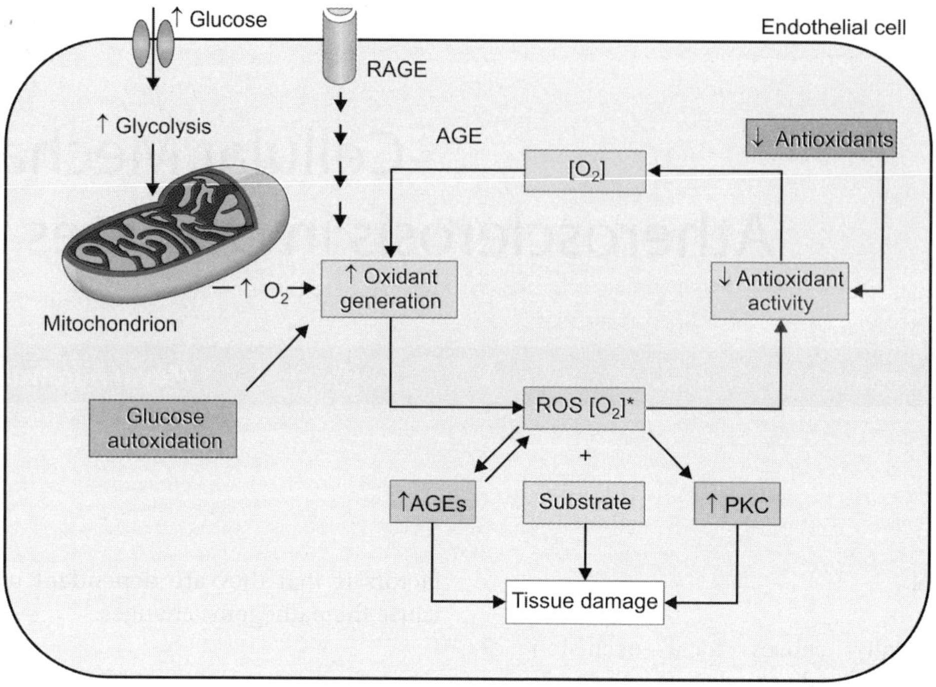

(AGE: advanced glycation end products; O_2: oxygen; PKC: protein kinase C; RAGE: receptor for advanced glycation end products; ROS: reactive oxygen species.)
$[O_2]^*$ represents various forms of reactive oxygen species (ROS)

Figure 1 Relationship between rates of oxidant generation, antioxidant activity, oxidative stress and oxidative damage in diabetes.
Source: Aronson D, Rayfield EJ. How hyperglycemia promotes atherosclerosis: molecular mechanisms. Cardiovas Diabetol. 2002;1:1.

factors.[5] Due to vastness of the topic and ever-increasing knowledge, it is impossible to cover all the things in this chapter, so we will be focusing mainly on cellular mechanism of atherosclerosis in diabetes (Figure 1).[6]

MECHANISMS OF HYPERGLYCEMIA-INDUCED ATHEROSCLEROSIS

Advanced Glycation End Products

Advanced glycation end products (AGEs) are harmful compounds that are formed when protein or fat combine with glucose in the bloodstream. This process is called glycation. Important factors crucial to the formation of AGEs include the rate of turnover of proteins for glycoxidation, the degree of hyperglycemia and the extent of oxidant stress in the environment. If one or more of these conditions is present, both intracellular and extracellular proteins may be glycated and oxidized. AGEs cause harmful effect by several mechanisms. One possibility is the purely mechanical dysfunction caused by AGE crossbridges among vessel wall macromolecules. A second form of damage promoting atherosclerosis is that AGE accumulation can cause circulating blood cells to adhere to the vessel wall. And lastly, nonmechanical source of damage is the perturbation of cellular function through binding to a variety of receptors that have been identified on various cell types, including macrophages, endothelial cells, smooth muscle cells, renal cells and neuronal cells. AGE formation may thus accelerate the atherosclerotic process through nonreceptor dependent and receptor mediated mechanisms.[7]

Protein Kinase C Pathway

Increased intracellular hyperglycemia causes de novo synthesis of diacylglycerol (DAG), an intracellular lipid messenger and this DAG activates PKC, a serine/threonine-related protein kinase, downstream in both endothelial and smooth muscle cells. PKC-b and PKC-g are most notable for pathogenesis of diabetes atherosclerosis. Hyperglycemia induces PKC upregulation, increases endothelial cell permeability, depresses nitric oxide (NO) production and increases production of vasoconstrictors, such as endothelin-1 (ET-1) and thromboxane A2 (TxA2). It is also seen that PKC increases the hypercoagulable and proinflammatory state seen in diabetes mellitus (DM) by upregulating plasminogen activator inhibitor type 1 (PAI-1) and nuclear factor-κ beta (NF-κβ), respectively, in endothelial and smooth muscle cells. Reactive oxygen species (ROS) levels are increased by PKC and it is because of activation of membrane-associated nicotinamide adenine dinucleotide phosphate (NADP H)-dependent oxidases and by inhibition of insulin-stimulated production of endothelial nitric oxide synthase (eNOS).[8]

Oxidative Stress

Oxidative stress is accepted as important mechanism for atherosclerosis. Among the sequence of hyperglycemia, oxidative stress has been suggested as the important potential mechanism of accelerated atherosclerosis. It is found that the hyperglycemia can increase the oxidative stress through several pathways. A major mechanism appears to be that hyperglycemia induces intracellular ROS, resulting in the increased production of the superoxide. Some other mechanisms also have been proposed that may explain how the hyperglycemia causes increased ROS formation. For example, one of the probable mechanisms is that it involves the transition metal catalyzed autoxidation of the free glucose as described in the cell-free system. Through this mechanism, glucose itself initiates auto-oxidative reaction and free radical production yielding superoxide anion and hydrogen peroxide.[9]

There is also evidence that hyperglycemia may compromise the natural antioxidant defense mechanism. It is well known that the under normal circumstances, free radical are rapidly eliminated by antioxidant such as vitamin C and vitamin E. But, in case of diabetes, the levels of these antioxidants are low, so levels of free radicals become high and they cause atherosclerosis. So, there appears to be a strong pathogenic link between the hyperglycemia-induced oxidative stress and hyperglycemia-dependent mechanism of vascular damage, namely the AGEs formation and PKC activation.[10]

Glycoxidation

Glycoxidation is a process when AGEs are produced by combined process of glycation and oxidation. It is seen that in some of the diabetic individual, advanced glycosylation product such as a carboxymethyl lysine and pentosidine are formed because of reaction of protein with glucose under the oxidative condition. It is also known that oxidation product of protein is irreversible and that is why, it is an integrative biomarker for accumulated oxidative stress of tissue exposed. It is also found that there is a strong correlation between levels of glycoxidation product of skin collagen and severity of diabetic retinal, renal and the vascular disease[11,12] (Flowchart 1).[13]

Endothelial Dysfunction

Endothelial cells synthesize multiple regulatory substances which help to regulate the vasodilation and vasoconstriction, homeostasis and inflammation on the vessel surface and within the wall. Endothelial cell injury and dysfunction is believed to be the important event in the development of atherosclerosis. These endothelial cells are particularly susceptible to accumulation of glucose seen in hyperglycemia and to many of the secondary side effects of the diabetes including the insulin resistance.[14]

Polyol Pathway

Aldo-keto reductase produces a variety of carbonyl compound to their respective sugar alcohol or also known as polyols. During hyperglycemia, glucose and glucose-derived compound are converted to sorbitol by aldose reductase which is then oxidized to fructose by sorbitol dehydrogenase with NAD+ as a cofactor. Because of this, there is an increased ROS and overall oxidative state.[8]

Hexosamine Pathway

Inhibition of GAPDH (glyceraldehyde-3-phosphate dehydrogenase) superoxide also diverts the glycolytic upstream metabolic fructose-6-phosphate into a hexosamine pathway. Post-translation liquidation and degradation of protective protein in the vasculature, such as eNOS and A20, tilt the balance towards atherogenesis while increasing the subscription of proatherogenic proteins, such as thrombospondin-1.[15]

High Sensitive C-reactive Protein

High sensitive C-reactive protein (hsCRP) is also one of the inflammatory markers and is associated with increased risk of atherlosclerosis. The hsCRP was found to be an independent predictor of diverse end points ranging from obesity, type 2 DM, Metabolic syndrome, increased carotid intima-media thickness, stable coronary artery disease (CAD), first acute coronary event and recurrent

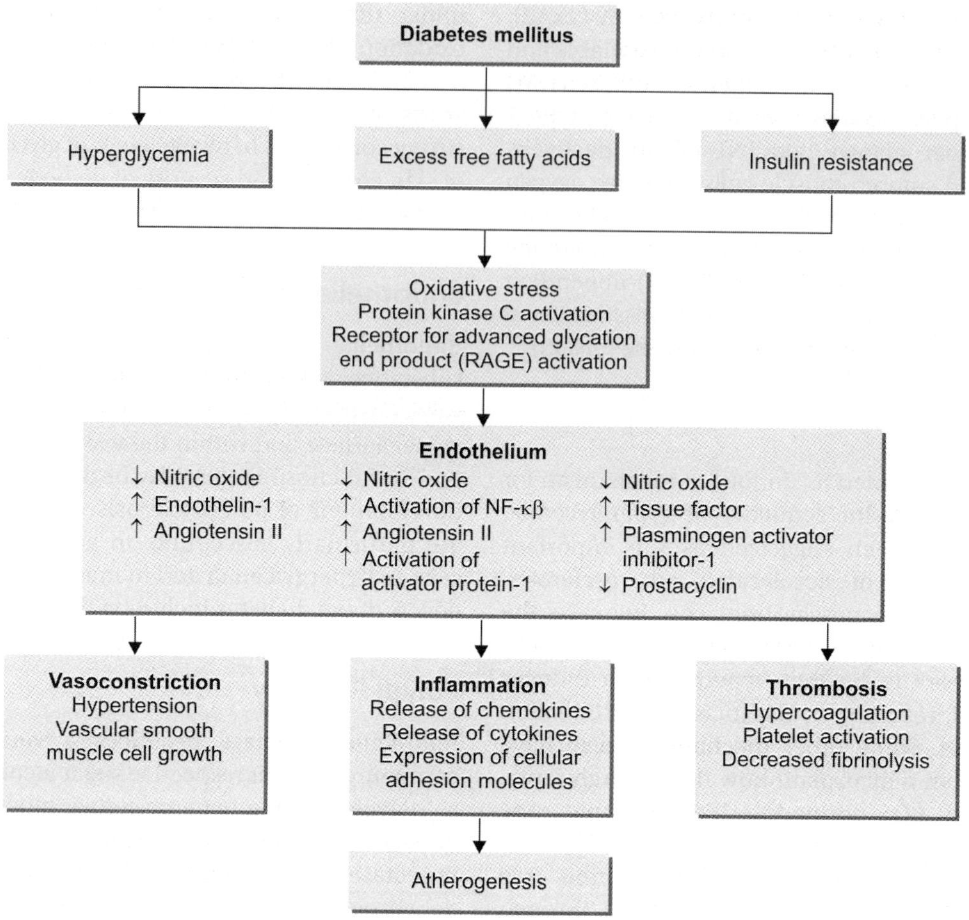

(NF-κβ: nuclear factor-kbeta.)

Flowchart 1 Endothelial dysfunction in diabetes.

Source: Beckman JA, Creager MA, Libby P. Diabetes and atherosclerosis: epidemiology, pathophysiology, and management. JAMA. 2002;287:2570-81.

cardiovascular disease (CVD) events. The hsCRP per se has also been found to increase the expression of vascular endothelial PAI-1 and other adhesion molecules and alter low-density lipoprotein (LDL) uptake by macrophages.[16]

Toll-like Receptor 4 Polymorphism

Toll-like receptor 4 (TLR4), part of innate immunity, regulates the inflammatory response to bacterial lipopolysaccharide. Subjects with the *Asp299Gly TLR4* allele had lower levels of proinflammatory cytokines and acute-phase reactants such as interleukin-6 and fibrinogen. Though there was increased risk of infection, risk of atherosclerosis was lower (odds ratio 0.54).[17]

Endothelin 1

Endothelin-1 is a potent vasoconstriction and stimulates the proliferation of the smooth muscle cells and it promotes the fibrosis and inflammation leading to thrombosis and plaque formation in the vessel wall.[18]

CONCLUSION

Atherosclerosis is a major factor responsible for the morbidity and mortality in diabetic patient. The development of atherosclerosis is not only because of the hyperglycemia but other secondary factors are also responsible like insulin resistance, dyslipidemia, hypercoagulability, altered secretion and function of the local regulatory substance and impaired response to the injury. So, because of this not only the strict glucose control is enough, but it also requires multifaceted approach targeting all the mechanism to achieve goal. A better understanding of complex cellular pathways of atherosclerosis is required for management and to improve the outcome.

REFERENCES

1. Laakso M. Hyperglycemia and cardiovascular disease in type 2 diabetes. Diabetes. 1999;48:937-42. [online] Available from: http://www.ncbi.nlm.nih.gov/pubmed/10331395 [Accessed September, 2018].
2. Grundy SM, Benjamin IJ, Burke GL, et al. Diabetes and cardiovascular disease: a statement for healthcare professionals from the American Heart Association. Circulation. 1999;100:1134-6. [online] Available from: http://www.ncbi.nlm.nih.gov/pubmed/10477542 [Accessed September, 2018].
3. Nishikawa T, Edelstein D, Du XL, et al. Normalizing mitochondrial superoxide production blocks three pathways of hyperglycaemic damage. Nature. 2000;404:787-90. [online] Available from http://www.nature.com/articles/35008121 [Accessed September, 2018].
4. Sun J, Sukhova GK, Wolters PJ, et al. Mast cells promote atherosclerosis by releasing proinflammatory cytokines. Nat Med. 2007;13:719-24. [online] Available from: http://www.nature.com/articles/nm1601 [Accessed September, 2018].
5. Colwell JA, Lopes-Virella M, Halushka PV. Pathogenesis of atherosclerosis in diabetes mellitus. Diabetes Care. 1981;4:121-33. [online] Available from: http://www.ncbi.nlm.nih.gov/pubmed/7009108 [Accessed September, 2018].
6. Aronson D, Rayfield EJ. How hyperglycemia promotes atherosclerosis: molecular mechanisms. Cardiovasc Diabetol. 2002;1:1
7. Sell DR, Monnier VM. Structure elucidation of a senescence cross-link from human extracellular matrix. Implication of pentoses in the aging process. J Biol Chem. 1989;264:21597-602. [online] Available from: http://www.ncbi.nlm.nih.gov/pubmed/2513322 [Accessed September, 2018].
8. Madonna R, De Caterina R. Cellular and molecular mechanisms of vascular injury in diabetes--part II: cellular mechanisms and therapeutic targets. Vascul Pharmacol. 2011;54:75-9. [online] Available from: http://linkinghub.elsevier.com/retrieve/pii/S1537189111000322 [Accessed September, 2018].
9. Baynes JW, Thorpe SR. Role of oxidative stress in diabetic complications: a new perspective on an old paradigm. Diabetes. 1999;48:1-9. [online] Available from: http://www.ncbi.nlm.nih.gov/pubmed/9892215 [Accessed September, 2018].
10. Yue DK, McLennan S, Fisher E, et al. Ascorbic acid metabolism and polyol pathway in diabetes. Diabetes. 1989;38:257-61. [online] Available from: http://www.ncbi.nlm.nih.gov/pubmed/2492477 [Accessed September, 2018].
11. Wells-Knecht MC, Thorpe SR, Baynes JW. Pathways of formation of glycoxidation products during glycation of collagen. Biochemistry. 1995;34:15134-41. [online] Available from: http://www.ncbi.nlm.nih.gov/pubmed/7578127 [Accessed September, 2018].
12. McCance DR, Dyer DG, Dunn JA, et al. Maillard reaction products and their relation to complications in insulin-dependent diabetes mellitus. J Clin Invest. 1993;91:2470-8. [online] Available from: http://www.ncbi.nlm.nih.gov/pubmed/8514859 [Accessed September, 2018].
13. Beckman JA, Creager MA, Libby P. Diabetes and atherosclerosis: epidemiology, pathophysiology, and management. JAMA. 2002;287(19):2570-81.
14. Brownlee M. Biochemistry and molecular cell biology of diabetic complications. Nature. 2001;414:813-20. [online] Available from: http://www.nature.com/articles/414813a [Accessed September, 2018].
15. Du XL, Edelstein D, Rossetti L, et al. Hyperglycemia-induced mitochondrial superoxide overproduction activates the hexosamine pathway and induces plasminogen activator inhibitor-1 expression by increasing Sp1 glycosylation. Proc Natl Acad Sci USA. 2000;97:12222-6.
16. Libby P. Mechanisms of acute coronary syndromes and their implications for therapy. N Engl J Med. 2013;368:2004-13. [online] Available from: http://www.nejm.org/doi/10.1056/NEJMra1216063 [Accessed September, 2018].
17. Kiechl S, Lorenz E, Reindl M, et al. Toll-like receptor 4 polymorphisms and atherogenesis. N Engl J Med. 2002;347(3):185-92.
18. Ergul A. Endothelin-1 and diabetic complications: focus on the vasculature. Pharmacol Res. 2011;63:477-82.

Chapter 45

Nondiabetic Ocular Complications in Diabetes

Chandrasekhar Valupadas

INTRODUCTION

Diabetes is a metabolic syndrome characterized by chronically elevated blood glucose levels in the body. It is a global epidemic, considered as lifestyle disease and its prevalence is continued to escalate constantly worldwide (Fig. 1). Currently, India represents 49% of the world's diabetes burden (8.8% in adults) in 2017 with an estimated 72 million cases[1] and its prevalence is anticipated to double to 134 million by 2025, approximately.

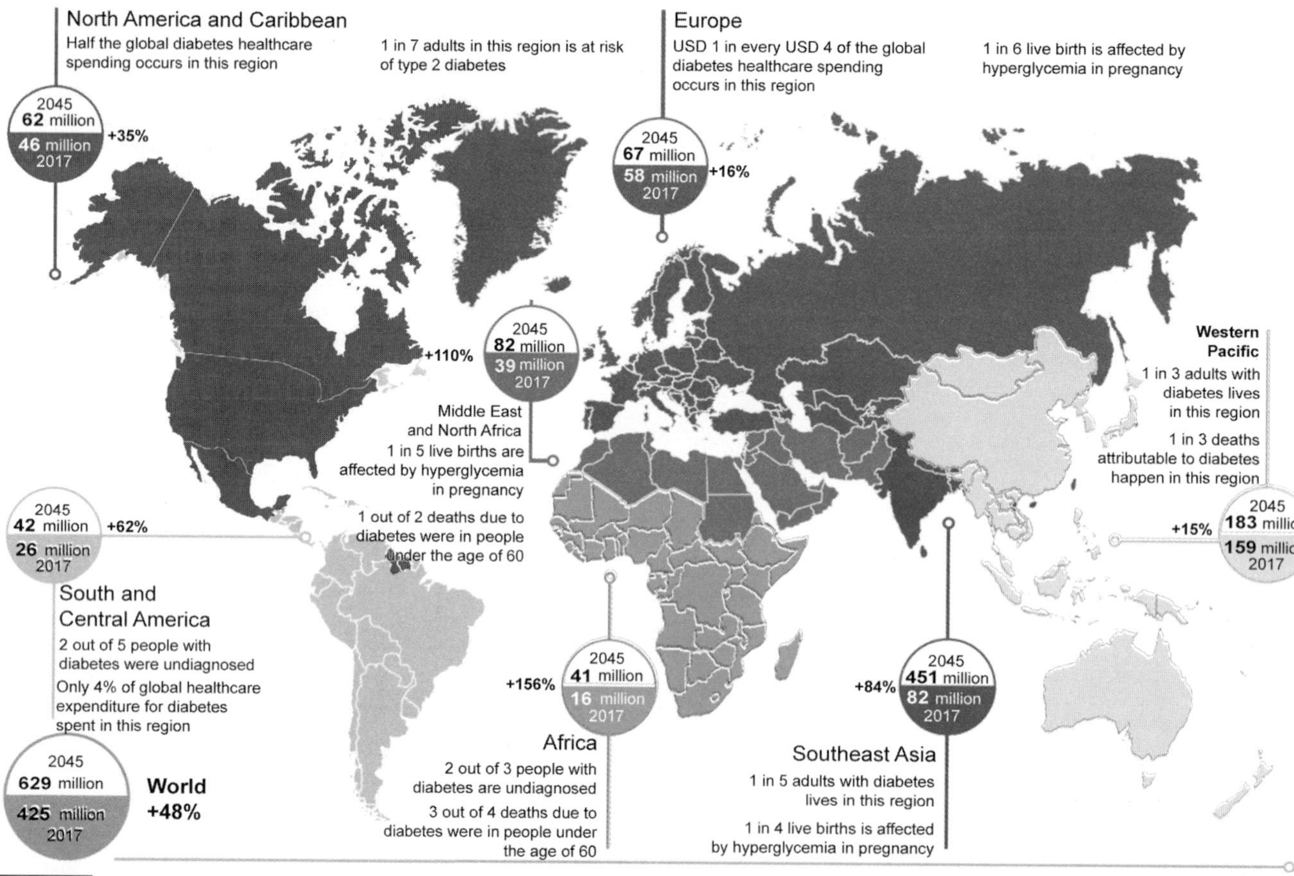

Figure 1 Prevalence of Diabetes in 2017 and prediction value for 2045.
Source: International Diabetic Federation Atlas (8th edition, 2017)]

Eye is a terminally differentiated highly specific sensory end organ by vessels and nerves in the human, and any subtle damage to it can lead to blindness. There are numerous ocular diseases which may develop due to various pathological mechanisms like environmental factors, trauma and chronic diseases, etc. Many chronic diseases can adversely affect the eye, among which diabetes and hypertension are high-flying ones.

Diabetic retinopathy (DR) is the most common microvascular complication of diabetes. There are other ocular complications, which tend to develop due to diabetes and the outcome varies in diabetics compared to nondiabetics. Therefore, this chapter focuses to enumerate the etiology, pathobiology and treatment options available for those nondiabetic complications of the eye in individuals with diabetes or who are at risk of developing diabetes in due course of time.

COMPLICATIONS ASSOCIATED WITH DIABETES

People with diabetes have an increased risk of developing numerable serious health problems affecting vital organs like heart and blood vessels, eyes, kidneys and nerves, due to consistent high-blood glucose levels (Fig. 2). These complications highly affect the quality of life causing increased disability physically and mentally.

OCULAR COMPLICATIONS ASSOCIATED WITH DIABETES

In general, it is temporary but consistent increase in glucose levels may cause irreparable damage to eye anatomically, thus developing serious complications unlike others. Table 1 describes how diabetes progressively manifests in ocular tissues at early-to-late stages of diabetes.[2] The complications are macular diseases, cataract, glaucoma and corneal dysfunction, etc.

Many ocular diseases are also associated with diabetes, which may lead to visual loss. Some of these ocular conditions may not be familiar to physicians treating diabetes listed in Table 2. Routine screening for retinopathy offers opportunity to detect these sight-threatening ocular diseases at the earliest.

Macular Disease

Macula, a small central area in the retina, contains special light-sensitive cells, allowing sharp-central vision which let's to see objects clearly that are straight ahead. There are two types of macular disease - (1) age-related macular degeneration (AMD) and (2) macular edema. AMD is an independent disease where the degeneration of macula increased with age. Its development and progression is rapid in diabetes compared to nondiabetes.

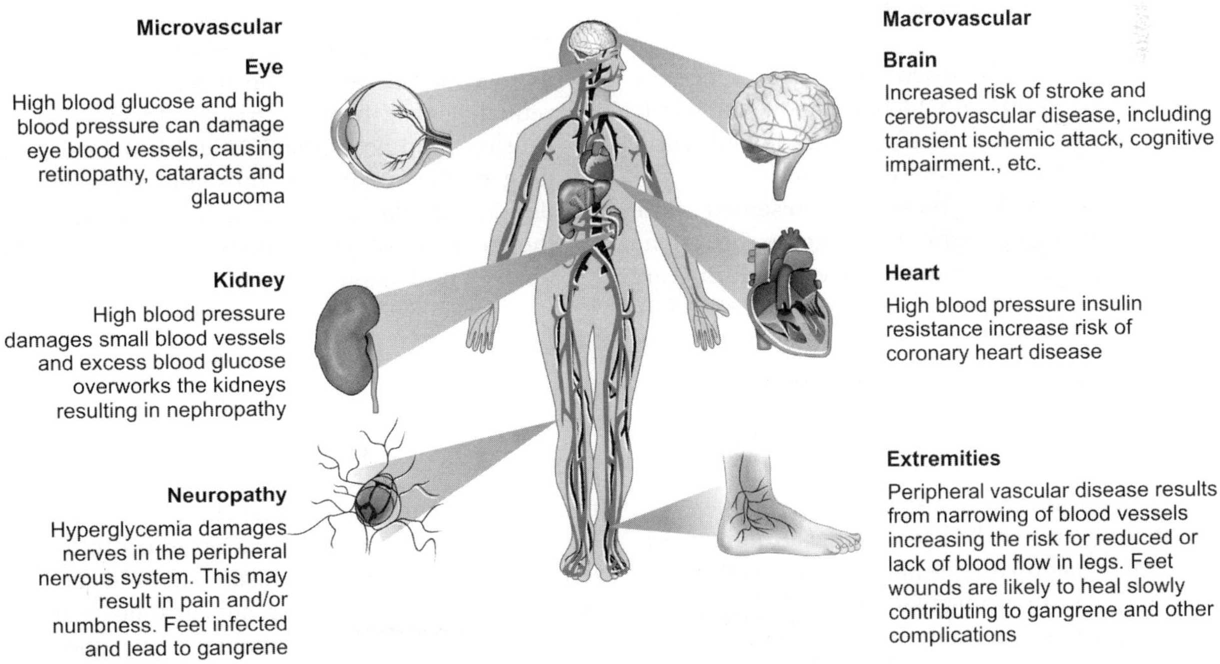

Figure 2 Complications of diabetes.

TABLE 1: Clinical manifestations of diabetes mellitus in ocular tissues.

Disease stage	Cornea	Ocular tissue nerve	Retina
Early/prediabetes	Ocular lens α-crystallin formation, increased central corneal thickness	Decreased corneal nerve fiber length	Microaneurysms, exudate, tortuosity of vessels, edema
Midpoint	Reduced corneal subbasal nerve density, increased corneal sensitivity and corneal erosion syndrome	Reduced subfoveal choroidal thickness, reduced comeal nerve density	Macular edema, hemorrhage, retinal detachment
Late-stage diabetes	Reduced tear meniscus parameters, lower nerve fiber and branch length	Optic neuropathy	Severe hemorrhage, retinal tearing/detachment, blindness

TABLE 2: List of ocular conditions associated with diabetes.

Ocular conditions directly associated with diabetes	Ocular conditions for which diabetes is a known risk factor	Ocular conditions where diabetes is possible risk factor	Ocular conditions mimicking as diabetic retinopathy
• Cataract and cataract surgery • Anterior ischemic optic neuropathy (AION) • Diabetic papillopathy • Extra ocularmotility disorders	• Glaucoma • Ocular ischemic syndrome (OIS)	• Retinal vein occlusion (RVO) • Retinal alveolar emboli • Retinal arterial • Retinal arterial occlusion (RAO) • Comeal diseases	• Age related macular degeneration • Hypertensive retinopathy • Radiation retinopathy • Miscellaneous like HIV, connective tissue diseases, retinal telangiectasias

- *Age-related macular degeneration*: AMD degeneration can develop in only one eye or possibly with a later stage in one eye compared to the other. There are three stages of AMD defined by the size and number of tiny yellow or white accumulations of extracellular material called *drusen* under the retina. They are as follows:
  1. *Early AMD* is diagnosed by the presence of medium-sized drusen which are about the width of an average human hair and people with early AMD typically do not have vision loss
  2. *Intermediate AMD* typically is presented with large-sized drusen, pigment changes in the retina, or both, which can only be detected during an eye examination. People with intermediate AMD may have some vision loss but mostly will not experience any significant symptoms
  3. *Late AMD* is manifested with drusen; people with late AMD have vision loss due to damage to the macula. Late AMD is further categorized into two types: dry AMD and wet AMD.

  In dry AMD, also called geographic atrophy, there is a gradual breakdown of the light-sensitive cells in the macula and the supporting tissue beneath the macula that convey visual information to the brain causing vision loss. *In wet AMD*, also called neovascular AMD, abnormal blood vessels grow underneath the retina. These vessels can leak fluid and blood, which may lead to swelling and damage of the macula. This damage may be rapid and severe, unlike the more gradual course of dry *AMD*. It is possible to have both dry and wet AMD in the same eye, and either condition can appear first.
- *Diabetic macular edema (DME)*: DME is the consequence of DR, where the macula swells and these retinal vessels become fragile. These vessels burst causing fluid accumulation which results in thickening of the retina and thus the retina is distorted developing blurry vision.[3] It has been observed that the incidence of DME is higher among type 2, but it is not well understood.[4]

Cataract, Cataract Surgery and Intraocular Lens Implantation

Cataract, clouding of the eye's lens, is one of the main causes of vision impairment in diabetes, which is two to five times more likely than those without diabetes. Deposition of advanced glycation end products in the lens is the possible mechanism. Anatomically, cataract is categorized as posterior subcapsular, cortical and nuclear cataracts, where diabetes has shown to be associated more with posterior subcapsular and cortical cataracts.

Although cataract surgery with intraocular lens implant (IOL) is relatively safe and has high success rates among healthy individuals, it is not the same with diabetics. Patients with diabetes may have poorer visual outcomes and is worsened in the operated eye of active DR. The most devastating postoperative complication is endophthalmitis. Studies also have reported greater foveal thickness and higher incidence of macular edema following cataract surgery in diabetic compared to nondiabetic patients.[5-7] Posterior capsular opacification (PCO) is a common finding following cataract surgery. In diabetes the prevalence of PCO is not well established. Also, cataract surgery accelerates progression of DR, following extracapsular cataract extraction. There are concerns that cataract surgery in diabetics may exacerbate the progression of macular edema.

Glaucoma

Glaucoma is a group of diseases that damage the eye's optic nerve. When aqueous humor does not properly drain through the trabecular meshwork and Schlemm's canal, it leads to increased pressure inside the eye. This could damage nerves and blood vessels, causing vision changes leading to glaucoma. In adults, diabetes nearly doubles the risk of glaucoma.

The World Health Organization has classified glaucoma as priority eye disease[8] and is categorized into "open-angle" and "closed-angle" glaucoma. Open-angle glaucoma is painless, chronic and generally asymptomatic until it progresses significantly. Closed-angle glaucoma, on the other hand, is known for sudden eye pain, redness, nausea and intraocular pressure spikes. Open-angle glaucoma can be treated with medications, while closed-angle glaucoma generally requires medical emergency care. People with diabetes tend to get open-angle glaucoma more than closed-angle glaucoma and are also more likely to get an uncommon type of glaucoma, called neovascular glaucoma, i.e. new blood vessels grow on the iris. These blood vessels block the normal flow of fluid out of the eye, raising pressure. This particular type is very difficult to treat, and the option to reduce the vessels is laser surgery. Surgeons are also looking into the use of implants to help drain the fluid, where injectable anti-vascular endothelial growth factor medications are widely used.[9]

Optic Neuritis and Ischemic Optic Neuropathy

Optic neuritis is inflammation of the optic nerve, caused by damage to and loss of the protective myelin sheath surrounding the nerve. Demyelinating optic neuritis is another term for this condition, which affects adults younger than 45 and mostly women. Vision symptoms include blurring and blind spots, distorted vision and reduced color vision; pain may also be noticed when eyes are moved. These symptoms develop prior to vision loss due to optic neuritis. The exact cause of optic neuritis is unknown, but it is believed to develop due to autoimmune disorders, infections, diseases, such as sarcoidosis and lupus, and drugs like quinine and antibiotics. There exists no positive association of diabetes with optic neuritis.

Ischemic optic neuropathy more generally describes optic nerve abnormalities or damage, including from causes, such as blocked blood flow or toxic exposure. Blockage can occur with inflammation of the arteries (called arteritic, typically as part of a disorder called giant cell arteritis) or without inflammation of the arteries (called nonarteritic). The only constant symptom is sudden painless vision loss. Risk factors for arteritic ischemic optic neuropathy is age over 70, and for nonarteritic neuropathy high blood pressure, smoking, diabetes and atherosclerosis are the causing ones.

Cornea, Contact Lens and Corneal Transplants

Common corneal dysfunctions in diabetics are corneal infections, poor wound healing, corneal edema and blindness. Around 70% of diabetics suffer from one or the other form of diabetic keratopathy. Corneal nerve alterations are now considered as surrogate marker of peripheral neuropathy and cardiac-autonomic neuropathy in diabetes. Advanced technologies like confocal microscopy and automated imaging are now possible to compare montages of subbasal nerve densities where epithelial nerve density of central cornea is higher than the periphery, which further results in reduced corneal sensitivity. These findings have implications in the use of contact lens and corneal transplants.

Several other problems with corneal transplantation in diabetics include recurrent corneal erosions, persistent epithelial defects and corneal endothelial damage. In diabetics, success of corneal transplantation is lower when compared with other diseases like keratoconus; reasons could be slower wound healing rates and corneal infections, such as fungal keratitis. There are several types of transplants, like Descemet's stripping automated endothelial keratoplasty, Descemet's membrane endothelial keratoplasty, anterior lamellar corneal transplant, LASIK (laser in situ keratomileusis), and PRK (photorefractive keratectomy), but LASIK and PRK are successful in vision correction. There are pros and cons for any new procedure and it is the surgeons' discretion to choose the best.

Diabetic Papillopathy

This is a rare complication of optic nerve characterized by acute disk edema and mild visual loss, which can precede the development of anterior ischemic optic neuropathy and is a risk factor for the progression of DR. This condition is differential diagnosis for papilledema and proliferative DR (mistaken for telangiectasia at disk for neovascularization) and is benign which resolves spontaneously within 1 year.

Ocular Movement Disorders

Extraocular motility disorders are common in diabetes secondary to peripheral neuropathy involving third, fourth and sixth cranial nerves. These patients' presents with binocular diplopia and pupil is spared. Usually, recovery is within 3 months, but recurrences can be common in same or other cranial nerves.

Ocular Ischemic Syndrome

Ocular ischemic syndrome (OIS) is rare vascular condition due to chronic hypoperfusion caused by ipsilateral internal carotid or ophthalmic artery occlusion which is secondary to glaucoma. The prevalence of OIS as part of macrovascular complication of carotid artery stenosis is higher in diabetes and 5-year all-cause mortality rate is almost 40%. Carotid ultrasonography can delineate carotid stenosis and carotid endarterectomy lowers the risk of visual loss and stroke.

Retinal Vein Occlusion

Retinal vein occlusion (RVO) is characterized by dilated tortuous retinal veins with retinal hemorrhages, cotton wool spots and macular edema. This can be central (at disk) and peripheral (at arteriovenous crossing); central is subdivided into nonischemic and ischemic where the latter is associated with poor vision outcomes. It is thought that diabetes is the major risk factor for RVO, but there is lack of robust data to prove this association. Retinal vein occlusion may lead to complications like neovascular glaucoma and macular edema. Treatment with panretinal laser photocoagulation can prevent the glaucoma.

Retinal Artery Occlusion

In contrast to RVO, retinal artery occlusion (RAO) or emboli is an ophthalmic emergency presented with the episodes of sudden onset, painless, unilateral, monocular vision loss associated with visual field defect. This condition mimics like transient ischemic attack/transient monocular blindness. There will be afferent papillary defect, diffuse retinal whitening with resultant classic "cherry spot" on the macula. The prevalence of diabetes in patients with RAO has been reported to be as high as 21%.

TREATMENT

There are numerous therapeutic modalities available both conventional and emerging methods to treat ocular complications in diabetes, which are described in Table 3.

CONCLUSION

Diabetes profoundly impacts ocular tissue by causing mechanical changes in microvasculature, resulting in increased permeability and ischemia. These changes can show effects in every part of the eye, particularly in cornea and retina. Though DR is the most familiar cause of blindness in diabetes, other ocular complications also play an important

TABLE 3: **Treatment options for ocular diseases in diabetes.**

Treatment option	Remarks
Blood glucose control	Six classes of OHA are used aiming at tight glycemic control, when these drugs are insufficient, insulin therapy is used
Insulin eye drops	Delivering insulin through ocular route is much easier and less expensive than insulin injections
Blood sugar contact lenses	Measures blood sugar levels in human tears, sensor chip in lens detects sugar level and transmits to external device wirelessly
Subconjuctival glucose sensors	As above, for longer duration monitoring by implants

Continued

Continued

Treatment option	Remarks
Treatment options for corneal diseases	1. Hypertonic drops/tear films 2. Bandage contact lenses 3. Anterior stromal puncture 4. Conreal implants: (a) penetrating keratoplasty (PKP) (b) deep anterior lamellar keratoplasty (DALK) (c) descement stripping automated endothelial keratoplasty (DSEAK)
Anti-steroidal implants	To improve drug delivery to retina, in lieu of intravitreal injections (a) OZURDEX (dexamethasone) (b) RETISERT (fluocinolone) (c) ILUVIEN (fluocinolone)
Antineovascular treatment	VEGF is key signalling molecule that stimulates neovascularisation and is target for treatment of diabetic ocular disease (a) PEGAPTANIB (b) BEVACIZUMAB (c) RANIBIZUMAB (d) AFLIBERCEPT
Nonsteroidal treatment options	Retinal detachment is due to growth of retinal vessels into vitreous that can pull the retina away from RPE cells. (a) Ocriplasmin (b) Flt23k—integrin receptor with RGD (c) RNA
Adipose derived stem cells	Concept of repairing terminally differentiated organ, the eye Single intravitreal injection of stem cells for treatment of DR
Anti-VEGF implants	Biodegradable polymer matrices to deliver anti-VEGF neutralization antibodies e.g. PLGA, PLA, PCM, poly-HEMA. Genetically modified RPE cells through NT 503 ECT implant.

(DR: diabetic retinopathy; VEGF: vascular endothelial growth factor; ECT: encapsulated cell technology; OHA: oral hypoglycemic agents; PCM: polycaprolactone dimethacrylate; PLA: polylactic acid; PLGA: poly lactic-co-glycolic acid; poly-HEMA: poly-hydroxyethyl methacrylate; RPE: retinal pigment epithelial.)

role in causing visual loss in general population, which has not gained much attention as warranted by physicians. Physicians treating diabetes are the first to encounter these complications at an early stage; therefore, the need of the hour is awareness among them and is best for public health strategy in prevention of vision loss.

The primary management of ocular complications in diabetes is prevention; hence, regular screening and timely ophthalmic referrals remain key strategy to reduce the impact of diabetes on vision loss.

REFERENCES

1. International Diabetes Federation. (2017). IFD SEA members. Available from: http://diabetesatlas.org/resources/2017-atlas.html.
2. Vieira-Potter VJ, Karamichos D, Lee DJ. Ocular complications of diabetes and therapeutic approaches. Biomed Res Int. 2016;2016:3801570.
3. Simó R, Carrasco E, García-Ramírez M, et al. Angiogenic and antiangiogenic factors in proliferative diabetic retinopathy. Curr Diabetes Rev. 2006;2(1):71-98.
4. Bandello F, Battaglia Parodi M, Lanzetta P, et al. Drug delivery to the posterior segment of the eye. Dev Ophthalmol. 2010;47:73-110.
5. Krepler K, Biowski R, Schrey S, et al. Cataract surgery in patients with diabetic retinopathy: visual outcome, progression of diabetic retinopathy, and incidence of diabetic macular oedema. Graefes Arch Clin Exp Ophthalmol. 2002;240(9):735-8.
6. Romero-Aroca P, Fernández-Ballart J, Almena-Garcia M, et al. Non-proliferative diabetic retinopathy and macular edema progression after phacoemulsification: prospective study. J Cataract Refract Surg. 2006;32(9):1438-44.
7. Squirrell D, Bhola R, Bush J, et al. A prospective, case controlled study of the natural history of diabetic retinopathy and maculopathy after uncomplicated phacoemulsification cataract surgery in patients with type 2 diabetes. Br J Ophthalmol. 2002;86(5):565-71.
8. Beynat J, Charles A, Soulié M, et al. Combined glaucoma and diabetic retinopathy screening in Burgundy. J Fr Ophtalmol. 2008;31(6):591-6.
9. Osaadon P, Fagan XJ, Lifshitz T, et al. A review of anti-VEGF agents for proliferative diabetic retinopathy. Eye. 2014;28(5):510-20.

Chapter 46

Nondiabetic Kidney Disease in Patients with Type 2 Diabetes Mellitus: When to Suspect?

Anuj Maheshwari, Mudit Khuranna, Anupma Kaul

INTRODUCTION

Type 2 diabetes is the most common cause of chronic kidney disease (CKD) and end-stage renal disease (ESRD) worldwide.[1] Patient with diabetes constitute 25–45% of all patients enrolled in ESRD program.[2] In view of its widespread prevalence and massive health and financial toll the diagnosis and management of diabetic kidney disease (DKD) are of great clinical and social relevance. Diabetic nephropathy occurs in type 1 and type 2 diabetes mellitus, and in other secondary forms of diabetes mellitus, in which the duration is long enough and level of glycemia high enough to result in complications.

Although patients with diabetes mellitus experience diabetic nephropathy, they can also develop other renal disease, pathologically unrelated to diabetes and known as nondiabetic kidney disease (NDKD).[3,4] Precise diagnosis of NDKD has obvious prognostic and therapeutic implications.[5,6]

DEFINITION OF DIABETIC KIDNEY DISEASE

Diabetic kidney disease (also termed "CKD" due to diabetes or diabetic nephropathy) is defined in both type 1 and type 2 diabetes as the presence of persisting severely elevated albuminuria of >300 mg/24-h (or >200 mg/min), or an albumin-to-creatinine ratio (ACR) of >300 mg/g, confirmed in at least two of three samples, with concurrent presence of diabetic retinopathy and absence of signs of other forms of renal disease.[7]

The broader term "kidney disease in diabetes" is used for patients with CKD [impaired renal function: estimated GFR (eGFR) <60 mL/min/1.73 m^2 or proteinuria] regardless of the background. Although impaired renal function with normal albuminuria (ACR <30 mg/g) is prevalent, particularly in elderly diabetic individuals, it is much less likely to progress if albuminuria is not present.[8,9]

THE EVOLVING PRESENTATION OF DKD

Diabetic kidney disease classically involves progressive stages of glomerular hyperfiltration, microalbuminuria, overt proteinuria and a decline in GFR, eventually leading to end-stage kidney disease (ESKD). In recent years there is enough evidence to challenge this concept.[10]

Several large cross-sectional studies have revealed that a large minority of patients with type 2 diabetes and reduced GFR present with normal levels of albuminuria.[11-14] Developing education on microalbuminuria for awareness of kidney and cardiovascular risk in diabetes study (DEMAND study) had concluded that large proportion of diabetic patients with completely normal urinary albumin excretion or microalbuminuria presented with significant kidney dysfunction. About 17% of this international cohort of 6,072 individuals with type 2 diabetes of mean duration of 8 years and eGFR <60 mL/min/1.73 m^2 had normoalbuminuria.[11] In one United States study this number of normoalbuminuric patient was reported to be as high as 33%.[12] The Italian Renal Insufficiency and Cardiovascular Events (RIACE) study of more than 15,000 participants with type 2 diabetes suggested that those with elevated albuminuria displayed the typical microvascular complications, whereas nonalbuminuric individuals with impaired renal function had a more cardiovascular or macrovascular phenotype.[15]

Whether these observations are a result of misdiagnosed DKD in patients who have another kidney disease, the effect of routine use of renin-angiotensin-aldosterone system (RAAS) blockers or other factors remains uncertain. Progressive decline in GFR occurs in normoalbuminuric patients, albeit slowly.[16]

The factors responsible for progressive decline in GFR in non-albuminuric DKD are not known. One possibility is intrarenal vascular disease. However, in a study of patients with type 2 diabetes and GFR below 60 mL/min, intrarenal vascular resistance on renal Doppler scan was elevated to a similar degree in patients with and without proteinuria.[17] Further, research is warranted into normoalbuminuric DKD, for selecting the appropriate treatment and identifying treatment success.

SCREENING FOR DKD

Annual screening of all individuals with diabetes is recommended to detect abnormal and/or changing levels of albuminuria and renal function (i.e. eGFR), so that early renoprotective treatment may be initiated.[18] Early-morning spot urine collections are enough for screening and monitoring and are convenient for the patient.[19] To take account of wide intraday variability (30–40%), two of three spot urine samples within 3–6 months must be elevated to confirm the diagnosis.

The second clinical variable to assess in screening for DKD is eGFR, using creatinine-based formulae such as the chronic kidney disease epidemiology collaboration (CKD-EPI) equation.[20] If untreated, the "natural" course of diabetic nephropathy displays a continuing annual decline in eGFR of between 2 and 20 mL/min/1.73 m^2 (mean 12 mL/min/1.73 m^2), but effective treatment targeting glycemia, control of blood pressure, blocking of the renin-angiotensin system (RAS), reduction of blood cholesterol levels, and improving lifestyle factors can limit progression to 2 to 5 mL/min/1.73 m^2 per year, demonstrating the importance of screening and intervention.[21]

Renal-retinal Relationship in Type 2 Diabetes Mellitus

Patients with nephropathy and type 1 diabetes almost always have other signs of diabetic microvascular disease such as retinopathy and neuropathy.[22,23] But conversely only minorities of patients with advanced retinopathy have histological changes in the glomeruli and increased protein excretion and most have little renal disease as assessed by renal biopsy and protein excretion.[24]

The relationship between diabetic nephropathy and retinopathy is less predictable in type 2 diabetes. Up to 30% of patients with proven diabetic nephropathy have no evidence of retinopathy in type 2 diabetes mellitus.[25,26] In a study by Schwartz et al. a close correlation was observed with the presence of severe retinopathy and Kimmelstiel-Wilson nodules on kidney biopsy.[27] Overall, severe retinopathy was more closely associated with nodules than with mesangial sclerosis.

Type 2 diabetics with marked proteinuria and retinopathy most likely have diabetic nephropathy, while those without retinopathy have a high frequency of nondiabetic glomerular disease.[28] Blockade of RAS slows the progression of diabetic nephropathy and may have similar benefit in diabetic retinopathy i.e. may decrease the odds of retinopathy progression.[29]

Features Differentiating DKD from NDKD

Retrospective studies of kidney biopsy specimens in cohorts of patient with type 2 diabetes mellitus have identify several clinical features that can help to differentiate DKD from other kidney disease.

- *Microscopic hematuria and active urinary sediments*: Urine sediment in diabetic nephropathy is usually bland, but microscopic hematuria can occur.[30,31] In a report from Japan glomerular hematuria was observed in 17% patients of diabetes mellitus and almost half of these had NDKD, but hematuria was also observed in a minority of DKD patients.[30] More severe diabetic nephropathic changes were observed on renal biopsy if hematuria was present.[30]
- Onset of proteinuria <5 years from documented onset of diabetes mellitus is suspicious of NDKD, since latent period of overt diabetic nephropathy is usually 10 to 15 years.[22,23] Time of onset is difficult to ascertain in type 2 diabetes
- *Rapid progression of disease*: Diabetic nephropathy is a slowly progressive disorder and rapid deterioration suggests NDKD
- *Absence of retinopathy*: In patients with type 1 diabetes mellitus, absence of retinopathy almost precludes the diagnosis of DKD, by contrast lack of retinopathy may be seen in patients with type 2 diabetes and underlying diabetic nephropathy.[25]
- *Heavy proteinuria*: Heavy proteinuria may be an indication of NDKD, but many studies suggest otherwise
- Signs and symptoms of other systemic disease[33]
- Significant reduction in GFR (>30%) within 2–3 months of administration of angiotensin converting enzyme (ACE) inhibitors or angiotensin II receptor blocker.[33]

The above-mentioned clinical features can help differentiate DKD from other kidney disease. In patient who have had type 2 diabetes for at least 10 years and who do not present with atypical findings, a tissue diagnosis is not usually necessary, but kidney biopsy is indicated in patients with atypical features (Box 1).

Histological Lesions of NDKD

A wide spectrum of nondiabetic histological lesions are reported in patients with NDKD patients, both glomerular and tubulointerstitial lesions have been reported in patients with type 2 DM (Box 2) which is to be differentiated from diabetic nephropathy (Box 3). Three patterns of histological lesions have been reported in these patients; (a) Isolated NDKD, (b) Pure diabetic glomerulosclerosis, (c) Concurrent NDKD and diabetic glomerulosclerosis.[34-46]

Various studies have found immunoglobulin A (IgA) nephropathy to be the most common cause of isolated NDKD[35,38,40,44-46] in the largest study by Sharma et al. 620 middle-aged patients from the United States with a median time from diagnosis of diabetes of 10 years, 37% of biopsy specimens were consistent with DKD, 36% had NDKD, and 27% showed coexisting DKD and NDKD. The most common causes of NDKD were focal segmental glomerulosclerosis (22%), hypertensive nephrosclerosis (18%), acute tubular necrosis (17%), IgA nephropathy (11%), membranous nephropathy (8%), and pauci-immune glomerulonephritis (7%). Duration of diabetes >12 years was the best predictor of DKD alone (sensitivity 58%, specificity 73%, positive predictive value 56%, negative predictive value 75%).

In a recent Spanish study by Bermejo et al. in 110 patients of type 2 DM - 61.8% showed non diabetic nephropathy, 34.5% showed diabetic nephropathy and 3.6% showed diabetic nephropathy plus non diabetic nephropathy. The most common NDN was IgA nephropathy (13.2%). In this study, the duration of diabetes, proteinuria, increased age and absence of retinopathy were risk factors for DKD.

Several studies have assessed the prevalence, causes and risk factors of NDKD, summarized in Table 1.

Box 1: Indications for renal biopsy in type 2 DM.

- Microhematuria
- Proteinuria with DM duration of <5 years
- Rapidly worsening renal failure
- Nephrotic syndrome/massive proteinuria
- Proteinuria in the absence of diabetic retinopathy
- Features of other systemic disease (like ANCA positivity, low C3 and low C4)

(DM: diabetes mellitus; ANCA: antineutrophil cytoplasmic antibodies.)

Box 2: Common histological lesions in Nondiabetic kidney disease.

Tubulo-interstitial disease
- Acute tubular Necrosis
- Interstitial nephritis

Glomerular causes
- FSGS (Focal Segmental Glomerulosclerosis)
- Hypertensive Nephrosclerosis
- IgA nephropathy
- Membranous Nephropathy
- Paucimmune Glomerulonephritis
- Post Infectious GN
- MPGN (Membrano-proliferative glomerulonephritis)

Approach to a Patient with Type 2 DM and Nephropathy

A simplified approach to diagnose NDKD in a diabetic patient is summarized in Flowchart 1. Kidney biopsy remains the gold standard to diagnose NDKD. Until such time when noninvasive biomarkers for DKD are available, the decision to biopsy a patient will remain a clinical judgment that should take into account, for each individual, the risk of the procedure and the likelihood that if another diagnosis should be uncovered then appropriate treatment will not only be offered but will influence the prognosis.

Future Perspectives

Alternative research has focused on hypothesis-free multiple marker approaches to find new markers or combinations of markers associated with progression of DKD. This has been described as the application of "-omics" platforms, including genomics, transcriptomics, metabolomics and proteomics.[46]

Box 3: Pathological classification of diabetic nephropathy.

- Class I: Isolated glomerular basement membrane thickening
- Class II: Mild (class IIa) or severe (class IIb) mesangial expansion
- Class III:At least one Kimmelstiel-Wilson lesion (nodularintercapillary glomerulosclerosis) is observed on biopsy and there is <50 percent global glomerulosclerosis
- Class IV: Advanced diabetic sclerosis. Thereis >50 percent global glomerulosclerosis thatattributable to diabetic nephropathy

TABLE 1: Important trials studying nondiabetic kidney disease

Author	Year	Number of participants	Most common diagnosis NDKD	NDKD risk factors	Factors that Do not Suggest NDKD
Mak et al.	1997	51	MPGN	Microhematuria	Proteinuria
Wong et al.	2002	68	IgA nephropathy	-	DR
Tone et al.	2005	97	-	-	DR, duration of DM
Chang et al.	2011	119	-		
Bi et al.	2011	220	IgA nephropathy	Microhematuria, Proteinuria	DR
Chong et al.	2012	110	Interstitial nephritis	Microhematuria	DR
Byun et al.	2013	110	IgA nephropathy	-	DR, duration of DM, proteinuria
Wilfred et al.	2013	93	Interstitial Nephritis	Microhematuria	DR
Sharma et al.	2013	620	ATN	-	DM duration
Horvatic et al.	2014	80	MN	-	DR, insulin
Liu et al.	2014	200	IgA nephropathy	Hb value, microhematuria	DM duration, BP reading, HbA1c
Bermejo et al.	2016	110	IgA nephropathy	Creatinine level	Proteinuria, DM duration, DR
Kritmetapak et al.	2017	101	IgA nephropathy	Short duration of DM, microhematuria, low HbA1c	DR

(ATN: acute tubular necrosis; DR: diabetic retinopathy; DM: diabetes mellitus; IgA: immunoglobulin A; HbA1c: glycated hemoglobin; Hb: hemoglobin; MN: membranous nephropathy; MPGN: membranoproliferative glomerulonephritis.)

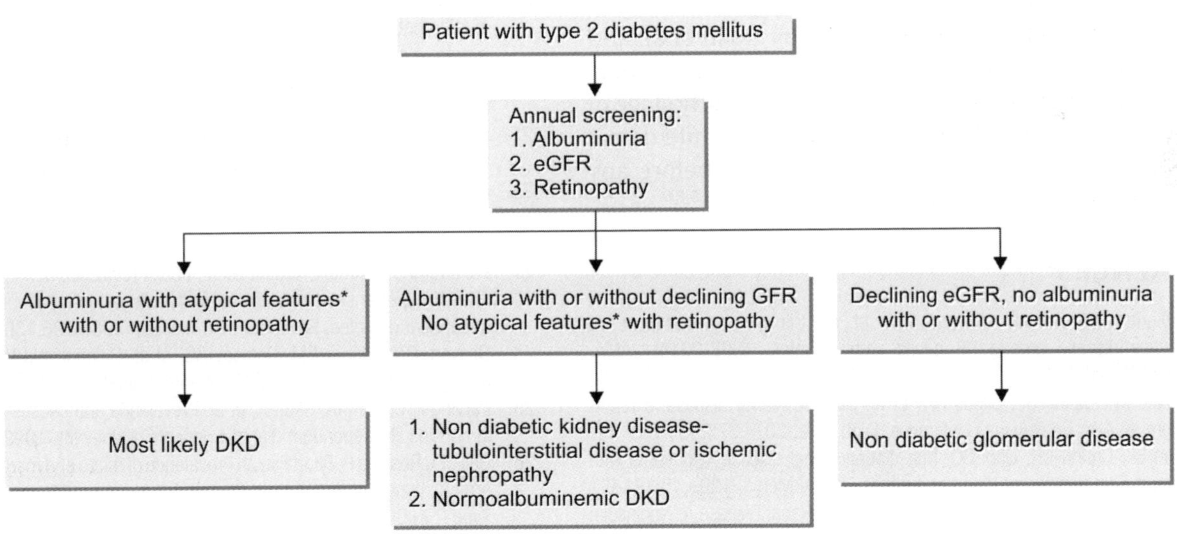

*Diabetes duration <5 years, microhematuria, rapid progression, massive proteinuria, low complements or features of other systemic disease.

(eGFR: estimated glomerular filtration rate; GFR: glomerular filtration rate; DKD: diabetic kidney disease.)

Flowchart 1 Approach to a patient with type 2 DM and nephropathy.

Genetics and Genomics

Familial clustering of DKD has been demonstrated. The ACE insertion or deletion polymorphism was found in some but not all studies to indicate risk of progression of DKD and interacted with the RAS-blocking intervention.[47] Further, the incites are required.

Transcriptomics

Transcriptomics is the study of transcriptosome - the complete set of RNA transcripts that are produced by the genome. Transcriptomic profiles of renal tissue from patients with DKD and animal models of DKD suggested the importance of the Janus kinase-signal transducer and activator of transcription (JAK-STAT) pathway as a key target.[48] A clinical study in diabetes intervening with a JAK-STAT inhibitor subsequently demonstrated reduced albuminuria.[49]

Metabolomics

Pena et al. demonstrated that a small number of metabolites in serum and urine could improve prediction of progression in albuminuria status in type 2 diabetes,[50] while Solini et al. demonstrated in patients with type 2 diabetes that serum but not urine metabolites could improve prediction of progression of albuminuria and decline in GFR.[51]

Urinary Proteomics

A CKD risk score based on a specific pattern of 273 peptides in urine has been developed by Good et al. and is associated with renal pathology and increased renal risk.[52] In cohorts that included patients at an early stage of diabetes with a long follow-up, this classifier could detect patients at renal risk at a mean of 1.5 years before any clinical sign (microalbuminuria) was detected.[53,54]

REFERENCES

1. Afkarian M, Zelnick LR, Hall YN, et al. Clinical manifestations of kidney disease among US adults with diabetes, 1998-2014. JAMA. 2016;316:602-10.
2. Tuttle KR, Bakris GL, Bilous RW, et al. Diabetic kidney disease: a report from an ADA Consensus Conference. Diab Care. 2014;37:2864-83.
3. Lee EY, Chung CH, Choi SO. Non-diabetic renal disease in patients with non-insulin dependent diabetes mellitus. Yonsei Med J. 1999;40:321-6.
4. John GT, Date A, Korula A, et al. Nondiabetic Renal Disease in Noninsulin Dependent Diabetics in a South Indian Hospital. Nephron. 1994;67:441-3.
5. Kleinknecht D, Bennis D, Altman JJ. Increased prevalence of non-diabeticrenal pathology in Type-II diabetes mellitus. Nephrol Dial Transplant. 1992;7:1258-9.
6. Pham TT, Sim JJ, Kujubu DA, et al. Prevalence of non-diabetic renal disease in diabetic patients. Am J Nephrol. 2007;27:322-8.
7. Parving HH, Mauer M, Fioretto P, et al. Diabetic nephropathy. In: Brenner B, ed. Brenner and Rector's The Kidney. Philadelphia, PA. Elsevier. 2012;1:1411-54.
8. Solini A, Penno G, Bonora E, et al. Diverging association of reduced glomerular filtration rate and albuminuria with coronary and noncoronary events in patients with type 2 diabetes: the renal insufficiency and cardiovascular events (RIACE) Italian multicenter study. Diab Care. 2012;35:143-9.
9. Thorn LM, Gordin D, Harjutsalo V, et al. The presence and consequence of nonalbuminuric chronic kidney disease in patients with type 1 diabetes. Diab Care. 2015;38:2128-33.
10. Adler AI, Stevens RJ, Manley SE, et al. UKPDS GROUP: Development and progression of nephropathy in type 2 diabetes: The United Kingdom prospective Diabetes Study (UKPDS 64). Kidney Int. 2003;63:225-32.
11. Dwyer JP, Parving HH, Hunsicker LG, et al. Renal dysfunction in the presence of normoalbuminuria in type 2 diabetes: Results from the DEMAND study. Cardiorenal Med. 2012;2:1-10.
12. Kramer HJ, Nguyen QD, Curhan G, et al. Renal insufficiency in the absence of albuminuria and retinopathy among adults with type 2 diabetes mellitus. JAMA. 2003;289:3273-77.
13. Penno G, Solini A, Bonora E, et al. Renal Insufficiency And Cardiovascular. J Hypertens. 2011 Sep;29(9):1802–9.
14. Penno G. Events (RIACE) Study Group: Clinical significance of non-albuminuric renal impairment in type 2 diabetes. J Hypertens. 2011; 29:1802-09.
15. Thomas MC, Macisaac RJ, Jerums G, et al. Nonalbuminuric renal impairment in type 2 diabetic patients and in the general population (national evaluation of the frequency of renal impairment co-existing with NIDDM [NEFRON] 11). Diab Care. 2009;32:1497-502.
16. Perkins BA, Ficociello LH, Ostrander BE, et al. Microalbuminuria and the risk for early progressive renal function decline in type 1diabetes. J Am Soc Nephrol. 2007;18:1353.
17. MacIsaac RJ, Panagiotopoulos S, McNeil KJ, et al. Is nonalbuminuricrenal insufficiency in type 2 diabetes related to an increase in intrarenal vascular disease? Diab Care. 2006;29:1560.
18. National Kidney Foundation. KDOQI clinical practice guideline for diabetes and CKD: 2012 Update. Am J Kidney Dis. 2012;60:850-86.
19. Lambers Heerspink HJ, Gansevoort RT, Brenner BM, et al. Comparison of different measures of urinary protein excretion for prediction of renal events. J Am Soc Nephrol. 2010;21:1355-60.
20. Levey AS, Stevens LA, Schmid CH, et al. A new equation to estimateglomerular filtration rate. Ann Intern Med. 2009;150:604-12.
21. Altemtam N, Russell J, El Nahas M. A study of natural history of DKD. Nephrol Dial Transplant. 2012;27(5):1847-54.
22. Orchard TJ, Dorman JS, Maser RE, et al. Prevalence of complications in IDDM by sex and duration. Pittsburgh Epidemiology of Diabetes complications Study II. Diabetes. 1990;39:1116.
23. Parving HH, Hommel E, Mathiesen E, et al. Prevalence of microalbuminuria, arterial hypertension, retinopathy and neuropathy inpatients with insulin dependent diabetes. Br Med J (Clin Res Ed). 1988;296:156.
24. Chavers BM, Mauer SM, Ramsay RC, et al. Relationship between retinal and glomerular lesions in IDDM patients. Diabetes. 1994;43:441.
25. Parving HH, Gall MA, Skøtt P, et al. Prevalence and causes of albuminuria in non-insulin-dependent diabetic patients. Kidney Int. 1992;41:758.
26. Gall MA, Rossing P, Skott P et al. Prevalence of micro and macroalbuminuria, arterial hypertension, retinopathy and large vesseldisease in European Type 2 (NIDDM) diabetic patients. Diabetologia. 1991;34:655-61.
27. Schwartz MM, Lewis EJ, Leonard-Martin T, et al. Renal pathology patterns in type II diabetes mellitus: relationship with retinopathy. The Collaborative Study Group. Nephrol Dial Transplant. 1998;13:2547.
28. Huang F, Yang Q, Chen L, et al. Renal pathological change in patients with type 2 diabetes is not always diabetic nephropathy: a report of 52 cases. Clin Nephrol. 2007;67:293.
29. Mauer M, Zinman B, Gardiner R, et al. Renal and retinal effects of enalapril and losartan in type 1 diabetes. N Engl J Med. 2009;361:40.
30. Matsumura N, Hanatani M, Nishino T, et al. The clinico-pathological significance of hematuria in diabetics. Nihon Jinzo Gakkai Shi. 1994;36: 1036.
31. O'Neill WM Jr, Wallin JD, Walker PD. Hematuria and red cell casts intypical diabetic nephropathy. Am J Med. 1983;74:389.

32. Kveder R, Kajtna-Koselj M, Rott T, et al. Nephrotic syndrome in patients with diabetes mellitus is not always associated with diabetic nephropathy. Nephrol Dial Transplant. 2001;16:86-7
33. KDOQI. KDOQI Clinical Practice Guidelines and Clinical Practice Recommendations for Diabetes and Chronic Kidney Disease. Am J Kidney Dis. 2007;49:S12-154.
34. Mak SK, Gwi E, Chan KW, et al. Clinical predictors of non-diabetic renal disease in patients with non-insulin dependent diabetes mellitus. Nephrol Dial Transplant. 1997;12:2588-91.
35. Wong TY, Choi PC, Szeto CC, et al. Renal outcome in type 2 diabetic patients with orwithout coexisting nondiabetic nephropathies. Diab Care. 2002;25:900-5.
36. Tone A, Shikata K, Matsuda M, et al. Clinical features of non-diabetic renal diseases in patients with type 2 diabetes. Diabetes Res Clin Pract. 2005;69:237-42.
37. Chang TI, Park JT, Kim JK, et al. Renal outcomes in patients with type 2 diabetes with or without coexisting non-diabetic renal disease. Diabetes Res Clin Pract. 2011;92:198-204.
38. Bi H, Chen N, Ling G, et al. Nondiabetic renal disease in type 2 diabetic patients: a review of our experience in 220 cases. Ren Fail. 2011;33:26-30.
39. Chong YB, Keng TC, Tan LP, et al. Clinical predictors of non-diabetic renal disease and role of renal biopsy in diabetic patients with renal involvement: a single centre review. Ren Fail. 2012;34:323-8.
40. Byun JM, Lee CH, Lee SR, et al. Renal outcomes and clinical course of nondiabetic renal diseases in patients with type 2 diabetes. Korean J Intern Med. 2013;28:565-72.
41. Wilfred DC, Mysorekar VV, Venkataramana RS, et al. Nondiabetic renal disease in type 2diabetes mellitus patients: a clinicopathological study. J Lab Physicians. 2013;5:94-9.
42. Sharma SG, Bomback AS, Radhakrishnan J, et al. The modern spectrum of renal biopsy findings in patients with diabetes. Clin J Am Soc Nephrol. 2013;8:1718-24.
43. Horvatic I, Tisljar M, Kacinari P, et al. Non-diabetic renal disease in Croatian patients with type 2 diabetes mellitus. Diabetes Res Clin Pract. 2014;104:443-50.
44. Liu M, Chen X, Sun X, et al. Validationof a differential diagnostic model of diabetic nephropathy and non-diabetic renal diseases and the establishment of a new diagnostic model. J Diabetes. 2014;6:519-26.
45. Bermejo S, Soler MJ, Gimeno J, et al. Predictive factors for non-diabetic nephropathy in diabetic patients. The utility of renal biopsy. Nefrologia. 2016;36:535-44.
46. Kritmetapak K, Anutrakulchai S, Pongchaiyakul C, et al. Clinical and pathological characteristics of non-diabetic renal disease in type 2 diabetes patients. Clin Kidney J. 2018;11(3):342-47.
47. Looker HC, Colombo M, Hess S, et al. Biomarkers of rapid chronic kidney disease progression in type 2 diabetes. Kidney Int. 2015;88:888-96.
48. Parving HH, de Zeeuw D, Cooper ME, et al. ACE gene polymorphism andlosartan treatment in type 2 diabetic patients with nephropathy. J Am Soc Nephrol. 2008;19:771-77
49. Komorowsky CV, Brosius FC III, Pennathur S, et al. Perspectives on systems biology applications in diabetic kidney disease. J Cardiovasc Transl Res. 2012;5:491-508.
50. Brosius FC, Tuttle KR, Kretzler M. JAK inhibition in the treatment of diabetic kidney disease. Diabetologia. 2016;59:1624-27.
51. Pena MJ, Lambers Heerspink HJ, Hellemons ME, et al. Urine and plasma metabolites predict the development of diabetic nephropathy in individuals with Type 2 diabetes mellitus. Diabet Med. 2014;31:1138-47.
52. Solini A, Manca ML, Penno G, et al. Prediction of declining renal function and albuminuria in patients with type 2 diabetes by metabolomics. J Clin Endocrinol Metab. 2016;101:696-704.
53. Good DM, Zurbig P, Argiles A, et al. Naturally occurring human urinary peptides for use in diagnosis of chronic kidney disease. Mol Cell Proteomics. 2010;9:2424-37.
54. Zurbig P, Jerums G, Hovind P, et al. Urinary proteomics for early diagnosis in diabetic nephropathy. Diabetes. 2012;61:3304-13.

Chapter 47

Management of Diabetes in Patients on Dialysis

Sanjay Agarwal, Ashwin Pillai

INTRODUCTION

The management of diabetes can be a challenging and nuanced task under the best of circumstances. The coexistence of end-stage renal disease (ESRD), however, tends to complicate matters significantly. A Pan-India survey[1] found that diabetes was the commonest cause of chronic kidney disease (CKD). Furthermore, 48% of cases presented in stage V. Up to 17% of diabetics progress to ESRD within 20 years of diagnosis.[2] From an Indian perspective, with an estimated diabetic population of 72.9 million, this would approximately translate to a staggering 10 million diabetics with ESRD. The economic ramifications of treating such a burgeoning population apart, the true burden of the coexistence of these diseases lies in the increased morbidity and mortality. Studies[3] have clearly shown the inferior survival rates in diabetics. Prominent factors responsible for inferior survival rates are hemodynamic instability, glucose intolerance with wide glycemic excursions and increased rates of hypoglycemia.

QUANTIFYING THE RISK OF HYPOGLYCEMIA

It is estimated that >40% of patients with CKD will experience significant hypoglycemia at some point during therapy.[4] The adapted Diabetes Complications Severity Index (aDCSI) scoring system is a useful tool to predict the risk of developing significant hypoglycemia (Fig. 1).[5] Higher scores were found to correlate with increased rates of hypoglycemia. This could guide the degree of aggression with which one would set glycemic targets.
The aDCSI scoring[6] (Tables 1 and 2).

DERANGEMENTS IN GLUCOSE HOMEOSTASIS

Diabetics on renal replacement therapy are prone to both hypo- and hyperglycemia due to renal dysfunction, uremia and the renal replacement modalities themselves.

Hypoglycemia[4]

The apparent normalization of HbA1c levels and resolution of hyperglycemia, independent of treatment, in diabetics with CKD is often referred to as "Burnt out diabetes". The increased susceptibility to hypoglycemia may broadly be attributed to reduced caloric load and insulin accumulation. Reduced renal gluconeogenesis, CKD-associated anorexia and diabetic gastroparesis all contribute to a reduced glycemic load. A schematic representation of contributory mechanisms is included in Flowchart 1(A).

Hyperglycemia

Renal failure is associated with impaired glycemic tolerance and high fasting sugars even in nondiabetic patients. Although the exact pathogenetic pathways are yet to be fully understood, the following factors are believed to be contributory (Flowchart 1B):

- Uremia,[7,8] it is believed that uremic toxins contribute to insulin resistance, through unclear mechanisms. This theory is supported by noticeable improvements in insulin sensitivity after dialysis, with peritoneal dialysis seeming to confer a greater improvement than hemodialysis (HD)

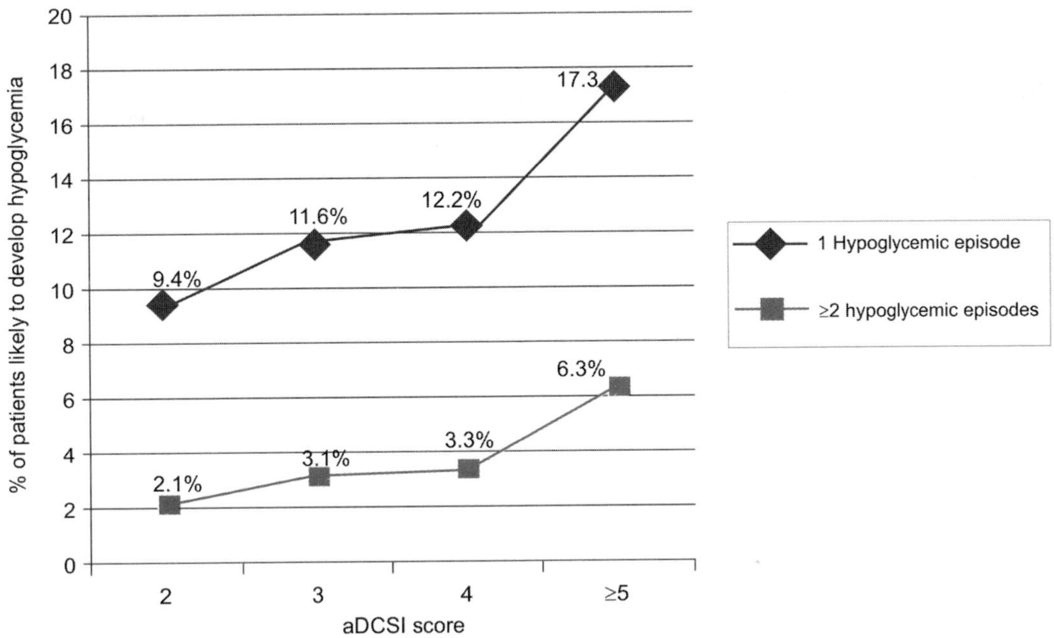

(aDCSI: adapted Diabetes Complications Severity Index.)

Figure 1 Correlation between aDCSI scores and hypoglycemic episodes.[5]

- *Reduced insulin secretion:* Renal failure is associated with decreased levels of activated vitamin D3 and secondary hyperparathyroidism. These metabolic derangements are believed to contribute to reduced insulin secretion. Supplementation of vitamin D3 has been shown to augment insulin production
- *Dialysate fluids:*[9,10] Fluids used in peritoneal dialysis (PD) are carbohydrate-replete, with glucose concentrations ranging from 1,360–3,860 mg/dL. These can provide up to 10–30% of a patient's total caloric requirement and thus contribute to the development of hyperglycemia.

MONITORING OF GLYCEMIC STATUS

Real-time Glycemic Status

Self-monitoring of Blood Glucose

Self-monitoring of blood glucose forms the cornerstone of glycemic monitoring, with a grade 1A recommendation (JBDS-IP 2016). Inter-instrument variability and occasionally inconsistent performance of point-of-care devices are notable limitations. Further, patients with ongoing dialysis are prone to rapid, asymptomatic, glycemic excursions that are likely to be missed with intermittent monitoring. In patients undergoing peritoneal dialysis with icodextrin-containing fluids, readings are likely to be falsely elevated for up to 2 weeks postexposure to such fluids. Despite the absence of clear guidelines regarding the frequency of monitoring, it may be prudent to assess glucose levels hourly in high-risk patients during dialysis sessions.

Continuous Glucose Monitoring

The use of continuous glucose monitoring (CGM) devices (grade 1C – JBDS-IP 2016) continues to increase. Standard devices provide an average of readings every 5 minutes. As such, the likelihood of missing sudden glycemic fluctuations decreases. However, a key limitation with this modality is that it measures glucose levels in interstitial fluid rather than plasma and that there may be a significant temporal delay in reflecting the true plasma level.

Potential Future Avenues

Studies are ongoing to explore the utility of infrared (IR) and near-infrared (NIR) technologies in estimating glucose levels. These optical-based modalities aim to estimate glucose levels in extra-corporeal blood. Potential benefits include real-time estimation of plasma glucose, minimal consumables, and limited need for human

TABLE 1: aDCSI scoring system.

Complications and ICD-9-CM diagnosis	ICD-9-CM code	aDCSI score	
		1	2
Retinopathy			
Diabetic ophthalmologic disease	250.5x	•	
Background retinopathy	362.01	•	
Other retinopathy	362.1	•	
Retinal edema	362.83	•	
CSME	362.53	•	
Other retinal disorders	362.81, 362.82	•	
Proliferative retinopathy	362.02		••
Retinal detachment	361.xx		••
Blindness	369.xx .00-.99		••
Vitreou shemorrhage	379.23		••
Nephropathy			
Diabetic nephropathy	250.4	•	
Acute glomerulonephritis	580	•	
Nephrotic syndrome	58 1	•	
Hypertension, nephrosis	581.81	•	
Chronic glomerulonephritis	582	•	
Nephritis/nephropathy	583	•	
Chronic renal failure	585		••
Renal failure NOS	586		••
Renal insufficiency	593.9		••
Neuropathy			
Diabetic neuropathy	356.9, 250.6	•	
Amyotrophy	358.1	•	
Cranial nerve palsy	951.0, 951.1, 951.3	•	
Mononeuropathy	354.0–355.9	•	
Charcot arthropathy	713.5	•	
Polyneuropathy	357.2	•	

(ICD-9-CM: International Classification of Diseases, Ninth Revision, Clinical Modification; aDCSI: adapted Diabetes Complications Severity Index; (CSME: clinically significant macular edema; NOS: nitric oxide synthase.)

TABLE 2: aDCSI scoring system (continued)

Complications and ICD-9-CM diagnosis	ICD-9-CM code	aDCSI score	
		I	2
Cerebrovascular			
TIA	435	•	
Stroke	431, 433, 434, 436		••
Cardiovascular			
Atherosclerosis	440.xx	•	
Other IHD	411	•	
Angina pectoris	413	•	
Other chronic IHD	414	•	
Myocardial infarction	410		••
Ventricular fibrillation, arrest	427.1, 427.3		••
Atrial fibrillation, arrest	427.4, 427.5		••
Other ASCVD	429.2	•	
Old myocardial infarction	412		••
Heart failure	428		••
Atherosclerosis, severe	440.23, 440.24		••
Aortic aneurysm/dissection	441		••
Peripheral vascular diseases			
Diabetic PVD	250.7	•	
Other aneurysm, LE	442.3	•	
PVD	443.81, 443.9	•	
Fool wound + complication	892.1	•	
Claudication, intermittent	443.9	•	
Embolism/thrombosis (LE)	444.22		••
Gangrene	785.4		••
Gas gangrene	0.4		••
Ulcer of lower limbs	707.1		••
Metabolic			
Ketoacidosis	250.1		••
Hyperosmolar	250.2		••
Other coma	250.3		••

(ICD-9-CM: International Classification of Diseases, Ninth Revision, Clinical Modification; aDCSI: adapted Diabetes Complications Severity Index; IHD: ischemic heart disease; TIA: transient ischemic attack; ASCVD: atherosclerotic cardiovascular disease; PVD: peripheral vascular disease;

intervention. However, trials[11] are ongoing and evidence of clinical utility is still limited.

Monitoring Glycemic Averages

The available modalities, i.e. HbA1c, fructosamine and glycated albumin are each prone to errors owing to certain confounding factors summarized in Table 3.[4]

Despite their individual shortcomings, the above modalities are complementary. HbA1c retains its utility in that it is widely available and that techniques for measurement are well standardized. A method to correct for altered hematocrit is suggested in Table 8. It is also

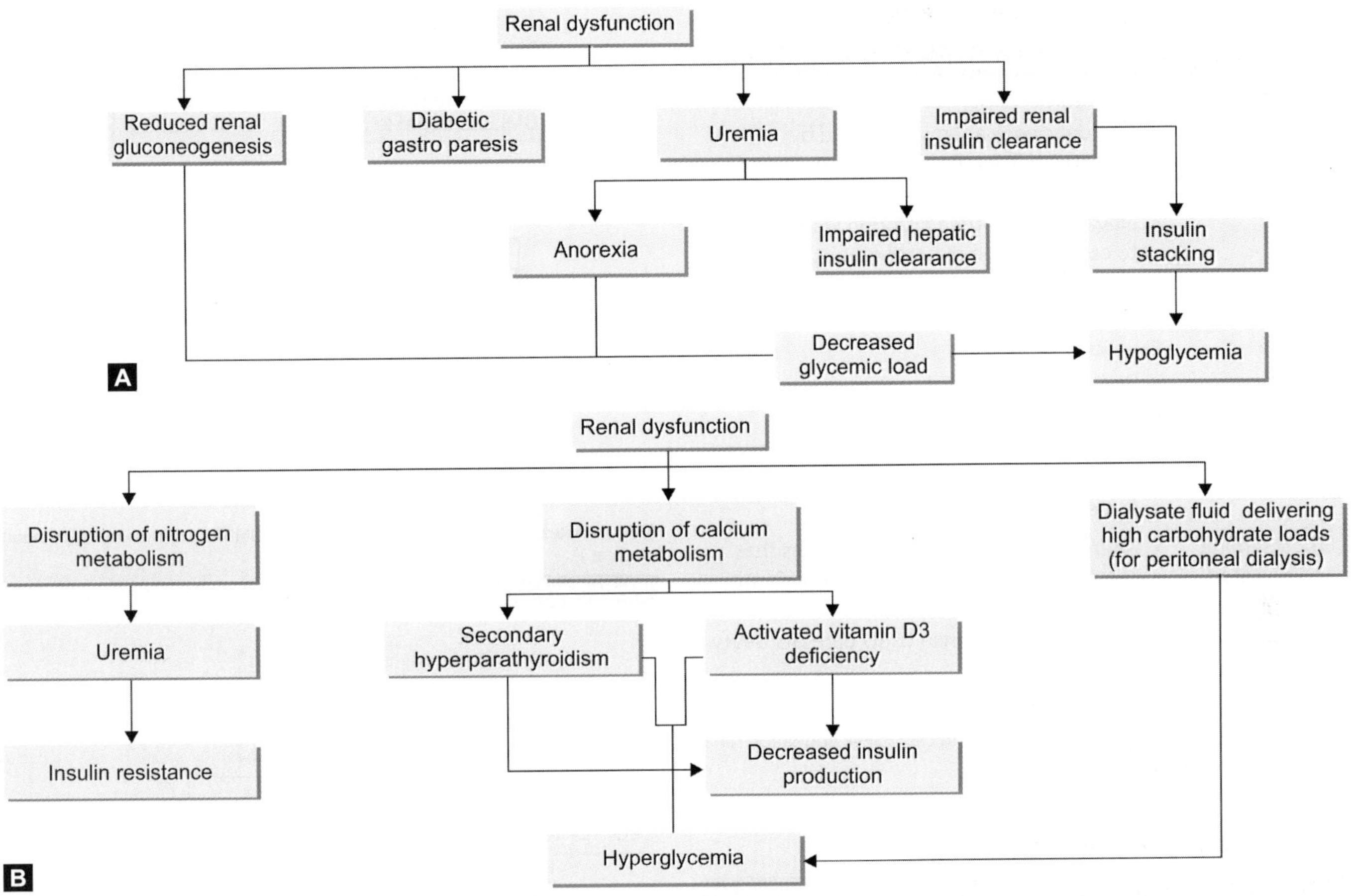

Flowchart 1 Proposed mechanisms of (A) Hypoglycemia; (B) Hyperglycemia.

more reliable in patients on PD. Fructosamine and glycated albumin are preferable in patients with significant erythrocyte disturbances.

GOALS OF TREATMENT

Hemoglobin A1c retains its utility as a yardstick of glycemic control. A U-shaped curve depicts the relationship between HbA1c levels and mortality. Mortality is seen to increase significantly both in burnt-out diabetes (HbA1c <6%) and in patients with higher values.

A meta-analysis of observational studies of diabetics on HD[12] found that maintaining HbA1c between 6.5% and 7.4% was associated with lower mortality than levels ≥8.5%. A cohort study[13] of 54,757 diabetics on HD found that HbA1c levels both <6% and >8% were associated with higher mortality.

It is vital to individualize targets on a risk-benefit basis. Studies suggest that liberal targets, within certain limits, may be superior in terms of reduced mortality. As a rule of thumb, it may be prudent to target HbA1c levels between 7% and 8%.

Therapeutics

Insulin[4,14]

Unlike endogenous insulin, exogenously administered insulin depends on the kidney rather than the liver for excretion. Insulin is freely filtered across the glomerulus, taken up by the proximal tubular epithelium, and enzymatically degraded. Additionally, peritubular endothelial cells also take up and degrade insulin. With a fall in glomerular filtration rate (GFR), the endothelial

TABLE 3: Potential pitfalls of modes of monitoring

Modality	Confounding variables in ESRD/on dialysis
HbA1c	False high: • Iron deficiency anemia (induced by repeated HD) leading to prolongation of RBC survival • Elevated blood-urea nitrogen leads to carbamylation of hemoglobin, and subsequent over-estimation of glycation • Metabolic acidosis False low: • Reduced RBC survival such as due to uremia • Increased rate of proliferation secondary to erythropoietin use • Protein-energy wasting
Fructosamine and glycated albumin	• Altered serum protein states such as that seen in peritoneal dialysis and proteinuria reduces utility • Hyperuricemia seen in ESRD pares its utility further • Malnutrition

(HbA1c: glycated hemoglobin; RBC: red blood cell; ESRD: end-stage renal disease; HD: hemodialysis.)

TABLE 4: Modification of insulin dose as per GFR

GFR (mL/min)	Reduction in insulin dose
10–50	By 25%
<10	By 50%

(GFR: glomerular filtration rate.)

degradation of insulin increases as a compensatory response. However, this can only compensate up to a GFR of 20 mL/min. Below that, insulin begins to accumulate.

Thus, when initiating insulin, patients with type 1 diabetes mellitus should be started at 0.3 IU/kg approximately half the standard dose and patients of type 2 diabetes mellitus should be started at 0.25 IU/kg. Doses may then be titrated based on individual responses and requirements.

Short-acting Insulin Preparations

Among the short-acting insulins, regular insulin is most affected by the alteration in metabolism, leading to a longer half-life and higher serum concentrations. This effect is less prominent with the newer rapid-acting analog insulins which may be preferred.

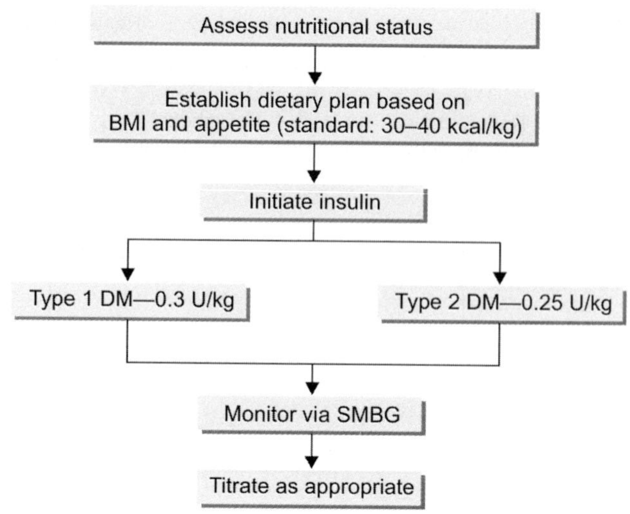

(DM: diabetes mellitus; BMI: body mass index; SMBG: self-monitoring of blood glucose.)

Flowchart 2 Suggested protocol for insulin initiation.

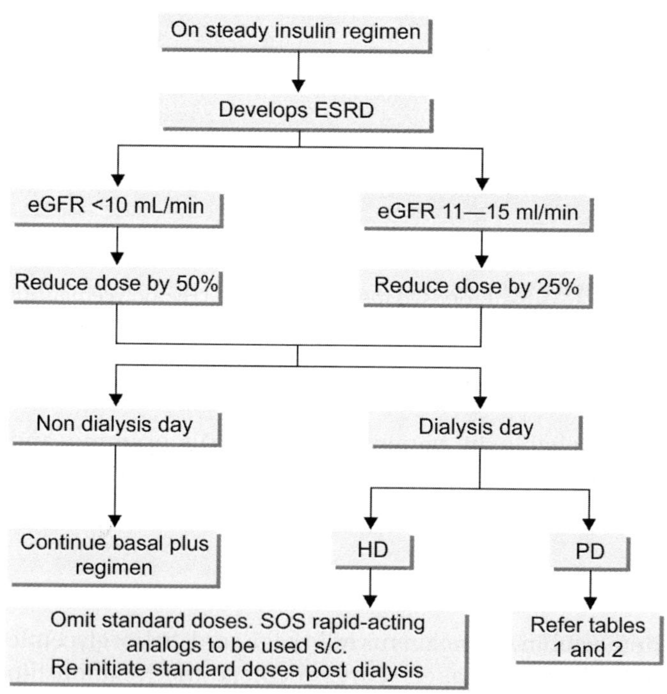

(HD: hemodialysis; PD: peritoneal dialysis; eGFR: estimated glomerular filtration rate; ESRD: end-stage renal disease.)

Flowchart 3 Suggested protocol for insulin use in patients on pre-existing stable regimens.

Long-acting Insulin Preparations

The use of long acting insulin requires caution. Glargine may be preferred over NPH. Detemir, due to its significant albumin-binding, undergoes unpredictable changes in pharmacokinetics and is better avoided. It is recommended to use a basal insulin with two or three doses of rapid acting analogs. No guidelines exist for modifying insulin doses in patients already on treatment. However, as a rule of thumb, the following may be considered (Table 4, Flowcharts 2 and 3).

Following initiation of dialysis, insulin resistance decreases with resolution of uremia. Thus, the insulin requirement is expected to correspondingly decrease. However, resolution of uremic symptoms can also lead to an improvement in appetite leading to an increased caloric load. Thus, careful titration of doses is necessary. The use of intravenous insulin in the ICU setting constitutes an area of special interest. A protocol is suggested in Table 7. Another interesting dynamic is the use of intraperitoneal (IP) insulin in patients on continuous ambulatory peritoneal dialysis (CAPD). IP administration has been found to stimulate endogenous insulin secretion while inhibiting ketogenesis and gluconeogenesis. IP-based regimens require higher doses of insulin to account for losses to both the dialysate fluid, and adsorption on to the plastic delivery systems. Potential drawbacks, however, include risk of bacterial contamination, peritoneal fibroblast proliferation and hepatic subcapsular steatonecrosis.

RECOMMENDATIONS FOR INSULIN USE ON PERITONEAL DIALYSIS

Insulin can be used both sub-cutaneously and intra-peritoneally. Regimens for use vary with the timing of PD and with the dialysate fluid (Tables 5 and 6). Four hourly glucose monitoring and dose adjustments are prudent.

TABLE 5: For Intraperitoneal insulin initiation.[15]

Dialysate fluid dextrose content	Initial Intraperitoneal Dose	
	For preprandial exchanges	For overnight exchanges
1.36% dextrose	0.2 IU/L/kg	0.1 IU/L/kg
3.86% dextrose	0.3 IU/L/kg	0.15 IU/L/kg

TABLE 6: For sub-cutaneous insulin regimens.[15]

For Patients on CAPD	Standard basal-bolus regimens
For overnight exchanges	70/30 or 75/25 premixed insulins at onset of cycle

ORAL HYPOGLYCEMIC AGENTS

Sulfonylureas

In general, sulfonylureas are preferably avoided in patients on dialysis. Glipizide, due to its predominant hepatic metabolism, may still be used cautiously.

Meglitinides

Repaglinide can be safely used in patients on dialysis due to its metabolism being primarily hepatic.

Thiazolidinediones

Pioglitazone can be used safely without dose modification in patients on dialysis. Evidence[17] suggests that the use of pioglitazone may be associated with improved survival in diabetics on dialysis. Care must be taken in cases with significant fluid retention, particularly in patients with incipient heart failure.

Dipeptidyl Peptidase-4 Inhibitors

All dipeptidyl peptidase-4 inhibitors, barring linagliptin, can be used with dose modification in patients with renal impairment. Linagliptin, despite being considered safe without dose adjustment in renal impairment is not recommended in dialysis due to limited studies.

TABLE 7: Recommendations for insulin infusion in AKI/CKD patients in ICU settings on enteral nutrition/parenteral nutrition/intravenous 5% dextrose[17] (algorithm for intravenous regular human insulin (RHI).

Blood glucose (mg/dL)	Intervention
<40	Stop RHI, give 25 g of 50% dextrose (D50W)*
40–70	Stop RHI, give 12.5 g of 50% dextrose (D50W)*
71–125	Decrease RHI by 50%
126–150	Continue the same dose
151–200	Increase RHI by 1 U/h
201–250	Increase RHI by 2 U/h
251–300	Increase RHI by 3 U/h
>300	Increase RHI by 4 U/h and re-evaluate plan

*Once >100 mg/dL, reinstitute RHI at half the previous infusion rate.

(AKI/CKD: acute kidney disease/chronic kidney disease; ICU: intensive care unit.)

Alpha-glucosidase Inhibitors

Acarbose and its metabolites undergo minimal renal excretion. However, due to inadequacy of studies, its use is not recommended in dialysis. Miglitol is renally excreted and is, thus, contraindicated. Biguanides, SGLT-2 inhibitors, amylin analogues and GLP-1 analogs are all to be avoided in dialysis.

Dialysate Fluid Choices

The dialysate fluid in patients undergoing PD is a major source of carbohydrate load. As such, a viable alternative is the use of carbohydrate-sparing dialytic regimens such as:

- *Icodextrin-based fluids:*[19] These fluids result in the carbohydrate absorption equivalent to that of a 2.5% dextrose-based fluid, while providing the ultrafiltration of a 4.5% dextrose-based fluid
- Amino-acid-based dialysate solutions.

Dietary Recommendations (as per the JBDS-IP 2016 Guidelines)

- Target caloric intake of 30–40 kcal/kg of ideal body weight (IBW) unless weight loss is desired and necessary
- Protein intake of 1.1 kg IBW
- Salt intake of <6 g/day
- Low-potassium fruits should be encouraged
- Small, frequent, low-fat, low-fiber diets for patients with gastroparesis
- Foods with high phosphate content should be discouraged.

APPROACH TO HYPERGLYCEMIA AND DIABETIC KETOACIDOSIS

When patients with ESRD develop severe hyperglycemia, there is significant expansion of the intravascular fluid compartment due to increased oncotic pressures. Further, as such patients are usually anuric, this fluid is retained intravascularly. Contrary to what is seen in nonrenally-impaired patients, this result in significant hypervolemia and dilutional hyponatremia. Hyperkalemia may also be a prominent feature. As such, therapy should be directed towards ensuring glycemic control using intravenous insulin infusions, rather than aggressive fluid administration which would be detrimental.

TABLE 8: **Correction factor for HbA1c on dialysis.**[20]

Hematocrit	Treatment with erythropoetin	Adjustment for HbA1c
≥30%	–	HbA1c x 1.14
<30%	Low dose	HbA1c x 1.19
<30%	High dose	HbA1c x 1.38

CONCLUSION

It is evident that the management of diabetes in patients on renal replacement therapies is complex, and fraught with vagaries. Constantly fluctuating insulin resistance, appetites as fickle as the weather, the challenges seem endless. That said, understanding the fundamental principles of each of the variables involved and flexibly adapting would enable us to muzzle this formidable beast. This is, veritably, a case of the devil being in the details.

REFERENCES

1. Rajapurkar MM, John GT, Kirpalani AL, et al. What do we know about chronic kidney disease in India: first report of the Indian CKD registry. BMC Nephrology. 2012;13:10.
2. Ghaderian SB, Hayati F, Shayanpour S, et al. Diabetes and end-stage renal disease; a review article on new concepts.J Renal Inj. Prev. 2015 Jun 1;4(2):28-33 doi: 10.12861/jrip.2015.07.eCollection 2015. Review
3. Beladi-Mousavi SS, Alemzadeh-Ansari MJ, Alemzadeh-Ansari MH, et al. Long-term survival of patients with end-stage renal disease on maintenance hemodialysis: a multicenter study in Iran. Iran J Kidney Dis. 2012;6(6):452-6.
4. Rhee CM, Leung AM, Kovesdy CP, et al. Updates on the management of diabetes in dialysis patients. Semin Dial. 2014;27(2):135-45.
5. Chu YW, Lin HM, Wang JJ, et al. Epidemiology and outcomes of hypoglycemia in patients with advanced diabetic kidney disease on dialysis: A national cohort study. PLoS One. 2017;12(3):e0174601.
6. https://www.researchgate.net/publication/298403868_040420_Fig_aDCSI
7. Mak RH. Impact of end-stage renal disease and dialysis on glycemic control. Semin Dial. 2000;13:4-8.
8. Kovesdy CP, Sharma K, Kalantar-Zadeh K. Glycemic control in diabetic CKD patients: where do we stand? Am J Kidney Dis. 2008;52(4):766-77.
9. Duong U, Mehrotra R, Molnar MZ, et al. Glycemic control and survival in peritoneal dialysis patients with diabetes mellitus. Clin J Am Soc Nephrol. 2011;6(5):1041-8.
10. Grodstein GP, Blumenkrantz MJ, Kopple JD, et al. Glucose absorption during continuous ambulatory peritoneal dialysis. Kidney Int. 1981;19(4): 564-7
11. Roth A, Dornuf F, Klein O, et al. Infrared spectroscopy in hemodialysis: reagent-free monitoring of patient detoxification by infrared spectroscopy. Analytical and Bioanalytical Chemistry. 2012;403(2):391-9.
12. Hill CJ, Maxwell AP, Cardwell CR, et al. Glycated hemoglobin and risk of death in diabetic patients treated with hemodialysis: a meta-analysis. Am J Kidney Dis. 2014;63:84.

13. Ricks J, Molnar MZ, Kovesdy CP, et al. Glycemic control and cardiovascular mortality in hemodialysis patients with diabetes: a 6-year cohort study. Diabetes. 2012;61(3):708-15.
14. Reilly JB, Berns JS. Selection and dosing of medications for management of diabetes in patients with advanced kidney disease. Semin Dial. 2010;23(2):163-8.
15. Beardsworth SF, Ahmad R, Terry E, et al. Intraperitoneal Insulin: A Protocol for Administration During CAPD and Review of Published Protocols. Peritoneal Dialysis International. 1988;8:145-51.
16. Hahr AJ, Molitch ME. Management of diabetes mellitus in patients with chronic kidney disease. Clin Diabetes Endocrinol. 2015;1:2.
17. Dickerson RN. Kidney Injury, Insulin Therapy, and Hypoglycemia. Journal of Pharmacy and Nutrition Sciences. 2012;2:43-9.
18. Lynch KE, Rhee CM, Brunelli SM. Thiazolidinedione use is associated with improved all-cause mortality compared with sulfonylureas among diabetic hemodialysis patients. J Diabetes. 2014;6(4):381-3.
19. Burkart J. Metabolic consequences of peritoneal dialysis. Semin Dial. 2004;17:498.
20. Uzu T, Hatta T, Deji N, Izumiya T, Ueda H, Miyazawa I et al. Target for glycemic control in type 2 diabetic people on hemodialysis: effects of anemia and erythropoietin on hemoglobin A(1c). Ther Apher Dial. 2009; 13:89-94.

Chapter 48

Charcot Foot—Overview and Latest Developments

Hamid Ashraf, Jamal Ahmed

INTRODUCTION

Diabetes mellitus (DM) is now one of the biggest global healthcare problems of the 21st century, 425 million people worldwide suffers from diabetes and this number is projected to increase to 629 million by 2045.[1] Diabetic polyneuropathy (DPN), is one of the most common chronic complication of diabetes and it has a lifetime prevalence of approximately 50%. DPN is associated with increased risk of foot ulceration, amputation and it is the leading cause for disability in patients with diabetes.[2]

One of the devastating complications of DPN, is the development of Charcot foot (CF) or Charcot neuropathic osteoarthropathy (CN). CF is named after the famous French neurologist Jean-Martin Charcot, who in 1868 first described neuroarthropathic changes in patients with tertiary syphilis.[3] William Riley Jordan in 1936, first described the link between DM and painless neuropathic arthropathy of ankle.[4] It is a rare disorder that is characterized by destruction of bones and joints leading to fractures, dislocations, deformities and amputation. CF is commonly associated with DM, alcoholic peripheral neuropathy, tertiary syphilis, leprosy, spinal cord injury, Charcot-Marie-Tooth disease and idiopathic neuropathy. Presently, the number of patients with diabetes is increasing throughout the world, and with improvement in the diabetes care these patients are living longer. This has led to a situation where DM is the most common cause of CN and the numbers of patients with CN are expected to increase. The reported incidence of CF varies widely in literature from 0.1–7.5%, because of different diagnostic criteria used, different inclusion criteria and different duration of diabetes.[5] Recently, a study from India revealed a high prevalence of CA (9.8%) in patients of type 2 DM with DPN.[6]

PATHOGENESIS

Exact pathogenesis of CF is still not clear, and there is no single factor for the development of CF, some patients of DM with neuropathy develop CF while others don't. There is multitude of factors which predisposes an individual to the development of CF. Conventional theories for the development of CF includes, the "neurovascular" theory proposed by Charcot himself which suggest, that because of underlying autonomic neuropathy there is loss of vasoregulation leading to high-flow state and opening of arteriovenous shunting.[3] This increased blood flow leads to greater flux of monocytes and osteoclast, leading to washout of structural calcium from the bone. The net result is localized osteopenia, and continued weight bearing leads to deformity. The "neurotraumatic" theory proposed by Volkmann and Virchow, suggested that repeated microtrauma to the foot, in absence of protective sensation causes an unregulated inflammatory cascade, resulting in the collapse and joint destruction observed in CN.[7] Most likely CF occurs because of combination of these factors. In presence of sensory neuropathy patients don't perceive the pain and repetitive microtrauma continues unabated. Motor neuropathy changes the pressure dynamics of the foot leading to abnormal plantar pressure and deformity. Autonomic neuropathy by increasing the blood, leads to local osteopenia. When fracture occurs in normal individuals, it leads to the release of proinflammatory cytokines including tumor necrosis factor-α (TNF-α), interleukin-1β (IL-1β), and IL-6, which in turn lead to enhanced expression of receptor activator of nuclear factor-kβ ligand (RANKL).[8] This proinflammatory cytokine profile favors the maturation and activation of osteoclast from the precursor cells. As the fracture will be accompanied by pain, and this leads to splinting of the bone, and the proinflammatory state will resolve with time. In contrast to normal person, when an individual with severe DPN develops an acute Charcot foot, loss of pain sensation, allows for continuous ambulation with repetitive trauma. This leads to uninterrupted proinflammatory state, causing persistent local osteolysis.[9] All these factors lead to bone destruction, fracture, dislocation at the foot and ankle joint.

Hyperglycemia leads to abnormal nonenzymatic glycation of collagen, and they reacts with the amino groups on other protein molecules, leading to formation of advanced glycation end products (AGEs). Binding of AGEs to their receptor (RAGE), inhibit differentiation of human mesenchymal stem cells.[10] They stimulate apoptosis of osteoblasts, also leads to augmented osteoclastogenesis via the RANKL/NF-κβ pathway. All these factors along with neuropathy help in perpetuating the inflammation and destruction.

Calcitonin gene-related peptide (CGRP), secreted normally from the nerve terminals, has been reported to be important for the maintenance of the integrity of joint capsules, and it also inhibits the synthesis of RANKL. Any decline in CGRP from the nerve terminals will be detrimental for the bone health and joint stability. Both peripheral and autonomic neuropathy has been found to be associated with reduced CGRP release, leading to uninterrupted RANKL activity.[11]

CLINICAL PRESENTATION

A high index of suspicion is needed for the diagnosis of CF in acute stages. Patients typically present in the sixth or seventh decade. CF can have both acute and chronic presentation. The initial manifestations of acute CF have includes pain which can be mild to moderate in intensity, swelling of the affected limb, increased local temperature and erythema.[12] Temperature difference between the two limbs is ≥2°C, which can be measured by infrared thermometer. Pain is less when compared to cellulitis.

The differential diagnosis at this stage includes cellulitis, deep vein thrombosis, or acute gout (Table 1). Systemic signs of inflammation like fever and tachycardia are absent, peripheral pulses are preserved in the affected limb or it can be bounding also.[13] Limb elevation leads to significant decline in the oedema and erythema. X-ray is not helpful at this stage as they may not show any changes, while magnetic resonance imaging can be helpful at an early stage of disease.[14] If proper diagnosis and treatment is not made at this stage, it can leads to additional destruction of bone and subsequent in permanent damage.

TABLE 1: Difference between cellulitis and acute Charcot foot.

Features	Cellulitis	Acute Charcot foot
Age	Any	5–7th decade
History of diabetes	+/–	+
Neuropathy	+/–	+
Deformity	–	+/–
Pedal pulses	Normal/reduced	Bounding
Pain	+++	+/–
Fever/tachycardia	+	–
Pus discharge	+/–	–
WBC Count	↑	Normal
MRI (low intensity on T1 and T2 hyperintensity)	Absent	present
Calcaneal BMD	Normal	Reduced

(BMD: bone mineral density; MRI: magnetic resonance imaging; WBC: white blood cells.)

After resolution of acute stage patients lands in chronic CF in which patients have established residual deformity. Rocker bottom deformity is the hallmark of chronic CF, and it develops secondary to collapse of mid foot arch. Clinical features at this stage are secondary to neurological, vascular, musculoskeletal and radiographic abnormalities.[15] All the patients of CF have established neuropathy, which can be diagnosed by five simple clinical tests, ideally two of these should be regularly performed during the screening exam-normally the 10 g monofilament and one other test. Other tests include, vibration test using 128 Hz tuning fork, ankle reflex, pinprick sensation and biothesiometry. Though patients have insensate foot, but up to 50% gives history of preceding trauma, which is often trivial.[16] Deformities in CF can be varying from trivial to grossly evident deformity (Fig. 1). Deformities result in abnormal high pressure areas on the weight bearing sites of the plantar surface, making it susceptible to ulceration.

Involvement in CF is unilateral in most of the cases, but bilateral presentation has also been reported in 9–75% of cases. An Indian study revealed bilateral presentation in 16% of cases.[6] Most commonly affected site is the midfoot in the literature, while an Indian study revealed midfoot involvement in 43% of patients. If sinus tract is present or probe test is positive than osteomyelitis should be strongly suspected.[13] The differences between chronic charcot foot and osteomyelitis has been enumerated in table 2.

IMAGING OF CHARCOT FOOT

Plain radiography (PR) is the primary imaging modality in the initial evaluation of CN, as they are freely available and economical, and provides information on bone density, joint structure and alignment. Anteroposterior, lateral and oblique nonweight–bearing X–rays of the foot and ankle should be taken. Localized demineralization is the earliest finding of CF on PR. Metatarsal head flattening is the first sign of diabetic neuroarthropathy on X-ray. Subchondral or periarticular changes in the midfoot with involvement of multiple joints without soft tissue involvement is highly suggestive of CF. Minor changes of CF like occult fractures and edema of marrow can't be visualized on PR. X-ray has got sensitivity and specificity rates of around 50% in early phase of CF.[16] Eichenholtz classification is based on radiography which divides CF into three stages: bone dissolution (stage I), bone coalescence (stage II) and bone remodeling (stage III) (Table 3). In chronic stages of CF, PR can reveal, decreased calcaneal inclination angle, destruction of talo-first metatarsal angle (Fig. 2). Calcification of intima media of arteries is common.[12] As the sensitivity and specificity of PR is low in acute CF, magnetic resonance imaging (MRI) is useful in initial stage of CF. MRI provides excellent details about the anatomy and pathology in both soft tissue and bone. MRI has a high sensitivity and specificity for osteomyelitis, and now it is the first line investigation for evaluation of the complicated foot in diabetic patients.[17] MRI is not required when the findings of CF are obvious on X-rays. In the early stages of CF, MRI reveals soft tissue edema, disruption of Lisfranc ligament, soft tissue edemas, joint effusions, subchondral bone marrow edema of involved. The specific feature of bone marrow edema on MR images is low signal intensity on T1W images and high signal intensity on T2W images. Differential signal enhancement of bone-marrow is characteristically present in the subchondral region.[17]

A number of different radionuclide studies are being used in CF. Triple phase technetium-99m methylene diphosphonate (Tc-99m MDP) is highly sensitive but

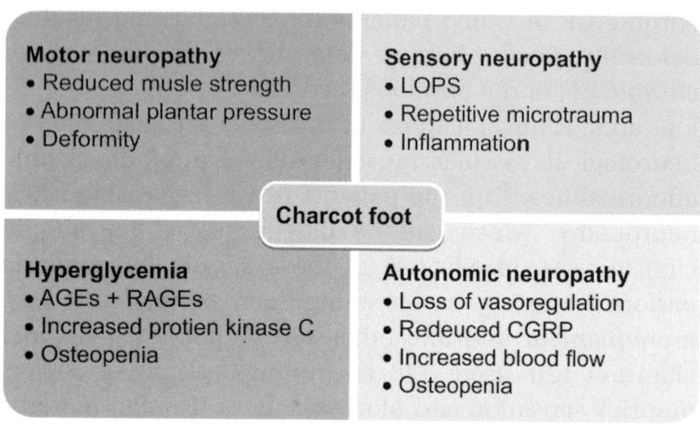

(AGEs: advanced glycation end products; CGRP: calcitonin gene-related peptide; LOPS: loss of protective sensation; RAGEs: receptor of advanced glycation end products.)

Figure 1 Pathogenesis of Charcot foot.

TABLE 3: **Classification of Charcot foot.**

Eichenholtz classification	Sanders and Frykberg
Natural history and radiological	**Anatomical**
Stage I: Developmental; erythema, edema and elevated temperature	Pattern 1: Phalanges, interphalangeal and the metatarsophalangeal joints
Stage II: Coalescence ; active period of the disease process when bony destruction and deformity occur	Pattern 2: Tarsometatarsal
Stage III: Stage of reconstruction; commencing when the destructive process "burns out" and the bone consolidates with the resulting deformity	Pattern 3: Cuneonavicular, talonavicular and calcaneocuboid articulations
	Pattern 4: Talocrural joint
	Pattern 5: Involves the posterior calcaneus

TABLE 2: **Difference between osteomyelitis and chronic Charcot foot.**

Features	Osteomyelitis	Chronic Charcot foot
Location	Toes and metatarsal heads	Commonly midfoot
Distribution	Multiple bones/joints	Focal
Deformity	Absent	Present
Soft tissue changes	Inflamed, sinus tracts, abscess formation	Subcutaneous tissue edema
Bone marrow edema	Periarticular	Around ulcers, fistula tracts

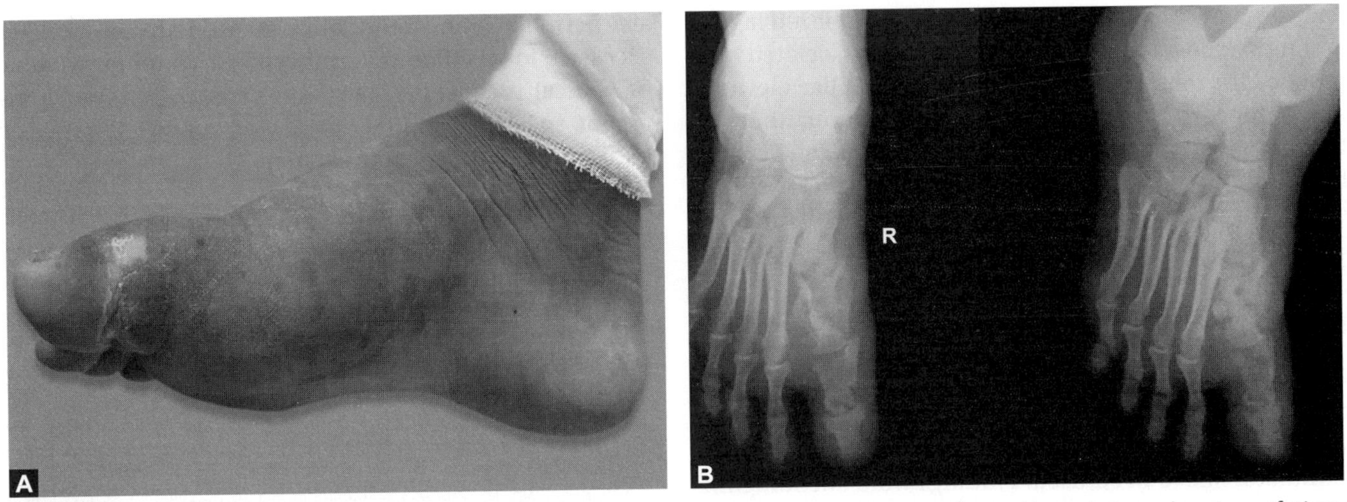

Figure 2 (A) Swelling and midfoot deformity in Charcot foot; (B) X-ray right foot anteroposterior and lateral views showing soft tissue swelling and destruction of bones. ***(For color version, see Plate 3)***

has got a low specificity for the detection of osteomyelitis (95–100% and 25–38%, respectively). As white blood cells (WBC) is recruited at the site of infection labeled white cell scans (In-WBC) are very accurate in the diagnosis of osteomyelitis with an accuracy level of 80–90%. In patient with high suspicion of osteomyelitis a combination of three phase Tc-99m MDP and In-WBC scans, can be performed. Nowadays positron emission tomography scanning has been utilized to differentiate Charcot foot from osteomyelitis. Few studies have reported better sensitivity and specificity than MRI, but still it remains investigational at this moment.[18]

MANAGEMENT OF THE CHARCOT FOOT

The aim of treatment of CF is to provide a plantigrade, steady foot which will fit into a shoe and to also prevent repeated ulceration. Factors that influence the treatment of CF includes phase of the disease, presence or absence of deformity, infection and comorbidities. The goals should be individualized depending upon the severity of the disease, and they should be realistic. Treatment of CF can be variable from modified foot wears to amputation of the limb.[17]

Medical Management

Medical management of CF includes offloading the foot, treating bony abnormalities and averting further foot fractures. Medical management is usually reserved for the acute stages of CF. These treatments are usually based on expert opinions because of lack of randomized control trials.

Offloading

Offloading is the most important part of management in acute CF. offloading could halt the progression to deformity. Total contact cast (TCC) is regarded as the gold standard for offloading. TCC decrease the mechanical pressure, reduces the inflammation and edema, thereby containing the bone and joint destruction. TCC should cover the whole foot including the ankle joint, with good cushion with cotton based bandages over bony prominence to prevent ulceration. The cast should be changed at regular interval of 3–7 days, and patients should be closely monitored.[19] The goal of TCC is to preserve a plantigrade foot, so that weight bearing in a shoe or brace can be achieved. Usually there is significant decline in the edema within the first few weeks of treatment. Repeated cast change is necessary, to avoid "pistoning" with declining edma. Weight bearing on the affected limb should be avoided, for this patient can use crutches or wheelchair. The casting is required till the edema has resolved and the temperature difference between the two limbs is <2°C. The average time of cast application in chronic CF with ulceration is 5 weeks, with progression to therapeutic footwear at 3 months. An alternative device for offloading the cute active stage of CF is a prefabricated removable walker braces. The advantage is the low cost in comparison to TCC, but it has problem of inability to fit severe deformities and possibly incomplete compliance.[17]

Antiresorptive Therapy

Bisphosphonate is an attractive treatment modality for acute CF, because of the increased osteoclastic activity.

Pamidronate has been most commonly utilized agent among bisphosphonates. Its use have been associated with reduced the markers of Charcot foot activity, like elevated skin temperature, edema and pain. However, there is lack of robust evidence in the literature. They can be used beside immobilization and offloading. The adverse effects of bisphosphonates and their contraindications for use should be kept in mind before prescribing them.[20]

Bone Growth Stimulation

In acute CF ultrasonic bone stimulation has been used for the healing of new fractures. In CF patients treated with arthrodesis, direct current electrical bone growth stimulators have been used. Findings were encouraging, but more evidence is required prior to its routine use, at this stage it is at best an adjuvant to the established treatment.[17]

Surgical Treatment

Surgical treatment of CF is primarily dependent on the expert opinion of treating surgeon. Surgery has been utilized for removal of infected bone in osteomyelitis, correction of prominent bony points so as to accommodate the foot in the therapeutic footwear. This decision is primarily based on expert opinion and small, uncontrolled retrospective case series. Prior to surgical treatment patient's other comorbidities, compliance, location and severity of deformity, infection or joint instability should be considered. The surgical procedure includes, release and augmentation of achilles tendon, plantar osteotomy, debridement of the osseous points, arthrodesis, and open reduction with various methods of internal fixation with or without external fixation. Currently, we don't have enough evidence for the superiority of any procedure. Now there is a group which has been advising earlier surgical correction of deformity and arthrodesis, based on the notion that it will lead to an improved patient-perceived quality of life.[21]

CONCLUSION

Charcot osteoarthropathy of the foot is not uncommon in patients with severe diabetic neuropathy. With increasing incidence of diabetes and aging population the burden of Charcot foot will increase. Delayed diagnosis and improper treatment can lead to amputation of the affected limb. Its main pathophysiological mechanisms are peripheral and autonomic neuropathy, as well as excessive local inflammatory response to minor trauma. In clinical practice, a high level of suspicion, including urgent specialist referral when appropriate, is required for timely diagnosis and treatment.

REFERENCES

1. IDF Atlas 2017. Available from https://www.idf.org/e-library/epidemiology-research/diabetes-atlas.html [Accessed on 20th September 2018].
2. Tesfaye S, Selvarajah D: Advances in the epidemiology, pathogenesis and management of diabetic peripheral neuropathy. Diabetes Metab Res Rev. 2012;28(Suppl 1):8-14.
3. Charcot JM. Sur quelques arthropathies qui paraiise d'ependre d' une l'esion du cerveau ou de la mouelle ´epini`ere. Arch Physiol Norm Pathol. 1868;1:161-78.
4. Jordan WR. Neuritic manifestations in diabetes mellitus. Arch Intern Med. 1936;57:307-66.
5. Rajbhandari SM, Jenkins RC, Davies C, Tesfaye S. Charcot neuroarthropathy in diabetes mellitus. Diabetologia. 2002;45:1085-96.
6. Salini D, Harish K, Minnie P, et al. Indian J Endocrinol Metab. 2018;22:107-11.
7. Ramanujam CL, Zgonis T. The Diabetic Charcot Foot from 1936 to 2016: Eighty Years Later and Still Growing. Clin Podiatr Med Surg. 2017;34:1-8.
8. Jeffcoate WJ, Game F, Cavanagh PR. The role of proinflammatory cytokines in the cause of neuropathic osteoarthropathy (acute Charcot foot) in diabetes. Lancet. 2005;366:2058-61.
9. Larson SA, Burns PR. The pathogenesis of Charcot neuroarthropathy: current concepts. Diabet Foot Ankle. 2012;3.
10. Katayama Y, Akatsu T, Yamamoto M, et al. Role of nonenzymatic glycosylation of type I collagen in diabetic osteopenia. J Bone Miner Res. 1996;11:931-37.
11. Jeffcoate WJ, Game FL. New theories on the causes of the Charcot foot in diabetes. In The Diabetic Charcot Foot: Principles and Management. Frykberg RG, Ed. Brooklandville, MD, Data Trace Publishing Company, 2010;29-44.
12. Eichenholtz SN. Charcot Joints. Springfield, IL, Charles C. Thomas, 1966.
13. Cofield RH, Morrison MJ, Beabout JW. Diabetic neuroarthropathy in the foot: patient characteristics and patterns of radiographic change. Foot Ankle. 1983;4:15-22.
14. Morrison WB, Ledermann HP. Work-up of the diabetic foot. Radiol Clin North Am. 2002;40:1171-92.
15. Caputo GM, Ulbrecht J, Cavanagh PR, et al. The Charcot foot in diabetes: six key points. Am Fam Physician. 1998;57:2705-10.
16. Morrison WB, Ledermann HP. Work-up of the diabetic foot. Radiol Clin North Am. 2002;40:1171-92
17. Rogers LC, Frykberg R G, Armstrong G, Boulton AJM, Edmonds M, Ha Van G.et al. The Charcot Foot in Diabetes. Diabetes Care. 2011;34(9):2123-29
18. Keidar Z, Militianu D, Melamed E, et al. The diabetic foot: initial experience with 18F-FDG PET/CT.J Nucl Med. 2005;46:444-9.
19. Armstrong DG, Lavery LA. Monitoring healing of acute Charcot's arthropathy with infrared dermal thermometry. J Rehabil Res Dev. 1997;34:317-21.
20. Harsh Durgia, Sahoo J, kamlanathan S, et al. Role of bisphosphonates in the management of acute Charcot foot. World J Diabetes. 2018;9(7):115-26.
21. Dhawan V, Spratt KF, Pinzur MS, et al. Reliability of AOFAS diabetic foot questionnaire in Charcot arthropathy: stability, internal consistency, and measurable difference. Foot Ankle Int. 2005;26:717-31.

Chapter 49

Rheumatological Complications in Diabetes

Harpreet Singh, Gaikwad Mahesh, Manoj Yadav

INTRODUCTION

Musculoskeletal complications are common disorders of the endocrine diseases especially diabetes. Diabetes spares no component—muscle, bone, and connective tissue of musculoskeletal system. Improved life expectancy in diabetes has increased the prevalence and clinical importance of the musculoskeletal complications associated with diabetes.

Diabetes may affect musculoskeletal system in a variety of clinical presentation (Table 1).[1-14]

The causative factor for rheumatological manifestations in diabetes may be due to impaired calcium metabolism, increased bone resorption, impaired parathyroid hormone function, and oxidative stress leading to low bone turnover status and also increased fat accumulation in muscle.[15] The collagen glycosylation, abnormal crosslinking of collagen, increased collagen hydration, microangiopathy, and neuropathy may result in the rheumatological manifestation with disease. The hands are most common site of involvement; other involved sites are shoulder, feet, muscle, and skeleton.

TABLE 1: Prevalence of musculoskeletal disorders in patients with or without diabetes.

Musculoskeletal disorder	With diabetes	Without diabetes
Adhesive capsulitis (frozen shoulder)[1-4]	11–30%	2–10%
Limited joint mobility[5-7]	8–50%	0–26%
Dupuytren's contracture[8-11]	20–63%	13%
Carpal tunnel syndrome[12,13]	11–16%	125/100,000*
Flexor tenosynovitis[14]	11%	<1%
Diffuse idiopathic skeletal hyperostosis[6,11]	13–49%	1.6–13%

*Incidence estimate over 5 years.

HAND

Diabetic HAND syndromes are reported more frequently in diabetes mellitus (DM) (type 1 >type 2) than the general population and is associated with increased duration of diabetes.[8]

In diabetic sclerodactyly, there is thickening and waxiness of skin most marked on the dorsum of fingers, and is often associated with limited joint mobility. Due to limited joint mobility, it is also known as diabetic stiff hand syndrome/diabetic cheiroarthropathy. It is more prevalent in patients with diabetic neuropathy.[12,13] Skin changes resembles those as of scleroderma but other features such as Raynaud's phenomenon and ulcerations calcinosis are absent as are autoantibodies. There are flexion deformities of the metacarpophalangeal and interphalangeal joints along with paresthesias/slight pain (Prayer's sign). The symptoms progress slowly and pain is aggravated by movement of the hands. Aim of therapy should be to improve glycemic control and hand care (including physiotherapy).

Dupuytren's contracture is the subcutaneous fibrosis of palmar aponeurosis of the hands leading to palmar/digital thickening, tethering, and contracture of the hands (especially involving the ring and middle finger). Limited joint mobility and Dupuytren's contracture are commonly found in the same patient in diabetes.[8,13,14]

The contractures are generally milder in diabetics and the prevalence increases with advancing age. Management should aim at optimizing glycemic control, physiotherapy, hand exercises, and surgery, if required.

Carpal tunnel syndrome (CTS) is characterized by abnormal sensations in the median nerve distribution in the hand and so involves the cutaneous area of the thumb, index, middle, and lateral half of the ring fingers. The symptoms are due to compression of the median nerve within the carpal tunnel or associated diabetic neuropathy or a combination of both.[16] The symptoms tend to be worse at night. Associations between CTS with age and the duration of diabetes have been suggested. Use of simple analgesics, splints, and possibly local steroid injections in the milder cases may help relieving the symptoms. Of those failing conservative measures surgery may be needed.

Flexor tenosynovitis present with sign and symptoms caused by fibrous tissue proliferation in the tendon sheath leading to limitation of the normal movement of the tendon; this leads to locking in flexion or extension with an audible crepitus during finger movement. This may also be associated with impaired glucose tolerance. A corticosteroid injection into the symptomatic flexor tendon sheath or surgical decompression (in severe cases) may be curative.

Reflex sympathetic dystrophy (regional pain syndrome type 1) is also referred as Sudeck's atrophy. This is associated with pain (localized or diffuse), swelling, trophic changes, and vasomotor disturbance resulting in impaired mobility in the involved hand.[17] It may also be associated with pain or limitation of the ipsilateral shoulder (shoulder hand syndrome). The presentation may be spontaneous or after a minimum trauma (postsurgery or fracture). Concurrent medical conditions including hyperthyroidism, hyperparathyroidism, and type 4 hyperlipidemia may predispose to reflex sympathetic dystrophy. The transcutaneous nerve stimulation (TENS) in early stages may help in relieving the symptoms supported by analgesics and physiotherapy. Bisphosphonates, calcitonin, oral corticosteroids (despite hyperglycemia), and sympathetic ganglion blocks or sympatholytic drugs have been reported to be useful.

SHOULDER

Frozen shoulder is a commonly disabling musculoskeletal problem associated with diabetes. It is also referred as adhesive capsulitis. The disablement may be due to shoulder periarthritis or obliterative bursitis. The thickened joint capsule is closely adherent to the humeral head, resulting in considerable reduction in the volume of the glenohumeral joint. There is progressive, painful restriction of shoulder movement, especially external rotation and abduction.[1] Diabetes generally have bilateral presentation and tends to have disease at young age. Intra-articular corticosteroid injections may be given in the painful early disease though regular analgesics help in relieving the symptoms. Regular graded physiotherapy program should be maintained especially after the pain relief.

FOOT

Charcot arthropathy is seen mostly in aged diabetic with prolonged history of diabetic neuropathy. Patient remains unaware of the underlying changes in foot structure due to poor sensations and hence continues to mobilize leading to painless progressive joint destruction. The weight-bearing joints are most commonly affected. The associated warmth and erythema may mimic osteomyelitis or septic arthritis. Regular foot care and review for impaired sensation helps in decreasing the associated morbidity. Orthotics and crutches for the relief of pressure during ambulation on affected joint may be used.[18] Surgery is indicated in those developing complicated fracture.

MUSCLE

Diabetic amyotrophy manifests as pain in large muscle groups. There is diffuse muscle weakness and wasting of proximal lower limb muscle. The shoulder girdle is less affected. It usually occurs in older men with type 2 diabetes, and is often associated with weight loss. Glycemic control and physiotherapy may help in reducing the progression of the disease. Most cases improve, but the improvement is gradual and often incomplete.[19]

Other uncommon muscular complications are:

- Diabetic muscle ischemia seen in chronic diabetic with microvascular complications. It often presents with acute pain and swelling of muscle which generally subsides with conservative treatment
- Diabetic muscle infarction (DMI) or diabetic myonecrosis has an abrupt clinical onset with severe thigh or calf pain followed by swelling that evolve over days or weeks, in the absence of leukocytosis and fever. It generally improves with conservative treatment. Surgical management is required if compartment syndrome develops

- *Infectious myositis*: Diabetic patients are vulnerable to infectious pyomyositis because of underlying immune dysfunction, a disease that results from the hematogenous spread of bacteria to muscle. It improves with good glycemic control and broad-spectrum antibiotics.

BONE

Diffuse idiopathic skeletal hyperostosis, also known as Forestier's disease, is characterized by new bone formation. Mechanism of causation of new bone is the prolonged insulin-like growth factors occurring in diabetic patients, which stimulates new bone growth. Obesity and diabetes seem to have independent contributions to the development of the condition.[10] It has higher prevalence in type 1 compared with type 2 diabetes (ratio 3:1).[15] It tends to involve spine, skull, pelvis, ligaments, or as large bony spurs at the heel or elbow. This may result in pain and stiffness of the affected part. Radiologically, diffuse idiopathic skeletal hyperostosis typically shows a line of calcification in the right anterolateral position of thoracic spine with preservation of disk space since new bone appears to "flow" to the next and is more prominent on the right side of thoracic vertebrae. Management consists of education, diabetic control, and physiotherapy.

MISCELLANEOUS

Osteoporosis is detectable early in the disease and is associated with increased incidence of fracture rates due to increase in bone porosity. The bone marrow density and bone mass are reduced in both DM, though the mechanism is not clear. Oral hypoglycemic agents (OHAs) especially pioglitazone may increase the risk for fracture in postmenopausal women.

CONCLUSION

Exercise is considered to be one of the three cornerstones of optimal diabetes treatment, along with diet and pharmacotherapy. Exercise training in patients with type 2 diabetes is valuable in its own right rather than being just an avenue to weight loss. Physical activity is therefore an attractive treatment for patients with diabetes given its low cost, nonpharmacological nature, and additional aerobic and cardiovascular benefits.

Based on the above discussion, people with DM are at increased risk for bone and muscle diseases. Poor glycemic control for longer duration causes higher complications rates and worsening of several musculoskeletal/rheumatological conditions. So early diagnosis, sensible pharmacotherapy, diet, and regular monitored physiotherapy program aid in maintaining the glycemic control and minimizing musculoskeletal problems and related morbidities.

REFERENCES

1. Reeves B. The natural history of the frozen shoulder syndrome. Scand J Rheumatol. 1975;4:193-6.
2. Forgács SS. Endocrine and hemoglobin arthropathies: diabetes mellitus. Rheumatology. London: Mosby-Year Book Europe Ltd; 1994.
3. Griggs SM, Ahn A, Green A. Idiopathic adhesive capsulitis. A prospective functional outcome study of nonoperative treatment. J Bone Joint Surg [Am]. 2000;82:1398-407.
4. Bridgman JF. Periarthritis of the shoulder and diabetes mellitus. Ann Rheum Dis. 1972;31:69-71.
5. Lequesne M, Dang N, Bensasson M, et al. Increased association of diabetes mellitus with capsulitis of the shoulder and shoulder-hand syndrome. Scand J Rheumatol. 1977;6:53-6.
6. Balci N, Balci MK, Tuzuner S. Shoulder adhesive capsulitis and shoulder range of motion in type II diabetes mellitus: association with diabetic complications. J Diabetes Complications. 1999;13:135-40.
7. Arkkila PE, Kantola IM, Viikari JS, et al. Shoulder capsulitis in type I and II diabetic patients: association with diabetic complications and related diseases. Ann Rheum Dis. 1996;55:907-14.
8. Gamstedt A. Hand abnormalities in patients with NIDDM. Prog Diabetes. 1993;4:1-6.
9. Buckingham BA, Uitto J, Sandborg C, et al. Scleroderma-like changes in insulin-dependent diabetes mellitus: clinical and biochemical studies. Diabetes Care. 1984;7:163-9.
10. Rosenbloom A. Connective tissue disorders in diabetes. International Textbook of Diabetes Mellitus, 2nd edition. Chichester: John Wiley; 1997. pp. 1517-31.
11. Crisp AJ, Heathcote JG. Connective tissue abnormalities in diabetes mellitus. J R Coll Physicians Lond. 1984;18:132-41.
12. Jennings AM, Milner PC, Ward JD. Hand abnormalities are associated with the complications of diabetes in type 2 diabetes. Diabet Med. 1989;6:43-7.
13. Starkman HS, Gleason RE, Rand LI, et al. Limited joint mobility (LJM) of the hand in patients with diabetes mellitus: relation to chronic complications. Ann Rheum Dis. 1986;45:130-5.
14. Eadington DW, Patrick AW, Frier BM. Association between connective tissue changes and smoking habit in type 2 diabetes and in non-diabetic humans. Diabetes Res Clin Pract. 1991;11:121-5.
15. Forgacs SS. Diabetes mellitus and rheumatic disease. Clin Rheum Dis. 1986;12:729-53.
16. Jung Y, Hohmann TC, Gerneth JA, et al. Diabetic hand syndrome. Metabolism. 1971;20:1008-1015.
17. Kozin F. Reflex sympathetic dystrophy syndrome: a review. Clin Exp Rheumatol. 1992;10:401-9.
18. Bayne O, Lu EJ. Diabetic Charcot's arthropathy of the wrist. Case report and literature review. Clin Orthop. 1998;357:122-6.
19. Sander HW, Chokroverty S. Diabetic amyotrophy: current concepts. Semin Neurol. 1996;16:173-8.

Chapter 50

Diabetic Hepatopathy

Anand Moses, S Charles Bronson, V Sanjay Moses

INTRODUCTION

Diabetes is a chronic metabolic cum vascular disease, which has risen as a major public health problem in modern times. Myriad are the complications of diabetes with almost no system that is spared. The effects of diabetes on the liver—collectively termed "diabetic hepatopathy"—are not being focused upon as extensively as the other complications.

DIABETIC HEPATOPATHY

Liver disease related to diabetes is termed as "diabetic hepatopathy". Unlike a complication like "diabetic retinopathy" which is etiologically specific for diabetes, diabetic hepatopathy is a broad and loose term that is usually considered to include the following:

- Nonalcoholic fatty liver disease (NAFLD)[1] and its spectrum
- Diabetic hepatosclerosis[1]
- Glycogenic hepatopathy[1]
- Acute liver failure[2]
- Hepatitis C infection in association with diabetes[2]
- Biliary disease[2] and
- Hepatogenous diabetes (HD)[2]

Nonalcoholic Fatty Liver Disease Associated with Diabetes Mellitus

The spectrum of NAFLD varies from a state of steatosis called nonalcoholic fatty liver (NAFL) to a more severe form of inflammation of liver, called nonalcoholic steatohepatitis (NASH), to fibrosis and cirrhosis (Fig. 1).

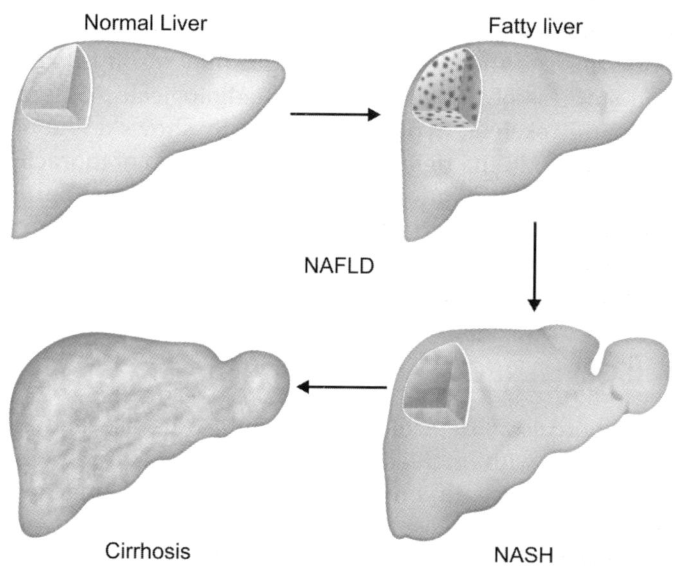

(NAFLD: nonalcoholic fatty liver disease; NASH: nonalcoholic steatohepatitis.)

Figure 1 The stages of nonalcoholic fatty liver disease.[3]

Diabetes leads to an increase in the severity as well as prevalence of nonalcoholic fatty liver disease (NAFLD).[1] NAFLD is considered to be the hepatic manifestation of the metabolic syndrome where the central pathophysiology is insulin resistance.[2] Kotronen et al.[1,4] showed that individuals with type 2 diabetes mellitus (T2DM) had 80% increased fat in the liver when compared to age-, sex- and weight-matched individuals without diabetes. In a study by McPherson et al.[5] it was seen that among those with NAFL who progressed to fibrosis, 80% had diabetes when compared to the nonprogressor group where only 25% were diabetic. Thus, NAFL can potentially progress to NASH with advanced fibrosis; especially in those with diabetes.[5] Portillo-Sanchez et al.[6] demonstrated in their study that the prevalence of NAFLD in T2DM patients with normal aminotransferases was 50%. In an Indian study by Prashanth et al.[7] it was observed that 127 of the 204 T2DM patients (62.25%) recruited had fatty infiltration of liver as seen by ultrasound. Of these ultrasound-detected fatty liver cases, among those on whom liver biopsy was performed, 87% had NAFLD. Of this, 62.6% patients had steatohepatitis and 37.3% had fibrosis. It is noteworthy that NASH and advanced fibrosis can occur in diabetes patients without any symptoms, signs and laboratory changes in liver functions.[7]

Nonalcoholic steatohepatitis and cirrhosis may lead to the development of hepatocellular carcinoma (HCC). In a population-based study done in the United States, NAFLD was found to be the most common underlying etiologic risk factor (59%) for HCC. A worrisome recent discovery is the fact that NAFLD-related-HCC could develop in noncirrhotic livers. HCC could even be the first presentation of an asymptomatic NASH.[8]

Treatment of Nonalcoholic Fatty Liver Disease

The treatment of NAFLD in diabetes primarily depends on lifestyle modification involving increased physical activity, exercise, reduction in body weight and a meal plan. Associated conditions like obesity, hypertension, and dyslipidemia need to be managed effectively.

Metformin, the first-line drug in the treatment of T2DM, decreases the incidence of HCC in diabetes patients in a dose-dependent manner.[1,9] The use of metformin, however, is contraindicated in a state of hepatic failure. Pioglitazone has been shown to reduce the severity of NASH, improve histological scores and reduce the hepatic triglyceride content.[1,10] In mouse models with diet-induced obesity, treatment with linagliptin significantly reduced liver fat content in a dose-dependent manner.[1,11] Other dipeptidyl peptidase-4 (DPP-4) inhibitors like vildagliptin and sitagliptin have also been shown to ameliorate the features of fatty liver.[12,13] In the LEAN (Liraglutide Efficacy and Action in NASH) trial, treatment with liraglutide led to histological resolution of NASH.[1,14] In animal models, sodium glucose co-transporter-2 (SGLT-2) inhibitors have been shown to reduce plasma aminotransferase levels, reduce the liver weight and decrease the hepatic triglyceride content.[15]

Diabetic Hepatosclerosis

In 2006, Stephen Harrison and coworkers described a noncirrhotic hepatic sinusoidal fibrosis which was not associated with NASH. They proposed the term "diabetic hepatosclerosis" for this entity. Most of the patients had a history of long-standing diabetes, a body mass index of <25 kg/m^2 and microvascular complications like retinopathy, nephropathy and neuropathy. Alkaline phosphatase was commonly elevated. Liver biopsy showed hepatic sinusoidal fibrosis (Fig. 2) and immunostaining demonstrated basement membrane components in a perisinusoidal pattern of distribution. Features

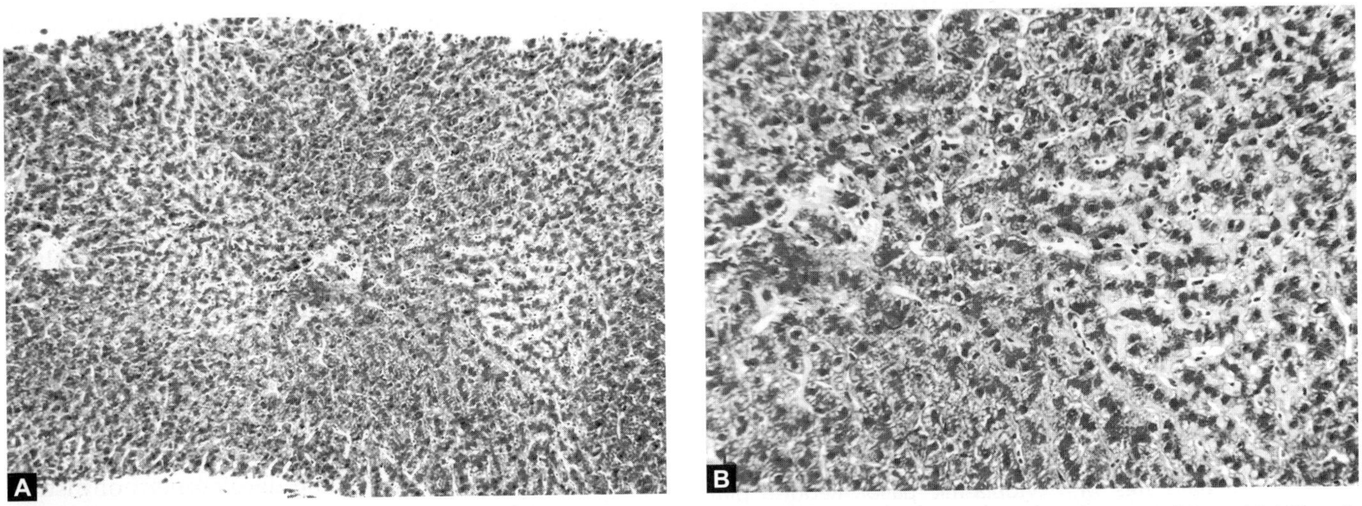

Figure 2 Diabetic hepatosclerosis: Masson's trichrome staining. The upper half is low power view that shows perisinusoidal fibrosis and lack of steatosis. The lower half is a higher power showing dense collagen deposition in the perisinusoidal spaces of the involved regions.[16] *(For color version, see Plate 3)*

of steatosis or steatohepatitis were not seen in these specimens. Diabetic hepatosclerosis is believed to be a form of diabetic microangiopathy that affects the liver.[16]

Glycogenic Hepatopathy

Glycogenic hepatopathy is a rare complication of diabetes and is characterized by the accumulation of excess glycogen in the hepatocytes leading to elevated transaminases and hepatomegaly. It is predominantly seen in patients with long-standing and poorly controlled type 1 diabetes and sometimes in patients with type 2 diabetes.[17]

In 1930, Pierre Mauriac described a condition of poorly controlled diabetes in a type 1 diabetes patient with associated hepatomegaly, poor growth and development and cushingoid features. This condition came to be known as Mauriac syndrome. Glycogenic hepatopathy was the hepatic manifestation of Mauriac syndrome. However, later on, many cases with glycogenic hepatopathy but without the extrahepatic features of Mauriac syndrome were reported. Subsequently the term glycogenic hepatopathy became a more unique pathologic entity.[17]

Glycogenic hepatopathy and NAFLD are clinically indistinguishable except for the setting in which they present, like type 1 diabetes or type 2 diabetes (Fig. 3). Gradient dual-echo magnetic resonance imaging (MRI) can distinguish between the two. However, liver biopsy is the definitive test to diagnose glycogenic hepatopathy.[17]

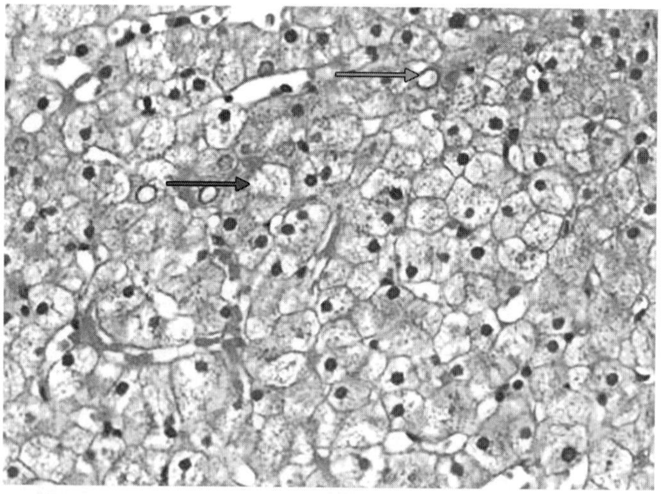

Figure 3 Glycogenic hepatopathy: Liver biopsy section. Hematoxylin and Eosin staining shows enlarged hepatocytes with cytoplasmic pallor. Reddish pink areas of glycogen accumulation (blue arrow) and prominent glycogenated nucleoli (green arrow) are seen.[17] *(For color version, see Plate 3)*

Adequate glycemic control can potentially result in a complete remission of clinical, biochemical and pathological parameters. Instances of hepatic fibrosis have been reported in patients with glycogenic hepatopathy in recent times.[17]

Diabetes and Acute Liver Failure

El-Serag and Everhart[18] analyzed a large cohort of people with and without diabetes, in the records of the Department of Veterans Affairs in the United States. They found out that diabetes was associated with an approximately 1.5-fold increased risk of acute liver failure and this increase in risk was not fully explained by underlying liver disease or the presence of risk factors like viral hepatitis, alcohol consumption, chronic liver disease (CLD) and congestive cardiac failure, etc. The reasons for the increased risk are not clear. A possibility of increased susceptibility to the toxic effects of drugs as well as an increased exposure to hepatotoxic drugs in the diabetic population ought to be considered.[2,18]

Hepatitis C, Diabetes and Liver Disease

Liver steatosis is a characteristic histological feature of chronic hepatitis C (CHC) as like as inflammation and fibrosis. Steatosis is seen in 42–73% patients with CHC and the prevalence of steatosis is about 2-fold higher than that seen with chronic hepatitis B.

Hepatitis C virus (HCV) is able to alter intracellular insulin signaling by various mechanisms. HCV can contribute to a wide array of metabolic abnormalities that include steatosis, insulin resistance, increased prevalence of impaired glucose tolerance and T2DM, abnormalities in lipid metabolism, and atherosclerosis.

Upregulation of the production of reactive oxygen species, increase in the production of proinflammatory and profibrotic cytokines and other mechanisms contribute to steatosis that occurs due to HCV. The relationship between HCV and insulin resistance is bidirectional. HCV causes steatosis which in turn may lead to insulin resistance. Further, many mechanisms that are involved in the development of steatosis due to HCV can also contribute to the development of insulin resistance (Fig. 4).

Figure 5 depicts the various metabolic disturbances associated with HCV infection.

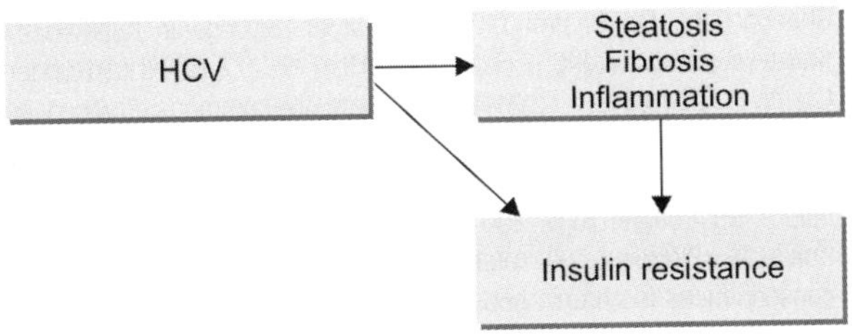

(HCV: hepatitis C virus.)

Figure 4 Pathogenesis of steatosis and insulin resistance in hepatitis C virus infection—a simplified representation.[19]

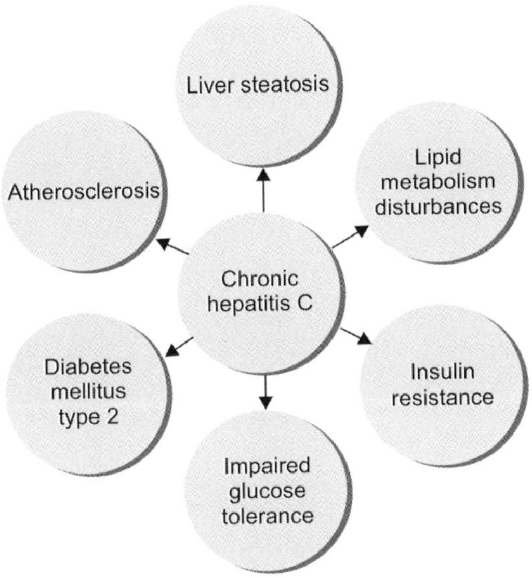

Figure 5 Metabolic abnormalities associated with hepatitis C virus infection.[19]

Biliary Diseases and Diabetes

The incidence of cholelithiasis appears to be higher in individuals with diabetes. However, it is not clear whether this is due to diabetes per se or due to associated features like obesity, dyslipidemia and old age.

Increased volume of the gallbladder and emptying abnormalities are observed in patients with diabetes due to autonomic neuropathy.[2]

Hepatogenous Diabetes

Diabetes that arises due to CLD is termed as HD.

Coexistent T2DM can occur in a patient with CLD. T2DM can in fact predispose to NAFLD and CLD. However, HD occurs after the onset of CLD and patients with HD usually do not have recognized risk factors of T2DM like obesity, family history of diabetes, etc.

Nearly 80–85% of such CLD patients may exhibit glucose intolerance or diabetes. Incidence of HD is especially higher in liver disease of alcoholic, HCV and cryptogenic etiology. The treatment of diabetes in HD is challenging due to liver insufficiency as well as the need for cautious usage of antidiabetic medications. The problem of HD is probably underestimated and is not yet recognized widely.[20]

CONCLUSION

In this brief discussion, we have seen the many facets of diabetic hepatopathy. The morbidity associated with diabetic hepatopathy is considerable. However, many of its components remain to be widely recognized and managed.

REFERENCES

1. Upadhyay R. Diabetic Hepatopathy. In: The Association of Physicians of India- Medicine Update 2017. Available from: http://www.apiindia.org/pdf/medicine_update_2017/mu_067.pdf.
2. Das S, Misra B, Bhattacharyy D. Diabetic Hepatopathy: A Syndrome In Evolution. 2013. Available from: https://www.researchgate.net/publication/261363426_Diabetic_Hepatopathy_A_Syndrome_In_Evolution.
3. Lonardo A, Nascimbeni F, Maurantonio M, et al. Nonalcoholic fatty liver disease: Evolving paradigms. World J Gastroenterol. 2017;23(36):6571-92. [Used under the Creative Commons License: http://creativecommons.org/licenses/by-nc/4.0/]
4. Kotronen A, Juurinen L, Hakkarainen A, et al. Liver fat is increased in type 2 diabetic patients and underestimated by serum alanine aminotransferase compared with equally obese nondiabetic subjects. Diabetes Care. 2008; 31:165-9.
5. McPherson S, Hardy T, Henderson E, et al. Evidence of NAFLD progression from steatosis to fibrosing steatohepatitis using paired biopsies, implications for prognosis and clinical management. J Hepatol. 2015;62(5):1148-55.
6. Portillo-Sanchez P, Bril F, Maximos M, et al. High Prevalence of Nonalcoholic Fatty Liver Disease in Patients With Type 2 Diabetes Mellitus and Normal Plasma Aminotransferase Levels. J Clin Endocrinol Metab. 2015;100(6):2231-8.
7. Prashanth M, Ganesh HK, Vima MV, et al. Prevalence of nonalcoholic fatty liver disease in patients with type 2 diabetes mellitus. J Assoc Physicians India. 2009;57:205-10.
8. Marengo A, Rosso C, Bugianesi E. Liver Cancer: Connections with Obesity, Fatty Liver, and Cirrhosis. Annual Review of Medicine. 2016;67(1):103-17.
9. Chen HP, Shieh JJ, Chang CC, et al. Metformin decreases hepatocellular carcinoma risk in a dose dependent manner: population-based and in vitro studies. Gut. 2013;62(4):606-15.
10. Cusi K, et al. Extended treatment with pioglitazone improves liver histology in patients with prediabetes or type 2 diabetes mellitus and NASH. Ann Intern Med. 2016;165(5):305-15.
11. Kern M, Klöting N, Niessen HG, et al. Linagliptin improves insulin sensitivity and hepatic steatosis in diet-induced obesity. PLoS One. 2012;7(6):e38744.
12. Hussain M, Majeed Babar MZ, Hussain MS, et al. Vildagliptin ameliorates biochemical, metabolic and fatty changes associated with non alcoholic fatty liver disease. Pak J Med Sci. 2016;32(6):1396-401.

13. Yilmaz Y, Yonal O, Deyneli O, et al. Effects of sitagliptin in diabetic patients with nonalcoholic steatohepatitis. Acta Gastroenterol Belg. 2012;75: 240-4.
14. Armstrong MJ, Gaunt P, Aithal GP, et al. Liraglutide safety and efficacy in patients with non-alcoholic steatohepatitis (LEAN): a multicentre, double blind, randomised, placebo-controlled phase 2 study. Lancet. 2016; 387(10019):679-90.
15. Logna Prat L, Tsochatzis EA. The effect of antidiabetic medications on non-alcoholic fatty liver disease (NAFLD). Hormones. 2018;17(2):219-29.
16. Harrison SA, Brunt EM, Goodman ZD, et al. Diabetic hepatosclerosis: diabetic microangiopathy of the liver. Arch Pathol Lab Med. 2006;130(1):27-32.
17. Sherigar JM, De Castro J, Yin YM, et al. Glycogenic hepatopathy: a narrative review. World J Hepatol. 2018;10(2):172-85. [Used under the Creative Commons License: http://creativecommons.org/licenses/by-nc/4.0/]
18. El-Serag HB, Everhart JE. Diabetes increases the risk of acute hepatic failure. Gastroenterology. 2002;122(7):1822-8.
19. Kukla M, Piotrowski D, Waluga M, et al. Insulin resistance and its consequences in chronic hepatitis C. Clin Exp Hepatol. 2015;1(1):17-29. [Used under the Creative Commons License: https://creativecommons.org/licenses/by-nc-sa/4.0/]
20. García-Compeán D, González-González JA, Lavalle-González FJ, et al. Hepatogenous diabetes: Is it a neglected condition in chronic liver disease? World J Gastroenterol. 2016;22(10):2869-74.

Chapter 51

Assessment of Cardiac Autonomic Neuropathy: How Relevant?

Benny Negalur

INTRODUCTION

Diabetes mellitus (DM) is a global health epidemic thought to be affecting 415 million people worldwide, with a further 318 million suffering with glucose intolerance and at increased risk of developing the disease.[1] Cardiac autonomic neuropathy (CAN) is a common underdiagnosed complication of DM. CAN is the impairment of cardiovascular (CV) autonomic control in the setting of diabetes after exclusion of other causes. Established risk factors for CAN are glycemic control in type 1 and a combination of hypertension, dyslipidemia, obesity and glycemic control in type 2 diabetes (T2D).[2]

CARDIOVASCULAR AUTONOMIC NEUROPATHY IN DIABETES MELLITUS

Cardiovascular autonomic neuropathy is a serious complication of DM that is strongly associated with approximately 5-fold increased risk of CV mortality.

Diabetic neuropathies, including CAN, are frequent chronic complications of type 1 and type 2 diabetes that influence quality of life and have potentially fatal outcomes. Prevalence of CAN around 31–73% in patients with T2DM. This large variation in CAN prevalence is thought to be due to discrepancies and variation in the criteria used to diagnose CAN, study populations, and variation in CAN risk factors in epidemiological studies.[3]

RISK FACTORS OF CARDIAC AUTONOMIC NEUROPATHY

The risk of developing CAN is dependent on several factors, which are discussed below.

Duration of Diabetes

Duration of diabetes is an important risk factor for CAN in both the type of diabetes. Patient at end of Diabetes Control and Complications Trial (DCCT) who were diagnosed with CAN experienced higher long-term risk of CV events during follow-up in the Epidemiology of Diabetes Interventions and Complications (EDIC) study.[4]

Study by Dimova et al. found CAN in 12.3% of normal glucose tolerance (NGT), 19.8% in prediabetes, and 32.2% in newly diagnosed T2D patients.[5]

Degree of Glycemic Control

Inadequate glucose control plays an important role in the initial pathophysiology.[6] Microcirculation dysfunction due to nitric oxide loss, oxidative stress and accumulation of free radicals with lesion of Schwann cell as well as in its progression causing neuronal apoptosis and axonal degeneration is likely.

Cardiovascular Risk Factors

The EURODIAB Prospective Complications Study evaluated the risk factors for the development of CAN apart from glycemic control. The study confirms importance of exposure to hyperglycemia as a risk factor for CAN and also found that glycated hemoglobin (HbA1c), hypertension, dyslipidemia, smoking and obesity can also predict the risk of CAN.[7] In the Steno-2 study, intensified multifactorial intervention reduced progression of CAN by 68%.

Microvascular Complications

Microvascular complications share common mechanisms, and several studies have shown that microvascular complications predict CAN development. For example, the EURODIAB study showed that the presence of retinopathy and albuminuria was associated with CAN.[8] Also age, gender and ethnicity are other factors that increase CAN. Possible factors associated with high mortality and sudden death due to autonomic neuropathy are CV arrest, silent myocardial ischemia, hypertension, ventricular arrhythmias, prolongation of the QT interval, resting tachycardia, orthostatic hypotension, exaggerated blood pressure (BP) responses with supine position and exercise.

CLASSIFICATION

- *Subclinical phase:* Decreased heart rate variability (HRV)
- *Early phase:* Resting tachycardia
- *Advanced phase:* Exercise intolerance, cardiomyopathy and left ventricular dysfunction, orthostatic hypotension, myocardial ischemia.

ASSESSMENT

Screening for High-risk Individuals

Screening is recommended for the following individuals:

- Type 2 DM at diagnosis
- Type 1 DM after 5 years
- Preoperative
- One major cardiovascular disease (CVD) risk factor
- Any chronic complications of DM
- Hypoglycemia unawareness.

DIAGNOSIS AND CLINICAL MANIFESTATIONS OF CARDIAC AUTONOMIC NEUROPATHY

Light headaches, palpitations, weakness, faintness and syncope are the most common symptoms of CAN. Development of orthostatic hypotension is associated with advanced disease stage and is easy to recognize in the office. There is no compensatory increase in heart rate, despite hypotension. CAN diagnosis includes evaluation of symptoms and signs of CAN.

Resting Tachycardia

One of the most important sign in CAN is the abnormality in heart rate. Later on, abnormal heart rate progresses to resting tachycardia (90–130 bpm). Fixed and unresponsive heart rate to breathing, moderate exercise, and sleep indicate complete cardiac denervation.[9]

Reduced Exercise Tolerance

Reduced heart rate and BP response to activity leads to impaired exercise tolerance as cardiac output does not increase with increase in exercise, so patients need to rely on their perceived exertion. In such scenarios, heart rate (HR) cannot be used as an indicator of exercise intensity.

Orthostatic Hypotension

Orthostatic hypotension is defined as a reduction in systolic blood pressure (SBP) >20 mm Hg or diastolic blood pressure (DBP) >10 mm Hg within 3 minutes of standing and a fall of 30 mm systolic when a person assumes a standing position following a postural change from supine to standing, and is deemed to be a late sign in CAN.[3] Fainting, dizziness, palpitations, blurred vision, and even nausea and syncope can be seen.

Orthostatic Tachycardia Syndrome

Symptoms compatible with orthostatic hypotension such as fainting, syncope, inappropriate sinus tachycardia, or abnormalities in baroreceptor function.

QT Interval Prolongation

Prolongation of QT interval has been defined as a QTc (corrected QT for HR >450 ms in men and >460 ms in women). Hyperinsulinemia can induce reversible prolongation in QT interval in healthy subjects. Hyperglycemia and acute hypoglycemia can do the same. Overnight hypoglycemia supports the arrhythmatic basis of "Dead in Bed" syndrome.

Impaired Heart Rate Variability

Decrease in HRV is the earliest sign and predicts increase in mortality after acute myocardial infarction.

Reverse Dipping and Nondipping Pattern

In normal people, BP is reduced at night secondary to predominance of vagal tone and decreased sympathetic activity. In CAN, this pattern is altered, resulting in predominance of sympathetic tone and nocturnal hypertension leading to left ventricular hypertension and increase in mortality.

Mortality

Cardiovascular autonomic neuropathy increases morbidity and mortality in diabetes through association with a high risk of cardiac arrhythmias and sudden death, possibly related to silent myocardial ischemia. During the subclinical stage, CAN can be detected through reduction in HRV.

BEDSIDE METHODS OF CARDIAC AUTONOMIC NEUROPATHY ASSESSMENT

Methods of CAN assessment in clinical practice include assessment of symptoms and signs, cardiac autonomic reflex tests (CARTs) based on heart rate and BP, and ambulatory blood pressure monitoring (ABPM). Before the symptoms appear, CAN remains subclinical. Subclinical CAN can be detected through a reduction in HRV. In healthy individuals, there is normal beat-to-beat variation during inspiration and expiration, which is driven by sympathetic and parasympathetic activity.[10,11]

Clinical Evaluation—Simple Bedside Tests

First Test: Heart Rate Response to Deep Breathing

Technique: Patient lies quietly and breathes deeply at a rate of six breaths per minute and ECG (electrocardiogram) is recorded. The difference between the maximum and minimum heart rate and expiration-to-inspiration (E:I) R-R interval ratio are calculated.

Interpretation: A difference in HR of <10 bpm and E:I ratio is >1.17 are abnormal.

Second Test: Heart Rate Response to Standing

Technique: ECG is recorded in lying followed by full upright position. The R-R interval is measured at beats 15 and 30 after the patient stands.

Interpretation: A 30:15 ratio of <1.03 is abnormal.

Third Test: Heart Rate Response to Valsalva

Technique: The patient forcibly exhales into the mouthpiece of a manometer, exerting a pressure of 40 mm Hg for 15 seconds. There are four phases during this maneuver. The longest and shortest R-R intervals are measured. The ratio is called Valsalva ratio.

Interpretation: Valsalva ratio of <1.2 is abnormal.

Fourth Test: Blood Pressure Response to Standing

Technique: BP is measured when the patient is lying down and 2 minutes after the patient stands.

Interpretation: SBP fall of ≥20 mm Hg or DBP fall of >10 mm Hg is abnormal.

Fifth Test: Blood Pressure Response to Isometric Exercise

Technique: The patient squeezes a handgrip dynamometer to establish his or her maximum. The patient then maintains the grip at 30% maximum for 5 minutes. BP is measured in the contralateral arm.

Interpretation: A DBP rise of <16 mm Hg is abnormal.

Cardiac Autonomic Reflex Tests

Cardiac autonomic reflex tests are time consuming and require patient cooperation for detecting CAN. HRV analysis requires less patient cooperation and is quicker to complete. Study by Herbert et al. concluded that HRV is suitable for clinical practice from ECG recordings of >90 seconds with high accuracy and repeatability within a session for each participant.[12,13]

Spectral Analysis of Heart Rate Variability

Spectral analysis is a spectrum of frequencies or related quantities of differing changes in heart rate. It is an advanced method to detect HRV in supine and standing position. The HRV signal is a chaotic signal of the influence of sympathetic and parasympathetic activity on sinus node.

CONCLUSION

Cardiovascular autonomic neuropathy is very common and often undiagnosed in patients with DM. Intensive multifactorial intervention targeting lifestyle, glycemic control and CVD risk factors prevents the development and slows the progression of CAN. Identifying patients with CAN is important, as CAN is associated with increased mortality, CVD, chronic kidney disease, perioperative morbidity, and lower-limb complications. As such, these patients should receive appropriate follow-up and preventive treatments to prevent or slow the progression of these complications. Further research into the pathogenesis of CAN is important, in order to identify novel treatment targets and develop new therapies.

REFERENCES

1. International Diabetes Federation. IDF Diabetes Atlas, 7th edition. Brussels: IDF; 2015.
2. Spallone V, Ziegler D, Freeman R, et al. Cardiovascular autonomic neuropathy in diabetes: clinical impact, assessment, diagnosis, and management. Diabetes Metab Res Rev. 2011;27(7):639-53.
3. Fisher VL, Tahrani AA. Cardiac autonomic neuropathy in patients with diabetes mellitus: current perspectives. Diabetes Metab Syndr Obes. 2017;10:419-34.
4. Pop-Busui R, Braffett BH, Zinman B, et al. Cardiovascular autonomic neuropathy and cardiovascular outcomes in the Diabetes Control and Complications Trial/Epidemiology of Diabetes Interventions and Complications (DCCT/EDIC) study. Diabetes Care. 2017;40(1):94-100.
5. Dimova R, Tankova T, Guergueltcheva V, et al. Risk factors for autonomic and somatic nerve dysfunction in different stages of glucose tolerance. J Diabetes Complications. 2017;31(3):537-43.
6. Pop-Busui R, Low PA, Waberski BH, et al. Effects of prior intensive insulin therapy on cardiac autonomic nervous system function in type 1 diabetes mellitus: the Diabetes Control and Complications Trial/Epidemiology of Diabetes Interventions and Complications study (DCCT/EDIC). Circulation. 2009;119(22):2886-93.
7. Witte DR, Tesfaye S, Chaturvedi N, et al. Risk factors for cardiac autonomic neuropathy in type 1 diabetes mellitus. Diabetologia. 2005;48(1):164-71.
8. Kempler P, Tesfaye S, Chaturvedi N, et al. Autonomic neuropathy is associated with increased cardiovascular risk factors: the EURODIAB IDDM complications study. Diabet Med. 2002;19(11):900-909.
9. Vinik AI, Erbas T, Casellini CM. Diabetic cardiac autonomic neuropathy, inflammation and cardiovascular disease. J Diabetes Investig. 2013;4(1): 4-18.
10. Chyun DA, Wackers FJ, Inzucchi SE, et al. Autonomic dysfunction independently predicts poor cardiovascular outcomes in asymptomatic individuals with type 2 diabetes in the DIAD study. SAGE Open Med. 2015;3:2050312114568476.
11. Razanskaite-Virbickiene D, Danyte E, Mockeviciene G, et al. Can coefficient of variation of time-domain analysis be valuable for detecting cardiovascular autonomic neuropathy in young patients with type 1 diabetes: a case control study. BMC Cardiovasc Disord. 2017;17(1):34.
12. American Diabetes Association. Classification and diagnosis of diabetes. Diabetes Care. 2017;40(Suppl 1):S11-24.
13. Jelinek HF, Adam MTP, Krones R, et al. Diagnostic Accuracy of Random ECG in Primary Care for Early, Asymptomatic Cardiac Autonomic Neuropathy. J Diabetes Sci Technol. 2017;11(6):1165-73.

Chapter 52

Pathophysiology of Macrovascular Impact of Psoriasis in Diabetes

Aastha Chawla

INTRODUCTION

Psoriasis is characterized by topical skin lesions as well as an increased risk for cardiovascular disease (CVD). Last two decades lot of evidence has emerged that patients with psoriasis have greater CVD risk factors (hypertension, diabetes, obesity and dyslipidemia) and tends to have higher risk of non-cardiac vascular diseases (carotid, peripheral artery and chronic kidney diseases), in comparison with the general population. These associations are even more significant in patients with severe psoriasis and those with psoriatic arthritis (PsA).[1]

What do psoriasis, a common chronic dermatological condition, and type 2 diabetes, a metabolic disorder of insulin resistance, have in common? On the surface, it may not appear to be very significant. Psoriasis' effect on new-onset diabetes is well documented, but its effect on course of diabetes is poorly understood. Patients with diabetes and psoriasis have an increased risk of developing vascular complications. Epidemiologic studies have revealed that patients with psoriasis are at risk for developing other immune mediated diseases (e.g. diabetes).[2] Patients with psoriasis have higher risk for developing new onset diabetes.[3–6]

Contrary to that in few studies new class of biologics, the tumor necrosis factor (TNF) inhibitors, not only improves psoriasis but reduces the risk of newonset diabetes among treated patients.[7,8] This could be a direct effect of TNF inhibitors on diabetes onset and/or a psoriasis-mediated indirect effect.

Inflammation is thought to play an important role in pathogenesis of Diabetes and results from metabolic stress through various mechanisms[9] and plays a role in the propagation of not only microvascular complications such as retinopathy,[10] neuropathy[11] and nephropathy,[12] but also the pathogenesis of macrovascular complications.[13] It is still poorly understood how psoriatic inflammation worsens these complications. Patients with psoriasis have more difficulty managing their hypertension than patients without psoriasis proving the fact that psoriasis effects progression of metabolic and cardiovascular (CV) diseases mediated through inflammation.[14]

RELATIONSHIP BETWEEN PSORIASIS AND CARDIOMETABOLIC FACTORS

Psoriatic arthritis occurs exclusively in the context of psoriasis. In few studies PsA was associated with increased mortality, with CVD being the leading cause of death. Patients with PsA were at greater risk for CV morbidity as compared with general population and more likely to develop hypertension, myocardial infarction and angina. Risk factors for CVD are commonly seen in psoriasis, including hypertension, dyslipidemia, elevated highly-sensitive C-reactive protein (hs-CRP), dysglycemia, obesity, metabolic syndrome and a history of coronary artery disease.[15] PsA itself is an independent risk factor for CVD. In patients with PsA without CV risk factors or clinically evident CVD also endothelial dysfunction and increased vascular intima/media thickness have been observed. It is well documented that severe psoriasis itself is an independent risk factor for myocardial infarction, stroke and CV mortality.[16,17]

Metabolic syndrome is a state of chronic inflammation and increased CV mortality. Severe psoriasis worsens metabolic syndrome, an emerging but variable health issue estimated to affect 25% of the population of the United States.[18] In a psoriasis patient there is systemic inflammation present associated with hyperhomocysteinemia, elevated blood inflammatory cytokines [e.g. interleukin (IL) 6, TNF-α, IL- 23, IL-17, IL-20, IL-22] and elevated hs-CRP, platelet hyperactivity which may contribute to the increased incidence of ischemic heart disease.[19] Inflammatory markers such as Th-1 cytokines (intracellular adhesion molecule-1, TNF-α) play a role not only in the pathogenesis of obesity, atherosclerosis, metabolic syndrome and myocardial infarction but also in pathogenesis of psoriasis. Patients with psoriasis have elevated levels of hs-CRP which increases risk of CVD[15].

OBESITY

Patients with severe psoriasis have higher body mass index (BMI) that increases risk of CV mortality.[20] Obesity with psoriasis both are associated with chronic inflammatory process which may exacerbate the process of atherosclerosis increasing CV risk.[21]

DIABETES

In a study by W Armstrong on 6,164 diabetic patients with psoriasis (27% moderate-to-severe) matched without psoriasis to find out psoriasis and risk of diabetes-associated microvascular and macrovascular complications revealed that patients with psoriasis were significantly more likely to develop microvascular events than patients without psoriasis overall [hazard ratio (HR) 1.14, p = 0.001] and by psoriasis severity (mild: HR 1.13, p = 0.004; moderate to severe: HR 1.16, p = 0.038). Risk of macrovascular events was seen to be higher for patients without psoriasis overall (HR 1.13, p = 0.001) and those with mild psoriasis (HR 1.15, p = 0.003), but not for moderate-to-severe cases (HR 1.10, p = 0.210). Psoriasis was generally associated with higher rates of microvascular and macrovascular complications among diabetic group. Severe psoriasis did not increase risk of diabetic complications. This study highlights an increased risk of microvascular and macrovascular complications among diabetic patients with psoriasis versus those without. This study suggests that patients having both diseases need to be given due care. While treating patients with psoriasis with diabetes, clinicians may consider a more aggressive screening for diabetic complications.

A study by Stovring et al. in Denmark found a prevalence of 2% amongst the participants aged 40–64 years and about 5% in those aged above 65 years while association between psoriasis and diabetes is underestimated because of low prevalence .

In a Danish nationwide cohort study[22] comprising a Danish population >10 years of age on 1 January, 1997 was followed until new-onset DM, death, or 31 December, 2009. The primary study end point was onset of diabetes mellitus (DM) requiring pharmacotherapy. Incidence rates for the development of DM events per 1,000 observational years were calculated and adjusted.

A total of 4,614,807 subjects were eligible for analysis, with a maximum follow-up of 13 years. In the study period, 52,613 patients with psoriasis, including 6,784 patients with severe psoriasis, were studies and followed. The overall incidence rates for new-onset DM were 3.67 [confidence interval (CI) 3.65–3.69], 6.93 (6.63–7.25) and 9.65 (8.68–10.73) for the reference population, mild psoriasis, and severe psoriasis, respectively. The incidence rate ratio (IRR) of new-onset DM was increased in all patients with psoriasis, i.e. IRR 1.49 (CI 1.43–1.56) and 2.13 (1.91–2.37) for those with mild and severe psoriasis compared with the reference population.

In this nationwide cohort, psoriasis was associated with increased incidence rates of new-onset DM significantly higher even after adjustment for confounding factors.

HYPERTENSION

The link between psoriasis and hypertension has been hypothesized to be related to increased levels of angiotensin-converting enzyme, endothelin-1 (ET-1) and rennin in patients with psoriasis.[23,24]

An increased risk of diabetes and hypertension in women with psoriasis, even after adjustment for age, BMI, alcohol intake and smoking status[25] has been seen in one prospective study.

CONCLUSION

It is presumed that psoriasis is associated with increased prevalence of CV risk factors. However, more prospective studies in the psoriatic population are needed to evaluate the true causal relationship between psoriasis and CVD. Screening practices and treatment aimed at CV risk factors and disease remain a challenge in the clinical practice. It is important to sensitize dermatologists, cardiologists and physicians on subclinical atherosclerosis in psoriasis patients, so as to reduce the burden of high mortality events such as acute myocardial infarction and stroke. Specific needs for follow-up are related to the natural history of psoriasis and the chronology of the association with the comorbidities.

REFERENCES

1. Katsiki N, Anagnostis P, Athyros V, et al. Psoriasis and vascular risk: an update. Curr Pharm Des. 2015;20:6114-25.
2. Reich K. The concept of psoriasis as a systemic inflammation: implications for disease management. J Eur Acad Dermatol Venereol. 2012;26(Suppl 2):3-11.
3. Gibson SH, Perry HO. Diabetes and psoriasis. AMA Arch Derm. 1956;74:487-8.
4. Shapiro J, Cohen AD, David M, et al. The association between psoriasis, diabetes mellitus, and a therosclerosis in Israel: a case-control study. J Am Acad Dermatol. 2007;56:629-34.
5. Qureshi AA, Choi HK, Setty AR, et al. Psoriasis and the risk of diabetes and hypertension: a prospective study of US female nurses. Arch Dermatol. 2009;145:379-82.
6. Solomon DH, Love TJ, Canning C, et al. Risk of diabetes among patients with rheumatoid arthritis, psoriatic arthritis and psoriasis. Ann Rheum Dis. 2010;69:2114-7.
7. Solomon DH, Massarotti E, Garg R, et al. Association between disease-modifying antirheumatic drugs and diabetes risk in patients with rheumatoid arthritis and psoriasis. JAMA. 2011;305:2525-31.
8. Cheng J, Kuai D, Zhang L, et al. Psoriasis increased the risk of diabetes: a meta-analysis. Arch Dermatol Res. 2012; 304:119-25.
9. Hotamisligil GS. Endoplasmic reticulum stress and the inflammatory basis of metabolic disease. Cell. 2010;140:900-17.
10. Zhang W, Liu H, Al-Shabrawey M, et al. Inflammation and diabetic retinal microvascular complical tions. J Cardiovasc Dis Res. 2011;2:96-103.
11. Vincent AM, Callaghan BC, Smith AL, et al. Diabetic neuropathy: cellular mechanisms as therapeutic targets. Nat Rev Neurol. 2011;7:573-83.
12. Navarro-Gonzalez JF, Mora-Fernandez C, Muros de Fuentes M, et al. Inflammatory molecules and pathways in the pathogenesis of diabetic nephropathy. Nat Rev Nephrol. 2011;7:327-40.
13. Libby P, Ridker PM, Hansson GK. Inflammation in atherosclerosis: from pathophysiology to practice. J Am Coll Cardiol. 2009;54:2129-38.
14. Armstrong AW, Lin SW, Chambers CJ, et al. Psoriasis and hypertensionseverity: results from a case-control study. PLoS One. 2011;6:e18227.
15. Qureshi AA, Choi HK, Setty AR, et al. Psoriasis and the risk of diabetes and hypertension: a prospective study of US female nurses. Arch Dermatol. 2009;145:379-82.
16. Gonzalez-Juanatey C, Llorca J, Miranda-Filloy JA, et al. Endothelial dysfunction in psoriatic arthritis patients without clinically evident cardiovascular disease or classic atherosclerosis risk factors. Arthritis Rheum. 2007;57:287-93.
17. Gonzalez-Juanatey C, Llorca J, Amigo-Diaz E, et al. High prevalence of subclinical atherosclerosis in psoriatic arthritis patients without clinically evident cardiovascular disease or classic atherosclerosis risk factors. Arthritis Rheum. 2007;57:1074-80.
18. Menter A, Griffiths C, Tebbey P, et al. Exploring the association between cardiovascular and other disease-related risk factors in the psoriasis population: the need for increased understanding across the medical community. J Eur Acad Dermatol Venereol. 2010;24:1371-7.
19. Nestle FO, Kaplan DH, Barker J. Psoriasis N Engl J Med. 2009;361: 496-509.
20. Sterry W, Strober BE, Menter A. Obesity in psoriasis: The metabolic, clinical and therapeutic implications. Report of an interdisciplinary conference and review. Br J Dermatol. 2007;157:649-55.
21. Willerson JT, Ridker PM. Inflammation as a cardiovascular risk factor. Circulation. 2004;109:II2-10.
22. Khalid U, Hansen PR, Hilmar G. Gislason: Psoriasis and New-Onset Diabetes A Danish nationwide cohort study Diabetes Care; 2013; 36:2402-7.
23. Ena P, Madeddu P, Glorioso N, et al. High prevalence of cardiovascular diseases and enhanced activity of the renin-angiotensin system in psoriatic patients. Acta Cardiol. 1985;40:199-205.
24. Das UN. Is angiotensin-II an endogenous pro-inflammatory molecule? Med Sci Monit. 2005;11:RA155-62.
25. Qureshi AA, Choi HK, Setty AR, et al. Psoriasis and the risk of diabetes and hypertension: a prospective study of US female nurses. Arch Dermatol. 2009;145:379-82.

Chapter 53

Osteoporosis—An Under-appreciated Complication of Diabetes

Sneha Kothari, Manoj Chadha

INTRODUCTION

The burden of diabetes is increasing as is the burden of osteoporosis.[1] The increase in life expectancy of people with diabetes will predispose them at risk of osteoporosis. Whether this reflects the coexistence of these two common diseases affected by aging, changes in lifestyle or whether skeleton involvement is a unique complication of diabetes, is a matter of debate.[1,2] One in three women and one in five men over the age of 50 years will experience an osteoporotic fracture at some point in life.[3]

FRACTURE RISK AND DIABETES MELLITUS

Type 1 Diabetes Mellitus

While both type 1 and 2 diabetes patients are at an increased risk of osteoporotic fractures, the probability is more profound in type 1 diabetes mellitus (T1DM).[4] The incidence of hip fractures in large prospective Nurses Health Study was 6-fold higher than the general population and 2.5-fold higher than in type 2 diabetes mellitus (T2DM).[5] The relative risk of hip fractures ranges from 1.7 to 12.3 and increases after age of 40 years. There is increased frequency of fractures at the spine and proximal humerus.[4-6]

Type 2 Diabetes Mellitus

The risk of hip fracture is increased in patients with T2DM. The risk is more in patients with long duration of diabetes (>10 years), poorly controlled diabetes and on treatment with insulin. In addition to hip fracture, wrist and foot fractures are more frequent in T2DM. The data regarding the risk of vertebral fractures are not concrete. In addition, diabetes has been shown to be predictive of increased mortality risk in patients with hip fracture.[2,4]

Mechanisms Underlying Bone Loss and Fractures in Diabetes Mellitus

Though investigated widely, the relationship between diabetes and osteoporosis remains controversial. Multiple mechanisms interplay to alter bone quantity [bone mineral density (BMD)] and bone quality.

Cellular and Molecular Mechanisms[2,7-9]

Hyperglycemia has direct and indirect deleterious effects on osteoblast function and bone formation (Flowchart 1). Diabetes mellitus (DM) increases osteoclast function but decreases osteoblast function, thereby leading to accelerated bone loss, osteopenia and osteoporosis. Hyperglycemia induces production of macrophage colony stimulating factor (MCSF), tumor necrosis factor (TNF)-α and receptor activator of nuclear factor-kB ligand (RANKL) which activates osteoclast proliferation and differentiation, and thereby leads to bone resorption. In addition, hyperglycemia suppresses osteoblast proliferation and function, by decreasing runt-related transcription factor (Runx)-2, osteocalcin and osteopontin expression. Reduced osteoblast function affects bone formation.

Hyperglycemia leads to adipogenic differentiation of mesenchymal stem cells by upregulating the expression of peroxisome proliferator-activated receptor (PPAR)-γ, adipocyte fatty acid binding protein (aP2), adipsin and resistin. A decrease in neovascularization further aggravates bone loss. Advanced glycation end products (AGE) reduces bone formation by inhibiting the

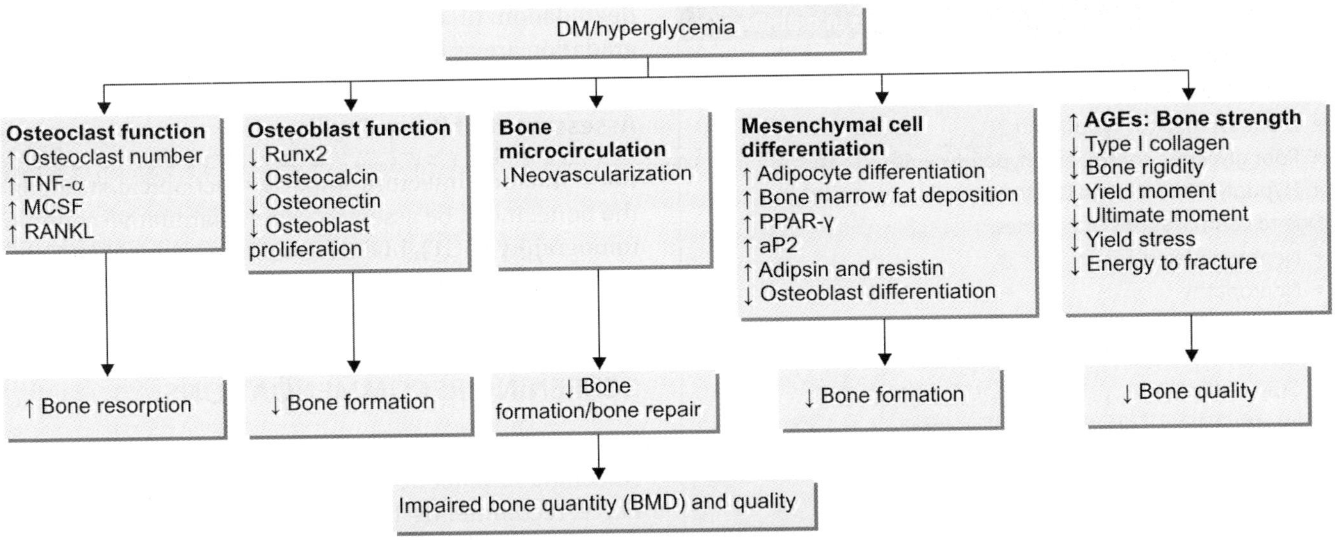

(aP2: acid binding protein; DM: diabetes mellitus; PPAR-γ: peroxisome proliferator-activated receptor-γ; RANKL: receptor activator of nuclear factor-kB ligand; Runx2: related transcription factor; MCSF: macrophage colony stimulating factor; TNF-α: tumor necrosis factor alpha.)

Flowchart 1 Possible deleterious effects of diabetes mellitus on bone metabolism and bone quality.[7]

synthesis of type 1 collagen and osteocalcin. Activation of the receptor for AGEs (RAGE) enhances inflammatory cytokine and reactive oxygen species (ROS) production, which leads to bone resorption.

Risk Factors for Osteoporotic Fractures in Diabetes[1,2,7-9]

Diabetes impacts bone through several mechanisms. Poor metabolic control is a risk for osteoporosis and fractures in diabetes.

In patients with T1DM, absolute deficiency of insulin and insulin-like growth factor-1 (IGF-1) leads to the impaired bone formation with lower values of peak bone mass. The low BMD predisposes them to risk of fracture. In addition, associated autoimmune diseases like Graves' disease and celiac sprue pose an additional risk.

In T2DM, obesity (increased load on bone) and insulin resistance resulting in hyperinsulinemia lead to increased bone formation and increased BMD. Bone microarchitecture is altered in T2DM patients. Increased cortical porosity and reduced cortical density impairs bone quality. Thiazolidinediones (TZDs) activate PPAR-γ leading to increased adipogenesis and impaired osteoblastogenesis. Sodium/glucose co-transporter 2 (SGLT-2) inhibitors like canagliflozin might cause bone loss at the hip and increase the risk of hip fractures. Dapagliflozin and empagliflozin do not seem to affect bone metabolism.

Almost all osteoporotic hip fractures result from fall. The risk of falling is increased by diabetic complications like retinopathy, cataracts, orthostatic hypotension, foot ulcers or amputations. Risk factors for osteoporotic fractures are listed in Box 1.

Flowchart 2 summarizes the complex interplay of cellular/molecular mechanism with risk factors for bone loss and fractures in diabetes.[4]

Evaluation of Fracture Risk in Diabetes

Bone Mineral Density and Fracture Risk Assessment

T1DM patients have lower (BMD) compared to healthy subjects. BMD is usually normal or increased in T2DM subjects.[10] Fracture risk assessment (FRAX) is a widely used online tool to calculate 10-year fracture risk probability; however, T2DM is neither currently included in the FRAX tool nor it is considered a secondary cause of osteoporosis. FRAX underestimates fracture risk in patients with T2DM, especially if disease duration is >10 years. In T2DM patients, the fracture risk is higher for a given T-score and age and for a given FRAX-score. For a similar fracture risk, patients with type 2 diabetes have nearly 0.5 higher T-score compared to nondiabetic people. Although BMD underestimates fracture risk in patients with type 2 diabetes, it does help to stratify fracture risk in them.[10,11]

Box 1: Risk factors for osteoporotic fractures in diabetes.[9]

Risk for osteoporosis

Directly due to diabetes:
- Diabetes mellitus type 1 and 2
- Poor glycemic control and hyperglycemia
- Hypoglycemia (due to DM treatment)

Due to complications of diabetes:
- Nephropathy
- Neuropathy
- Diabetic diarrhea

Due to diseases associated with diabetes:
- Graves' disease
- Intestinal bowel disease and celiac sprue
- Amenorrhea
- Delayed puberty
- Eating disorders

Risk of falls:
- Episodes of hypoglycemia due to medication (mostly insulin)
- Episodes of nocturia (during uncontrolled DM)
- Poor vision due to retinopathy or cataracts
- Poor balance due to neuropathy, foot ulcers, or amputations of diabetic foot
- Orthostatic hypotension (due to autonomic neuropathy)
- Impaired joint motility

(DM: diabetes mellitus.)

Trabecular Bone Score

Trabecular bone score (TBS) is a noninvasive modality designed to assess the trabecular microarchitecture parameters derived from DXA images. TBS reflects pixel gray level variations in DXA images. TBS measures degradation of trabecular structure.[1,9,10] Levels of degradation are as described below in Table 1.[9]

Assessment of Bone Quality

Bone microarchitecture imparts mechanical strength to the bone. It can be assessed using quantitative computed tomography (QCT), high resolution peripheral QCT, high resolution magnetic resonance imaging (MRI) and micro-computed tomography (micro-CT).[9]

SCREENING RECOMMENDATIONS[2]

There are no specific recommendations for osteoporosis screening in diabetic patients. The US Preventative Task Force recommends that screening should be routinely provided in all women over age 65 years and in those women between 60 and 64 years with increased risk. The National Osteoporosis Foundation also recommends screening for postmenopausal women younger than age 65 years who have had a fracture or who have one or more risk factors for osteoporosis. There are no evidence-based guidelines for screening. However T1DM patients with any complications and thin women with other extensive complications of diabetes should undergo BMD screening.

MANAGEMENT OF OSTEOPOROSIS IN DIABETES

Management recommendations in diabetic patients with osteoporosis are mostly based on good clinical practice rather than from evidence obtained from randomized controlled trials.[1,10]

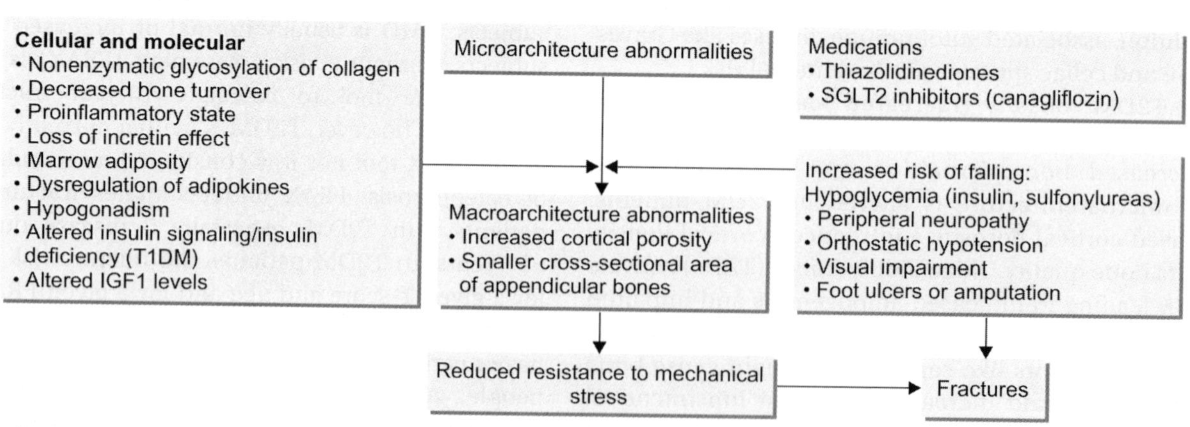

(IGF1: insulin-like growth factor 1; SGLT2: sodium-glucose cotransporter 2; T1DM: type 1 diabetes mellitus.)

Flowchart 2 Interplay of mechanisms underlying bone loss and fractures in type 2 diabetes mellitus.[4]

TABLE 1: Degradation of trabecular structure and its description.

Degradation	Description	TBS range
Normal	–	>1.350
Moderate	Grade 1	1.300–1.350
	Grade 2	1.250–1.300
	Grade 3	1.200–1.250
Degraded	Severe	1.100–1.200
	Highly degraded	<1.100

(TBS: trabecular bone score.)

General Measures

Lifestyle intervention[1,10]

Lifestyle intervention with medical nutrition therapy and exercise forms the cornerstone of therapy of diabetes and coexistent osteoporosis.

Components of medical nutrition therapy include:

- Modest weight loss
- Mediterranean-style diet rich in monounsaturated fats and long-chain ω-3 fatty acids
- Nuts and seeds
- At least 1,000 mg of calcium/day, 800–1,000 IU of vitamin D per day
- Limited intake of alcohol (to <3 units/day) and sodium
- Quit smoking

Physical Activity[1,10]

Regular physical activity is the best way to build up peak bone mass and strength especially in T1DM who have difficulty in achieving peak bone mass. About 150 minutes per week of intense walking is recommended along with weight bearing exercise.

Optimizing Metabolic Control[1,10]

The American Diabetes Association and European Association for the Study of Diabetes guidelines recommend HbA1c target of ≈7%. However in patients with longer duration of diabetes, with cardiovascular disease, recurrent severe hypoglycemia episodes, or hypoglycemia unawareness, HbA1c target (7.5–8%) is set at a higher level to avoid hypoglycemia and falls, which predisposes to the increase the risk of fracture.

After lifestyle intervention, most patients require pharmacologic therapy for optimal glycemic control.

TABLE 2: Effect of antidiabetic agents on BMD and fragility fractures in humans.[10]

Antidiabetic agent	BMD	Fractures
Thiazolidinediones		
Rosiglitazone	↓	↑ ↔ (in men in some studies)
Pioglitazone	↓	↑ ↔ (in men in some studies)
Metformin	↔ ↑	↔ ↑
Sulfonylureas	–	↔ ↓
Incretin therapies		
GLP-1 analogues	↑ ↔	↔
DPP-4 inhibitors	–	↓ ↔
Insulin	↔	↑ ↔
SGLT2 inhibitors		
Canagliflozin	↓ (total hip)	↑
Dapagliflozin	↓	↑ ↔

(BMD: bone mineral density; GLP-1: glucagon like peptide-1; DPP-4: dipeptidyl peptidase-4; SGLT2: sodium/glucose co-transporter 2; ↓: decreased; ↑: increased; ↔: no change noted.)

It is evident from the clinical studies that diabetes medications modulate bone loss and fracture risk. The effect of hypoglycemic agents on fracture risk in T2DM is summarized in Table 2.[1,2,10]

Metformin is the first-line pharmacologic therapy for T2DM patients. If HbA1c remains over target after 3 months, then a second agent should be added. The sulfonylureas, dipeptidyl peptidase-4 (DPP-4) inhibitors, or glucagon like peptide-1 receptor agonist (GLP-1RA) should be rather preferred add on agents as against basal insulin, SGLT2 inhibitors and TZDs.[1,10]

ANTIOSTEOPOROSIS TREATMENTS IN DIABETIC PATIENTS

An osteoporosis range BMD in postmenopausal women and men over age of 50 years and presence of typical fragility fracture merits treatment either with anabolic agents or anti-resorptive agent. Since T2DM patients fracture at higher BMD, an areal BMD intervention threshold at T-score-2 at the spine or hip may be considered appropriate to initiate intervention.[10]

The existing data shows no real effect of antiosteoporotic medications on the incidence of T2D and on glucose metabolism. Intact, bisphosphonates may reduce the risk of developing diabetes. There is currently no data exists on the use of medications such as denosumab and

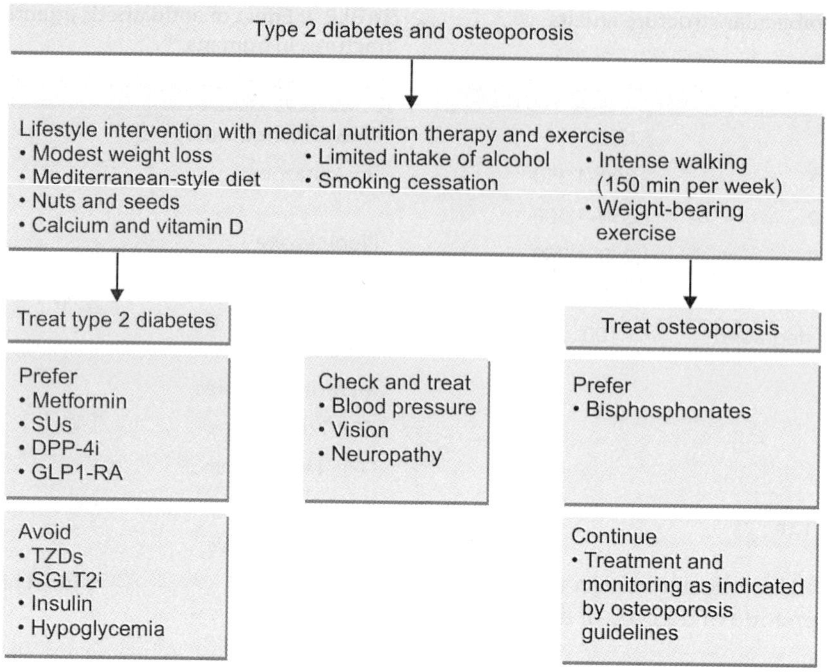

(SUs: sulfonylureas; DPP-4i: dipeptidyl peptidase-4 inhibitor; GLP1: glucagon like peptide-1; RA: receptor agonist; TZDs: Thiazolidinediones; SGLT2i: sodium/glucose co-transporter 2 inhibitor)

Flowchart 3 Algorithm for optimal management of patients with diabetes mellitus (DM) and coexisting osteoporosis.

strontium in the management of osteoporosis in diabetes. The treatment and the monitoring of osteoporosis should be continued as per international guidelines without any changes due to concomitant diabetes. Currently, bisphosphonates are among the first choices for osteoporosis treatment in diabetic as in nondiabetic subject.[1,10]

MANAGEMENT OF COMORBIDITIES[1]

Most patients with T2DM present with hypertension and are treated with several antihypertensive agents. Proper control of blood pressure and avoiding hypotension is important to prevent falls.

Patients should be subjected to annual fundoscopy to assess vision and at least annual neuropathy assessment.

Algorithm for optimal management of patients with DM and coexisting osteoporosis is summarized in Flowchart 3.

MANAGEMENT OF HOSPITALIZED PATIENTS WITH FRACTURE[1]

Insulin therapy should be used for achieving glycemic control in hospitalized patients with T2DM and fracture. The treatment option of choice is basal bolus scheduled subcutaneous insulin.

CONCLUSION

- Patients with T1DM or T2DM diabetes are at increased risk for fractures
- Longstanding DM, poor glycemic control, β-cell failure, chronic complications and treatment with insulin are some of the factors which increase the fracture risk
- Bone mineral density underestimates the risk in T2DM patients
- Care of patients with diabetes should include assessment of bone health. However, how to properly assess fracture risk and manage osteoporosis in patients with diabetes is not clear and guidelines do not exist
- The effect of oral anti-diabetic agents on skeletal fragility should be considered when treating diabetes in osteoporotic patients.

REFERENCES

1. Paschou SA, Dede AD, Anagnostis PG, et al. Type 2 Diabetes and Osteoporosis: A Guide to Optimal Management. J Clin Endo Metab. 2017;102:3621-34.
2. Brown SA, Sharpless JL. Osteoporosis: An Under-appreciated Complication of Diabetes. Clin Diabetes. 2004;22:10-20.
3. International Osteoporosis Foundation. (2017). The global burden of osteoporosis: a fact-sheet. [online] Available from: https://www.iofbonehealth.org/data-publications/fact-sheets/global-burden-osteoporosis. [Accessed Oct., 2018].

4. Napoli N, Chandran M, Dominique D, et al. Mechanisms of diabetes mellitus-induced bone fragility. Nat Rev Endo. 2017;13:208-19.
5. Janghorbani M, Feskanich D, Willett WC, et al. Prospective study of diabetes and risk of hip fracture: the Nurses' Health Study. Diabetes Care. 2006;29:1573-8.
6. Janghorbani M, Van Dam RM, Willett WC, et al. Systematic review of type 1 and type 2 diabetes mellitus and risk of fracture. Am J Epidemiol. 2007;166:495-505.
7. Wongdee K, Charoenphandhu N. Osteoporosis in diabetes mellitus: Possible cellular and molecular mechanisms. World J Diabetes. 2011;2(3):41-8.
8. Dhaon P, Shah VN. Type 1 diabetes and osteoporosis: A review of literature. Ind J Endo Metab. 2014;18:159-65.
9. Jackuliak P, Payer J. Osteoporosis, Fractures, and Diabetes. Int J Endo. 2014;ID 820615.
10. Chandran M. Clinical aspects and management of osteoporosis and fragility fractures in patients with diabetes. Osteopor Sarcopenia. 2017;3: 123-7.
11. Schwartz AV, Vittinghoff E, Bauer DC, et al. Association of BMD and FRAX score with risk of fracture in older adults with type 2 diabetes. JAMA. 2011;305:2184-92.

Chapter 54

Diabetes, Hypertension and Atherosclerosis—Common Soil Hypothesis—Fighting Against the Deadly Trio

A Muruganathan, M Gowri Sankar

INTRODUCTION

In India, diabetes, hypertension and atherosclerosis are the growing health problems. As we all know hypertension is a major risk factor for cardiovascular (CV), cerebrovascular and renal disease. Moreover, when hypertension occurs in diabetes, it accelerates the progression of both microvascular and macrovascular complications. Mortality also gets increased by more than seven-fold. This deadly duo is a well-known risk factor for cardiovascular disease (CVD). Atherosclerotic cardiovascular disease (ASCVD) is the costliest complication, which accounts for rapidly increase in the prevalence in developed as well as in developing countries and have emerged as the leading cause of premature mortality.[1]

INCIDENCE OF DIABETES AND HYPERTENSION[2]

Hypertension is twice as prevalent in diabetics as in nondiabetic individuals. In patients with type 1 diabetes mellitus (DM), hypertension develops at the onset of diabetic nephropathy while in type 2 DM, more than 50% patients are hypertensive at the time of diagnosis.

The estimated number of people with hypertension is increasing worldwide and is expected to increase from 972 million in 2000 to 1.56 billion by 2025. In diabetes, estimated number of people worldwide is expected to increase from 382 million in 2012 to 592 billion in 2030. Forty-eight percent of the anticipated absolute global increase of 186 million people with diabetes is projected to occur in India and China alone.

EVIDENCE

Studies Related to Diabetes, Hypertension and Atherosclerosis Worldwide[2]

- In the UKPDS (UK Prospective Diabetes Study) study, each 10 mm Hg decrease in mean systolic blood pressure (SBP) was associated with relative risk reduction of 12% for any complication of diabetes, 15% for deaths related to diabetes, 11% for myocardial infarction and 13% for microvascular complications. The study also shows improved insulin resistance with metformin and decreased macrovascular events
- The HOT (Hypertension Optimal Treatment) study showed that diabetics with high blood pressure (BP) will need two to three drugs to control their BP
- The Systolic Hypertension in the Elderly Program (SHEP) and other studies like Hypertension Detection and Follow-up Program (HDFP), Systolic Hypertension in Europe (Syst-Eur), HOT, normotensive Appropriate Blood pressure Control in Diabetes (ABCD) and Heart Outcomes Prevention Evaluation (HOPE) provide firm evidence that even small BP reductions translate to significant decrease in both micro- and macrovascular complications in persons with type 2 diabetes
- The ADVANCE (Action in Diabetes and Vascular Disease; Preterax and Diamicron MR Controlled Evaluation) study showed that intensive control of BP resulted in reduction in composite micro- and macrovascular complications by 9%, coronary events by 14% and renal events by 21%
- The ADVANCE Collaborative Group study demonstrating the benefit of an angiotensin-converting

enzyme inhibitor (ACEI) and indapamide in a fixed combination, strongly suggesting that the BP goal (<130/80 mm Hg) was beneficial

- The ACCORD (Action to Control Cardiovascular Risk in Diabetes) trial was unable to find a significant reduction in incidence of major CV events in patients with diabetes whose SBP was lowered to an average of 119 mm Hg compared with patients whose SBP remained at an average of 133 mm Hg
- The Reduction of Atherothrombosis for Continued Health (REACH) Registry, which collected global data on atherosclerosis risk-factors from around 68,000 patients aged older than or equal to 45 years in 44 countries, found that classic CV risk-factors such as hypertension, diabetes, dyslipidemia, obesity and smoking are consistent and common in diverse ethnic populations
- The ONTARGET (telmisartan, ramipril, or both in patients at high risk for vascular events) study compared between telmisartan and ramipril in patients with diabetes and vascular events.

How are Diabetes, Hypertension and Atherosclerosis related?

Atherosclerosis is a complex multifactorial disease resulting from both genetic and environmental factors. The DM, hypertension and dyslipidemia are considered as the accepted risk factors, which are responsible for the development and acceleration of atherosclerosis (Box 1).

METABOLIC SYNDROME[3]

Metabolic syndrome also known as insulin resistance syndrome or syndrome X is a global epidemic with increasing prevalence from 10% in the 30–39 year age group to 45% in the 60–69 year age group.

Box 1: Risk factors for the development of atherosclerosis.

- Age
- Male gender
- Family history of early onset of vascular events
- Insulin resistance syndromes
- Systemic hypertension
- Diabetes mellitus
- Increased LDL cholesterol
- Decreased HDL cholesterol
- Cigarette smoking
- Low physical activity

(LDL: low-density lipoprotein; HDL: high-density lipoprotein.)

TABLE 1: Criteria for diagnosing metabolic syndrome.

S. no	Criteria for diagnosing metabolic syndrome
1	Waist circumference >35 inches (88 cm) in women >40 inches (102 cm) in men
2	Triglycerides >150 mg/dL
3	HDL <40 mg/dL in men and <50 mg/dL in women
4	Blood pressure >130/85 mm Hg or treated hypertension
5	Fasting glucose >100 mg/dL

Note: Three of five of these conditions is diagnostic.

(HDL: high-density lipoprotein.)

Box 2: Risk factors of metabolic syndrome.

- Advanced age
- Genetic inheritance
- Sedentary lifestyle
- Obesity
- Impaired glucose tolerance
- Hyperglycemia
- Hyperinsulinemia
- Altered fibrinolysis
- Hypertension
- Increased triglycerides
- Increase in small dense LDL
- Decreased HDL
- Chronic stress
- Sleep deprivation

(LDL: low-density lipoprotein; HDL: high-density lipoprotein.)

According to National Cholesterol Education Program-Adult Treatment Panel III (NCEP-ATP III) guidelines, metabolic syndrome may be diagnosed when a patient has three or more of the five clinically identifiable risk factors (Table 1).

These clusters of metabolic syndrome risk factors are associated with increased risk of development of ASCVD and type 2 DM. The central core of metabolic syndrome is insulin resistance, which is associated with following risk factors (Box 2).

PATHOPHYSIOLOGY OF DIABETES, HYPERTENSION AND ATHEROSCLEROSIS—COMMON SOIL HYPOTHESIS[2]

The common pathophysiological mechanisms contributing to both occurrence as well as exacerbation of these conditions are insulin resistance hypothesis. It is gaining more acceptance as a common etiological factor for these diseases as "the common soil hypothesis", a term coined to point out that these diseases originate from the same soil rooting from insulin resistance. Box 3 shows causes of insulin resistance.

Box 3: Causes of insulin resistance.

- Obesity/overweight (especially excess visceral adiposity)
- Autoantibodies to the insulin receptor
- Mutations of insulin receptor
- Mutations of the peroxisome proliferators-activated receptor-γ (PPAR-γ)
- Mutations that cause genetic obesity (e.g. melanocortin receptor mutations)
- Pregnancy, gestational diabetes
- Polycystic ovary disease
- Excess glucocorticoids (Cushing's syndrome or steroid therapy)
- Excess growth hormone (acromegaly)
- Lipodystrophy (acquired or genetic, associated with lipid accumulation in liver)
- Hemochromatosis (a hereditary disease that causes tissue iron accumulation)

Source: Guyton and Hall.

Role of Insulin Resistance in Diabetes and Hypertension[2,4]

- The abnormal metabolic state in diabetes and in hypertension causes endothelial cell dysfunction. The insulin resistance and the resultant hyperinsulinemia in diabetes cause various pathological consequences in nitric oxide pathway, activates sympathetic drive, increases in vascular smooth muscle cell (VSMC) cytosolic calcium, induction of endothelin secretion and enhancement of vascular lipid deposition, sodium and fluid retention, all contributing to the pathogenesis of hypertension (Flowchart 1)

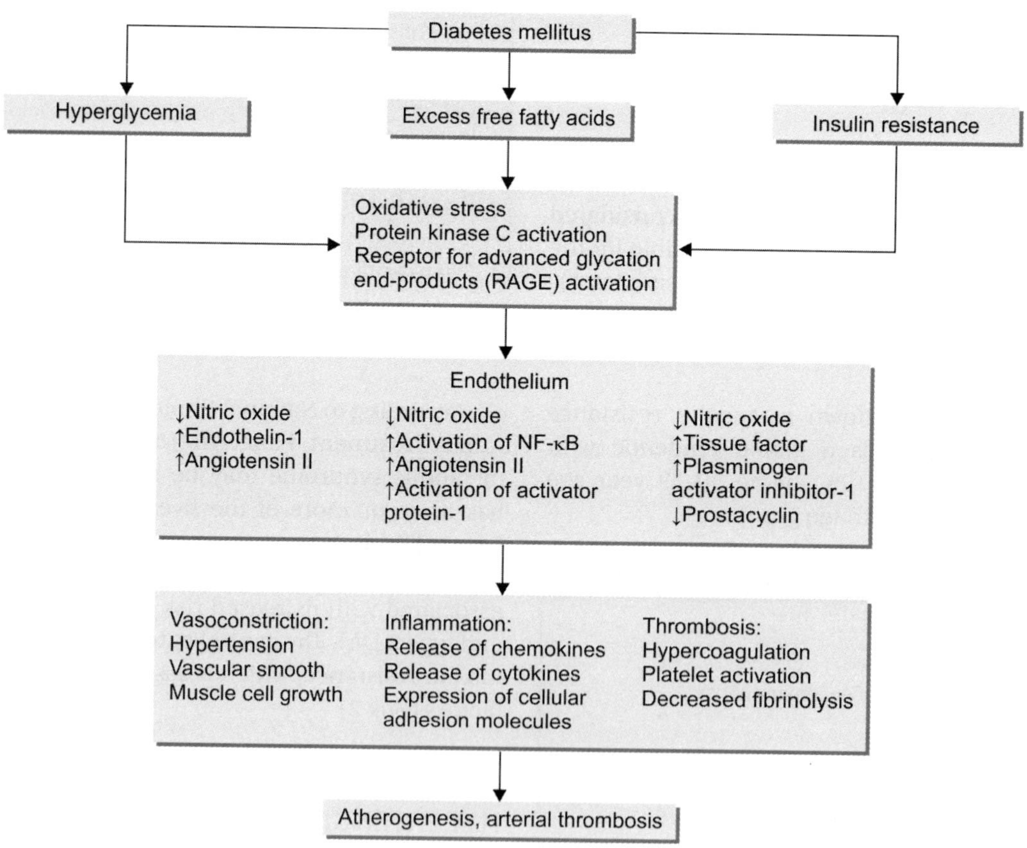

(NF-κB: nuclear factor-κB.)

Flowchart 1 Common pathophysiological mechanism of diabetes, hypertension and atherosclerosis.

- Hyperglycemia inhibits the production of endothelium-dependent nitric oxide release by blocking endothelial nitric-oxide synthase (eNOS) activation and increases the production of reactive oxygen species (ROS) in endothelial and VSMCs, thereby it reduces vasodilation effect
- Hyperglycemia also increases other endothelium-derived substances such as prostanoids and angiotensin II which cause vasoconstriction. The advanced glycation end-products (AGEs) in circulation and vessel wall are associated with impaired endothelial-dependent vasodilatation and increased vessel wall stiffness
- Hyperinsulinemia leads to excess flux of free-fatty acids from adipose tissue, which activates the signaling enzyme protein kinase C (PKC), inhibit phosphatidylinositol-3 (PI-3) kinase (an eNOS agonist pathway), and increases the production of ROS. Thereby, it impairs nitric oxide production and its vasodilatation effect
- Hyperinsulinemia also increases the production of endothelin-1, which in turn activates endothelin-A receptors on VSMC to induce vasoconstriction. Endothelin-1 also increases renal sodium and water retention and also stimulates the renin–angiotensin–aldosterone system (RAAS) and induces VSMC hypertrophy. Activation of the RAAS results in unregulated angiotensinogen II activity through its angiotensin I receptor leading to the formation of ROS. RAAS activation also leads to uninhibited production of aldosterone, which in turn induces sodium retention, enhanced sympathetic and decreased parasympathetic activity and increased extracellular matrix deposition
- Insulin resistance prevents intracellular magnesium transport into VSMCs and diminishes Na^+/K^+-ATPase activity resulting in elevated cytosolic calcium and increased vascular tone
- Increased sympathetic activity has been observed in people with insulin resistance and obesity
- High serum leptin levels (hyperleptinemia) from the increased fat mass or secondary to leptin receptor resistance are further potentiated by hyperinsulinemia. This increases sympathetic drive via central and peripheral mechanisms, thus contributing to increased BP and heart rate
- Adiponectin (an adipocyte derived peptide has anti-inflammatory, insulin-sensitizing and endothelium-protective properties) is lower in obese subjects and inversely related to systolic and diastolic pressure
- Insulin promotes renal tubular reabsorption of sodium via Na/H antiport system or the Na^+/K^+-ATPase in the renal tubule leads to sodium and water retention, thus contributing to increased BP
- Erythrocyte sodium-lithium countertransport, which represents sodium reabsorption in the proximal tubule, has been found to be overactive in persons with diabetes and hypertension
- Hyperglycemia activates the nuclear transcription factor-κB (NF-κB) through a PKC dependent pathway and activator protein 1 induces inflammatory gene expression, with liberation of leukocyte-attracting chemokines, increased production of inflammatory cytokines, and augmented expression of cellular adhesion molecules. Increased plasminogen activator inhibitor-1 (PAI-1) expression creates a prothrombotic milieu and augments atherosclerotic lesions.

Role of Insulin Resistance in Obesity

- Central obesity reflects increased visceral adipose tissue, i.e. intra-abdominal fat around the intestines and in liver. These adipose tissue produces proinflammatory cytokines like tumor necrosis factor-α (TNF-α), C-reactive protein, interleukins 6 and PAI-1. TNF-α acts by inhibiting intracellular insulin signaling in adipocytes and hepatocytes and also inhibits peroxisome proliferation-activated receptor-γ function leads to insulin resistance. The insulin resistance resulting in lipolysis by adipocyte-derived free fatty acids promoting triglyceride accumulation. Obesity also associated with RAAS activation leads to higher levels of angiotensin II, renin, aldosterone and ACE leading to hypertension. Proinflammatory and prothrombotic factors in turn enhance CV risk. Obesity is also characterized by high levels of leptin consistent with leptin resistance
- Enhanced activity of enzyme 11 β-hydroxysteroid dehydrogenase type 1 leading to increased fat tissue-specific cortisol production, and reduced inactivation of cortisol by altered 11 β-hydroxysteroid dehydrogenase type 2 in fat cells has been demonstrated in insulin-resistant obese subjects
- The ACE-D (angiotensin-converting enzyme-D) isoform is associated with an increase in the circulating ACE activity and has recently been shown to be a significant predictor of weight gain and abdominal adiposity in men.

Role of Insulin Resistance in Atherosclerosis

- The atherosclerotic lesions are proposed by "response to injury" hypothesis to the vascular endothelium. Endothelial cell injury may occur in the form of mechanical forces like hypertension or by metabolic conditions, such as DM and dyslipidemia, or by environmental agents like tobacco smoke directly injures the endothelium and causes endothelial dysfunction, which precedes the development of morphological atherosclerotic changes
- Insulin resistance and hyperinsulinemia are also involved in atherogenic lipid profile. Hyperinsulinemia enhances very low-density lipoprotein (VLDL) synthesis leads to hypertriglyceridemia. From VLDL there is an increased formation of atherogenic low density lipoprotein. Insulin stimulates cholesterol transport into arteriolar smooth muscle cells and thereby enhances endogenous lipid synthesis, also stimulates the smooth muscle proliferation, collagen synthesis in vessel wall and the subsequent inflammatory response result in atheroma formation
- Thus, diabetes, hypertension and atherosclerosis share the common soil hypothesis of endothelial dysfunction, insulin resistance and RAAS system.

Genetic Causes

- Genetic variants in the gene encoding angiotensinogen, adrenomedullin, apolipoprotein, and α-adducin have been associated with common conditions such as diabetes, hypertension or metabolic syndrome
- A missense mutation of the β3 adrenergic receptor gene (*ADRB3*) is associated with low resting metabolic rate, weight gain, early onset of type 2 diabetes and hypertension
- Polymorphisms of the glucocorticoid receptor gene, particularly those which alter the receptor's sensitivity to cortisol, have been associated with central obesity and hypertension.

Assessment Methods of Insulin Resistance

- Fasting insulin and serum triglycerides levels can be used as a screening in clinical practice
- Homeostatic model assessment (HOMA)
- Euglycemic clamp—gold standard
- Frequently Sampled Intravenous Glucose Tolerance Test (FSIVGTT)—standard method in research field
- Short insulin tolerance test (ITT)
- Continuous infusion of glucose with model assessment (CIGMA)
- Insulin suppression test (IST).

DIABETIC NEPHROPATHY AND HYPERTENSION

- In type 1 diabetes, hypertension begins with the onset of nephropathy (microalbuminuria stage). A history of hypertension in the parents and increased erythrocyte sodium-lithium countertransport and DD isoform of the *ACE* gene, which is linked to increased ACE generation are markers of genetic susceptibility to hypertension and nephropathy
- In type 2 diabetes, about 50% already have obesity and age-related essential hypertension. Hypertension is present in more than 90% of diabetics with impaired renal function. Increased SBP is a significant risk factor for microalbuminuria and rapid progression of nephropathy
- Overall diabetic kidney disease is a potent risk factor for macrovascular disease, namely atherosclerosis, myocardial infarction, heart failure and cerebro-vascular events.

Risk Assessment

All modifiable and nonmodifiable risk factors to be assessed by quick 15-minute evaluation (Box 4).

Strategy for Management of Hypertensive Diabetic Patients[2]

- Proper blood sugar control
- Achieve target level of BP control for diabetic patients
- Early detection of both diabetes and hypertension complications, manage them to delay their progression and improve patient's quality of life.

Non-drug Therapy

The multifactorial approaches, based on the following nonpharmaco-therapeutic interventions, are:

Nutrition

Blood pressure of diabetic patients more sensitive to salt intake and this sodium sensitivity is found even in absence of nephropathy. A decreased salt intake is important for diabetic patients with hypertension.

Box 4: Quick 15-minute evaluation.

Ask history of:
- Age
- Diet habits
- Level of physical activity
- Smoking
- Family history of premature CV events
- Past history of diabetes mellitus, hypertension and dyslipidemia
- History of psychosocial stress
- Drug history of growth hormones, steroids, nicotinic acid, etc.
- Menstrual history in PCOS

Examination:
- Look for external markers of insulin resistance like acanthosis nigricans
- Measure blood pressure
- Examination of peripheral arteries
- Measure waist circumference, calculate body mass index
- Systemic examination

(CV: cardiovascular; PCOS: polycystic ovary syndrome.)

Reducing Salt (Sodium) Intake

Aim for less than 3–5 g/day. However, the daily average salt consumption in Indian scenario is 8–9 g/day.

Ways to Reduce Sodium Intake

- Food items without added salts
- Unsalted nuts, seeds, beans
- Avoid adding salt and canned vegetables to homemade dishes
- Unsalted and sodium free, fat-free broths and soups
- Use fresh poultry, lean meat and fish
- Rinse canned foods to reduce sodium
- Low sodium, low fat cheeses
- Add spices and herbs to enhance taste
- Add fresh lemon juice instead of salt to fresh vegetable salad.

Benefits of Moderate Sodium Reduction (Box 5)

Box 5: Benefits of moderate sodium reduction.
- Improvement in large artery compliance (Gates et al. 2004)
- Enhancement of efficacy of antihypertensive drugs (Slagman et al. 2011; Aziza et al. 2013)
- Reduction of diuretic-induced potassium loss (Ram et al. 1981)
- Regression of left ventricular hypertrophy (Rodriguez et al. 2011)
- Reduction in proteinuria (Agarwal, 2012)
- Reduction in urine calcium excretion (Carbone et al. 2003)
- Decrease in osteoporosis (Martini et al. 2000)
- Decreased prevalence of stomach cancer (Fock et al. 2008)
- Decreased prevalence of stroke (Joossens and Kesteloot, 2008)
- Decreased prevalence of cataract (Cumming et al. 2000)
- Protection against onset of hypertension (Whellton PK, 2014)

Know what to eat:

Dietary Approaches to Stop Hypertension *(DASH)* diet is an eating plan, rich in fruits, vegetables, whole grains, fish, poultry, nuts, legumes and low-fat dairy. These foods are high in key nutrients such as potassium, magnesium, calcium, fiber and protein. The DASH diet can lower BP because it has less salt and sugar.

4–5 servings of fruits and vegetables/6–8 servings of whole grain/saturated fat 6% of total calories/total cholesterol of less than 150 mg/day.

WEIGHT REDUCTION

The prevention and correction of overweight/obesity [body mass index (BMI) >25 kg/m^2] is a prudent way of reducing the risk of hypertension and indirectly reducing coronary artery disease; it goes with dietary changes. Loss of weight by 1 kg decreases BP by approximately 1 mm Hg.

EXERCISE PROMOTION

Physical activity:

F Frequency	—at least 5 days/week
I Intensity	—Moderate
T Time	—30–45 minutes
T Type	—Cardiorespiratory activity
	—Walking, jogging
	—Cycling
	—Noncompetitive swimming

Exercise should be prescribed as an adjunctive to pharmacological therapy.

BEHAVIORAL CHANGES

Reduction of stress, cessation of smoking, moderation of alcohol drinking, modification of personal lifestyle, yoga and transcendental meditation could be beneficial.

SELF-CARE

Blood Pressure Monitoring

In order to overcome the limitations of the office blood pressure (OBP) measurement, two methods are widely used in clinical practice:

1. Home blood pressure monitoring (HBPM)
2. Twenty-four hours ambulatory blood pressure monitoring (ABPM).

The patient is taught about self-care, i.e. HBPM and to keep a log-book of his BP readings. Twenty-four hours ABPM monitoring is a precise method to quantify BP levels and to diagnose hypertension and also it is used as a marker of CV morbidity and mortality.

Glucose Monitoring

Self-monitoring of blood glucose (SMBG) is becoming an important component in improving glycemic control in diabetes. It helps in adjustment of a treatment regimen in response to blood glucose level and provide information on glucose excursions and hypoglycemia related to drugs, insulin and lifestyle changes like dietary intake and exercise.

Role of Ambulatory Blood Pressure Monitoring in Diabetic Patients[5,6]

- Ambulatory BP monitoring is advisable in all diabetic patients with high-normal BP
- Diabetic patients are more likely to have:
    - White-coat hypertension
    - Masked hypertension
    - Non-dipping
    - Reverse dipping
    - Morning BP surge.
- High prevalence of masked hypertension in diabetic patients is associated with higher risk of brain and kidney damage and possible cardiac damage, which further increase CV complications
- White-coat hypertension in diabetic patients appears to be associated with a lower risk than sustained hypertension
- Non-dipping and reverse dipping may reflect autonomic dysfunction and it might be used as a clinical marker of diabetic autonomic neuropathy
- Ambulatory BP monitoring provides information on heart rate at the time of BP measurements all over the 24 hours, and a rough estimate of heart rate variability. The reduced heart rate variability is the index of diabetic neuropathy
- Ambulatory BP monitoring also provides information on pulse pressure (difference between systolic and diastolic BP), when increased is considered as a surrogate marker of stiffening of arterial walls.

Target Blood pressure in Diabetes Mellitus

- Most patients with diabetes and hypertension should be treated with a BP goal of less than 130/80 mm Hg
- In patients with high risk of CVD BP should be less than 130/80 mm Hg[7]
- The aim is to maintain low BP which the patient can tolerate without postural hypotension and without compromise on critical vascular beds as well as quality of life.

Ideal Antihypertensive Drug in Diabetes Mellitus[2]

- Must decrease BP to less than or equal to 130/80 mm Hg
- Must reduce the RAAS activity, improve endothelial dysfunction
- Must prevent, improve or arrest proteinuria
- Must prevent and protect from coronary artery disease, chronic kidney disease, congestive heart failure
- Must be favorable on glycemic control
- Must improve the dyslipidemia—not worsen it
- Must not worsen peripheral arterial disease
- Must not cause impotence
- Must not decrease estimated glomerular filtration rate and increase serum creatinine
- Must not increase uric acid, serum potassium
- Can be easily combined with other drugs
- An ideal agent should not increase insulin resistance
- Well-tolerated, cost-effective.

Effects of Antihypertensives on Diabetes

- There are three classes of RAS modulating agents are available ACE inhibitors, angiotensin receptor blockers (ARBs) and renin inhibitors. ACEIs and ARBs are suitable first-line antihypertensive in diabetics. It has renal protective effect in incipient nephropathy, reduces insulin resistance and may improve glycemia in diabetics and patients with the metabolic syndrome
- Why ACEI is preferred in DM?
    - *Improves insulin sensitivity:*
        - Reverse vascular and ventricular remodeling.
    - *Reverse left ventricular hypertrophy:*
        - Cardioprotection
        - Renal protection.

- Favorable glucose lipid metabolism.
- Thiazide diuretics and β-blockers have metabolic side-effects such as increasing insulin resistance or direct diabetogenesis, which make them less appropriate as first-line agents
- The use of calcium channel blockers (CCBs) was not significantly associated with incident diabetes compared to other antihypertensive agents: the association with diabetes was lowest for ACEIs and ARBs, followed by CCBs, β-blockers and diuretics.

Antidiabetic drugs

- The antidiabetic agents like metformin and thiazolidinediones reduce insulin resistance
- Sodium-glucose cotransporter 2 inhibitors cause osmotic diuresis leading to BP reduction and reduced the rate of CV events
- Glucagon-like peptide-1 agonists and dipeptidyl peptidase-4 inhibitors have been demonstrated to exert their effects directly through the activation of their receptors on the cardiac and vascular tissues or centrally positioned receptors to reduce the BP
- Insulin causes salt and water retention, increases body weight and it causes growth of tissues as an anabolic hormone.

Statin Treatment Recommendations[7]

See Tables 2 and 3.

Bariatric Surgery

Metabolic surgery is the only treatment modality for morbid obesity with a BMI of 40 kg/m^2 or greater. It may also be suggested for the patient with a BMI between 35 and 40 kg/m^2 in presence of obesity-related disease and the patient failed to lose weight despite lifestyle and optimal medical therapy. In the appropriate patient, metabolic surgery results in resolution of diabetes, hypertension, hyperlipidemia and sleep apnea.

TABLE 2: Statin treatment recommendations.

Diabetes patients of all ages + ASCVD	LSM + high-intensity statin
Diabetes patients aged <40 years + ASCVD risk factor	LSM + moderate-intensity statin
Diabetes patients aged 40–75 years without ASCVD	LSM + moderate-intensity statin
Diabetes patients with ASCVD with LDL cholesterol ≥70 mg/dL on maximally tolerated statin dose	LSM + high-intensity statin + LDL lowering therapy (ezetimibe or PCSK9 inhibitor)

(LDL: low-density lipoprotein; LSM: lifestyle modifications; ASCVD: atherosclerotic cardiovascular disease; PCSK9: proprotein convertase subtilisin/kexin type 9.)

TABLE 3: High-intensity and moderate-intensity statin therapy.

High-intensity statin therapy	Moderate-intensity statin therapy
• Atorvastatin 40–80 mg • Rosuvastatin 20–40 mg	• Atorvastatin 10–20 mg • Rosuvastatin 5–10 mg • Simvastatin 20–40 mg • Pravastatin 40–80 mg • Lovastatin 40 mg • Fluvastatin XL 80 mg • Pitavastatin 2–4 mg

CONCLUSION

Diagnose the disease, detect its root cause,
Discern its cure and then act aptly.
—Saint Thiruvalluvar (300–700 BCE)

Diabetes mellitus, hypertension and dyslipidemia are comorbid illnesses, in both developing and developed countries. The presence of one increases the risk of having the other. All three increase the risk of ASCVD events. So, every diabetes patient needs measuring of BP in every visit. Hypertensive patients need to be screened for diabetes and dyslipidemia regularly. HBPM could be an ideal way in monitoring BP in hypertensive patients in general and diabetic patients in particular to ensure that the patient does not progress to develop CV and renal complications.

REFERENCES

1. Reddy KS, Yusuf S. Emerging epidemic of cardiovascular disease in developing countries. Circulation. 1998.
2. Muruganathan A. Diabetes and hypertension—Common soil hypothesis, cardiodiabetes update. 2017.
3. Codario RA. Type 2 diabetes, pre-diabetes, and the metabolic syndrome, 2nd edition. 2011;68-78.
4. Beckman JA. Diabetes and Atherosclerosis Epidemiology, Pathophysiology, and Management. JAMA. 2002;287(19):2570-81.
5. Grossman E. Ambulatory Blood Pressure Monitoring in the Diagnosis and Management of Hypertension. Diabetes Care. 2013;36 (suppl 2): S307-S311.
6. Leitão CB, Canani LH. Ambulatory Blood Pressure Monitoring and Type 2 Diabetes Mellitus: Arq Bras Cardiol. 2007;89(5):315-21, 347-54.
5. American Diabetes Association. (2018). American Diabetes Association Standards of Medical Care in Diabetes-2018. [online] Available from: http://care.diabetesjournals.org/content/41/Supplement_1 [Accessed Oct., 2018].

Chapter 55

Diabetes Care in Elderly—Clinical Care Issues

Jugal Kishor Sharma

INTRODUCTION

The incidence and prevalence of diabetes is progressively increasing worldwide and latest population data from International Diabetes Federation (IDF) atlas released in 2017 is not only alarming but disturbing as well. The burden of diabetes is rising; more and more people worldwide are getting affected with diabetes at a younger age and at the same time average life span of world population is also increasing,[1] which may be attributed to better access to food, education and healthcare system. As a result of this, we are going to witness a boom in population which was diagnosed with diabetes at a much earlier age and is also likely to live longer because of the average increase in life span. This is contrary to usual trend where diabetes was diagnosed at a later age and average life span was shorten than what it is used to be today. This is also going to pose a challenge to medical community as elderly diabetic patients will also be more susceptible to complications and will increase the burden on healthcare infrastructure and at the same time will also require a geriatric diabetes care team which can understand the unique challenges of the elderly population. Elderly patients with diabetes are unique because of likelihood of coexistence of many age-related complications, thus increasing the possibility of polypharmacy. Also the most common geriatric problems like depression in elderly, tendency to fall, cognitive and behavioral changes and urinary incontinence, inability to carry out tasks of daily living because of joint pains and musculoskeletal diseases, increased susceptibility to infections limited self-care abilities apart from social challenges which may include but not limited to finances and care by children and caregivers. I would briefly discuss the aspects in which diabetes care in elderly may differ from diabetes care in young.

INDIAN PERSPECTIVE

According to the official World Health Organization (WHO) data, India tops the list of countries with the highest number of diabetics; China America, Indonesia, Japan, Pakistan, Russia, Brazil, Italy and Bangladesh follow. In the year 2000, the total number of diabetics in India stood at 31.7 million and is expected to rise by >100% in the year 2030 to account to a whopping 79.4 million.

Hyperglycemia in Elderly—Is it Different?

As we know spontaneous fall is a significant concern in elderly patients, dehydration secondary to uncontrolled blood glucose levels can lead to visual impairment as well as cognitive impairment[2]—accelerating the functional decline and further increasing the risk of fall. Elderly patients may have less osmotic symptoms and can tolerate even higher degree of hyperglycemia without osmotic symptoms. This can be explained by age-related decline in glomerular function and estimated glomerular filtration rate (eGFR) (decreased glucose load to the tubules for reabsorption). Action to control cardiovascular risk in diabetes (ACCORD) trial has shown that polypharmacy in patients with high risk for cardiovascular disease (CVD) may increase the risk of adverse CV outcomes including cardiovascular (CV) death.[3] Hemoglobin A1c (HbA1c) estimation may not be that accurate because of frequent coexistence of comorbid conditions like anemia, chronic kidney disease (CKD), chronic liver disease (CLD), recent illness and hospitalizations. Risk of sarcopenia which is defined as decrease in muscle mass is significantly higher in elderly population.[4]

Hypoglycemia—Challenges in Elderly

Elderly people are more susceptible to hypoglycemia,[5] but contrary to young patients they have more neuroglycopenic symptoms and less adrenergic symptoms.[6] This means less tremors and sweating (autonomic dysfunction) and more atypical symptoms like altered sensorium, dizziness, headache and confusion and sometimes symptoms may mimic a transient ischemic attack and needs high degree of suspicion for hypoglycemia. Studies have shown that hypoglycemia is an independent risk factor for adverse CV outcomes, increases autonomic dysfunction[7] and frequent hypoglycemic episodes also increase the risk of dementia. So, in a frail elderly patient even an episode of minor hypoglycemia can lead to events which can be fatal. So it is important to address the risk of hypoglycemia in the specific population by choosing drugs and therapeutic approaches which minimizes the risk of hypoglycemia.

TREATMENT GOALS

Treatment goals in elderly patients with diabetes are not any different as in young patients and are directed towards management of hyperglycemia, complications as well as comorbidities and risk factors. However, a personalized and individualized approach may be more suitable as it is important to address the social structure (living alone, at old age home or in a nursing home), existing medical conditions (coronary artery disease and heart failure, chronic obstructive lung disease, dementia, depression to name a few), comorbid conditions (frail, structural and functional disabilities), cognitive impairment (missed doses, multiple doses), multiple drugs and possibility of drug-drug interactions and inability to perform self-management tasks.

Glycemic Targets in Elderly

There are limited studies and data to actually define specific glycemic goals in elderly but the limited data suggest that one should assess the risk factors, overall health status and expected or projected survival before defying the glycemic goals in a patient as many of the expected complications of diabetes are dependent on its duration. Table 1 based on various recommendations and guidelines[8-10] by American Diabetes Association (ADA), American geriatric society, IDF and various International and European working groups summarizes the various glycemic goals including HbA1c, fasting and prandial sugar while considering the overall health status, average life expectancy and risk of hypoglycemia may be a suitable guide for deciding treatment strategy in diabetic patients at the same time improving quality of life.

Cardiovascular Risk Management

Coronary heart disease (CHD) is the leading cause of death in patients with diabetes. Age again is an independent risk factor for CHD, so it is not a surprise that an elderly diabetic patient is at much higher risk of morbidity and mortality due to CHD than their younger counterparts.[11] Studies like Steno-2 and Veterans Affairs Diabetes Trial (VADT) has taught us that CV risk reduction requires a multipronged approach and more benefit being derived with focus on aggressive lipid lowering, smoking cessation, blood pressure management and aspirin for primary prevention. Strict blood glucose control can actually worsen the CV outcomes in elderly and frail patients.

TABLE 1: Glycemic targets in elderly patients with diabetes.

HbA1c target (%)	Fasting/prandial targets (mg %)	Overall health	Life expectancy	Risk of hypoglycemia
<7.5	140–150	Fit	>10 years	Low
7.5–8	160–170	Frail	<10 years	High
8–8.5	190–200	Very old	Limited life expectancy	Very high

(HbA1c: hemoglobin A1c.)

TREATMENT

Lifestyle modification[1,10,12] should not be overlooked in elderly as Diabetes Prevention Program (DPP) has shown that the following lifestyle intervention the oldest age group (>60 years) had the highest benefit in terms of glycemic improvement, so again proving beyond doubt that lifestyle intervention can be done at any age and age should not be a barrier in advising lifestyle interventions. Physical activity prescription must consider all the comorbidities before beginning of the activity and must include aerobic activities as well as weight training. Medical nutrition therapy (MNT) must consider age-specific issue like altered taste perception, poor dentition, altered bowel movements and limited ability to procure and prepare specific food. In general simple food and dietary regimens in elderly may be more beneficial than complex and difficult to follow dietary regimens. Any unintentional weight loss in elderly patient warrants further evaluation.

Drug Therapy

Pharmacotherapy and drugs available for the management of diabetes in elderly are no different from those used in management of diabetes in younger population. A summary[13] of the various class of drugs, there main advantages and potential disadvantages are listed in Table 2. It is important to realize that while choosing the medication for the elderly diabetic patient, due emphasis should be given to special attributes as discussed above in this population. Every effort should be made to achieve realistic glycemic goals while at the same time minimizing the risk of hypoglycemia and other potential adverse effects which may compound the other existing comorbidities.

Monitoring of Glycemic Goals

The HbA1c monitoring[1] may be done twice in a year in patients who are regularly on targets while once in 3 month A1c estimation is required, if therapy is altered or changed or if patient is not meeting the glycemic targets. Self-monitoring of blood glucose (SMBG)[12] is indicated in a motivated patient who is on drugs with high risk of hypoglycemia like insulin, or requires intensification or down titration of insulin. SMBG may also help the patient in modifying and changing eating patterns.

Microvascular Complications of Diabetes in Elderly

All elderly patients should be screened for presences of microvascular complications namely retinopathy, nephropathy and neuropathy. Patient must be screened for presence of cataract, glaucoma and retinopathy and a dilated fundus examination is indicated once a year. Screening for diabetic nephropathy and estimation of eGFR will also help in guiding therapy. Foot problems are extremely common in elderly subjects and present of neuropathy[14] can further increase the risk of fall. A foot examination must be carried out at every visit in all diabetic patients.

VACCINATION AND IMMUNIZATION

As universal standard of diabetes care all elderly patients must be vaccinated against vaccine preventable diseases[10] like flu, pneumococcal infection and other diseases as per local vaccination guidelines.

Geriatric Syndromes and Diabetes-impact on Care

Elderly diabetic patients suffer increased morbidity and mortality when compared to their nondiabetic elderly counterpart. Diabetes increases the risk of dementia. Dementia and cognitive impairment can interfere with self-management ability and behavior. Depression is present very commonly but is often under diagnosed[15] and underrated further compromising the quality of life.[16] Patients are often taking multiple drugs; this can lead to compounding of side effects. A review of medication list at every visit will help in removing unwanted or nonessential medications. Functional and structural disabilities with osteoarthritis and joint problems, neuropathy and frequent hypoglycemic episodes and poor vision increase the tendency to fall.[17]

CONCLUSION

Elderly patients require special and individualized care based on certain facts and evidences as discussed above. A sincere effort can go a long way in improving the glycemic complications and hence quality and productivity of life in an elderly patient with diabetes.

TABLE 2: **Classes of drugs and its advantages.**

Drug	Advantages	Disadvantages/caution
Metformin	• Low cost • Low risk of hypoglycemia • Weight neutral or minimal weight loss • Anti-aging effects	• To be discontinued when eGFR <30 mL/min • Lactic acidosis • Gastric intolerance to metformin
Thiazolidinediones (pioglitazone)	• Insulin sensitizer • Low risk of hypoglycemia	• Weight gain • Heart failure • Osteoporosis and bone fracture • Bladder cancer
Sulfonylureas Glimepiride/gliclazide/glipizide Glibenclamide	• Low cost • Highly efficacious/potent drugs	• Weight gain • Risk of hypoglycemia
Glinides Meglitinides, repaglinide	• Dose adjustment not required in patients with CKD	• Weight gain • Hypoglycemia
Alpha glucosidase inhibitors (acarbose/voglibose)	• Weight neutral	• Thrice daily dosing • GI side effects like diarrhea, flatulence, pain abdomen
DPP-4 inhibitors Linagliptin/sitagliptin/saxagliptin/vildagliptin, teneligliptin and others	• Weight neutral • Low risk of hypoglycemia • Less side effects	• High cost • Headache, pancreatitis • Nasopharyngitis • Arthralgia (rare) • Heart failure with saxagliptin
GLP-1 agonist Liraglutide/dulaglutide/lixisenatide	• Weight loss • Cardiovascular Benefit	• Expansive • Injectable therapy • GI side effects
SGLT2 inhibitors Empagliflozin, canagliflozin, dapagliflozin	• Weight loss • Reduction in systolic blood pressure • Reduced cardiovascular mortality in patients with established CVD	• Vulvovaginal candidiasis • Urinary tract infections • Bone fractures • Lower limb amputations • Acute kidney injury • DKA • Long-term safety not established
Insulin therapy	• No dose limitation • Rapidly effective	• One to four daily injections • Requires monitoring with SMBG • Weight gain • Hypoglycemia • Analogs-expensive

(CKD: chronic kidney disease; CVD: cardiovascular disease; DKA: diabetic ketoacidosis; eGFR: estimated glomerular filtration rate; GI: gastrointestinal; GLP-1: glucagon-like peptide 1; SGLT2: sodium glucose cotransporter 2; SMBG: self-monitoring of blood glucose; DPP-4: dipeptidyl peptidase 4.)

REFERENCES

1. Sue Kirkman M, Briscoe VJ, Clark N, et al. Diabetes in older adults: a consensus report. J Am Geriat Soc. 2012;60(12):2342-56.
2. Mooradian AD, Perryman K, Fitten J, et al. Cortical function in elderly noninsulin dependent diabetic patients: Behavioral and electrophysiologic studies. Arch Intern Med. 1988;148(11):2369-72.
3. Action to Control Cardiovascular Risk in Diabetes Study Group. Effects of intensive glucose lowering in type 2 diabetes. New Engl J Med. 2008;358(24):2545-59.
4. Kalyani RR, Saudek CD, Brancati FL, et al. Association of diabetes, comorbidities, and A1C with functional disability in older adults: results from the National Health and Nutrition Examination Survey (NHANES), 1999-2006. Diabetes Care. 2010;33:1055-60.

5. Geller AI, Shehab N, Lovegrove MC, et al. National estimates of insulin-related hypoglycemia and errors leading to emergency department visits and hospitalizations. JAMA Intern Med. 2014;174(5):678-86.
6. Matyka K, Evans M, Lomas J, et al. Altered hierarchy of protective responses against severe hypoglycemia in normal aging in healthy men. Diabetes Care. 1997;20(2):135-41.
7. Khunti K, Davies M, Majeed A, et al. Hypoglycemia and risk of cardiovascular disease and all-cause mortality in insulin-treated people with type 1 and type 2 diabetes: a cohort study. Diabetes Care. 2015;38(2):316-22.
8. Inzucchi SE, Bergenstal RM, Buse JB, et al. Management of hyperglycaemia in type 2 diabetes, 2015: a patient-centred approach. Update to a position statement of the American Diabetes Association and the European Association for the Study of Diabetes. Diabetologia. 2015;58(3):429-42.
9. Sinclair AJ, Paolisso G, Castro M, et al. European Diabetes Working Party for Older People 2011 clinical guidelines for type 2 diabetes mellitus. Executive summary. Diab Metabol. 2011;37:S27-38.
10. Herman WH, Donner TW, Dudl RJ, et al. Professional Practice Committee of the American Diabetes Association. Standards of medical care in diabetes-2016: Summary of revisions. Diabetes Care. 2016;39(Suppl 1):S4-5.
11. Bethel MA, Sloan FA, Belsky D, et al. Longitudinal incidence and prevalence of adverse outcomes of diabetes mellitus in elderly patients. Arch Intern Med. 2007;167(9):921-7.
12. Abbatecola AM, Paolisso G. Diabetes care targets in older persons. Diab Res Clin Prac. 2009;86:S35-40.
13. Neumiller JJ, Setter SM. Pharmacologic management of the older patient with type 2 diabetes mellitus. Am J Geriat Pharmacotherapy. 2009;7(6):324-42.
14. Franklin GM, Kahn LB, Baxter J, et al. Sensory neuropathy in non-insulin-dependent diabetes mellitus: the San Luis Valley Diabetes Study. Am J Epidemiol. 1990;131(4):633-43.
15. Anderson RJ, Freedland KE, Clouse RE, et al. The prevalence of comorbid depression in adults with diabetes: a meta-analysis. Diabetes Care. 2001;24(6):1069-78.
16. Maraldi C, Volpato S, Penninx BW, et al. Diabetes mellitus, glycemic control, and incident depressive symptoms among 70 to 79-year-old persons: the health, aging, and body composition study. Arch Intern Med. 2007;167(11):1137-44.
17. Schwartz AV, Vittinghoff E, Sellmeyer DE, et al. Diabetes-related complications, glycemic control, and falls in older adults. Diabetes care. 2008;31(3):391-6.

Chapter 56

Biomarkers in Type 1 Diabetes Mellitus

Meena Chhabra

INTRODUCTION

Type 1 diabetes (T1D) is characterized by autoimmune-mediated infiltration and destruction of insulin-producing β-cells of pancreatic islets. It basically results from the mistaken recognition of islets of Langerhans, as a foreign entity by the individual's own immune system. So, this T cells mediated destruction of the pancreas results in insulin deficiency. But researches in the past have proved that a clinical T1D is preceded by an asymptomatic phase that can be identified by serum islet autoantibodies. Thus, this perspective proposes that there is now sufficient evidence to allow a broader use of islet autoantibodies as biomarkers to predict T1D that is already at an asymptomatic stage and also to prevent its initiation and further progression which may lead to complete destruction of β-cells.

Furthermore, genetic and environmental influences are important in the etiology. There is a strong association between the HLA region in the short arm of chromosome 6. Human leukocyte antigen (HLA) class II (DR, DQ) regions have the strongest influence on T1D.

Besides, family history of diabetes and other autoimmune diseases are also considered important for risk assessment. Thus, biomarkers are required for achieving this level of sophistication and dissemination.

WHAT ARE BIOMARKERS ?

Biomarkers are measurable indicators of any biological state which can influence or predict the incidence of outcome or disease. Biomarkers can be detected by molecular biological techniques. However, in individuals with T1D, antibodies act as biomarkers as these can be detected by a technique called "immunohistochemistry".

Hence, a biomarker can be any substance, a cell, a molecule, a gene, a protein, an enzyme coded by a gene, or it could be an antibody. These biomarkers help in the detection of T1D.[1] Metabolic markers like C-peptide level can also help in diagnosing T1D, for instance, low or absence of metabolic marker C-peptide indicates that there is "low" or "absolutely no" residual insulin secretion in a diabetic patient. So, these biomarkers aid in evaluation and diagnosis of the targeted disease.

AUTOANTIBODIES AS BIOMARKERS

Autoantibodies against β-cell proteins and peptides are often used to diagnose T1D. In fact, prediction of T1D is greatly enhanced by islet autoantibodies. The four islet autoantibodies that appear to be the most useful T1D markers are antibodies to insulin (IAA),[2] glutamic acid decarboxylase (GAD),[3] protein tyrosine phosphatase (IA2) and zinc transporter 8 (ZnT8).[4]

It has been found that the risk of developing diabetes is strongly correlated to the number of autoantibody markers found, like, the presence of two or more autoantibodies gives a higher probability of developing the disease than the presence of a single antibody, regardless of genetic susceptibility.[5] Though sometimes the progression from antibody positive pre-symptomatic to the clinical T1D may vary greatly from a few weeks to decades, in multiple-autoantibody positive children.

Usually, the progression of T1D depends on which antibody turns positive. For instance, if IAA and IA2 are positive in a patient, T1D will progress slowly, but if GAD and ZnT8 are positive, they will progress quickly to T1D.

Secondly, being positive only for one antibody can be a transient event which means having only one antibody positive, may not necessarily make someone a clinical case of T1D in the future. In fact, subjects who are positive with only one antibody have a meager 10% chance to develop T1D within 5 years, even if there's a positive family history of T1D.

Similarly, individuals who are positive for three antibodies, have a greater chance of developing T1D that approaches 90% within 8 years.

Furthermore, in a study known as DAISY (Diabetes Autoimmunity Study in the Young), autoantibodies were checked in offspring of a diabetic parent who had HLA DR3/4 DQ8. If antibodies were positive there was a greater chance of developing T1D. There was a higher frequency of false or transiently positive antibody tests in those whose parents did not express this high-risk haplotype.

To summarize, these biomarkers in form of antibodies certainly help to establish if an individual is at an increased risk to develop T1D, but their positivity does not appear to mean that the patient is already diabetic and is not correlated with progression of the disease.

APPEARANCE WITH PATHOLOGY

The etiopathology of T1D may be divided into three clinical stages:

1. *Stage 1:* Beta-cell autoimmunity normoglycemia Pre-symptomatic
2. *Stage 2:* Beta-cell autoimmunity dysglycemia pre-symptomatic
3. *Stage 3:* Beta-cell autoimmunity dysglycemia symptomatic.

Stage 1 represents the presence of β-cell autoimmunity as evidenced by the presence of two or more islet autoantibodies with normoglycemia and is pre-symptomatic. Stage 2, on the other hand, has the presence of β-cell autoimmunity with dysglycemia and is presymptomatic. This means despite the destruction of beta cells and the development of autoantibodies, the patient is still not diabetic. And, stage 3 highlights the onset of symptomatic disease. It's the stage when all the β-cells of an individual are destroyed and the patient is now hyperglycemic and needs treatment for his/her survival.

Adoption of this staging classification provides a standardized taxonomy for T1D and aids in the development of therapies and the design of clinical trials to prevent symptomatic disease, promote precision medicine and adopt measures that would intervene in the early stages of T1D to prevent symptomatic disease.

RELATIONSHIP BETWEEN DIFFERENT ANTIBODIES IN TYPE 1 DIABETES

In India, there have been several cases of T1D who are antibody negative. The T1D with at least one antibody positive are labeled as type 1A and those with all four antibodies negative are labeled as type 1B. There isn't much data from India on biomarkers though. Very recently to understand the prevalence of T1B (islet antibody negative) diabetes among recently diagnosed (<12 weeks) T1D children and adolescents, a study was conducted at the Sanjay Gandhi Postgraduate Institute of Medical Sciences, Lucknow. The study is first of its kind to be conducted in India with focus on all four major islet autoantibodies at the onset of the disease. However, it was found that there is a high prevalence of type 1B diabetes in the study, with 28% of children studied being negative for all four major islet antibodies and 25% negative for three antibodies, i.e. GADA, IA2A and ZnT8A - which is much high in comparison to caucasians (3.5–5%). Also, the study highlighted that patients with type 1B diabetes were similar in their clinical profile to those with islet antibodies (both at onset and after 1 year of follow-up).[6]

Methodology

- A cross-sectional study of 110 T1D patients was studied
- GADA, IA2A and ZnT8A were measured by radio binding assay using in vitro transcribed and translated islet antigen labeled [^{35}S] methionine
- IAA was measured only in patients with duration of diabetes <2 weeks again using radiobinding assay
- Fasting C-peptide was measured at the onset and at 1 year of follow-up using immunoradiometric assays (IRMA).

Results

- All antibodies were negative (type 1B diabetes) in 17 patients. At least one antibody was positive in the remaining patients
- Clinical and biochemical parameters, including plasma C-peptide, were not different between antibody positive and type 1B diabetes
- Islet antibody positive patients revealed risk association for *DRB1*0301* [OR = 5.10 (CI =1.61–16.16) p = 0.003]

- The prevalence of antibodies against IA2 and IAA were considerably lower than children of caucasian origin
- The prevalence of ZnT8 in the studied population was 29%, low as compared to studies in other caucasians (63–65%).

Thus, it was concluded that there is a high proportion of type 1B diabetes among Indian children and adolescents. However, clinical features and β cell-reserve does not differ significantly from islet antibody positive patients. The *HLA-DR3* allele was more frequent in antibody positive patients. And, the measurement of ZnT8A was useful in decreasing proportion of type 1B diabetes.

Clinical Characteristics of Different Islet Autoantibodies

- IAAs are the first to appear
- IA2 are very specific for the development of T1D
- GAD and IAA are most frequent antibodies in childhood
- GADA is the hallmark of adult-onset T1D
- IAAs and GAD are heterogeneous
- ZnT8 is detected in individuals who are found negative with GAD, IAA and IA2
- ZnT8 increases with age and so, the antibody has high value in predicting T1D in older children
- ZnT8 were positive in 29% patients, with a higher frequency in females
- ZnT8 positive patients had a higher frequency of diabetic ketoacidosis and a lower fasting plasma C-peptide after 1 year of follow-up
- ZnT8 was alone positive in four patients and its inclusion reduced the frequency of islet-antibody negative patients from 34 to 28%
- The frequency of the allele *DRB1*0301* was increased in ZnT8A positive patients.

ROLE OF T-CELL MARKERS IN TYPE 1 DIABETES

When it comes to biomarkers that also reflect pancreas-specific changes, autoreactive T cells are often the first choice. Both autoreactive CD4+ and CD8+ T cells can be detected in blood.[7] Moreover, the tools to measure these have improved in recent years and it has been highlighted in multiple clinical studies. However, the practical use of biomarkers that are expected to reside mainly in or around the pancreas and are only seen in high numbers in the circulation during discrete periods seem to be limited. So, while counting islet-specific T cells in peripheral blood is interesting, it is probably unsuitable as a biomarker for estimating the rate of progression to clinical diabetes.

GOAL OF BIOMARKERS

As discussed above, biomarkers of T1D are important for assessing the risk of developing disease, monitoring disease progression and determining responses to clinical treatments, especially in patients who have a genetic susceptibility, i.e. first-degree relationship (son, daughter, brother or sister/twin or parent) with a type 1 diabetic.

CLINICAL SIGNIFICANCE

Application of biomarker plays a vital role in predicting that if an individual is at a risk of developing T1D, despite being a first-degree relative (FDR) case. And, if an individual is found positive with autoantibodies, i.e. the biomarkers are positive, a suitable and specific line of treatment can be offered so that hyperglycemia can be prevented or delayed.

However, biomarkers are not recommended in the general population for screening purpose and should be performed on high-risk patients; children who are born to T1D mother, father or a sibling diagnosed with T1D. Besides, biomarkers help in distinguishing various types of diabetes. In a young diabetic patient if antibodies are positive and C-peptide is low or absent, then an individual is definitely T1D. However, if antibodies are negative and C-peptide is low or absent, the patient can be antibody negative or type 1B diabetes. And, if the patient is antibody positive but there are enough insulin reserves in the form of a normal C-peptide level, the patient is diagnosed as latent autoimmune diabetes in adults (LADA), which is considered as a slowly progressive T1D. But, if antibodies are negative and C-peptide is normal and the patient has a stigma of metabolic syndrome in the form of abdominal obesity, generalized obesity, increased waist circumference, acanthosis, dyslipidemia or hypertension, then he/she is type 2 diabetes. So, biomarker helps to follow-up cases with clarity while adhering to specific treatment. Besides, follow-up of infants who are genetically susceptible and antibody negative at birth can be helpful as seroconversion to antibody positivity can occur as early as 6 months.

FUTURE PERSPECTIVE

The TEDDY study (The Environmental Determinants of Diabetes in the Young) is hopeful of finding the environmental triggers of T1D in children with higher risk genes. The ongoing trial will provide an opportunity to fill important gaps in the understanding of the events leading to T1D by studying from birth high-risk general population children and relatives and by systematic screening of candidate environmental and genetic factors. In the future, through this information, diabetes in children can be prevented.[8]

Flowchart 1 shows risk assessment stage 1 and risk assessment stage 2.

CONCLUSION

Biomarkers in the asymptomatic genetically susceptible individual can predict T1D. This approach may permit prevention of diabetes, especially if a person is at a high genetic risk or secondary prevention in those individuals who are β-cell antibody positive.

Even after the clinical diagnosis, further loss of functional β-cells can be averted by giving timely and type 1 specific treatment, like immunomodulation, though this line of treatment is not promising at the moment. Additionally, early diagnosis of T1D can prevent severe hyperglycemia in a patient and avert serious complications like ketoacidosis and ketoacidotic coma.

However, several longitudinal studies are required, starting right from the birth of a newborn to detect antibodies and predict β-cells autoimmunity in offspring and the FDR of the T1D patient.

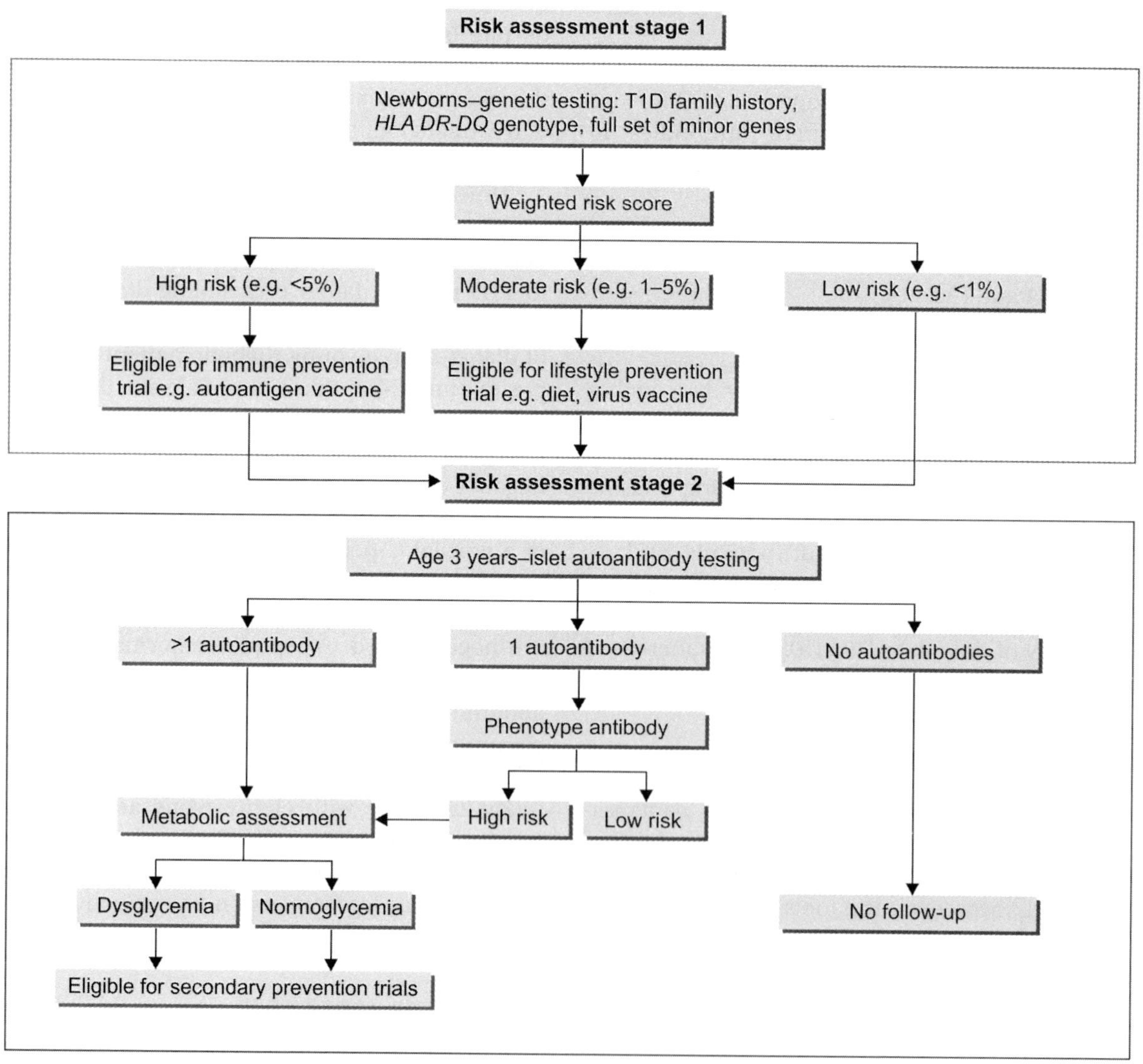

(T1D: type 1 diabetes; HLA: human leukocyte antigen.)

Flowchart 1 Effects of maternal fuels on fetal and offspring development.

Thus, biomarkers are important because both prevention and prediction of T1D is a very high priority.

REFERENCES

1. Strimbu K, Tavel JA. What are biomarkers? Curr Opin HIV AIDS, 2010;5:463-6.
2. Palmer JP, Asplin CM, Clemons P, et al. Insulin antibodies in insulin-dependent diabetics before insulin treatment. Science. 1983;222: 1337-9.
3. Baekkeskov S, Aanstoot HJ, Christgau S, et al. Identification of the 64K autoantigen in insulin-dependent diabetes as the GABA-synthesizing enzyme glutamic acid decarboxylase. Nature. 1990;347:151-6.
4. Rabin DU, Pleasic SM, Shapiro JA, et al. Islet cell antigen 512 is a diabetes-specific islet autoantigen related to protein tyrosine phosphatases. J Immunol. 1994;152:3183-8.
5. Ziegler AG, Bonifacio E; BABYDIAB-BABYDIET Study Group. Age-related islet autoantibody incidence in offspring of patients with type 1 diabetes. Diabetologia. 2012;55:1937-43.
6. Vipin VP, Zaidi G, Watson K, et al. Department of Endocrinology and Medical Genetics, Sanjay Gandhi Post Graduate Institute of Medical Sciences, Lucknow. (Poster at ISPAD 2018, Hyderabad).
7. Eugster A, Lindner A, Catani M et al. High diversity in the TCR repertoire of GAD65 autoantigen-specific human CD4+ T cells. J Immunol. 2015;194:2531–8.
8. Krischer JP, Lynch KF, Schatz DA, et al. The 6 year incidence of diabetes-associated autoantibodies in genetically at-risk children: the TEDDY study. Diabetologia. 2015;58(5):980-7.

Chapter 57

Diabetes in Children and Adolescents—Challenges and Way Forward

KM Prasanna Kumar

INTRODUCTION

Diabetes mellitus in children is one of the common endocrine diseases in children.

Diabetes in children and adolescent could be of many types—like type 1 diabetes (A and B), type 2 diabetes, maturity-onset diabetes of young, monogenic diabetes, genetic syndromes associated with diabetes, polycystic ovarian disease, latent autoimmune diabetes of adults and pancreatic diabetes. Though there are many types of diabetes in children and type 1 diabetes is the most common type of diabetes seen in children and adolescent.

Type 1 diabetes is usually diagnosed in children and young adults. Only 1–5% of people with diabetes have this form of the disease, and rest of people have type 2 or other types of diabetes. Although, it is one of the most common chronic diseases in children and adolescents, even today many children die because of undiagnosed diabetes, where in some cases, children die within few years of diagnosis, and those who eventually survive are poorly controlled and have a poor quality of life.

CURRENT BURDEN AND CHALLENGE OF TYPE 1 DIABETES IN INDIA

It is estimated that India has approximately 125,000 cases of type 1 diabetes mellitus (T1DM), with an annual increase rate of 3–5%. Clearly, there are major challenges in the management of T1DM in India; this includes primarily, diagnosis, healthcare delivery and availability of trained physicians, infrastructure and availability of insulin, monitoring and providing psychosocial support. This calls for support not just from family but from school and society too.

Healthcare, in India, is primarily financed through out-of-pocket payments by households, and since taking care of type 1 diabetes is continuous and expensive, many children from economically poor background have to lose their lives because of no or inadequate treatment.

Psychosocial aspect of management of diabetes in children is the biggest challenge. Lack of education, motivation and access to quality of healthcare delivery is a big challenge as the children with diabetes living at remote rural areas of India do not have access to the best of the care, and the physicians in periphery lack proper training and knowledge in managing children with diabetes.

COMMITMENT FOR HOLISTIC CARE—CHANGING DIABETES® IN CHILDREN IN INDIA

In an attempt to address the critical gap in the management of children with type 1 diabetes in India, Novo Nordisk Education Foundation, in collaboration with leading government institutions, private hospitals, nongovernmental organizations and key doctors have launched Changing Diabetes® in Children (CDiC) program with the objective of giving children with type 1 diabetes <18 years coming from below the poverty line families, access to comprehensive diabetes care and management.

Vision

To initiate and strive for comprehensive diabetes care for children <18 years with type 1 diabetes from the economically underprivileged families in India.

The program was launched in India by Late Dr APJ Abdul Kalam on September 7, 2011, in Bangalore. There are currently 21 CDiC main and 45 satellite centers spread across the country with more than 4,000 children under its care, thus creating a pan-India footprint.

The Karnataka model—Primer Academy of Medical Sciences (PAMS)—has established 30 satellite centers of CDiC in Karnataka, covering almost all districts of Karnataka. In addition, we have established satellite centers at neighboring states such as Tamilnadu, Telangana, Andhra Pradesh and Puducherry. Apart from 840 children under CDiC-India PAMS is taking care of another 600 children and adolescent up to 25 years of age proving the same quality of care as CDiC-India.

Main Components of the Changing Diabetes® in Children Program

The CDiC program integrates a number of mutually reinforcing components, which together add to the uniqueness and comprehensiveness of the program, namely:

- Infrastructure and equipment
- Capacity building of healthcare professionals
- Provision of insulin
- Patient education
- Diabetes registry
- Equipment and supplies
- Learnings and outcome
- Improvement of existing infrastructure—Twenty-one CDiC main and 45 subcenters spread across the country, equipped with dealing type 1 diabetes have been made functional reaching to more than 4,000 children
- Capacity building—As a capacity building initiative, with the support from doctors, managing the CDiC centers across India, continuing medical educations on management of children with type 1 diabetes have been conducted reaching out to >6,000 doctors and other health care professionals
    - Systematic initiative for doctors and other health-care professional through specially created modules on type 1 diabetes, accredited by State Medical Councils and implemented with the support of CDiC center directors
    - Creation of a CDiC textbook on pediatric diabetes (diabetes educator handbook and Hindi translation of International Society for Pediatric and Adolescent Diabetes textbook on diabetes in children and adolescents).
- Care of children—The key benefits for each child registered in the program are enlisted below, covers medication, monitoring, diagnostics, consultation and understanding to manage their diabetes:
    - Doctor consultation
    - Human insulin vials
    - Insulin syringes
    - Glucose meter
    - Glucose meter strips
    - HbA1c—twice a year
    - Complete blood count, creatinine and micro-albuminuria once a year
    - Thyroid-stimulating hormone at recruitment
    - Fundus once a year
    - Keto-Diastix strips
    - Diabetes educator counseling
    - Children camps.

Care of chronic disease not only requires medical treatment but also information, education, counseling and holistic support, which includes insulin, lifestyle changes, monitoring, diabetes education and behavioral interventions. Coping skills for this lifelong disorder requires diabetes self-management education appropriate to age and environment, empathy, insight, counseling, and supporting relationships. The CDiC program is trying to provide all these in resource-limited settings as all are essential for holistic care of child with type 1 diabetes. This is done with the help of regular children camps and periodic release of children-friendly supportive literatures and tools. Many of these printed materials are made in nine Indian languages apart from English.

- *Diabetes education for children:*

    This is achieved through periodic, systemic children camps. As part of program, >600 camps have been conducted across the country.

    These camps are meant to provide comprehensive care, mass education and social support for the children enrolled in the program. Most of these camps consist of these three elements:

    i. Diabetes education
    ii. Experience sharing
    iii. Fun activities.

    The children learn what is being taught to them for managing their diabetes well in these groups. These camps are generally led by doctor or diabetes educator and have minimum 15–250 children with their parents at one place. Basics of management of diabetes in day-to-day life, namely, self-injection techniques, injection site selection, technique for drawing the insulin from the vials, awareness about hypoglycemia, managing simple hypoglycemia's, knowing what are the essentials while traveling, at school, during holidays, while in parties or examination, etc. are discussed during these camps

- Innovative patient education material like Novo Nordisk teaches to take insulin doll, Mishti books and videos, snakes and ladders, make a healthy change, make your own plate poster, HbA1c calculator, HypoKit, diabetes foot, door knob hanger and healthy eating plate are made and distributed to all the participating children during these programs
  - Most of these inputs are made available in nine Indian languages. There are many such education materials. Given below is the list of few such educative children materials
    - *Novo Nordisk teaches to take insulin*: A soft toy, which demonstrates insulin sites selection and helps in learning self-injection. The target population are people who need insulin and healthcare professionals for education purpose
    - *HbA1C wheel and chart*: It is educative monitor which helps in understanding average blood glucose levels from HbA1c value and thus diabetes control for people with diabetes and healthcare professionals
    - *Posters on diabetes awareness and management*: Pictorial representation of key aspects of diabetes prevention and management, e.g. know your symptoms, hypoglycemia and hyperglycemia
    - *Visual aid binder*: Detailing on the basics of diabetes and its management made for use of the diabetes nurse educators while they are interacting with the children their parents and siblings or other relatives
    - *Diabetes educators handbook*: It is a book meant to help educators for management of type 1 diabetes in children, adolescents, and guardian
    - *Mishti*: Means "sweet" in Hindi, it is series of story books and videos of a little girl with type 1 diabetes. It touches multiple aspects of living with type 1 diabetes like basics of diabetes management, attending a party, while traveling and sick day rules. Now we are coming with Mishti Digest—a comic book and video series which touches various aspects of living with diabetes
    - *Know about carbohydrates:* It is a leaflet prepared to give understanding about carbohydrates in Indian context
    - *Snakes and ladders*: It is a board game to understand both good and bad habits for healthy life with and without diabetes. Snake and ladder has also been adapted as online game
    - *Children educational scholarship*: For long-term self-reliance, >400 eligible children have been awarded educational scholarships, and around 25 of them are pursuing professional courses.
- Diabetes registry—One of the largest registries has been created to understand the health status, needs, and requirements of children with type 1 diabetes from economically underprivileged families
- Equipment and supplies—Continuous supplies of all the essential supplies for management of type 1 diabetes for all the registered children is a true achievement of the program
- Learnings and outcome—Learnings from this comprehensive program has been worked upon in three ways:
  - i. *Bringing out scientific publications*: To share this impact and learning with medical fraternity
  - ii. *Bringing out real-life children insights*: These compilations of real-life stories of children have helped stakeholders from governments and others to understand that the problem is real and needs urgent attention. On the other hand, it also shows that when taken care of children with type 1 diabetes can live long healthy lives and be useful citizens of the country
  - iii. *Awareness creation*: Through World Diabetes Day, World Health Day, and Insulin Day campaign and "Talking Diabetes in school", an emailer campaign for school teachers. This is resulting in improving of overall awareness and acceptance on type 1 diabetes among general public.
- *Advocacy*: It is to sensitize and increase the attention of policy makers and governments on the specific needs of children with type 1 diabetes. So far, four national-level and five state-level advocacy programs have been conducted. These programs had the participation of key stakeholders from the Government of India, state governments, key doctors, policy makers, media and patient groups.

All these efforts to support the CDiC children with type 1 diabetes coming from poor families are really making a difference to them. This is evident from the positive health outcomes, and after a long time, no child died of diabetes in the last 2 years in the CDiC program. Child first and diabetes next is our motto.

SUMMARY

Diabetes in children and adolescent is an increasing challenge in India. There is an urgent need to develop infrastructure for management of children with diabetes and resources in our country. The CDiC is one of the large programs in India as well as other Afro Asian countries in meeting this challenge.

REFERENCES

1. Ahuja M, Talwar G, Varma V, et al. Diabetes mellitus in young Indians. Indian J Med Res. 1965;53:1138.
2. Dharmalingam M, Kumar KMP, Aravind SR, et al. IDDM Registry-data from Bangalore. In: Prasanna Kumar KM, Thakur SS Associate (Eds). Endocrinology metabolism and diabetes, proceedings, pp. 85-90. Mumbai: Print Communications (P) Ltd; 1997.
3. John M, Koledova E, Kumar KM, et al. Challenges in the diagnosis and management of growth hormone deficiency in India. Int J Endocrinol. 2016;2016:2967578.
4. Kalra S, Kalra B, Sharma A. Prevalence of type 1 diabetes mellitus in Karnal district, Haryana state, India. Diabetol Metab Syndr. 2010;2:14.
5. Kalra S, Sridhar GR, Balhara YP, et al. National recommendations: psychosocial management of diabetes in India. Indian J Endocrinol Metab. 2013;17(3):376-95.
6. Kumar KMP, Azad K, Zabeen B, et al. Type 1 diabetes in children: fighting for a place under the sun. India J Endocrinol Metab. 2012;16(Suppl. 1):S1-3.
7. Kumar KMP, Prabhu Dev N, Raman KV, et al. Consensus statement on diabetes in children. Indian J Endocrinol Metab. 2014;18(3):264-73.
8. Kumar KMP. Improving diabetes care for children with type 1 diabetes from poor families: Changing Diabetes® in children program, India. Indian J Endocrinol Metab. 2014;18(1):116-7.
9. Kumar KP, Shah N, Viswanathan V, et al. Best practices from Changing Diabetes® in children India. J Soc Health Diabetes. 2016;4(2):137.
10. Kumar P, Krishna P, Reddy SC, et al. Incidence of type 1 diabetes mellitus and associated complications among children and young adults: results from Karnataka Diabetes Registry 1995–2008. J Indian Med Assoc. 2008;106:708-11.
11. Ly TT1, Maahs DM, Rewers A, et al. ISPAD Consensus guidelines for the management of type 1 diabetes mellitus in children and adolescents with diabetes. Pediatr Diabetes. 2014;15 Suppl 20:180-92.
12. Mylariah K, Kumar P. Incidence trends for childhood type 1 diabetes in India. Indian J Endocrinol Metab. 2015;19(Suppl. 1):S34-5.
13. Ramachandran A, Snehalatha C, Abdul Khader OM, et al. Prevalence of childhood diabetes in an urban population in south India. Diabetes Res Clin Pract. 1992;17:227-31.
14. Shivaprasad C, Mittal R, Dharmalingam M, et al. Zinc transporter-8 autoantibodies can replace IA-2 autoantibodies as a serological marker for juvenile onset type 1 diabetes in India. Indian J Endocrinol Metab. 2014;18(3):345-9.
15. Sridhar GR. Diabetes mellitus in children below the age of five. Indian J Endocrinol Metab. 1997;1:13-5.
16. Srikanta SS. Insulin "dependent" diabetes mellitus in India: classical versus atypical. Int J Diabetes Dev Ctries. 1993;13:29-35.
17. Sudhir PM, Kumaraiah V, Munichoodappa C, et al. Management of children with diabetes mellitus—psychosocial aspects. Int J Diabetes Dev Countries. 2001;21:69-76.
18. Udani PM, Shah PM, Karani AN. Diabetes in children. Clinical and biochemical aspects. Indian Pediatr. 1968;5:391-400.

Chapter 58

Monogenic Diabetes—India Specific

Ranjit Unnikrishnan

INTRODUCTION

The term "monogenic diabetes" refers to diabetes caused by mutations or variations in a single gene. There are several subtypes of monogenic diabetes, the majority of which involve genes concerned with insulin secretion. Diagnosis of the monogenic diabetes may have important implications for therapy and prognosis in some cases and is an excellent example of precision medicine. While most of the information on monogenic diabetes comes from western populations, there is an increasing body of literature describing the prevalence and characteristics of these syndromes in India. This chapter will briefly summarize the available literature on monogenic diabetes from India.

TERMINOLOGY

The term "monogenic diabetes" is applied to those individuals in whom the diabetes phenotype can be directly attributed to mutations or variations in a single gene, in contrast to the polygenic inheritance of type 1 and 2 diabetes. Depending on the genes involved, there are several subcategories of monogenic diabetes. However, most of these conditions arise from mutations in the genes responsible for pancreatic islet cell development and function, and are therefore associated with the insulin secretory defect. Many of these forms of diabetes were described under the umbrella term "MODY" (maturity onset diabetes of the young) in the past. However, it is now known that the different types of MODY are actually quite dissimilar to one another and that it is not appropriate to clump them all together as a single entity. Hence, the use of the term "MODY" is no longer recommended and the diagnosis should instead mention the specific gene involved [e.g. monogenic diabetes due to hepatocyte nuclear factor (HNF)-1A mutation, neonatal diabetes due to *ABCC8* mutation, etc.].[1]

Based on the clinical phenotype, four subcategories of monogenic diabetes due to insulin secretory defect have been described:[1]

1. Youth-onset diabetes with affected parent
2. Isolated nonprogressive fasting hyperglycemia
3. Neonatal diabetes
4. Familial diabetes with extrapancreatic features.

As per the Western literature, monogenic forms of diabetes represent around 1–2% of all patients with diabetes.[1]

YOUTH-ONSET DIABETES WITH AFFECTED PARENT

The most common genes associated with this genotype are *HNF-1A* and *HNF-4A*. These patients present with diabetes before the age of 25 years and usually demonstrate transmission of diabetes across three generations. They are usually nonobese and lack the markers of insulin resistance, such as acanthosis nigricans and skin tags. These patients can usually be treated with sulfonylureas, to which they are often exquisitely sensitive. However, in many cases, the diabetes is progressive necessitating the addition of insulin. They are also as prone to micro- and macrovascular complications as patients with type 1 and 2 diabetes. Mutations in several other genes have been reported to cause youth-onset diabetes, but they are rare and incompletely characterized. Table 1 shows an incomplete list of these genes.

TABLE 1: List of genes associated with the phenotype of youth-onset diabetes with affected parent.

Former terminology	Gene involved	Specific features
MODY1	*HNF-4A*	Mild – moderate fasting and postprandial plasma glucose
		Respond well to sulfonylurea agents (low dose)
MODY3	*HNF-1A*	Same as *HNF-4A*
MODY4	*IPF1*	Phenotypes ranging from impaired glucose tolerance to overt diabetes; homozygous or compound heterozygous mutations of PDX1 are associated with pancreatic agenesis
MODY6	*NEUROD1*	Rare, with phenotype characterized by obesity and insulin resistance
MODY7	*KLF11*	Very rare, phenotype ranges from impaired glucose tolerance or impaired fasting glucose to overt diabetes
MODY8	*CEL*	Very rare, associated with both exocrine and endocrine pancreatic deficiency and with demyelinating peripheral neuropathy
MODY9	*PAX4*	Very rare, crucial transcription factor for β-cell development
MODY10	*INS*	Very rare, usually associated with neonatal diabetes (<1% cases)
MODY11	*BLK*	These adapter proteins contribute to the qualitative and quantitative control of B-cell signaling
MODY12	*KCNJ11*	Very rare, usually associated with neonatal diabetes (<1% cases)
		Responds to sulfonylurea (high dose)
MODY13	*ABCC8*	Very rare, usually associated with neonatal diabetes (<1% cases)
		Responds to sulfonylurea (high dose)
MODY14	*APPL1*	Very rare, reported in a single family

(MODY: maturity onset diabetes of the young.)

As per the Western literature, HNF-1A monogenic diabetes is the most common cause of this phenotype, closely followed by HNF-4A. There is a paucity of data from India on the prevalence of these forms of diabetes. Studies from a tertiary diabetes care center in Southern India attempted to assess the prevalence of various forms of monogenic diabetes among patients with young-onset diabetes identified by the clinical criteria of Tattersall and Fajans.[2] In a series of 96 unrelated patients with clinically suspected monogenic diabetes, 9 (9.3%) were found to have mutations in HNF-1A.[3] Out of the remaining 87, 3 (3.4% of clinically diagnosed patients) had HNF-4A mutations.[4] Therefore, the two most commonly cited causes of monogenic diabetes in the Western population only accounted for around 12% of cases in this south Indian population. Another hospital-based study from Southern India showed that only 19% of patients with clinically suspected monogenic diabetes had mutations in any of the genes studied.[5] In a more recent study of 289 individuals with young-onset diabetes (152 with a clinical diagnosis of monogenic diabetes), HNF-1A mutations were found to be most frequent (7.2%) followed by *ABCC8* (3.3%).[6] In addition to the already known genes, mutations were also identified in *RFX6*, *WFS1*, *AKT2* and *NKX6-1*, and functional analysis of the NKX6-1 revealed functional impairment, implicating it as a cause of diabetes.

ISOLATED NONPROGRESSIVE FASTING HYPERGLYCEMIA

This phenotype is caused by mutations in the glucokinase (*GCK*) gene and was earlier termed MODY2. GCK acts as the glucose sensor of the pancreatic β-cell, enabling it to respond to rising plasma glucose concentrations by increasing the output of insulin. In patients with inactivating mutations of GCK, the set point for initiation of insulin release is raised, but once initiated, secretion proceeds in a normal fashion thereafter. Therefore, these patients present with mild fasting hyperglycemia that is present from birth and stable over time. There is a minimal increment in blood glucose after a meal or a glucose load. These patients require no treatment as they are not at increased risk of diabetes complications.

In the Western population, mutations in GCK are said to be the most common cause of monogenic diabetes. However, clinic-based studies from India have failed to reproduce these findings. Even in population studies, the prevalence of GCK mutations has been found to be lower than expected.[7]

NEONATAL DIABETES

Diabetes developing before 6 months of life is termed neonatal diabetes. Autoimmune type 1 diabetes is virtually unknown at this age, and nearly all cases of neonatal diabetes are monogenic in origin. Neonatal diabetes can be classified as transient neonatal diabetes, and permanent neonatal diabetes (PNDM) depending on whether the diabetes spontaneously resolves or persists with time. The majority of cases of PNDM are due to mutations in the *KCNJ11* and *ABCC8* genes, which encode the Kir 6.2 and sulfonylurea receptor (SUR) subunits, respectively, of the adenosine triphosphate (ATP)-sensitive potassium (K) channel of the β-cell. The presence of the mutation impairs ATP binding to the channel, rendering it unable to close in response to rising plasma glucose levels and thereby impairing insulin secretion. Most patients with these mutations can be successfully transitioned from insulin injections to sulfonylureas, as these oral drugs bypass the block in the K-ATP channel by binding to a distinct site on the SUR subunit.[8]

The exact prevalence of neonatal diabetes is unknown, even in Western countries. In a series from Southern India, 205 patients with onset of diabetes below 1 year of age were evaluated for mutations in several candidate genes. A total of 70 mutations were identified. Mutations were identified in 51 out of 165 cases (30.9%) where the onset of diabetes was below 6 months, 5 out of 21 cases (23.8%) where the onset was between 6 months and 1 year, and in 14 out of 19 (73.6%) cases where diabetes was associated with extrapancreatic features. The genes involved were *KCNJ11*, *ABCC8*, and *INS* in the majority of cases in the first two categories.[9] Many of these patients with *KCNJ11* and *ABCC8* mutations have been shifted to sulfonylureas from insulin and continue to do well on follow-up.

FAMILIAL DIABETES WITH EXTRAPANCREATIC FEATURES

There are several monogenic syndromes associated with diabetes, including Wolfram syndrome, Wolcott-Rallison syndrome and the thiamine responsive megaloblastic anemia syndrome. The clinical diagnosis of these conditions is usually straightforward, and the prognosis is determined by the extrapancreatic features.

An interesting monogenic syndrome associated with diabetes is the renal cysts and diabetes syndrome, earlier called MODY5. This condition arises from defects in the *HNF-1B* gene and is characterized by defects in the genitourinary system, in addition to diabetes. The common defects include renal cysts, renal agenesis, horseshoe kidney, and ureteric duplication. Pancreatic atrophy is also seen, and most of these patients require insulin treatment. The exact prevalence of this condition is unknown; in a series of 40 patients with renal disease (renal cysts, hyperechogenicity, hypoplasia, horseshoe kidney, and renal aplasia) and diabetes, four were found to have mutations in the *HNF-1B* gene.[10]

PECULIARITIES OF MONOGENIC DIABETES IN INDIA

The exact prevalence of monogenic diabetes in India is unknown. Studies in multiethnic populations in the United Kingdom suggest that the prevalence rates of monogenic diabetes are much lower in Asian Indians compared to the white population. It has also been shown that the clinical criteria for monogenic diabetes have low sensitivity and specificity in identifying candidates for genetic testing in this population (Table 2). Even the newer risk scores used in the West for identifying monogenic diabetes fare poorly when applied to Asian Indians.[11] A major hurdle to the use of these criteria and risk scores is the high prevalence of young-onset type 2 diabetes in this population, which often mimics the clinical features of monogenic diabetes.

Another major issue is nonavailability of genetic testing in India and its cost. Testing for the entire monogenic diabetes gene panel remains prohibitively expensive for most patients and hence we cannot recommend blanket screening of all patients with young-onset diabetes in India.

It is therefore clear that a great deal of clinical acumen is necessary in identifying those patients in India who would benefit the most from the results of genetic testing, so that we can make the best possible use of the available resources. Three such categories of patients are mentioned below, along with the benefits anticipated should the screening return positive:

TABLE 2: Clinical criteria for diagnosing maturity onset diabetes of the young and their shortcomings in the Indian scenario.

Criterion	Remarks
Autosomal dominant inheritance with multiple generations affected	Family history is usually positive in type 2 generations and may show three-generation transmission
Early age at onset (<25 years)	Age of onset is lower in Asian Indians with type 2 diabetes
Usually no obesity or insulin resistance	Many Asian Indians with type 2 diabetes are nonobese or even lean
Characterized by the absence of ketosis and β-cell autoimmunity	Applies to type 2 diabetes also
Controllable without insulin for at least 5 years	

1. Patients with "type 1 diabetes" who have a positive family history of diabetes, who are autoantibody negative, and who have evidence of preserved β-cell function (C-peptide) >5 years after diagnosis (detection of *HNF-1A* or *HNF-4A* mutations can enable transfer to sulfonylurea)
2. Patients with stable fasting hyperglycemia (detection of *GCK* mutation can enable cessation of therapy)
3. Patients with onset of diabetes below 6 months of age, being treated with insulin (detection of *KCNJ11* or *ABCC8* mutations can facilitate transfer to sulfonylurea).

CONCLUSION

Diagnosis and treatment of monogenic diabetes is an excellent example of precision medicine. Provision of accurate diagnosis can prove life changing for many patients and lead to improved glycemic control and quality of life. However, preliminary reports suggest that the diagnosis of monogenic diabetes is not as straightforward in India as in Western countries. The cost and unavailability of genetic testing is also an issue. There is an urgent need to frame population-specific guidelines for identification of candidates for genetic testing and to provide facilities for provision of such testing at reasonable cost. Till such time, physicians should use their clinical judgment to identify those patients who would benefit the most from genetic testing, and direct diagnostic efforts to them.

REFERENCES

1. Murphy R, Ellard S, Hattersley AT. Clinical implications of a molecular genetic classification on monogenic β-cell diabetes. Nat Clin Pract Endocrinol Metab. 2008;4:200-13.
2. Tattersall RB, Fajans SS. A difference between the inheritance of classical juvenile-onset and maturity-onset type diabetes of young people. Diabetes. 1975;24:44-53.
3. Radha V, Ek J, Hansen T, et al. Identification of novel variants in the hepatocyte nuclear factor-1 gene in south Indian patients with maturity onset diabetes of young. J Clin Endocrinol Metab. 2009;94:1959-65.
4. Anuradha S, Radha V, Mohan V. Association of novel variants in the hepatocyte nuclear factor 4A gene with maturity onset diabetes of the young and early onset type 2 diabetes. Clin Genet. 2011;80:541-9.
5. Chapla A, Mruthyunjaya MD, Asha HS, et al. Maturity onset diabetes of the young in India—a distinctive mutation pattern identified through targeted next-generation sequencing. Clin Endocrinol (Oxf). 2014;82:533-42.
6. Mohan V, Radha V, Thong N, et al. Comprehensive genomic analysis identifies pathogenic variants in maturity-onset diabetes of the young (MODY) patients in south India. BMC Med Genet. 2018;19:22.
7. Kanthimathi S, Jahnavi S, Balamurugan K, et al. Glucokinase gene mutations in Asian Indians. Diabetes Technol Ther. 2014;16:180-5.
8. Pearson ER, Flechtner I, Njolstad PR, et al. Switching from insulin to oral sulfonylureas in patients with diabetes due to Kir 6.2 mutations. N Engl J Med. 2006;355:467-77.
9. Jahnavi S, Poovazhagi V, Mohan V, et al. Clinical and molecular characterization of neonatal diabetes and syndromic diabetes in Asian Indian children. Clin Genet. 2012;83:439-45.
10. Kanthimathi S, Balamurugan K, Mohan V, et al. Identification and molecular characterization of HNF1B gene mutations in Indian diabetic patients with renal abnormalities. Ann Hum Genet. 2015;79:10-9.
11. Misra S, Shields B, Colclough K, et al. South Asian individuals with diabetes who are referred for MODY testing have lower mutation pick-up rate than white European people. Diabetologia. 2016;59:2262-5.

Chapter 59

Diabetes Management in Chronic Liver Disease

Soumitra Ghosh

INTRODUCTION

The prevalence of diabetes mellitus and chronic liver disease (CLD) is rising fuelled by the obesity epidemic. Obesity is a risk factor for nonalcoholic fatty liver disease (NAFLD), the most common CLD and type 2 diabetes through complex pathogenetic mechanisms that involve peripheral and hepatic insulin resistance (IR); release of inflammatory adipokines and hepatokines; and accelerated β-cell failure.

The entire spectrum of CLD ranging from abnormal liver enzymes; nonalcoholic steatosis and steatohepatitis; and cirrhosis and hepatocellular carcinoma is seen in diabetes. Coexistence of both conditions adversely affects the course of the other and brings complexities in their management.

In patients with CLD due to other causes, the presence of diabetes results in higher progression to cirrhosis and hepatocellular carcinoma.[1,2] CLD is a risk factor for hyperglycemia. Approximately 80% of CLDs have impaired glucose intolerance and 30–60% have frank diabetes.[3,4] In patients with pre-existing diabetes, CLD worsens morbidity and mortality outcomes. In the Verona Diabetes Study, cirrhosis was the fourth leading cause of death in diabetes.[5] In diabetes mellitus, the standardized mortality rate (the relative rate of a condition compared to background rate) is higher for cirrhosis (2.52) than for coronary artery disease (1.34).

Numerous challenges are faced when managing diabetes patients with CLD. The chapter highlights these and discusses appropriate management options.

ROLE OF LIVER IN GLUCOSE HOMEOSTASIS

The liver is an important organ involved in regulation of whole body nutrient supply and glucose homeostasis. In concert with a number of hormones involved in nutrient metabolism, the liver functions as an organ for glucose supply or as an organ for glucose consumption in the fasted and fed state, respectively. Hormones like insulin; counter-regulatory hormones, most importantly glucagon; and hepatokines ensure that this function is accomplished. In the fasted state, the liver ensures a steady blood glucose concentration by releasing glucose via glycogenolysis and gluconeogenesis. However, after prolonged fasting glycogenolysis no longer takes place as glycogen stores are depleted and gluconeogenesis occurs from gluconeogenic amino acids and glycerol which are breakdown products of protein and triglycerides, respectively. The converse happens in the fed state. In the fed state, insulin-mediated uptake of glucose via glucose transporter-2 (GLUT2) in the liver promotes glycolysis. The glycolytic intermediates promote glycogen and lipid synthesis which is stored in the liver to be utilized in times of calorie needs. In CLD, this fine balanced is lost.

LIVER—AN IMPORTANT ORGAN FOR METABOLISM OF INSULIN AND OTHER AGENTS

The liver is an important site for insulin metabolism. About 60% of endogenously secreted insulin is removed by first-pass metabolism in the liver and the kidney clears remaining 40%. The concentration of insulin in portal vein is two- to four-fold higher than in peripheral circulation and plays an important role in suppressing hepatic glucose production. When given exogenously insulin, it bypasses the portal circulation. Therefore, more exogenous insulin is needed to suppress hepatic glucose output. The kidney removes more than 80% of the exogenous insulin and the liver clears another 20–30%.

Many antidiabetic agents and other agents used for diabetes are metabolized by the liver. Dose modifications or avoidance of certain drugs becomes necessary.

A TWO-WAY COMMUNICATION IS INVOLVED IN PATHOGENESIS OF DIABETES MELLITUS AND CHRONIC LIVER DISEASE

There is an extensive interconnected mechanism by which type 2 diabetes mellitus and CLD engage and accelerate each other. The core defect is IR. IR results in hyperglycemia and release of free fatty acid (FFA) from the adipose tissue. Accumulation of FFA as triglycerides in the liver and hyperglycemia-induced de novo lipogenesis causes ectopic fat in the liver. Release of inflammatory adipokines from the adipose tissue along with hepatic steatosis promotes mitochondrial oxidative stress. Oxidative stress increases free radical formation with subsequent inflammation and hepatic necrosis. Inflammation promotes the stellate cells of the liver to produce collagen and consequent fibrosis and cirrhosis.

Cirrhosis, a chronic inflammatory state, worsens IR and cause hyperglycemia by impairing oxidative and nonoxidative glucose utilization. IR, portosystemic shunting and decreased hepatic insulin clearance cause hyperinsulinemia with resultant mitogenic effects of insulin. Beta-cell IR, impaired clearance of the advanced glycation end products and direct effects of hepatitis C virus (HCV) core protein cause β-cell failure. Interferon treatment for chronic hepatitis increases incidence of type 1 and type 2 diabetes.

CHALLENGES TO MANAGEMENT OF DIABETES IN CHRONIC LIVER DISEASE

Poor nutritional status in CLD due to the disease or dietary restrictions imposed by the disease; and disease associated physical activity limitations represent major challenges in the therapeutic life style measures in diabetes management. The liver is a vital organ involved in glucose homeostasis and its dysfunction increases hypoglycemia risk. However, IR and β-cell failure due to CLD-associated inflammation causes hyperglycemia. Monitoring of diabetes control like glycated hemoglobin (HbA1c) and fructosamine assay can be a problem due to altered red blood cell (RBC) lifespan and changes in serum albumin. Drug dosage modification is frequently needed.

MANAGEMENT OF DIABETES MELLITUS IN CHRONIC LIVER DISEASE

Define Liver Disease and Assess Comorbidities

When faced with a diabetes patient with altered liver function, the first step is define the liver disease as acute or chronic. Once chronicity is established, staging of the liver disease is necessary to determine therapeutic targets. The Child-Pugh staging helps to stage the liver disease (Table 1). It is important to assess comorbidities like coexisting renal disease which can further limit pharmacotherapy choice. Coexisting alcohol use needs to be assessed and advised against.

Glycemic Targets and Monitoring

A relaxed HbA1c target (7.5–8%) is preferred especially in advanced CLD. However, in patients with CLD, HbA1c can be inaccurate due to altered RBC lifespan. Patients with CLD have anemia, hypersplenism, variceal bleeding and antiviral therapy which can alter the lifespan of the RBC. Nutritional anemia increases RBC lifespan and gives a falsely high HbA1c value. Anemia due to RBC destruction due to hypersplenism and ribavirin-induced hemolysis falsely lowers the HbA1c by decreasing RBC lifespan. Fructosamine assay can be erroneous due to altered albumin concentration and lifespan. Frequent self-monitoring of blood glucose (SMBG) is helpful. Downloading glucose memory from readings can help determine the average blood glucose through computer programs. Continuous glucose monitoring (CGM) is indicated in insulin treated patient at risk of hypoglycemia which includes CLD. It is expensive and can be used as a supplement to SMBG.

Choice of Pharmacotherapy

The choice of pharmacotherapy becomes restricted in advanced CLD (Child-Pugh class C) due to altered metabolism and risk of hepatotoxicity. However, in early stages like class A and B, treatment is essentially the same as in those without liver disease with some dose modification.

TABLE 1: Child-Pugh score for severity of liver disease.

Encephalopathy	Ascites	Bilirubin	Albumin	Prothrombin time prolongation
1 point: None	1 point: Absent	1 point: <2 mg/dL	1 point: >3.5 mg/dL	1 point: <4 s above control/INR <1.7
2 points: Grade 1: Altered mood/confusion 2 points: Grade 2: Inappropriate behavior, impending stupor, somnolence	2 points: Slight 3 points: Moderate	2 points: 2–3 mg/dL 3 points: >3 mg/dL	2 points: 2.8–3.5 mg/dL 3 points: <2.8 mg/dL	2 points: 4–6 s above control/INR 1.7–2.3 3 points: >6 s above normal/INR >2.3
3 points: Grade 3: Markedly confused, stuporous, arousable 3 points: Grade 4: Comatosed/unresponsive				

Child-Pugh score interpretation:
- Child-Pugh class A: 5–6 points
- Child-Pugh class B: 7–9 points
- Child-Pugh class C: 10–15 points.

(INR: international normalized ratio.)

Biguanides (Metformin)

Metformin is not hepatotoxic, does not cause hypoglycemia, and is beneficial in patients with NAFLD. It can be used in patients with mild CLD and can be used with caution and dose reduction in moderate CLD. It should be avoided in advanced CLD and binge drinkers due to risk of lactic acidosis as metformin decreases lactate clearance by suppressing the conversion of lactate to glucose.[6] It should be avoided in any acute illness and hepatic decompensation.

Alpha-Glucosidase Inhibitor

Alpha-glucosidase inhibitors (AGIs) are promising agents in the treatment of type 2 diabetes mellitus and compensated CLD because they inhibit carbohydrate absorption decreasing postprandial hyperglycemia. Studies have shown that they decrease the ammonia level.[7] The postulated mechanism is that AGI-induced increased bowel mobility increases the saccharolytic bacteria while decreasing the proteolytic bacteria. However, acarbose can cause elevation in the alanine transaminase (ALT) and or rare occasions cause severe liver disease.

Sulphonylureas

Sulphonylureas (SUs) are protein bound and metabolized in the liver. Levels are increased in CLD due to impaired metabolism and poor protein binding due to hypoalbuminemia. They should be avoided in advanced CLD. Shorter-acting SUs like glipizide, gliclazide and glimepiride can be used in mild and moderate CLD with caution and dose reduction. But SUs are not preferred agents in CLD, as they can cause hypoglycemia. Moreover, SUs do not address the IR that is significant in CLD. Glinides too should be used with caution only in mild CLD.

Thiazolidinediones

Thiazolidinediones (TZDs) improve peripheral and hepatic insulin sensitivity. They are one of the treatment options for NAFLD. Troglitazone (no longer used) was associated with acute liver failure; but pioglitazone and rosiglitazone do not share such risks. However, it is currently recommended that serum ALT should be evaluated before starting. They are not to be used when the serum ALT exceeds 2.5 times the upper limit of normal (ULN). Monitoring is advised periodically and not every 2 months as previously advised. TZDs can be thus used in Child-Pugh class A but are to be avoided in class B and class C, or in anyone who has edema.

Dipeptidyl Peptidase-4 Inhibitors

Sitagliptin and vildagliptin are excreted unchanged via the kidneys or metabolized by hydrolysis at other sites; a small percentage undergoes hepatic metabolism.[8] However, prescribing information (PI) of vildagliptin suggests that it should not be used in patients with hepatic impairment, including those with ALT or aspartate transaminase (AST) more than three times the ULN. Linagliptin undergoes enterohepatic cycling but little hepatic metabolism and is excreted through the hepatic and renal routes. Saxagliptin, however, undergoes hepatic metabolism and is excreted by both the kidneys and the liver.[8]

Dipeptidyl peptidase 4 inhibitors have not been studied in patients with advanced CLD. They can be used without dose modification (except vildagliptin and probably saxagliptin) in class A CLD and used with caution in class B CLD. They should be avoided in class C CLD.

Sodium-Glucose Cotransporter-2 Inhibitors

Sodium-glucose cotransporter-2 inhibitors are metabolized in the liver. PI suggests canagliflozin use without dose modification in class A and class B and avoidance in class C CLD. PI of dapagliflozin suggests no dose adjustment but use with caution if initiating in severe impairment. Empagliflozin PI suggests no dose adjustment even if systemic exposure is increased in CLD as those changes are not considered clinically significant. Thus, the information on use of these agents in CLD is inconclusive. They may, therefore, be used in class A CLD without dose modification, used with caution in class B, and avoided in class C.

Glucagon-like Peptide 1 Receptor Agonists

Liraglutide and dulaglutide are metabolized by protein catabolism pathways to amino acids. PI of liraglutide, dulaglutide and exenatide suggests no dose adjustment in hepatic impairment but advises caution due to limited experience. Due to lack of sufficient data, it would be wise to use this class of drugs in class A CLD only.

Insulin

Insulin is indicated in any stage of CLD with acute complications, can be used in conjunction with other agents (which may have insulin sparing effect and other benefits) in early CLD, and frequently remains the only option along with lifestyle measures in advanced CLD. It is important to start insulin low and titrate slow. Frequent SMBG is vital as insulin requirement can change due to impaired insulin metabolism and clearance, and IR. Rapid-acting analogs may be preferred as they provide good postprandial coverage, have shorter duration and decrease postprandial and nocturnal hypoglycemia. Basal peakless insulin can be combined with relatively safe oral agents.

Prevention of Long-term Complications

Management of other risk factors to prevent long-term diabetes complications remains the same in diabetes patients with and without CLD. Statins not only improve dyslipidemia but have pleiotropic effects. The pleiotropic properties include improving endothelial dysfunction, and antioxidant, antifibrotic, anti-inflammatory, anti-proliferative, proapoptotic or immunomodulation properties. However, they can cause myositis, rhabdomyolysis and dose-dependent elevation of hepatic enzymes. Recommendations from the National Lipid Association Statin Liver Safety Assessment Task Force state that presence of CLD or compensated cirrhosis is not a contraindication for the use of statins.[9] They should, however, be avoided in decompensated cirrhosis and acute liver failure.

In patients with advanced CLD and diabetes, the risk of cirrhosis complications is higher than the risk of diabetes complications. Hepatologists frequently treat diabetes and cirrhosis due to the complication profile. A team effort is a necessity for proper patient management. The liver is an important endocrine organ and it is indispensable to understand the liver from an endocrine perspective.

CONCLUSION

Diabetes mellitus and CLD frequently coexist and their incidence is rising as a fallout of the obesity epidemic. IR lies at the heart of the problem. The natural history of the disease is adversely affected by the other. There are numerous challenges in treating diabetes patients with CLD. This is because the liver is an important endocrine organ and an important organ for metabolism of many pharmacotherapeutic agents. Frequent monitoring of blood glucose levels by SMBG, relaxed HbA1c targets and cautious use of drugs are important to improve outcome.

REFERENCES

1. Harrison SA, Torgerson S, Hayashi PH, et al. The natural history of nonalcoholic fatty liver disease: A clinical histopathological study. Am J Gastroenterol. 2008;98:2042-7.
2. Targher G, Byrne CD. Clinical review: Nonalcoholic fatty liver disease: A novel cardiometabolic risk factor for type 2 diabetes and its complications. J Clin Endocrinol Metab. 2013;98:483-95.
3. Petrides AS: Liver disease and diabetes mellitus. Diabetes Rev. 1994;2:1-18.
4. García-Compean D, Jaquez-Quintana JO, Maldonado-Garza H. Hepatogenous diabetes: Current views of an ancient problem. Ann Hepatol. 2009;8:13-20.
5. de Marco R, Locatelli F, Zoppini G, et al. Cause-specific mortality in type 2 diabetes. The Verona Diabetes Study. Diabetes Care. 1999;22(5):756-61.
6. Brackett CC. Clarifying metformin's role and risks in liver dysfunction. J Am Pharm Assoc. 2010;50:407-10.
7. Gentile S, Guarino G, Romano M, et al. A randomized controlled trial of acarbose in hepatic encephalopathy. Clin Gastroenterol Hepatol. 2005;3:184-91.
8. Golightly LK, Drayna CC, McDermott MT. Comparative clinical pharmacokinetics of dipeptidyl peptidase-4 inhibitors. Clin Pharmacokinet. 2012;51:501-14.
9. Bays H, Cohen DE, Chalasani N, et al. The National Lipid Association's Statin Safety Task Force. An assessment by the Statin Liver Safety Task Force: 2014 update. J Clin Lipidol. 2014;8(3 Suppl):S47-57.

Chapter 60

Diabetes Management in Cancer Patients

Sambit Das, Mahesh Rath, Sunil Kumar Kota

INTRODUCTION

Type 2 diabetes mellitus (T2DM) has been one of the major public health problems around the world and in the past decade, the prevalence of T2DM is seen to be increasing rapidly among the Asian populations.[1] Certain cancers carry a higher risk and poor outcomes when associated with diabetes.[2] The risk of mortality due to diabetes is increased by around 40% in cancer patients, as compared to nondiabetics.[3] Presently, around 20% of cancer patients concurrently have diabetes,[4] and thus are at risk of worse outcomes.

The adverse outcomes, poor prognosis and increased mortality among cancer patients with diabetes have been attributed to lower cancer screening rates, more advanced stage at diagnosis and less aggressive cancer treatments being offered.[5,6] In addition to that, insulin resistance and compensatory hyperinsulinemia, in turn increase tumor proliferation rates and contribute to cancer progression and metastases.[7-9]

CANCER: GLOBAL ESTIMATES AND ASSOCIATION WITH DIABETES

Cancer has become one of the most important threats to human health and life all over the world. The latest GLOBOCAN 2018 reported that globally there were 18.1 million new cancer cases, 9.6 million cancer deaths and 43.8 million people living with cancer. India had around 1.1 million new cases of cancer cases, 0.78 million cancer deaths and around 2.2 million people living with cancer.[10] In the early 20th century, various studies have shown possible interactions between DM and cancer.[1,11]

Diabetes if not well controlled can lead to stroke, heart disease and disabilities, such as vision problems, kidney failure, or amputations of the foot or leg. Diabetes has been strongly associated with the development of pancreatic, liver and endometrial cancer; while breast, colorectal and bladder cancer have shown to have a moderate association. In case of prostate cancer, diabetes has shown to have contributed to a decreased incidence [glycated hemoglobin (HbA1c) >7.0%).[12] Increased colon cancer incidence in women has been associated with insulin use, but not with colon cancer in men or breast or prostate cancer risk. There has been reduced incidences breast and prostate cancer with metformin use, but no association with colon cancer risk has been shown. On the contrary, sulfonylurea exposure has not been associated with risk of any type of cancer.[13] Morphine in turn has been linked with a 1.24-fold risk of T2DM in breast cancer women. The risk rises with morphine dosage and tamoxifen or aromatase inhibitors, but is not significant in breast cancer women receiving megestrol acetate.[14]

CANCER AND DIABETES MANAGEMENT

A negative impact has been noted on the performance of diabetes self-management activities in adults with both diabetes and cancer due to chemotherapy and associated adverse effects thus increasing the risk for hyperglycemia and development of complications.[15]

The treatment of a patient with cancer in general depends on various factors, primary being the prognosis.[16] Depending on whether the patient is expected to live for several months or only days to weeks, the management needs to be planned. On diabetes perspective, close and optimum glucose monitoring must be ensured in be palliative care patients who are still active and enjoying a relatively good quality of life, to ensure that physical activities are not impaired by lack of energy due to glycemic derangements. The goal for terminally ill patients should be to minimize interventions and thus maximize comfort. On a whole the goal of diabetic therapy should be to maintain patient comfort and quality of life, rather than simply the control of blood sugar. Thus less strict monitoring and glycemic control and lesser dietary restrictions, thereby encouraging patients to enjoy eating should be advocated in terminally ill patients.

The management of both type 1 and type 2 diabetes in patients with advanced cancer is complicated by a number of factors. A balance between hypoglycemic therapies and food intake needs to be done to ensure a good glycemic control. It is a challenge to ensure the glycemic control, due to the anorexia, nausea and vomiting usually associated with the disease, which may be precipitated by opioid analgesics. Insulin is usually administered as a basal bolus or basal plus and the dose is predicated upon expected energy consumption. The insulin requirements are greatly increased in stress conditions such as infection primarily in immunologically suppressed and bedridden patients who are highly prone to develop them.[17]

The diabetic control can be adversely affected by certain medications used in treating advanced cancer. Glucocorticoids must be used with caution in patients with known glucose intolerance as they frequently precipitate marked hyperglycemia.[18] Any patient taking steroids for longer than 3 weeks should have intermittent monitoring for hyperglycemia.

Development of hepatic or renal failure has affected the metabolism and duration of action of oral hypoglycemic agents. Due to their long duration of action, hypoglycemia may persist 48–72 hours following discontinuation of these drugs and up to 96 hours, if renal or hepatic failure is present.[18] In sick patients, metformin and sodium-glucose cotransporter-2 (SGLT2) inhibitors need to be avoided. Sulfonylureas can lead to hypoglycemia. In patients of hepatic and renal failure and those who have a poor and irregular appetite, oral hypoglycemic agents need to be avoided. Dipeptidyl peptidase 4 (DPP-4) inhibitors can be used selectively in such patients.

Thiazide diuretics and furosemide which are used to control ascites may produce hyperglycemia[18] while potassium-sparing diuretics (such as spironolactone) may cause hyperkalemia. Patients with longstanding diabetes are particularly predisposed to this effect, as they have an increased incidence of type 4 renal tubular acidosis, or hyporeninemic hypoaldosteronism.[18] This form of renal tubular acidosis results in decreased potassium excretion and hyperkalemia.

It has been shown that scheduled insulin (basal bolus) is effective in attainment of glucose targets in diabetic cancer patients.[19] But, it has also been observed in studies that there has been a higher prevalence of nonadherence to oral antidiabetic medications as well as negative consequences associated with nonadherence, among patients with cancer.[20]

CONCLUSION

In persons with diabetes and cancer, tight control of blood glucose is not important and may be undesirable in terminally ill patients, but optimum control can be ensured in patients who have a better prognosis. There is no added benefit to the patient to have glucose more tightly controlled than 8 mmol/L (150 mg/dL). In cases of hyperglycemia requiring institution of insulin therapy, satisfactory control is most readily achieved by administering short-acting insulin every 6–8 hours in doses determined by result of blood sugar determinations. Institution of basal insulin [neutral protamine Hagedorn (NPH), glargine U100 or U300 and degludec] is important to prevent frequent glucose excursions and nocturnal hypoglycemia. In the initial 24–48 hours, these glucose determinations and insulin injections may have to be done every 6 hours. As soon as the glucose is reduced into the range of 10-15 mmol/L, the patient may be started on once or twice daily injections of an intermediate-acting insulin such as NPH or a 70/30 preparation. Patients with T1D must continue to receive insulin daily to prevent the development of fatal ketoacidosis. Tight control is not necessary, and blood glucose in the range of 140–200 mg/dL is acceptable unless the patient is symptomatic.

REFERENCES

1. Wolf I, Sadetzki S, Catane R, et al. Diabetes mellitus and breast cancer. Lancet Oncol. 2005;6:103-11.
2. Vigneri R. Diabetes: diabetes therapy and cancer risk. Nat Rev Endocrinol. 2009;5:651-2.
3. Barone BB, Yeh HC, Snyder CF, et al. Long-term all-cause mortality in cancer patients with pre-existing diabetes mellitus: a systematic review and meta-analysis. JAMA. 2008;300:2754-64.
4. Richardson LC, Pollack LA. Therapy insight: Influence of type 2 diabetes on the development, treatment and outcomes of cancer. Nat Clin Pract Oncol. 2005;2:48-53.
5. Lipscombe LL, Hux JE, Booth GL. Reduced screening mammography among women with diabetes. Arch Intern Med. 2005;165:2090-5.

6. Peairs KS, Barone BB, Snyder CF, et al. Diabetes mellitus and breast cancer outcomes: a systematic review and meta-analysis. J Clin Oncol. 2011;29:40-6.
7. Dowling RJ, Niraula S, Stambolic V, et al. Metformin in cancer: translational challenges. J Mol Endocrinol. 2012;48:R31-43.
8. Goodwin PJ, Ennis M, Pritchard KI, et al. Fasting insulin and outcome in early-stage breast cancer: results of a prospective cohort study. J Clin Oncol. 2002;20:42-51.
9. Pollak M. Insulin and insulin-like growth factor signalling in neoplasia. Nat Rev Cancer. 2008;8:915-28.
10. Global Cancer Statistics 2018 (online) Available at: http://www.iarc.fr/en/media-centre/iarcnews/2018/gco_globocan2018.php [Accessed October, 2018].
11. Chodick G, Zucker I. Diabetes, gestational diabetes and the risk of cancer in women: epidemiologic evidence and possible biologic mechanisms. Womens Health (Lond Engl). 2011.7;227-37.
12. Kasper JS, Giovannucci E. A meta-analysis of diabetes mellitus and the risk of prostate cancer. Cancer Epidemiol Biomark Prev. 2006;15:2056-62.
13. Onitilo AA, Stankowski RV, Berg RL, et al. Type 2 diabetes mellitus, glycaemic control, and cancer risk. Eur J Cancer Prev. 2014;23(2):134-40.
14. Yang SP, Muo CH, Wang IK, et al. Risk of type 2 diabetes mellitus in female breast cancer patients treated with morphine: A retrospective population-based time-dependent cohort study. Diabetes Res Clin Prac. 2015;110(3):285-90.
15. Hershey DS, Given B, Given C, et al. Predictors of Diabetes Self-Management in Older Adults Receiving Chemotherapy. Cancer Nurs. 2014;37(2):97-105.
16. Heber D, Byerly LO, Chlebowski RT. Metabolic abnormalities in the cancer patient. Cancer. 1985;55:225-9.
17. National Diabetes Data Group. Classification and diagnosis of diabetes mellitus and other categories of glucose intolerance. Diabetes 1979; 28:1039-1057.
18. Wilson JD, Isselbacher KJ, Braunwald E, Martin JB, Fauci AS, Kasper DL. Harrison's principles of internal medicine, 12th edition. New York: McGraw Hill, 1991.
19. Brady VJ, Grimes D, Armstrong T, et al. Management of Steroid-Induced Hyperglycemia in Hospitalized Patients with Cancer: A Review. Oncol Nurs Forum. 2014;41(6)E355-65.
20. Tan X, Feng X, Chang J, et al. Oral antidiabetic drug use and associated health outcomes in cancer patients. J Clin Pharm Ther. 2016;41(5):524-31.

Chapter 61

Diabetes in the Lean Indian

Sanjay Reddy AC, Nagaraj

INTRODUCTION

Diabetes mellitus (DM), the most common metabolic condition, is associated with substantial disease burden, including increased mortality risk and significant long-term morbidity.[1-4]

It is increasing in epidemic proportions across the globe.

According to the Diabetes Atlas published by the International Diabetes Federation (IDF), there are an estimated 82 million people with diabetes in India in 2017 and it is predicted to increase to 134.3 million by 2045, which makes every fifth diabetic patient in the world to be an Indian and also it is estimated that around 57.9% patients are undiagnosed.

Epidemiological data in India over the past decades have shown that the pattern and profile of DM are disparate.

Evidence show that obesity has been a notable risk factor for diabetes. However, beyond the classical obesity related type 2 diabetes and other well-defined types of diabetes like type 1 DM, maturity onset diabetes of the young (MODY), gestational diabetes, etc. there is a renewed interest in the underweight or normal weight/lean diabetes that is emerging.

Paradoxically, nearly 80% of Indian type 2 diabetic patients are nonobese, whereas 60–80% of such diabetics in the West are obese.[5,6]

Lean or low bodyweight includes >20% below the ideal bodyweight for height and gender and such noninsulin-dependent diabetic patients constitute a very heterogeneous group, although they present with similar clinical characteristics.

Therefore, leanness was the inherent characteristic and unrelated to the diabetic state as such.[7]

Analysis of dietary intake has revealed that they were neither protein deprived nor poor, as the mean daily intake was over 50 g.

The prevalence of DM-lean varies depending on type of population, ethnic origin and geopolitical situation.

LEAN TYPE 2 DIABETES MELLITUS

Diabetes in low-bodyweight group [body mass index (BMI) <18.5 kg/m^2].

Prevalence

Though recognized as a distinct entity early on, very little attention has been paid to the qualitative changes associated with it.

The preferred cut-off for Indians to define as lean is a BMI of 18.5 kg/m^2 (International Diabetes Institute, 2000).

Studies have reported a prevalence rate of lean diabetes ranging from 3.5 to 27%.

Risk Factors

Lean diabetics are predominantly males and are more likely to be older at the time of diagnosis.

This category of people is more often current smokers and also has history of alcohol consumption over 20 g/day and associated with sedentary lifestyle.

Even though smoking has an effect on bodyweight reduction, it is observed that smoking is conducive to visceral fat accumulation and insulin resistance, and it increases the risk of type 2 DM (T2DM).

Alcohol consumption is almost 2-fold higher in lean DM when compared to obese DM and chronic alcoholism induces pancreatic β-cell dysfunction and apoptosis.

A region of chromosome 21q has been linked to T2DM in lean individuals. Further examination of this region led to identification of KCNJ15 (potassium inwardly-rectifying channel, subfamily J, member 15) as a susceptibility gene.

This KCNJ15 is linked to dysfunctional glucose-stimulated insulin secretion in lean type 2 diabetics.

Metabolic Mechanics

Glucose storage is severely impaired in lean type 2 diabetes. Changes in glycogen synthase action, which result in dysregulation of glucose storage in skeletal muscle after meal, are probably the main alteration of glucose metabolism in lean type 2 diabetics. Lean-T2DM patients have moderately-severe to severe basal hyperglycemia.[5,8] Levels of glycated hemoglobin (HbA1c) are significantly higher than others.

Unlike in most classical diabetics, treatment requires the advice to increase calorie intake, as the daily intake is often lower than desirable for physical activity and lifestyle of the patient with lean-T2DM. Although there was a slight gain in bodyweight with the change in BMI, the mean value remained within the definition of low bodyweight in both males and females.[9-12]

It is found that hepatic enzymes concerned with CHO cycles operate differently and at higher levels in lean-T2DM and such increase in levels of glucokinase could be their inherent characteristic.

Hepatic glucose uptake is normal in T2DM, while hepatic glucose output (HGO) is high, which indicates that such a hyperactive metabolic state observed in the liver of these diabetics with lean habitus is probably responsible for excess utilization of insulin during its first pass.[10,13]

The C-peptide levels are similar in lean as well as obese T2DM with no significant difference in the fasting or stimulated C-peptide levels, suggesting a good β-cell reserve in the lean with probably excess extraction of insulin in the portohepatic circulation leading to lower levels of circulating insulin.[14-16]

These lean diabetics have a favorable lipid profile that could be a consequence of hepatic handling of high-density lipoprotein (HDL) and CHO metabolism and lack of hyperinsulinemia–insulin resistance in the peripheral bed with low prevalence of macrovascular diseases as well.

Homocysteine which is an independent marker/ risk factor of macrovascular disease[17-19] was found to be significantly lower in the lean-T2DM, which also contributes to low macrovascular complications in these patients.

Proteinuria in the lean-T2DM was more related to poor glycemic control rather than a predictor for developing further deteriorating nephropathy as proteinuria improved rapidly with good glycemic control.[9]

Also, islet cell antibodies (ICAs) are absent in the serum of lean-T2DM and 74% of lean subjects with adult onset diabetes were anti-GADA (glutamic acid decarboxylase) negative.[9,15]

Principally, lean subjects with diabetes have good β-cell function, insulin resistance but express severe hyperglycemia despite adequate serum insulin levels.

Clinical Features

There is a definite male preponderance in lean-T2DM with mean age of lean-T2DM ranging from 45 to 58 years among the Indians at the time of diagnosis.

Mean fasting, postprandial, or 2-hour postchallenge blood glucose is higher among lean diabetics. HbA1c levels are significantly higher in the lean diabetics in comparison to obese.

Hypertension is seen in only up to 12–16% of lean-T2DM when compared to 40–60% among obese. Both systolic and diastolic blood pressures are lower in lean-T2DM.

Lipid profile is more favorable in lean diabetics. Serum cholesterol and triglycerides levels are lowest among the lean diabetics and contrastingly higher than in normal weight and obese patients with serum triglyceride (TG)/ HDL ratio lower in lean-T2DM. Also, glycemic control does not have much influence on lipid metabolism in lean diabetics.

Complications

Lean diabetics have a higher prevalence of peripheral neuropathy, retinopathy, nephropathy and infections compared to macrovascular complications.

In most lean-type 2 diabetics, peripheral neuropathy was the presenting feature.

Prevalence of these microvascular complications ranged from 50 to 70% for peripheral neuropathy, 19 to 25% for retinopathy, 13 to 28% for nephropathy and infections 14 to 26%.

Among the infections, tuberculosis was high in up to 16–26.6% followed by foot and systemic infections. Bronchopneumonia contributes to about 11.6% of respiratory infections followed by urinary tract infection (14%).

Macrovascular complications like coronary artery disease (CAD) and stroke are low in lean diabetics ranging from 1 to 2.7% and 2 to 3.6%, respectively.

Management

It is found that 48–80.5% of lean-T2DM patients were well controlled on oral hypoglycemic agents (OHAs). It is well established that lean-T2DM patients have good β-cell reserve for insulin and are sulfonylurea responsive.[5,8,20]

Metformin continues to be the recommended first-line treatment independent of bodyweight. Dipeptidyl peptidase 4 inhibitors are also a good choice among lean diabetics.

Insulin requirement is high among the lean-T2DM with secondary OHA failure.

SUMMARY

Low-bodyweight type 2 DM/T2DM-lean are neither latent autoimmune diabetes of adulthood (LADA) nor forme fruste of Type 1 DM but variants of classical T2DM having absence of markers for autoimmune destruction of β-cells and good insulin C-peptide reserve for a prolonged period of life. They constitute an independent variant of T2DM with inherent peculiarities in insulin kinetics in the liver along with altered profile and behavior of key enzymes related to CHO metabolism which are marked by excess extraction of insulin in hepatic bed, hyperactive cytochrome system, and nonsuppressible glucokinase activity. These peculiarities are reflected in the peripheral circulation as states of hypoinsulinemia, hyperglycemia, dyslipidemia without low HDL cholesterol (HDL-C), raised triglycerides, and fewer other markers for atherosclerosis which make diabetics less prone to develop macrovascular disease.

Peripheral neuropathy and the consequences of hyperglycemia like infections and proteinuria dominate the clinical picture. However, due to presence of insulin resistance and good β-cell reserve for insulin, despite of lean habitus, most of them respond well to OHA for long periods of life as may be comparable with any other phenotype of type 2 diabetes.

An early focus on multiple metabolic defects may provide an optimal approach to treating the lean patient with type 2 diabetes in clinical practice, and combination therapy that addresses both insulin secretory dysfunction and insulin resistance would seem a rational approach.

REFERENCES

1. UK Prospective Diabetes Study Group. Tight blood pressure control and risk of macrovascular and microvascular complications in type 2 diabetes: UKPDS 38. BMJ. 1998;317(7160):703-13.
2. Beckman JA, Creager MA, Libby P. Diabetes and atherosclerosis: epidemiology, pathophysiology, and management. JAMA. 2002;287(19): 2570-81.
3. Heron M, Hoyert DL, Murphy SL, et al. Deaths: final data for 2006. Natl Vital Stat Rep. 2009;57(14):1-134.
4. Riddle MC. Glycemic control and cardiovascular mortality. Curr Opin Endocrinol Diabetes Obes. 2011;18(2):104-9.
5. Das S. Identity of lean-NIDDM: Clinical, metabolic and hormonal status. In: Kochupillai N (Ed). Advances in Endocrinology, Metabolism and Diabetes, 2nd volume. Delhi, India: Macmillan; 1994. pp. 42-53.
6. Sahay BK. Profile of lean-NIDDM as seen in Hyderabad. In: Kapur A (Ed). Proceedings of the Second Novo-Nordisk Diabetes Update. Bombay: Health Care Communication; 1993. pp. 161-4.
7. Das S. Lean-NIDDM: An independent entity. In: Kapur A (Ed). Proceedings of the Second Novo- Nordisk Diabetes Update. Bombay: Health Care Communication; 1993. pp. 153-9.
8. Tripathy BB, Kar BC. Observations on clinical patterns of Diabetes Mellitus in India. Diabetes. 1965;14:404-12.
9. Das S. Low body weight NIDDM: An independent entity. In: Das AK (Ed). Medicine Update. Mumbai: Assn Phys India; 1998. pp. 595-602.
10. Nigam A. Lean-NIDDM a definite entity: In: Das S (Ed). Brochure on Problems, Practical Aspects, Publications and Questionnaire. Cuttack: International Workshop on Types of Diabetes Peculiar to the Tropics; 1995. pp. 54-6.
11. Mohan V, Vijayaprabha R, Rema M, et al. Clinical profile of lean NIDDM in South India. Diabetes Res Clin Pract. 1997;38:101-8.
12. Ahuja MM. Diabetes care in India the reality and a dream. In: Kapur A (Ed). Proceedings of the second Novo-Nordisk Diabetes Update. Bombay: Health Care Communication; 1993. pp. 15-20.
13. Malnutrition and Diabetes in the Tropics. Report of the International Workshop on Types of Diabetes Peculiar to the Tropics. Diabetes Care. 1996;19:1014-7.
14. Kanan K. Lean Type II diabetes mellitus-a distinct entity. In: Kapur A (Ed). Proceedings of the Second Novo-Nordisk Diabetes Update. Bombay: Health Care Communication; 1993. pp. 147-51.
15. Unnikrishnan AG, Singh SK, Sanjeevi CB. Prevalence of GAD65 antibodies in lean subjects with type 2 diabetes. Ann NY Acad Sci. 2004;1037:118-21.
16. Das S, Samal KC, Baliarsinha AK, et al. Lean (underweight) NIDDM-peculiarities and differences in metabolic and hormonal status. J Assoc Physicians India. 1995;43:339-42.
17. Das S, Sotaniemi EA. Hepatic microsomal enzymes and Cyto P450 activity. In: Das S (Ed). Technical Series on "Low Bodyweight Type 2 Diabetes Mellitus". Mumbai: Indian College of Physicians (Academic Wing of Association of Physicians of India); 1999. pp. 54-8.
18. Clarke R, Daly L, Robinson K, et al. Hyperhomocysteinemia: an independent risk factor for vascular disease. N Eng J Med. 1991:324;1149-55.
19. Munshi MN, Stone A, Fink L, et al. Hyperhomocysteinemia following methionine load in patients with non-insulin dependent diabetes mellitus and macrovascular disease. Metabolism. 1996;45:133-5.
20. Punyakrit DB, Ranabir S, Prasad L, et al. Clinical and biochemical profile of lean type 2 diabetes mellitus. Indian J Endocrinol Metabol. 2011;15 (Suppl 1):S40-S43.

Chapter 62

Alzheimer Disease in Diabetes Mellitus

P Jabbar, Geena Suasa

INTRODUCTION

Type 2 diabetes mellitus (T2DM) and Alzheimer disease (AD) are age-related conditions, with increased incidence and prevalence with aging in both.[1,2] Besides, the development of one increases the risk of the other.[3] Moreover, epidemiological studies have shown an association of DM and AD. It was estimated in a population-based historical cohort study that the risk of acquiring AD increased with adult onset DM.[4] Similarly, patients with AD were at risk in developing impaired fasting glucose and T2DM.[5] A variety of mechanisms have been put forward in the risk of AD and T2DM–metabolic abnormalities of insulin resistance (dyslipidemia, hypertension), hyperglycemia per se or insulin, by disturbing synaptic plasticity, learning and memory.[6]

EPIDEMIOLOGICAL EVIDENCES

Epidemiological and biological evidences prove without doubt the link between these two aging-related diseases. First and foremost, DM is associated with changes in perception and cognitive dysfunction.

There is a reportedly higher incidence of AD and cognitive decline in persons with diabetes. There is an increased risk of developing all types of dementia, including AD in patients with DM.[2,4-6] A systematic review of eligible longitudinal population-based studies of variable methodological quality found that in most studies the incidence of "any dementia" was higher in persons with diabetes than in those without diabetes.[7] Even though there are defects in the studies, the association holds strong. Some studies have relied on self-reported diagnosis of diabetes, and many patients with diabetes may remain undiagnosed especially the elderly people. For the same reason, the duration of diabetes is difficult to determine in older adults.[8]

In a community-based controlled study (Mayo Clinic Alzheimer Disease Patient Registry), the prevalence of glucose intolerance and diabetes was examined in patients with AD against control participants without AD. The study suggested that frank diabetes (35%) or glucose intolerance (46%) might be present in up to 80% of patients with AD.[5] In a longitudinal cohort study for a duration of 9 years, the risk of developing AD was 65% higher in persons with diabetes than in persons without diabetes.[9]

Even with the limitations discussed above, several studies have suggested that prevalence of diabetes is generally associated with a higher risk of developing dementia.[10,11] Cognitive deficits in T2DM mainly affects the areas of psychomotor efficiency, attention, learning and memory, mental flexibility and speed and executive function.[12,13] In random effects models, T2DM was associated with lower levels of global cognition, episodic, semantic and working memory, and visuospatial ability at baseline.[5]

Recently, studies have also shown a positive association between T2DM and mild cognitive impairment (MCI), and an accelerated progression from MCI to dementia in T2DM.[14]

PHYSIOPATHOLOGICAL LINK

The strong epidemiological association has suggested the existence of a physiopathological link. However, the contributing factors of the accelerated cognitive decline in T2DM are less clear. The most studied hypothesis proposes that the primary cause of the association may be linked to the inadequate cerebral circulation and diabetic vascular disease, with subsequent silent ischemic damage induced by diabetes. However, even after controlling the cardiovascular risk factors, several studies on the cerebral structure of patients with diabetes have evidence of increased cortical and subcortical atrophy and increased leukoaraiosis, which were associated with impaired cognitive performance.

The only way to diagnose AD with certainty is by postmortem demonstration of abundant neurofibrillary tangles and neurotic plaques with accompanying accumulation of amyloid precursor protein, amyloid beta (APP-Aβ) deposits in plaques and vessel walls in selected regions of the brain. Neuronal cytoskeletal collapse and accumulation of hyperphosphorylated and polyubiquitinated microtubule-associated proteins, such as tau, are the cause of dementia-associated structural lesions resulting in the formation of neurofibrillary tangles, dystrophic neuritis and neuropil threads.[15-17] Disconnection of synaptic circuitry and progressive loss of fibers and cell mediate the cerebral atrophy that worsens over time.

The molecular, biochemical and cellular abnormalities that precede or accompany AD neurodegeneration, including increased activation of pro-death genes and signaling pathways, mitochondrial dysfunction, impaired energy metabolism, chronic oxidative stress and DNA damage, are virtually stereotypical yet they lack a clear etiology.[18-20] For nearly three decades of intense research on AD, the inability to interlink this constellation of abnormalities under a single primary pathogenic mechanism resulted in the emergence and propagation of various profoundly debated theories, each of which focused on how one particular component of AD could trigger a cascade that contributes to the development of all other known abnormalities.

Most recent studies have focused on the possible role of insulin, and insulin action. Insulin resistance has been strongly implicated as a possible link between T2DM and AD. T2DM, the most common form, is caused by insulin resistance in peripheral tissues and is most frequently associated with aging, obesity, a family history of diabetes, and failure to exercise. Individuals with T2DM have hyperinsulinemia and hyperglycemia.

Insulin resistance in T2DM is partly mediated by reduced insulin receptor expression, insulin receptor tyrosine kinase activity, insulin receptor substrate (IRS) type 1 expression, and/or phosphatidylinositol-3 (PI3) kinase activation in skeletal muscle and adipocytes. A condition of hyperinsulinemia, regardless of the presence of T2DM, seems to be associated with a worse cognitive performance. There is a rapid growth in the literature pointing toward insulin resistance and insulin deficiency as mediators of AD-type neurodegeneration. De la Monte has even suggested that AD may be termed as "type 3 diabetes", indicating that AD may represent a form of diabetes that selectively involves the brain with molecular and biochemical features overlapping with DM.

Interest in clarifying the roles of T2DM, hyperinsulinemia, insulin resistance, and in relation to cognitive impairment, AD-associated neuronal cytoskeletal lesions, or APP-Aβ deposits in the brain began around 2000, but since around 2005, this field literally exploded with new information and a new concept, i.e. the primary brain insulin resistance and insulin deficiency mediate cognitive impairment and AD.[21] This idea was fueled by evidence that phosphorylation and *tau* gene expression are regulated through insulin and insulin-like growth factor (IGF) signaling cascades. In addition, research performed in our laboratory demonstrated that many key aspects of the central nervous system (CNS) degeneration that occur in AD can be effectuated by impaired insulin signaling.[22]

The importance of the role of insulin in brain aging has long been known. Insulin has significant neurotrophic properties in the brain. The hormone is rapidly transported to the level of the CNS through the blood-brain barrier by a transport mechanism mediated by insulin receptors. It is interesting to note that these receptors are mainly localized at the level of the entorhinal cortex, hippocampus, and frontal areas known to be involved in functions such as memory and learning. Insulin is also involved in the production of important neurotransmitters such as acetylcholine and norepinephrine. It is known that an acute increase in circulating levels of insulin, as it occurs in the postprandial period, determines a physiological parallel increase of the concentrations of the hormone in the brain. A state of chronic hyperinsulinemia, as it occurs in insulin-resistance conditions and in T2DM may determine a downregulation of the insulin receptors at the blood-brain barrier, thus reducing the transport of insulin in the brain.

Evidence is growing to link an alteration of metabolism and the deposition of precursors of amyloid in the brain that may occur in persons with diabetes, which is suggested as the pathogenesis of AD in T2DM. The amyloid precursor protein is a transmembrane protein consisting of 770 amino acids; it is known to be the precursor of the amyloid beta involved in the etiopathogenesis of AD. Although the role of amyloid beta and its isoforms has yet to be elucidated, it seems to take part in numerous physiological processes. How can clinical hyperinsulinemia be a risk factor for AD even though insulin is an important neurotrophic factor? These two apparent paradoxical findings may be resolved by the notion of insulin resistance. Whereas insulin is a neurotrophic factor at moderate concentrations, hyperinsulinemia with elevated concentrations of insulin in the brain may be associated with reduced amyloid-beta clearance due to competition for their common and main degrading mechanism—the "insulin-degrading enzyme" (IDE). Metabolism of amyloid precursor protein is modulated by insulin decreasing intracellular accumulation. Insulin is degraded by the IDE, which is also involved in the metabolism and degradation of amyloid beta. This multifunctional enzyme degrades insulin and amylin, peptides related to the pathology of T2DM, together with amyloid beta peptide in the AD brain. Through insulin's competition with amyloid beta for IDE, hyperinsulinemia may elevate amyloid beta.[19] Therefore, it has been suggested that the link between hyperinsulinemia and AD may be the IDE. Since IDE is much more selective for insulin than for amyloid beta, brain hyperinsulinemia may deprive amyloid beta of its main clearance mechanism, favoring its accumulation in the brain and its consequent neurotoxic effects.[23]

Disturbances in brain insulin signaling mechanisms represent early and progressive abnormalities and could account for the majority of biochemical, molecular and histopathological lesions in AD. Increasing insulin resistance and hyperinsulinemia were associated more with hippocampal and amygdaloid atrophy on magnetic resonance imaging (MRI) in persons with T2DM when compared to matched nondiabetic controls, regardless of vascular pathology. Given these links, it has been suggested that may be a common underlying mechanism predisposes to amyloid deposition in the brain and in the pancreatic islet.

Glucose levels itself are a risk factor for cognitive dysfunction and dementia. In a prospective, community-based cohort study, higher plasma glucose concentrations were associated with an increased risk of dementia in populations with and without diabetes, suggesting that higher levels of glucose may have deleterious effects on the aging brain.

Although there is still limited knowledge concerning the association between impaired fasting glucose and/or impaired glucose tolerance and cognitive impairment, there is increasing evidence that these prediabetic conditions may increase the risk of AD in elderly patients. The risk of incident dementia increased in diabetic and in nondiabetic persons according to the average glucose concentrations during the preceding 5 years. Hyperglycemia and hyperinsulinemia may accelerate brain aging also by inducing amyloid oligomerization and *tau* hyperphosphorylation, as well as by leading to widespread brain microangiopathy. Persons with diabetes are more prone to develop accelerated leukoaraiosis (white matter high-intensity lesions).[24,25]

GLYCEMIC CONTROL AND THE ROLE OF HYPOGLYCEMIA

The effect of diabetes treatment and glycemic control on dementia risk are not clear. It has been suggested that glycemic control may have a role in preserving cognitive performance among patients with T2DM. Using baseline cognitive measures collected in the Memory in Diabetes, substudy of the Action to Control Cardiovascular Risk in Diabetes trial, the authors found that a 1% higher glycated hemoglobin (HbA1c) value was associated with a significant lower test performance and memory score in patients with diabetes.[26]

The HbA1c was also identified as an additional risk factor for a greater rate of brain atrophy. Enzinger et al. measuring the annual brain volume changes over 6 years with MRI in 201 participants in the Austrian Stroke Prevention Study, found significant differences in brain atrophy rates by quartiles of HbA1c level. Clustering of factors associated with the so-called metabolic syndrome in persons with high HbA1c suggests a link between this syndrome, which is associated with insulin resistance and hyperinsulinemia, with late-life brain tissue loss. An inverse relationship was found, in diabetic patients, between serum HbA1c and working memory, executive functioning, learning, and complex psychomotor performance, supporting the hypothesis that an inadequate glucose control may be associated with deteriorating cognitive function.[27]

However, an excessively tight glycemic control in older persons with T2DM, and its related increased risk of hypoglycemia, may also have deleterious effects on cognitive function.[28] In the presence of hypoglycemia, several responses occur within the brain, including activation of the central sympathetic nervous system; hypoglycemic symptoms include alterations of cognitive function, such as difficulty in concentrating and drowsiness, among others. Recurrent symptomatic and asymptomatic hypoglycemic episodes have been suggested to cause permanent cognitive impairment and subclinical brain damage. In addition, hypoglycemic states may increase the action of the receptors through an arteriolar vasodilatation. Since chronic hyperglycemia in T2DM is associated with endothelial alterations, this may cause in case of hypoglycemia, a reduced vasodilation effect at the level of the blood-brain barrier, with a possible amplification of the brain damage due to hypoglycemia itself.

Older patients with type 2 diabetes with a history of severe hypoglycemic episodes collected and reviewed using hospital discharge and emergency department diagnoses from 1980 to 2002 were associated with a greater risk of dementia.[29] More recently, a 12 years prospective population-based study of 783 older adults who were participating in the Health, Aging and Body Composition Study, found a bidirectional association between hypoglycemia and dementia. During the 12-year follow-up period, the participants who experienced at least one hypoglycemic event had a 2-fold increased risk for developing dementia, while older adults with T2DM who developed dementia had a greater risk for having a subsequent hypoglycemic event compared with participants who did not develop dementia.[30]

Therefore, it has been suggested that drugs that cause lower postprandial glucose excursions and minor risk of hypoglycemia may prevent cognitive decline in older diabetic persons. This data needs to be confirmed by future trials.

RESEARCH AND CLINICAL IMPLICATIONS

Cognitive function has not been included as an outcome in large-scale randomized controlled trials of type 2 diabetes, and screening for dementia and cognitive impairment is still not included in routine diabetic patient care. There are sufficient epidemiological and clinical data to include an evaluation of cognitive complications in the clinical practice of persons with diabetes, in particular in those older than 70–75 years, and those with a long-lasting history of diabetes.

There are some barriers in implementing a screening and diagnostic program for dementia in patients with diabetes. Neurocognitive testing in which an expert examiner administers a battery of tests to assess different aspects of cerebral function is still the gold standard for the diagnosis of dementia, and a computed tomography (CT) scan or an MRI may be required. This evaluation requires substantial financial and human resources. CT scans are expensive and screening cognitive tests are time consuming. However, diagnosis is even more important in older populations, because many older persons with diabetes nowadays live alone and self-manage their drugs. A mistake due to cognitive impairment may be extremely dangerous in particular in patients who need insulin, and self-practice insulin injections. Many hypoglycemic episodes may be due to errors in self-administration in undiagnosed subclinical demented patients.

CONCLUSION

There is convincing epidemiological evidence showing an increased risk of dementia in people with diabetes, but there are few mechanistic studies that provide a clear pathophysiological link too, although the cause may be multifactorial. Cerebrovascular alterations, insulin resistance, insulin action, altered amyloid metabolism, chronic hyperglycemia and recurrent hypoglycemic episodes seem to play a major role. Future trials are required to clarify the mechanistic link and to address the question whether cognitive decline may be prevented by an adequate metabolic control, and to better define the role of drugs that may cause hypoglycemic episodes. Clinicians treating older persons with diabetes should start to routinely search for cognitive impairment as well as search for cardiovascular, renal or other common complications of diabetic disease. There is sufficient evidence to support the view that time has probably arrived to incorporate cognitive evaluation in future national and international diabetic guidelines.

REFERENCES

1. Centres for Disease Control and Prevention. Estimates of diabetes and its burden in the United States. National Diabetes Statistics Report. Atlanta, GA: US Department of Health and Human Services; 2014.
2. Kukull WA, Higdon R, Bowen JD, et al. Dementia and Alzheimer disease incidence: a prospective cohort study. Arch Neurol. 2002;59:1737-46.
3. Llorente MD, Urrutia V. Diabetes, psychiatric disorders, and the metabolic effects of antipsychotic medications. Clin Diabetes. 2006;24:18-24.
4. Leibson CL, Rocca WA, Hanson VA, et al. Risk of dementia among persons with diabetes mellitus: a population-based cohort study. Am J Epidemiol. 1997;145:301-8.
5. Janson J, Laedtke T, Parisi JE, et al. Increased risk of type 2 diabetes in Alzheimer disease. Diabetes. 2004;53:474-81.
6. Biessels GJ, Kappalle LJ. Increased risk of Alzheimer's disease in Type II diabetes: insulin resistance of the brain or insulin-induced amyloid pathology? Biochem Soc Trans. 2005;33:101-4.
7. Biessels GJ, Staekenborg S, Brunner E, et al. Risk of dementia in diabetes mellitus: a systematic review. Lancet Neurol. 2006;5:64-74.

8. Allen KV, Frier BM, Strachan MW. The relationship between type 2 diabetes and cognitive dysfunction: longitudinal studies and their methodological limitations. Eur J Pharmacol. 2004;490:169-75.
9. Arvanitakis Z, Wilson RS, Bienias JL, et al. Diabetes mellitus and risk of Alzheimer disease and decline in cognitive function. Arch Neurol. 2004;61:661-6.
10. Bruce DG, Davis WA, Casey GP, et al. Predictors of cognitive decline in older individuals with diabetes. Diabetes Care. 2008;31:2103-7.
11. Bruce DG, Davis WA, Casey GP, et al. Predictors of cognitive impairment and dementia in older people with diabetes. Diabetologia. 2008;51: 241-8.
12. Convit A. Links between cognitive impairment in insulin resistance: an explanatory model. Neurobiol Aging. 2005;26(Suppl 1):31-5.
13. Kodl CT, Seaquist ER. Cognitive dysfunction and diabetes mellitus. Endocr Rev. 2008;29:494-511.
14. Alagiakrishnan K, Sclater A. Psychiatric disorders presenting in the elderly with type 2 diabetes mellitus. Am J Geriatr Psychiatry. 2012;20:645-52.
15. Jalbert JJ, Daiello LA, Lapane KL. Dementia of the Alzheimer type. Epidemiol Rev. 2008;30:15-34.
16. Jellinger KA. Neuropathological aspects of Alzheimer disease, Parkinson disease and frontotemporal dementia. Neurodegener Dis. 2008;5(3-4): 118-21.
17. Wang XP, Ding HL. Alzheimer's disease: epidemiology, genetics, and beyond. Neurosci Bull. 2008;24(2):105-9.
18. Steen E, Terry BM, Rivera EJ, et al. Impaired insulin and insulin-like growth factor expression and signaling mechanisms in Alzheimer's disease—is this type 3 diabetes? J Alzheimers Dis. 2005;7(1):63-80.
19. de la Monte SM, Wands JR. Molecular indices of oxidative stress and mitochondrial dysfunction occur early and often progress with severity of Alzheimer's disease. J Alzheimers Dis. 2006;9(2):167-81.
20. Moreira PI, Santos MS, Seiça R, et al. Brain mitochondrial dysfunction as a link between Alzheimer's disease and diabetes. J Neurol Sci. 2007;257(1-2):206-14.
21. Craft S. Insulin resistance and cognitive impairment: a view through the prism of epidemiology. Arch Neurol. 2005;62(7):1043-4.
22. Schubert M, Gautam D, Surjo D, et al. Role for neuronal insulin resistance in neurodegenerative diseases. Proc Natl Acad Sci USA. 2004;101(9):3100-5.
23. Qiu WQ, Folstein MF. Insulin, insulin-degrading enzyme and amyloid-beta peptide in Alzheimer's disease: review and hypothesis. Neurobiol Aging. 2006;27:190-8. [PMID: 16399206 DOI: 10.1016/j.neurobiolaging. 2005.01.004].
24. Crane PK, Walker R, Hubbard RA, et al. Glucose levels and risk of dementia. N Engl J Med. 2013;369:540-8.
25. S Roriz-Filho J, Sá-Roriz TM, Rosset I, et al. (Pre)diabetes, brain aging, and cognition. Biochem Biophys Acta. 2009;1792:432-43.
26. Cukierman-Yaffe T, Gerstein HC, Williamson JD, et al. Relationship between baseline glycemic control and cognitive function in individuals with type 2 diabetes and other cardiovascular risk factors: the action to control cardiovascular risk in diabetes-memory in diabetes (ACCORD-MIND) trial. Diabetes Care. 2009;32(2):221-6.
27. Enzinger C, Fazekas F, Matthews PM, et al. Risk factors for progression of brain atrophy in aging: six-year follow-up of normal subjects. Neurology. 2005;64:1704-11.
28. Warren RE, Frier BM. Hypoglycaemia and cognitive function. Diabetes Obes Metab. 2005;7:493-503.
29. Whitmer RA, Karter AJ, Yaffe K, et al. Hypoglycemic episodes and risk of dementia in older patients with type 2 diabetes mellitus. JAMA. 2009;301:1565-72.
30. Yaffe K, Falvey CM, Hamilton N, et al. Association between hypoglycemia and dementia in a biracial cohort of older adults with diabetes mellitus. JAMA Intern Med. 2013;173:1300-6.

Chapter 63

Cognitive Disorder in Diabetes: Effect of Hypoglycemia and Hyperglycemia

Man Mohan Mehndiratta, Shahla Shafique, Abhijit Das

INTRODUCTION

Diabetes mellitus is a complex metabolic disease that can have devastating effects on multiple organs in the body. The long-term complications of diabetes mellitus on the retinal, renal, cardiovascular and peripheral nervous systems are widely known. Less attention has given to the effect of diabetes on the cognitive system. Apart from the well known major complications of diabetes, cognitive dysfunction is one of the least acknowledged and lesser recognized complications of diabetes. Both type 1 diabetes mellitus (T1DM) and type 2 diabetes mellitus (T2DM) have found to have multiple cognitive deficits that can be attributed to the disease. Cognitive dysfunction in diabetes can be the result of both hyperglycemia and hypoglycemia and many patients fear that recurrent hypoglycemia will impair their memory over time. Despite so much of extensive research, the pathophysiology underlying this complication is not completely understood and the most appropriate methods that can diagnose, treat and prevent cognitive dysfunction in diabetes have not yet been fully defined.

COGNITIVE DISORDERS—DEFINITION

Cognitive disorders are considered mental health disorders that primarily affect learning, memory, perception and problem solving, which include amnesia, dementia and delirium. It significantly impairs the cognitive function of an individual to the point where its normal functioning is impossible within a society without treatment.[1]

CLASSIFICATION

Mild and Major Neurocognitive Disorders

Mild and major neurocognitive disorders are differentiated based on the severity of their symptoms. Previously known as dementia, major neurocognitive disorder is characterized by significant cognitive decline and interference with independence, while mild neurocognitive disorder is characterized by moderate cognitive decline and does not interfere with independence. When severe acquired cognitive impairment compromises social and/or occupational functioning, it typically signifies dementia. On the other hand, mild cognitive impairment (MCI) is characterized by a state in between normal cognition and dementia, when the functional abilities are essentially preserved.

The previous edition of American Psychiatric Association's, Diagnostic and Statistical Manual of Mental Disorders (DSM-IV) included a section entitled "Delirium, Dementia and Amnestic and Other Cognitive Disorders", which was revised in the (DSM-V) (Table 1) to the broader "neurocognitive disorders". Neurocognitive disorders are described as those with "a significant impairment of cognition or memory that represents a marked deterioration from a previous level of function". Briefly, the DSM-V diagnosis of major neurocognitive

TABLE 1: Neurocognitive disorders as diagnosed in DSM-V.[1]

Diagnostic criteria	Major neurocognitive disorder/dementia	Minor Neurocognitive Disorder/Dementia
A	Significant cognitive decline in one or more cognitive domains, based on:	Modest cognitive decline in one or more cognitive domains, based on:
	• Concern about significant decline, expressed by individual or reliable informant, or observed by clinician	• Concern about mild decline, expressed by individual or reliable informant, or observed by clinician
	• Substantial impairment, documented by objective cognitive assessment	• Modest impairment, documented by objective cognitive assessment
B	Interference with independence in everyday activities	No interference with independence in everyday activities, although these activities may require more time and effort, accommodation or compensatory strategies
C	Not exclusively during delirium	
D	Not better explained by another mental disorder	
E	Specify one or more etiologic subtypes, "due to": • Alzheimer's disease • Frontotemporal lobar degeneration (frontotemporal neurocognitive disorder) • Dementia with Lewy bodies (neurocognitive disorder with Lewy bodies) • Cerebrovascular disease (vascular neurocognitive disorder) • Traumatic brain injury • Parkinson's disease • Huntington's disease • HIV Infection • Prion disease • Multiple etiologies • Another medical condition	

(HIV: human immunodeficiency virus.)

disorder, which corresponds to dementia, requires substantial impairment to be present in one or (usually) more cognitive domains.[1]

PATHOPHYSIOLOGY OF COGNITIVE DYSFUNCTION IN DIABETES

The exact etiopathology of cognitive dysfunction in patients with diabetes has not been fully understood. Many hypotheses have been postulated along with various supportive evidences. Causative factors implicated in the pathogenesis are—role of hyperglycemia and hypoglycemia, insulin resistance, amyloid deposition and vascular damage (Flowchart 1).[1]

Type 1 Diabetes Mellitus

Patients with type 1 diabetes mellitus have found to have multiple cognitive impairments (Box 1).[1] Cognitive dysfunction in patients with diabetes mellitus first came to limelight in 1922. It was noticed that, on performing cognitive function tests on these subjects they were found to have impaired memory and attention as compared to the control subjects. Hence, these subjects were "free from acidosis but usually not sugar free".[3] Patients with diabetes mellitus tend to show early onset of cognitive impairment. Deficits in cognitive function have been detected as early as 2 years after diagnosis in children with type 1 diabetes. The age of onset of type 1 diabetes may also contribute to the presence of cognitive dysfunction, because those who developed type 1 diabetes at less than 4 years of age had severely impaired executive skills, attention and processing speed when compared with those that were diagnosed after 4 years of age.[4]

Type 2 Diabetes Mellitus

Many studies have shown that T2DM is a risk factor for cognitive dysfunction and dementia in the elderly population. With the increase in the number of elderly individuals with T2DM, the number of diabetic patients with cognitive dysfunction also tends to increase.

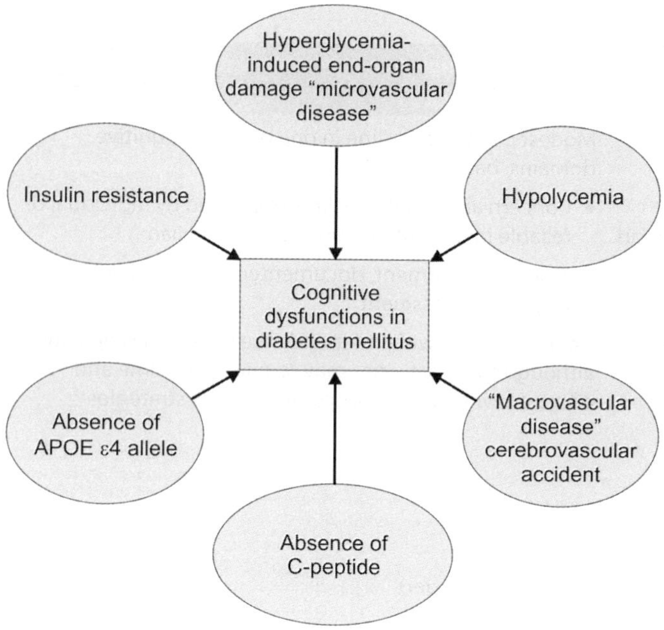

(APOE: apolipoprotein E.)

Flowchart 1 Pathophysiology of cognitive dysfunction in diabetes mellitus.[1]

Patients with T2DM suffer from multiple cognitive impairments as enlisted (Box 2).[1] It has been found that patients with type 2 diabetes have an increased risk of developing depressive symptoms as compared to nondiabetic persons. Clinically, relevant depressive symptoms were found to be present in only a small portion of population suffering from diabetes. Although, it has been found out that depressive symptoms can affect cognitive performance, and might have a role to play in the etiology of diabetes-associated cognitive decrements.[5] But the exact nature of the relation between development of depression and type 2 diabetes is not completely understood. Studies reveal that disturbance in the levels of cerebral neurotransmitter due to metabolic consequence of type 2 diabetes could be the possible etiology leading to depression. Depression can also be the result from difficulties in coping with chronic disease.[6] In addition, vascular damage in the brain can also lead to depression.[7,8] It is important to consider that, the relation between diabetes and depression may be bidirectional (Flowchart 2), as depression can predispose to development of type 2 diabetes and vice versa.[9] Therefore, it is very unlikely to say that depression would be the sole explanation for the association between cognitive dysfunction and diabetes mellitus.

Box 1: Summary of cognitive domains that have been found to be negatively affected by type 1 diabetes mellitus.[1]

- Slowing of information processing*
- Psychomotor efficiency*
- Problem solving
- Learning
- Attention*
- Memory
- Motor speed
- Visuoconstruction*
- Visual perception
- Vocabulary
- General intelligence
- Executive function
- Mental flexibility*
- Somatosensory examination
- Motor strength

Domains marked by asterisks have particularly strong supporting data.

Box 2: Summary of cognitive domains that have been found to be negatively affected by type 2 diabetes mellitus.

- Memory*
  - Verbal memory
  - Working memory
  - Visual retention
  - Immediate recall
  - Delayed recall
- Executive function*
- Psychomotor speed*
- Processing speed
- Verbal fluency
- Complex motor function
- Depression
- Attention

Domains marked by asterisks have particularly strong supporting data.

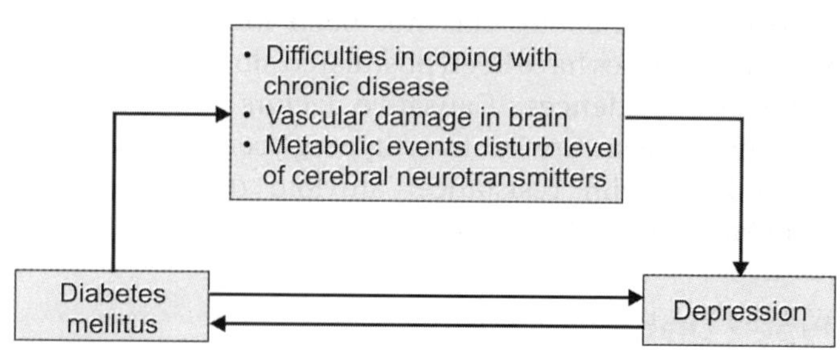

Flowchart 2 Bidirectional relation between diabetes mellitus and depression.

COGNITIVE DYSFUNCTION IN PATIENTS OF DIABETES

Effect of Hyperglycemia

The acute and chronic effects of hyperglycemia affecting our cognitive function are as important as that due to hypoglycemia. In majority of the cases, it has been observed that patients with diabetes fail to achieve the desired therapeutic targets, which is potentially significant. Recognizing the risk factors, self monitoring of blood glucose and management interventions should target not only toward avoidance of any disability due to hypoglycemia but, also toward any unwanted hyperglycemia. There is always a potential risk of development of dementia over a long-term due to hyperglycemia. Acute episodes of hyperglycemia, above 15 mmol/L have shown to affect cognitive motor tasks. Evidence suggests that optimization the blood glucose levels in the middle-aged diabetic can attenuate or possibly revert some of the cognitive deficits found to be associated with hyperglycemia and insulin resistance. Various tests have been developed and validated for recognizing different domains of cognitive functioning, such as verbal and nonverbal memory, executive function, processing speed and mental state. Processing speed, verbal memory, and visuospatial performance are found to be more affected than other domains in patients suffering from diabetes mellitus.[10]

In general, the etiology of cognitive dysfunction in the aging population is likely to be a combination of ischemic and degenerative pathology. In vascular dementia (VD), small vessel disease exacerbated by diabetes affects cognitive function. It is also believed that insulin regulates neurons in the central nervous system and affects amyloid β-metabolism, in addition to many other effects, which accelerates Alzheimer-related pathology.[11] Recent studies have indicated that older people with T2DM have a higher risk of cognitive dysfunction or dementia.[12] Ample evidence has indicated that T2DM is related not only to VD but also to the clinical diagnosis of Alzheimer's disease (AD—type dementia.[13]

Acute hyperglycemia is not a benign event for many individuals with diabetes, but it is associated with mild cognitive dysfunction. Patients with diabetes often report acute and transient cognitive disruptions associated with hyperglycemia. Such effects could influence quality of life and daily functioning, as well as helps patients in better recognizing the presence of hyperglycemia. However, diabetes alone cannot be held responsible for the cognitive decline. Hyperglycemia may also lead to acute changes in cognitive functioning. Patients with type 1 and 2 diabetes showed acute psychomotor slowing and an increase in the amount of errors over a 4-week period as soon as blood glucose levels increased above 15 mmol/L.[14] Mild cognitive decrements in patients with type 2 diabetes have been associated with longer diabetes duration and elevated glycated hemoglobin (HbA1c) levels.[15]

Research suggests that blood-brain barrier microvascular dysfunction may occur as a result of transient hyperglycemia.[16] Altered synthesis or reuptake of monoamine neurotransmitters as a result of altered availability of precursor to the brain or changes in insulin availability to the brain are other possible explanations.[17] Complex effects on peptide neurotransmitters may be produced by uncontrolled diabetes.[18]

Genetic predisposition may play a role in the association between type 2 diabetes, cognitive decrements and dementia. The most widely examined risk factor is the apolipoprotein E (APOE) ε4 allele, an important risk factor for cardiovascular disease and late-onset AD. Several studies have shown interaction effects between type 2 diabetes and the APOE ε4 allele, further increasing the diabetes-associated risk of cognitive decline and cognitive impairment or dementia.[19]

Effect of Hypoglycemia

It is well proven fact that the human brain depends on glucose as its energy source. The most common side effect of glucose-lowering therapy is hypoglycemic, which is proven to have deleterious effects on the brain. Recurrent episode of acute hypoglycemia results in neuroglycopenia leading to cognitive impairment in future. According to various studies, it has been observed that individuals with type 1 diabetes are exposed to an average of two episodes of self-treated hypoglycemia per week. It has been observed that cognitive function rapidly deteriorates when blood glucose falls below 3.0 mmol/L (54 mg/dL) and improves again after restoration of blood glucose levels.[20] Memory, attention, information processing, psychomotor function and spatial ability are the most common cognitive domain affected by hypoglycemic episode. There are numerous case reports of hypoglycemia-induced brain damage and cognitive deterioration attributed to repeated severe hypoglycemia. As per the study done by Deary IJ, it was found that patient with T2DM showed rapid cognitive decline after a hypoglycemic episode. It also emphasized that people suffering from dementia were at increased risk of severe hypoglycemic episodes in future over the subsequent 5 years.[21]

Bidirectional relationship has been found between dementia and the risk of hypoglycemia. The impact on cognitive dysfunction due to hypoglycemia has found to be more critical in the older population. As per a prospective population-based study, it was found that there was twofold higher risk of developing dementia in patients after any hypoglycemic episode.[22] On the other hand, patients with dementia had a three times higher risk of developing hypoglycemic episode in future. It has been observed that there is a strong association between cognitive dysfunction and the risk of hypoglycemia in patients with both T1DM and T2DM.[23]

CONCLUSION

There has been a marked gain in our understanding of the effect of diabetes on cognitive dysfunction. Evidence from various studies conducted on neurocognitive disorders signifies that cognitive dysfunction should also be enlisted as one of the major complications of diabetes, along with retinopathy, nephropathy, neuropathy and cardiovascular disease. The pathogenesis of cognitive dysfunction in diabetes is still under evolution and much need to be done before arriving at a final conclusion. Although, according to many studies the major culprits that lead to changes in the cerebral structure and function in diabetes are due to hyperglycemia-induced end organ damage, role of hypoglycemia, insulin resistance, amyloid lesions and macrovascular diseases. More studies should be undertaken in upcoming days for better understanding the natural history of diabetes and its related complications and the mechanisms responsible for its development. Hopefully advancement of newer knowledge can be applied to develop new and improved ways to prevent and treat all the diabetes related cognitive disorders in near future.

REFERENCES

1. American Psychiatric Association. Diagnostic and Statistical Manual of Mental Disorders. Fifth Edition. Arlington, VA: American Psychiatric Association; 2013.
2. Kodl CT, Seaquist ER. Cognitive Dysfunction and Diabetes Mellitus: Endocrinology and Diabetes. Endocr Rev. 2008;29(4):494-511.
3. Chan RCK, Chen EYH. Assessment of executive functions for schizophrenia in Hong Kong. Hong Kong J Psychiatry. 2005;15:23–8.
4. Northam EA, Anderson PJ, Jacobs R, et al. Neuropsychological profiles of children with type 1 diabetes 6 years after disease onset. Diabetes Care. 2001;24:1541-6.
5. Krabbe KS, Nielsen AR, Krogh-Madsen R, et al. Brain-derived neurotrophic factor (BDNF) and type 2 diabetes. Diabetologia. 2007;50:431-8.
6. Baldwin RC, O'Brien J. Vascular basis of late-onset depressive disorder. Br J Psychiatry. 2002;180:157-160.
7. Bruce DG, Casey G, Davis WA, et al. Vascular depression in older people with diabetes. Diabetologia. 2006;49:2828-36.
8. Knol MJ, Twisk JWR, Beekman ATF, et al. Depression as a risk factor for the onset of type 2 diabetes mellitus. A meta-analysis. Diabetologia. 2006;49:837-45.
9. Anderson RJ, Freedland KE, Clouse RE, et al. The prevalence of comorbid depression in adults with diabetes: a meta-analysis. Diabetes Care. 2001;24:1069-78.
10. Cox DJ, Kovatchev BP, Gonder-Frederick LA, et al. Relationship between hyperglycemia and cognitive performance among adults with type 1 and type 2 diabetes. Diabetes Care. 2005;28(1):71-7.
11. Masters CL, Multhaup G, Simms G, et al. Neuronal origin of a cerebral amyloid: neurofibrillary tangles of Alzheimer's disease contain the same protein as the amyloid of plaque cores and blood vessels. EMBO J. 1985;4:2757-63.
12. Stewart R, Liolitsa D. Type 2 diabetes mellitus, cognitive impairment and dementia. Diabet Med. 1999;16(2):93-112.
13. Li L, Hölscher C. Common pathological processes in Alzheimer disease and type 2 diabetes: a review. Brain Res Rev. 2007;56(2):384-402.
14. Cox DJ, Kovatchev BP, Gonder-Frederick LA, et al. Relationships between hyperglycemia and cognitive performance among adults with type 1 and type 2 diabetes. Diabetes Care. 2005;28:71-77.
15. Manschot SM, Brands AM, van der Grond J, et al. Brain magnetic resonance imaging correlates of impaired cognition in patients with type 2 diabetes. Diabetes. 2006;55:1106-13.
16. Mooradian A. Central nervous system complications of diabetes mellitus: a perspective from the blood-brain barrier. Brain Res Brain Res Rev.1997;23:210-8.
17. Wurtman RJ. Effects of their nutrient precursors on the synthesis and release of serotonin, the catecholamines, and acetylcholine: implications for behavioral disorders. Clin Neuropharmacol. 1998;11 (Suppl. 1):S187-93.
18. Sipols AJ, Baskin DG, Schwartz MW. Effect of intracerebroventricular insulin infusion on diabetic hyperphagia and hypothalamic neuropeptide gene expression. Diabetes. 1995;44:147-51.
19. Dore GA, Elias MF, Robbins MA, et al. Presence of the APOE epsilon4 allele modifies the relationship between type 2 diabetes and cognitive performance: The Maine-Syracuse Study. Diabetologia. 2009;52:2551-60.
20. Peila R, Rodriguez BL, Launer LJ. Type 2 diabetes, APOE gene, and the risk for dementia and related pathologies: The Honolulu-Asia Aging Study. Diabetes. 2002;51:1256-62.
21. Deary IJ. Symptoms of hypoglycaemia and effects on mental performance and emotions. In: Frier BM, Fisher M (Eds). Hypoglycaemia in Clinical Diabetes, 2nd edition. Chichester: John Wiley & Sons;, 2007. p. 25.
22. Bruce DG, Davis WA, Casey GP, et al. Severe hypoglycaemia and cognitive impairment in older patients with diabetes: The Fremantle Diabetes Study. Diabetologia. 2009;52:1808-15.
23. Yaffe K, Falvey CM, Hamilton N, et al. Health ABC Study. Association between hypoglycemia and dementia in a biracial cohort of older adults with diabetes mellitus. JAMA Intern Med. 2013;173:1300-6.

Chapter 64

Can Integument be a Curtain Raiser of Poor Glycemic Control?

Rajesh Dutt Mehta, Aastha Chawla

INTRODUCTION

Bulgarian dermatologist Krum Balabanov's sayings in Latin goes as "*Dermatologia mater medicinae est*";[1] the English translation of which may be quoted, "Specialty of dermatology statures as mother of medical science or medicine". Is it the megalomanic gesture by a dermatology expert for his own specialty or the evidence-based medicine which affirms and reaffirms that cutaneous changes reflect the mirror image of milieu interior? It holds absolutely true for diabetes mellitus, where glycemic levels can be predicted and titrated by dermatological signs and symptom complex.

The clinical findings may be categorized as follows:

- Predictive indicators
- Affirmative indicators.

Mehta and Chawla's dermatological criteria for diabetes[2] are described in Boxes 1 and 2.

Cutaneous markers of diabetes may be grouped as shown in Box 3.

Flowchart 1 shows the etiopathogenesis of cutaneous markers of Diabetes.

Box 1: Predictive indicators.

- Candidal balanoposthitis
- Diffuse alopecia
- Extensive dermatophytosis
- Fulminant herpes zoster
- Recurrent bacterial infections

Box 2: Affirmative indicators.

- Acanthosis nigricans
- Acquired perforating dermatoses
- Diabetic dermopathy
- Diabetic foot
- Scleredema

Box 3: Cutaneous markers of diabetes mellitus,

- Cutaneous manifestations of diabetes mellitus
- Cutaneous concurrences of diabetes mellitus
- Diabetes association with dermatological pathologies
- Diabetic therapy causing cutaneous complication

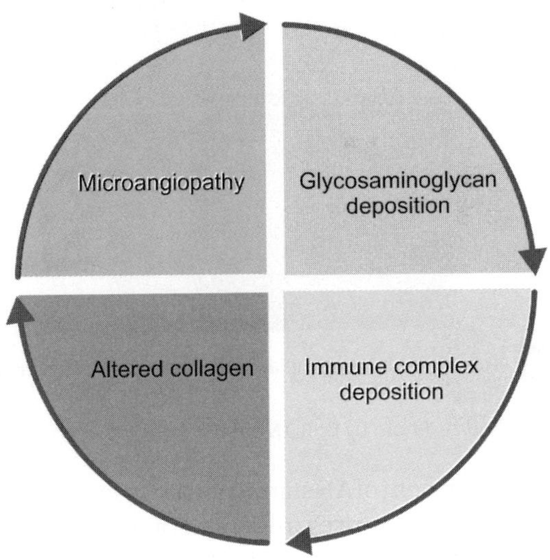

Flowchart 1 Etiopathogenesis of cutaneous markers.

CUTANEOUS MANIFESTATIONS OF DIABETES MELLITUS

- *Acanthosis nigricans*: Clinical presentation of acanthosis nigricans (AN) is a velvety or verrucous plaque or patch of dark brown or black color. The sites of predilection are the intertriginous or the flexural surfaces of body (Figs. 1 and 2).[3]

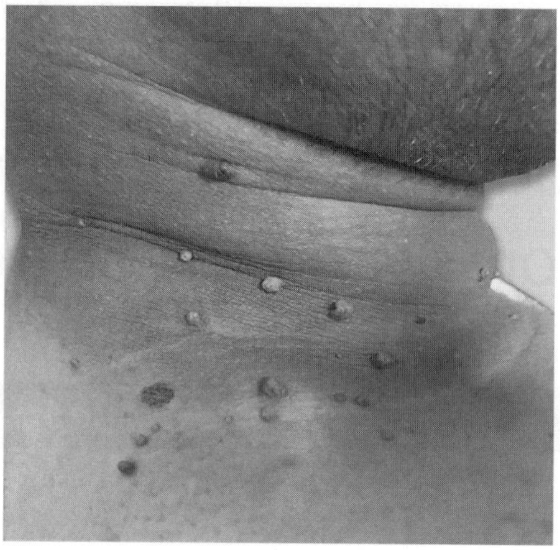

Figure 1 Acrochordons with acanthosis nigricans. ***(For color version, see Plate 4)***
Source: Photo by Dr RD Mehta.

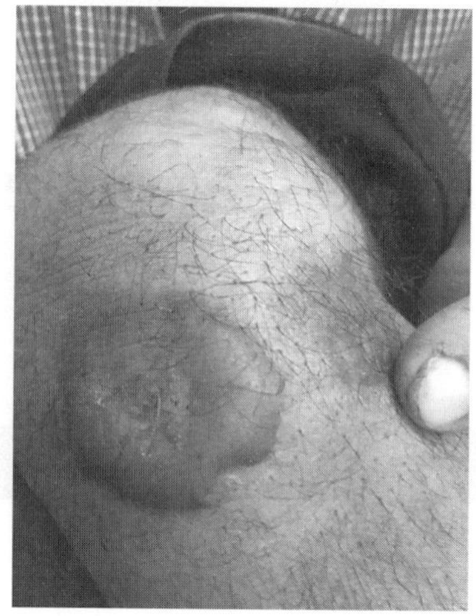

Figure 3 Bullosis diabeticorum over the extensor surface of the knee. ***(For color version, see Plate 4)***
Source: Photo by Dr RD Mehta.

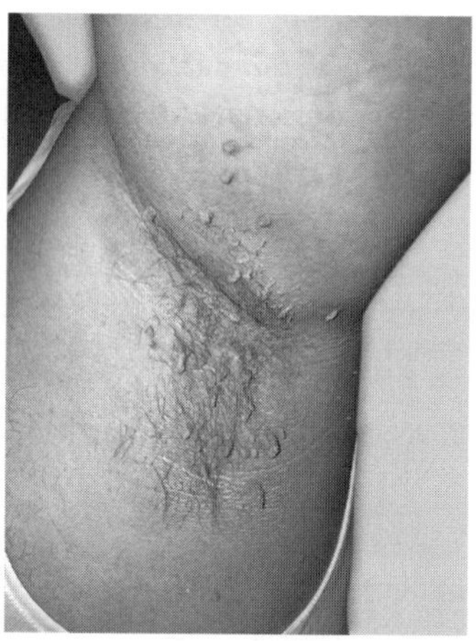

Figure 2 Acrochordons in the axillary fold. ***(For color version, see Plate 4)***
Source: Photo by Dr RD Mehta.

Management of AN starts with lifestyle modification. Second step comprises treatment of insulin resistance and optimization of glycemic control.

Dermatological therapy includes application of keratolytic agents, e.g. salicylic acid, tretinoin and potent steroids with ammonium lactate

- *Acquired perforating dermatoses*: Clinical presentation of acquired perforating dermatoses (APD) includes perifollicular dome-shaped papulonodular lesions with central darker keratin plugs. These lesions may be seen on legs, trunk or head. Severe pruritus may lead to excoriation and koebnerization (appearance of newer lesions over traumatized sites).

  Management includes topical retinoids, potent corticosteroids (clobetasol/halobetasol), intralesional corticosteroid triamcinolone, psoralen and ultraviolet A (PUVA) therapy and cryotherapy. Systemic retinoids, oral corticosteroids and allopurinol have been used successfully
- *Bullosis diabeticorum*: Clinical presentation is painless, including noninflamed blisters on normal looking skin with sterile contents. These are mainly on the limbs (Fig. 3), but sometimes trunk may get involved.[4]

  Management of bullosis diabeticorum includes sterile drainage and topical antibiotics
- *Diabetic dermopathy*: Clinical presentation of diabetic dermopathy is asymptomatic pretibial macules,[5] scaly papulo-plaques of red/brown color; these are also named as "shin spots" or "pigmented pretibial patches"(Fig. 4).

  Management of diabetic dermopathy is to prevent the superadded bacterial infection; it is otherwise a self-limiting condition where the lesions heal with hyperpigmentation and atrophy
- *Diabetic foot*: Clinical presentation of diabetic foot and ankle shows thick callus over trauma-prone bony areas with repeated injuries causing ulceration. Consequently, microbial infection of ulcerated lesions may culminate into gangrene warranting amputation.

  Management of diabetic foot is based on avoidance of triggering factors. Wound debridement, offloading prosthesis (contact cast), use of healing promoters,

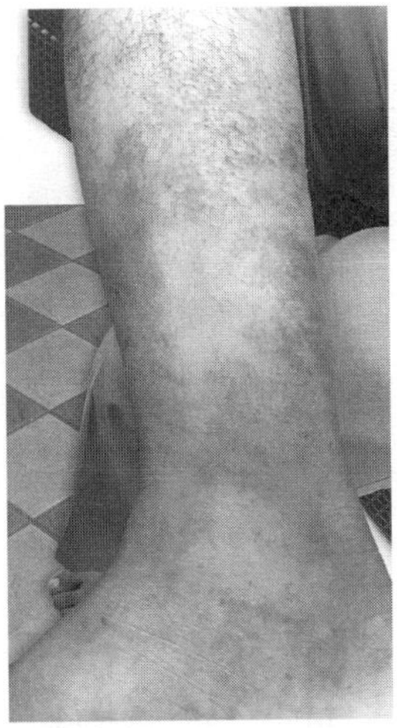

Figure 4 Diabetic dermopathy. ***(For color version, see Plate 4)***
Source: Photo by Dr Aastha Chawla.

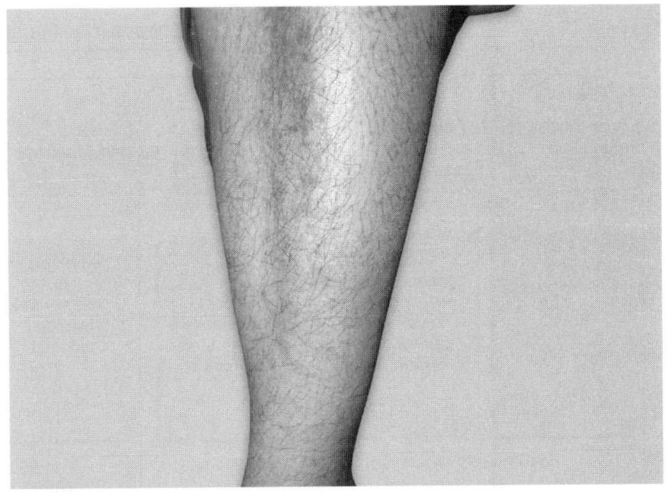

Figure 5 Evoluting necrobiosis lipoidica diabeticorum over the shin. ***(For color version, see Plate 4)***
Source: Photo by Dr RD Mehta.

surgical revascularization methods, applicable growth factors, bioengineered skin grafts and oral antibiotics for bacterial secondary infection are the pillars of managing indolent diabetic ulcer.[6]

Wound-healing agents in practice are saline dressings, silver salts, calcium alginate in various formulations, i.e. hydrogel, hydrocolloids, impregnated gauze pieces, and even hyperbaric oxygen are found to be beneficial.

- *Eruptive xanthomas*: Clinically, eruptive xanthomas (EX) present as yellowish red papules observed over extensors and buttocks. The lesions are pruritic, tender and tend to happen at trauma-prone sites.

  Management revolves around glycemic control and controlling hypertriglyceridemia. Statin and fibrate therapy helps to improve the xanthomatosis
- *Necrobiosis lipoidica diabeticorum*: Clinical presentation of this necrotizing granulomatous dermatological condition is yellowish brown, usually bilaterally symmetrical painless plaques with ulceration. The area is demarcated with erythematous borders, often over pretibial area (Fig. 5).[7]

  Management requires topical corticosteroids and tacrolimus. Oral systemic therapy with pentoxifylline, low-dose aspirin, immunomodulators and biologics promote the healing process. Compression therapy and phototherapy are also used as adjuvants
- *Scleredema diabeticorum*: Clinical presentation of scleredema diabeticorum (SD) is diffuse asymptomatic symmetrical nonpitting erythematous lesion over neck, shoulder and interscapular area.[8]

  Management of scleredema includes ultraviolet A1, PUVA therapy and physiotherapy. The severe variants may require intravenous immunoglobulin therapy
- *Sclerodermatoid changes*: Clinical presentation includes thickened, waxy, indurated painless areas of skin. Most commonly proximal interphalangeal (IP) and metacarpophalangeal (MCP) joints show bilaterally symmetrical involvement. It does have distinguishable absence of pain, telangiectasias, atrophic changes, edematous feel and Raynaud's phenomenon.[9]

  Diabetic hand syndrome with "prayer's sign" refers to decreased ROM (range of movements) of IP and MCP joints and incomplete extension of fingers. It leads to inability to press the palmar surfaces in opposition to each other, resulting in a gap between hands. Dupuytren's contracture could be an additional sclerodermatoid diabetic change.

  Management in the form of physiotherapy may improve the restricted joint mobility. Amongst pharmacotherapeutic agents, aldose reductase inhibitor has shown good result.

  Cutaneous manifestations are summarized in (Flowchart 2).

CUTANEOUS FINDINGS OF DIABETES MELLITUS

- *Acquired ichthyosiform changes*:
  - Clinically, skin of tibia shows dry, fish-like scales. In most of the cases, condition is bilaterally symmetrical[10]

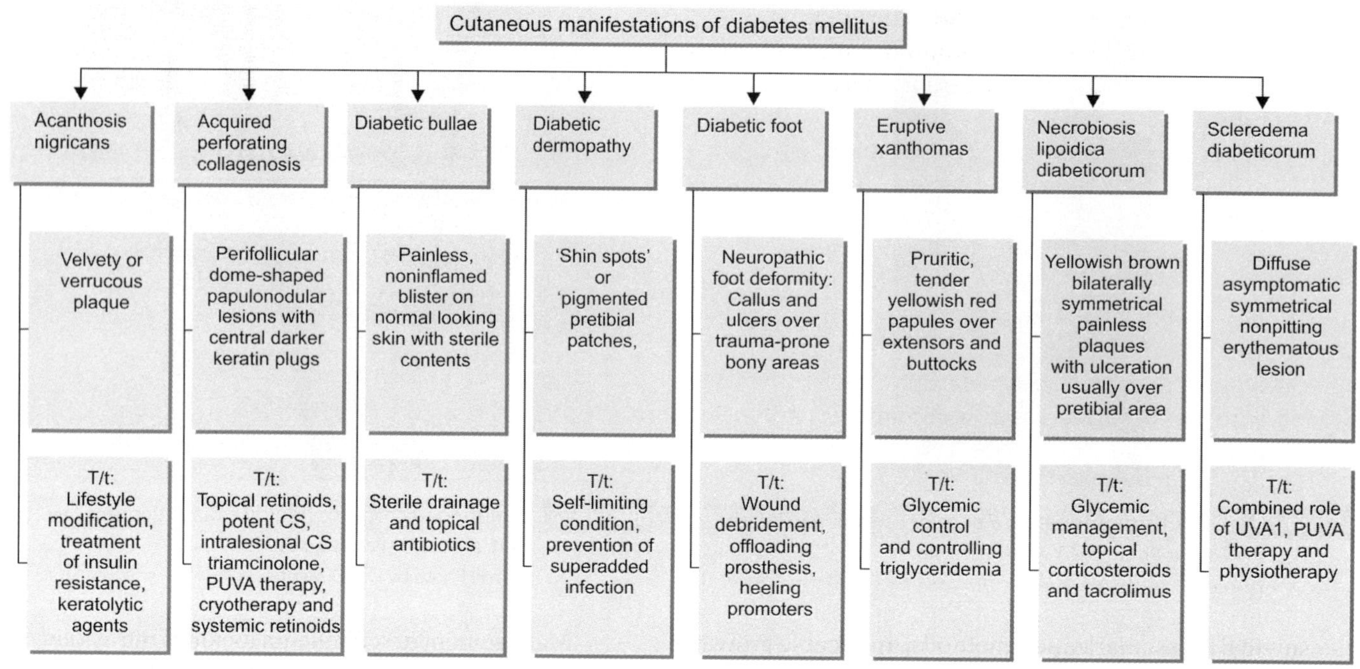

(T/t: treatment; CS: corticosteroid; UVA: ultraviolet A; PUVA: psoralen and ultraviolet A.)

Flowchart 2 Cutaneous manifestations of diabetes mellitus.[2]

- Management includes topical emollients and moisturizers.

- *Diabetic cheiroarthropathy*:
  - Clinically, the decreased ROM of IP and MCP joints culminate into stiffened joints[12]
  - Management is improving the ROM through physiotherapy.
- *Diabetic thick skin*:
  - Clinically, the skin of hands and feet has the sclerodermatous changes. This asymptomatic waxy thickening of skin is diagnosed by ultrasonography
  - Management is topical use of natural moisturizing factors and emollients.
- *Diabetic pruritus*:
  - Clinically, the diabetics suffer from generalized itching, which is perceived on mainly scalp, trunk and limbs[13]
  - Management is oral gabapentin and pregabalin and topical emollients and capsaicin.
- *Diabetic carotenemia*:
  - Clinically, asymptomatic yellow discoloration of skin and nail is known as diabetic carotenemia. It is seen in the areas with increased sebum production (face) and the areas of thick stratum corneum, i.e. nails, palms and soles[14]
  - Management of diabetic carotenemia is ensuring a good glycemic control.
- *Finger pebbles*:
  - Clinically, it presents as diabetic, thick skin on various parts of dorsum of hand, over knuckles and periungual areas. It is also labeled as Huntley's papules, which conglomerate to form bigger plaques. The lesions are usually hypopigmented[15]
  - Management of finger pebbles includes emollients or keratolytics to combat the thick roughened area.
- *Follicular keratosis*:
  - Clinically, the lesions of follicular keratosis are thorny, spinous micropapules. These are present mainly on the extensor aspects (Fig. 6)
  - Management of follicular keratosis is frequent use of emollients, keratolytics and moisturizing agents. Commonly used preparations contain corticosteroids, salicylic acid, lactic acid, α-hydroxy acid, tretinoin and urea in different combinations.
- *Infections*: Skin and soft tissue infections are more severe and prevalent amongst diabetics. The mechanism behind cutaneous infections stands as deranged microcirculation which causes decreased phagocytosis[16]

- *Viral infections*: The most common of viral infections can be in the form of fulminant herpes zoster (Fig. 7) or recurrent herpes simplex infections
- *Mycological infections*: The common etiological agents are *Candida albicans*, dermatophytes (*Trichophyton*, *Epidermophyton*, and *Microspora* species) (Fig. 8), and rarely Mucormycosis.

Clinically, the most common feature may be candidal balanoposthitis (Fig. 9) and vulvo-vaginitis. Angular cheilitis, stomatitis and recurrent paronychia, finger/toe cleft intertrigo, with hyperhidrosis and submammary intertrigo amongst obese have been attributed to different candidal species.

Diabetic ketoacidosis pushes the host to suffer from mucormycosis, as phycomycetes cause angiocentric necrotizing infection of nasopharyngeal area, which may culminate into life-threatening cerebral involvement.

Management starts with simple preventive steps of keeping higher levels of personal hygiene. Topical management includes antifungal dusting powders for intertriginous areas (clotrimazole, terbinafine and itraconazole, etc.) and bedtime medicament can be in the form of cream or gel formulations of the same. Amongst oral antifungals, terbinafine happens to be the drug of choice. The rest of the antifungals may have an agonist action with most of the oral hypoglycemic

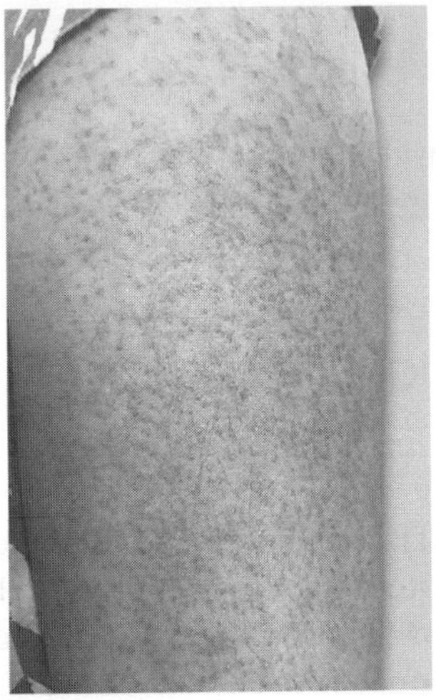

Figure 6 Follicular keratosis over the extensor surface of the arm. ***(For color version, see Plate 4)***
Source: Photo by Dr Aastha Chawla.

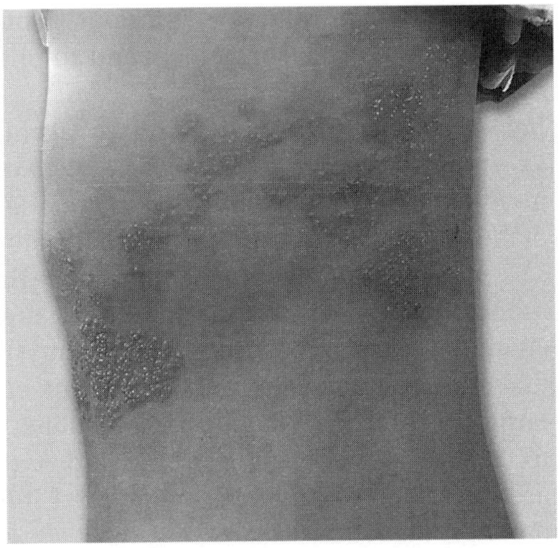

Figure 7 Herpes zoster along the thoracic dermatome. ***(For color version, see Plate 5)***
Source: Photo by Dr Aastha Chawla.

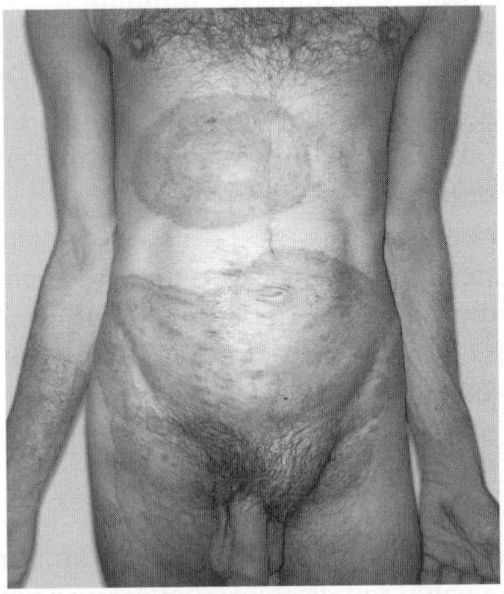

Figure 8 Extensive tinea. ***(For color version, see Plate 5)***
Source: Photo by Dr RD Mehta.

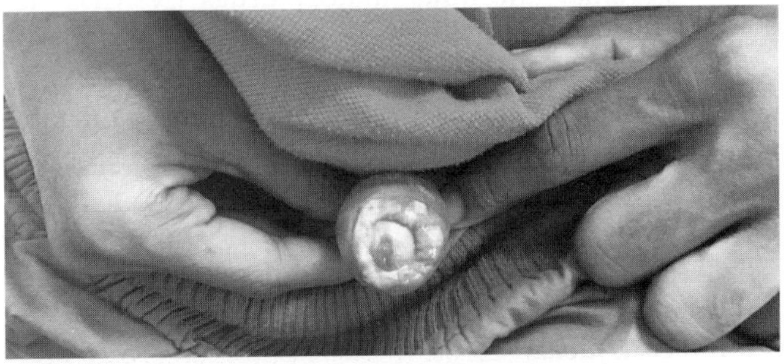

Figure 9 Candidal balanoposthitis. ***(For color version, see Plate 5)***
Source: Photo by Dr RD Mehta.

agents. Mucormycosis warrants lifesaving measures, surgical debridement and amphotericin B through parenteral route.
- *Bacterial infections*: Polymicrobial agents such as gram-negative *Pseudomonas aeruginosa* and methicillin-resistant *Staphylococcus aureus* make diabetic bacterial infections very challenging.

  Clinically, *P. aeruginosa* happens to be the commonest etiological bacteria to cause gangrenous changes (Fig. 10), ecthyma gangrenosum (Fig. 11), diabetic foot infection, and malignant otitis externa. Recurrent furunculosis, folliculitis, cellulitis, erysipelas, necrotizing fasciitis and erythrasma are the other commonly encountered infections amongst diabetics.

  Management of bacterial infections includes topical antibacterial preparations (mupirocin, retapamulin and fusidic acid) for mild cases. Systemic β-lactamase inhibitors, clindamycin, quinolones, and linezolid are to be judiciously used depending upon the severity. Necrotizing fasciitis and severe malignant otitis externa may require hyperbaric oxygen therapy and surgical debridement.

- *Palmar erythema*:
  - Clinically, palmar erythema manifests as asymptomatic bilaterally symmetrical appreciable redness of thenar and hypothenar eminences of the palm[17]
  - Management of palmar erythema is reassurance to the patient
- *Periungual telangiectasia*:
  - Clinically, patients would present as asymptomatic noticeable red discoloration around proximal nail folds. Sometimes, it may be associated with ragged cuticles and tender fingertips also[18]
  - Management is simple reassurance and non-steroidal anti-inflammatory drugs (NSAIDs) for tender fingertips.
- *Pigmented purpuric dermatosis*:
  - Clinically, the brownish-orange non-blanchable patches over skin mark the presence of pigmented purpuric dermatosis[19]
  - Management is only reassurance and preventive measures to retard its progression to stasis dermatosis.
- *Rubeosis faciei*:
  - Clinically, the persistent pinkish-red flushing of face and neck is termed as rubeosis faciei[20]
  - Management of rubeosis can be achieved with dietary restrictions of alcohol and caffeine.

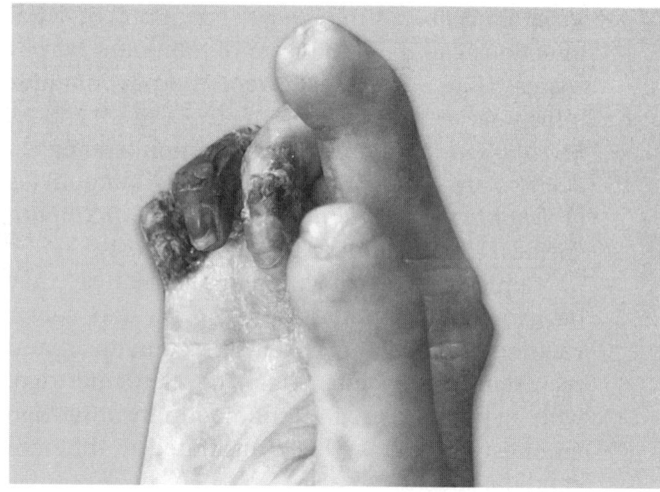

Figure 10 Gangrenous changes of the fingers. ***(For color version, see Plate 5)***
Source: Photo by Dr RD Mehta.

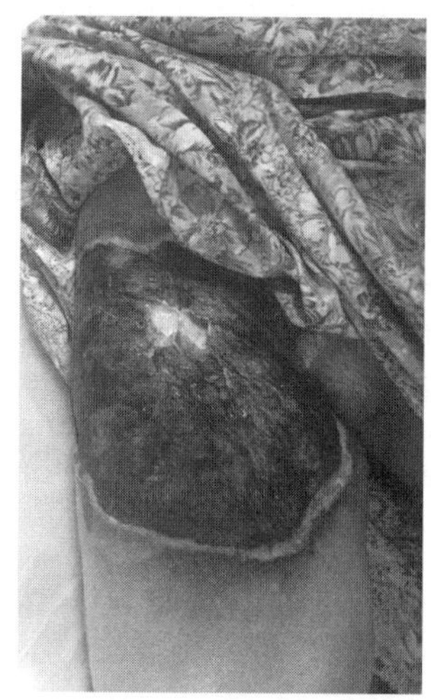

Figure 11 Ecthyma gangrenosum. ***(For color version, see Plate 5)***
Source: Photo by Dr Aastha Chawla.

DIABETES' ASSOCIATION WITH DERMATOLOGICAL DISEASES

- *Granuloma annulare*:
  - Clinically, disseminated form of granuloma annulare (GA) is associated with diabetes, and presents as asymptomatic "skin colored" to brownish papulonodular lesions (Fig. 12). The adjoining lesions form plaques with central clearing.[21]
- *Lichen planus*:
  - Clinically, these are violaceous to gray itchy papular lesions at trauma-prone sites with Koebner's phenomenon being positive[22] (Fig. 13).

- *Psoriasis vulgaris*:
  - Clinically, it is a papulosquamous condition presenting as plaques studded with silvery white scales over trauma-prone sites[23] (Fig. 14).
- *Vitiligo (leukoderma)*:
  - Clinically, it is a depigmented, socially stigmatizing, asymptomatic cosmetic disorder having localized stable variant and an extensive universal form[24] (Fig. 15).

DIABETIC THERAPY AND CUTANEOUS REACTIONS

- Oral hypoglycemic agents of various groups may lead to mild-to-severe *cutaneous adverse drug reactions*, which may manifest as generalized pruritus, urticaria, non-blanchable erythema and rarely erythema multiforme minor and lichenoid drug rash[25]
  - Tolbutamide and chlorpropamide may induce photoallergic rash.
- *Insulin therapy*: The major component of diabetic therapy, i.e. insulin, may cause both lipoatrophy and hypertrophy.
  - *Lipoatrophy*:
    - Clinically, it manifests at injection site as depressed circumscribed areas around thighs
    - It is due to the lipolytic component of the various insulin formulations
    - Management of lipoatrophy is to opt for rotational injection sites, even though it may not be of much benefit. Better option would be to switch to nonlipolytic preparations, such as rapidly acting purified and recombinant human insulin.

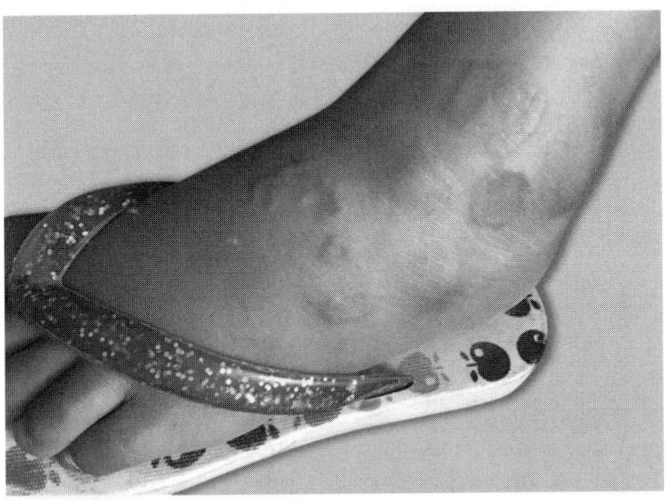

Figure 12 Granuloma annulare. ***(For color version, see Plate 5)***
Source: Photo by Dr Aastha Chawla.

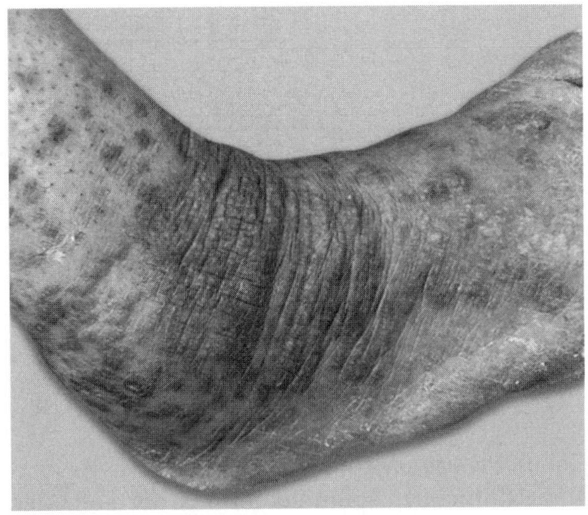

Figure 13 Lichen planus over foot. ***(For color version, see Plate 6)***
Source: Photo by Dr RD Mehta.

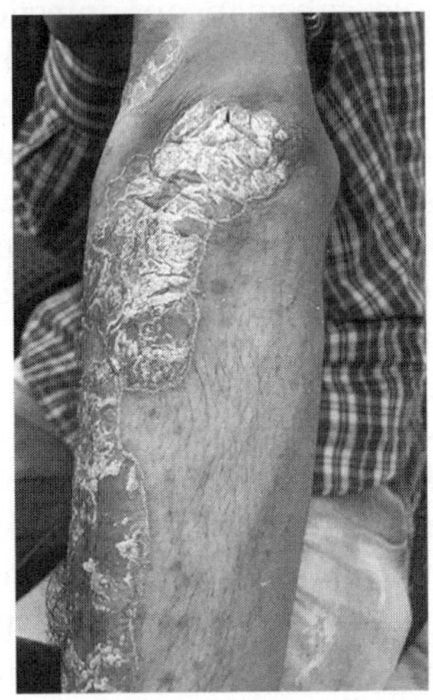

Figure 14 Psoriasis vulgaris. ***(For color version, see Plate 6)***
Source: Photo by Dr RD Mehta.

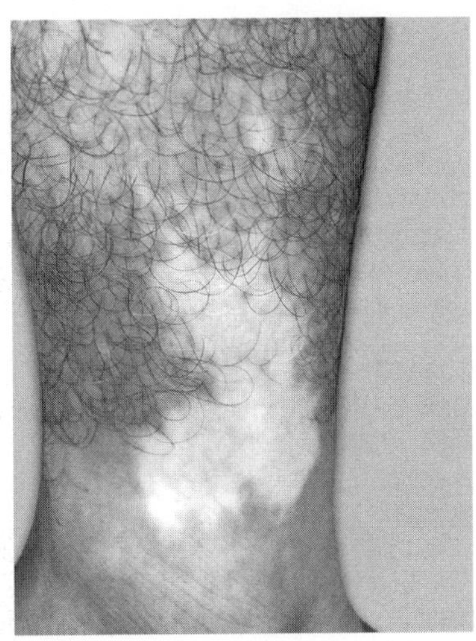

Figure 15 Localized vitiligo. ***(For color version, see Plate 6)***
Source: Photo by Dr Aastha Chawla.

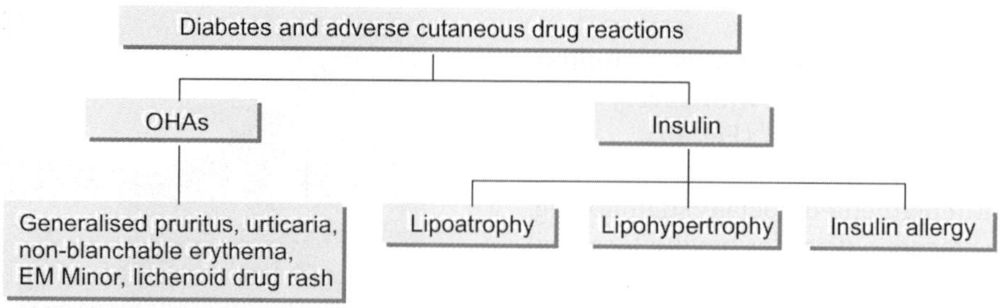

(EM: erythema multiforme; OHA: oral hypoglycaemic agents.)

Flowchart 3 Diabetic therapy and cutaneous reactions (CADRs).[2]

- *Lipohypertophy*:
  - Clinically, lipomoid lesions are soft, dermal, slippable, nodular swellings at the injection sites
  - Multiple subcutaneous injections of human insulin lead to lipohypertrophy. The corroborating factors are reuse of insulin syringes, very high total insulin dose per day and not following the site rotation principle for therapy
  - Management of lipohypertrophy comprises of counseling the patient with correct therapy technique.
- *Insulin allergy*:
  - Clinically, it is more prevalent with bovine insulin as compared to porcine variant. It may present as urticaria, serum sickness, purpuric vasculitis, or rarely nodular lesions may be seen as a result of delayed type of hypersensitivity
  - Management comprises of changing to cutaneous-friendly insulin preparations (Flowchart 3).

REFERENCES

1. Tsankov N, Kazandjieva J, Darlenski R. The skin as a target organ in multisystemic diseases II. Clin Dermatol. 2015;33(5):509-11.
2. Mehta RD, Chawla A. Skin disorders in diabetes. In: Kamlakar T, Banshi S (Eds). Sadikot's international textbook of diabetes. New Delhi: Jaypee Brothers Medical Publishers (P) Ltd; 2018. pp. 530-40.
3. Kutlubay Z, Engin B, Bairamov O, et al. Acanthosis nigricans: a fold (intertriginous) dermatosis. Clin Dermatol. 2015;33(4):466-70.
4. Ghosh SK, Bandyopadhyay D, Chatterjee G. Bullosis diabeticorum: a distinctive blistering eruption in diabetes mellitus. Int J Diabetes Dev Ctries. 2009;29(1):41-42.
5. Morgan A, Schwartz R. Diabetic dermopathy: pathognomonic of diabetes mellitus. J Am Acad Dermatol. 2011;64(2):AB34.
6. Singh N, Armstrong DG, Lipsky BA. Preventing foot ulcers in patients with diabetes. JAMA. 2005;293(2):217-28.
7. Sibbald C, Reid S, Alavi A. Necrobiosis lipoidica. Dermatol Clin. 2015;33(3):343-60.
8. Dinato SL, Costa GL, Dinato MC, et al. Scleredema of Buschke associated with diabetes mellitus type 2: case report and review of the literature. Arq Bras Endocrinol Metabol. 2010;54(9):852-5.
9. Wielosz E, Kurowska M, Suszek D, et al. Coexistence of diabetes mellitus type 1 with diffuse systemic sclerosis—case report and literature review. Rheumatologia. 2017;55(2):104-7.
10. Seité S, Khemis A, Rougier A, et al. Importance of treatment of skin xerosis in diabetes. J Eur Acad Dermatol Venereol. 2011;25(5):607-9.
11. Sudy E, Urbina F, Maliqueo M, et al. Screening of glucose/insulin metabolic alterations in men with multiple skin tags on the neck. J Dtsch Dermatol Ges. 2008;6(10):852-6.
12. Gerrits EG, Landman GW, Nijenhuis-Rosien L, et al. Limited joint mobility syndrome in diabetes mellitus: a mini review. World J Diab. 2015;6(9):1108-12.
13. Ko MJ, Chiu HC, Jee SH, et al. Postprandial blood glucose is associated with generalized pruritus in patients with type 2 diabetes. Eur J Dermatol. 2013;23(5):688-93.
14. Suzuki K, Ito Y, Nakamura S, et al. Relationship between serum carotenoids and hyperglycemia: a population-based cross-sectional study. J Epidemiol. 2002;12(5):357-66.
15. Guarneri C, Guarneri F, Borgia F, et al. Finger pebbles in a diabetic patient: Huntley's papules. Int J Dermatol. 2005;44(9):755-6.
16. Joshi N, Caputo GM, Weitekamp MR, et al. Infections in patients with diabetes mellitus. N Engl J Med. 1999;341(25):1906-12.
17. Serrao R, Zirwas M, English JC. Palmar erythema. Am J Clin Dermatol. 2007;8(6):347-56.
18. Van Hattem S, Bootsma AH, Thio HB. Skin manifestations of diabetes. Cleve Clin J Med. 2008;75(11):772-7.
19. Piérard GE, Seité S, Hermanns-Lê T, et al. The skin landscape in diabetes mellitus. Focus on dermocosmetic management. Clin Cosmet Investig Dermatol. 2013;6:127-35.
20. Namazi MR, Jorizzo JL, Fallahzadeh MK. Rubeosis faciei diabeticorum: a common, but often unnoticed, clinical manifestation of diabetes mellitus. ScientificWorldJournal. 2010;10:70-1.
21. Piette EW, Rosenbach M. Granuloma annulare: pathogenesis, disease associations and triggers, and therapeutic options. J Am Acad Dermatol. 2016;75(3):467-79.
22. Seyhan M, Ozcan H, Sahin I, et al. High prevalence of glucose metabolism disturbance in patients with lichen planus. Diabetes Res Clin Pract. 2007;77(2):198-202.
23. Armstrong AW, Harskamp CT, Armstrong EJ. Psoriasis and the risk of diabetes mellitus: a systematic review and meta-analysis. JAMA Dermatol. 2013;149(1):84-91.
24. Raveendra L, Hemavathi RN, Rajgopal S. A study of vitiligo in type 2 diabetic patients. Indian J Dermatol. 2017;62(2):168-70.
25. Nolte Kennedy MS, Masharani U. Chapter 41. Pancreatic hormones and antidiabetic drugs. In: Katzung BG, Masters SB, Trevor AJ (Eds). Basic and clinical pharmacology, 13th edition. New York, NY: McGraw-Hill Education; 2015.

Chapter 65

Vascular Complications in Diabetic Pregnancy

Sunil Gupta

INTRODUCTION

Worldwide, 199.5 million of women have diabetes, which is expected to increase to 313.3 million in 2035.[1] Hyperglycemia is an important and common medical disorder women encounter during pregnancy. The International Diabetes Federation (IDF) highlighted that one in six live births (16.8%) born of women with some form of hyperglycemia in pregnancy (20–49 years), of them 84% of hyperglycemia in pregnancy is due to gestational diabetes mellitus (GDM), which appears during pregnancy and disappears after delivery. The other 16% are pregestational diabetes mellitus (pre-GDM), i.e. either pre-existing type 2 diabetes mellitus (T2DM) or type 1 diabetes mellitus (T1DM) with pregnancy or the hyperglycemia first detected at any time during the course of pregnancy, if meets the criteria for diagnosis of diabetes in the nonpregnant state. The International Federation of Gynecology and Obstetrics (FIGO) has classified this category as DIP (Diabetes In Pregnancy).[2]

The high prevalence of obesity and sedentary lifestyle in the population, compounded by later child bearing, has led to an increase in the prevalence of T2DM predating pregnancy. In some centers, pregnant women with T2DM now outnumber those with T1DM. The T1DM complicates approximately 0.3–0.5% of all pregnancies and both are associated with an increased risk of adverse outcome to the mother and fetus.[3] Rates of perinatal mortality (25/1,000) and congenital malformation (99/1,000) are significantly greater than those in background populations and at least as poor as those in T1DM. The rates of hypertension (HT), preeclampsia, and postpartum hemorrhage are greater than the general maternity population, as is the rate of operative delivery.[4] Although women with prevalent vascular disease are often older and had a longer duration of diabetes, the maternal vascular disease significantly and adversely affects pregnancy outcome. Macrosomia is the expected outcome in babies born to women with uncomplicated T1DM. In contrast, in women with vascular disease, the babies have more often problems related to intrauterine growth retardation (IUGR) most often associated to preeclampsia. This suggests that maternal diabetes and vascular disease provide an even poorer intrauterine environment—a double hit that restricts macrosomia to "falsely normalize growth". This reinforces the need for frequent assessment of fetal well-being.

MICRO- AND MACROANGIOPATHY NEXUS IN DIABETIC PREGNANCY

Pregnancy accelerates renal insufficiency in patients with pre-existing renal impairment when blood pressure (BP) is not controlled. At baseline, parous women had a lower prevalence of retinopathy and a similar prevalence of microalbuminuria when compared with nulliparous women. However, glycemic control was better in the parous women. The authors examined prospectively the relationship between pregnancies and the incidence or progression of microvascular complications over a mean follow-up period of 7.3 years. The study confirmed earlier studies that pregnancy itself (first or subsequent) was not a risk factor for developing microalbuminuria, any retinopathy, proliferative retinopathy or neuropathy, several years postpartum. These findings have practical implications for planning a pregnancy by young women.

However, in current practice, women having experienced a worsening of their retinopathy during pregnancy are often counseled not to have another pregnancy. Endothelial dysfunction, an early marker of macrovascular disease, is present in pregnancies complicated by T2DM, glucose intolerance and gestational diabetes. This alteration seems to be directly related to glycemic levels but also to dyslipidemia and HT, which can precede the T2DM. Interestingly, hypertensive pregnancy disorders are strongly associated with subsequent T2DM and HT, the latter independent of subsequent T2DM. The severity, parity, and recurrence of these hypertensive pregnancy disorders increase the risk of subsequent cardiovascular events.[5]

Determining the risks of maternal T1DM and T2DM in pregnancy requires a full assessment of maternal vascular disease, including examination for microangiopathies (nephropathy, retinopathy and neuropathy) mainly for T1DM and macroangiopathies (coronary artery disease, HT) mainly for T2DM. Although there is controversy as to whether T2DM is associated with worse outcomes than T1DM in pregnancy, modern reports clearly acknowledge the seriousness of this condition.

DOES PREGNANCY AFFECT THE ONSET AND PROGRESSION OF DIABETIC RETINOPATHY?

Strict glycemic control during pregnancy is expected to have beneficial effect on diabetic retinopathy (DR), as intensified glycemic control is associated with significantly slower development and progression of DR in T1DM and T2DM,[6,7] but studies have shown that rapid normalization of blood glucose can cause acute progression of retinopathy.[8] Thus, institution of strict glycemic control during pregnancy may actually be associated with deterioration of DR. The progression of DR occurs at least temporarily during pregnancy and postpartum. Several factors related to metabolic changes (hyperglycemia), diabetes itself (duration of diabetes before conception, baseline status of DR), pregnancy physiology (hypervolemia and hypercoagulation, impaired retinal autoregulation) and pregnancy complications seem to play important roles in the advancement of DR. One of the largest prospective studies to assess the effect of pregnancy on the development and progression of DR showed that in both intensive and conventional treatment groups, there was a short-term increase in the level of retinopathy during pregnancy that persisted into the first year postpartum. The conventional group was somewhat more affected by pregnancy than the intensive group. A minor effect of rapid improvement of glycemic control on worsening of retinopathy confirmed earlier findings. Good glycemic control, normotension, lack of nephropathy as well as lack of preproliferative/proliferative changes of DR are good prognostic factors as regards the progression of DR during pregnancy.[9] Risk factors for retinopathy progression include chronic and pregnancy-induced HT, preeclampsia, more severe pre-existing DR and a greater decrease in A1C between the first and third trimester of pregnancy.

A retrospective study on 193 women with type 1 diabetes, 63 with an active second-stage delivery (3 with proliferative DR) found no impact of expulsive efforts in the second stage of labor on retinopathy progression in women with stable retinopathy.[10] Data from the Diabetes Control and Complications Trial (DCCT) has suggested that pregnancy does not affect the long-term outcome of mild-to-moderate retinopathy.[11] More recently, preeclampsia and pregnancy-induced HT in women with T1DM has been shown to be associated with an increased risk of severe DR later in life.[12] Still, the abrupt increases in BP, that occur with maternal expulsive efforts during delivery may cause acute retinal hemorrhages in mothers with preproliferative changes. The adverse effect of pregnancy on retinal status persists into the first year postpartum, and increased retinal surveillance by a retina specialist should be continued during the first year. Fortunately, the effect of pregnancy is relatively transient and most changes revert to prepregnancy levels after a year or more.

The evidence is not sufficient to confirm the safety or harm from the use of intravitreal anti-vascular endothelial growth factor (anti-VEGF) injections for diabetic macular edema or proliferative DR during pregnancy. Potential adverse events include HT, proteinuria, defective embryogenesis and fetal loss. It is not known whether these medications cross the placenta or if they are secreted in breast milk. Thus, gestational timing of exposure should be considered in situations where potential benefit to the woman justifies the potential fetal risk. Until more safety evidence is available, it is recommended: (1) to warrant a negative pregnancy test and contraception use during intravitreal anti-VEGF therapy, and (2) to consider delaying conception for 3 months after the last intravitreal injection. During first trimester, intravitreal anti-VEGF therapy should be avoided. Second and third trimester use should be done only if absolutely necessary after explaining potential risks and benefits of procedure. Postpregnancy, diabetic macular edema may often regress without specific therapy. No specific data exists to guide treatment recommendations for diabetic macular edema during pregnancy.[13]

Recommendation

Women with T1DM and T2DM should ideally have ophthalmological assessments before conception, during the first trimester, as needed during pregnancy, and within the first year postpartum. Laser photocoagulation for severe nonproliferative or proliferative retinopathy prior to pregnancy reduces the risk of visual impairment in pregnancy; if not performed prior to pregnancy, it is still considered safe to receive during pregnancy.[13]

DOES DIABETIC NEPHROPATHY AFFECT THE COURSE AND OUTCOME OF PREGNANCY?

Nephropathy complicates 5–10% of pregnancies in women who have diabetes mellitus and is associated with increased risk of preeclampsia, nephrotic syndrome, preterm delivery, fetal growth restriction and perinatal mortality. In early pregnancy, the degree of renal impairment and proteinuria predict pregnancy complications in women with diabetic nephropathy. The risk for preeclampsia increases with severity of proteinuria; diabetic women with microalbuminuria and macroalbuminuria have preeclampsia in 42% and 64% of the cases, respectively.[14] Many of these women have pre-existing chronic HT and even in those that do not, preeclampsia is a common complication. It appears that preeclampsia develops in up to 50% women with nephropathy.[15-17] Approximately, 25–30% of these pregnancies are delivered prior to 34 weeks gestation and approximately 50% are delivered before 37 weeks. Increased risk of fetal distress and IUGR occurs in approximately 20% of pregnancies.

All women aspiring for pregnancy should be screened for chronic kidney disease, prior to conception. Proteinuria and overt nephropathy are associated with increased risk of maternal and fetal complications in pregnancy. An estimated glomerular filtration rate (eGFR) should be used prior to pregnancy to determine risk of adverse outcomes.[13] During pregnancy, serum creatinine instead of eGFR should be used, as eGFR will underestimate glomerular filtration rate (GFR) in pregnancy. Proteinuria is likely to increase during pregnancy, but, in women with a normal GFR, pregnancy has no adverse effects on long-term renal function as long as BP and blood glucose are well controlled. BP elevations in the first trimester and protein excretion are associated with delivery before 37 weeks, usually due to preeclampsia.[18] Few of the cohort studies have proposed that antihypertensive therapy for BP more than 135/85 mm Hg in women with diabetes and albuminuria during pregnancy may reduce the risk of preeclampsia and preterm delivery without adversely impacting other pregnancy outcomes.[19,20]

There is conflicting evidence on whether first-trimester exposure to angiotensin-converting enzyme inhibitors (ACEIs) and angiotensin receptor blockers (ARBs) is associated with an increased risk of congenital malformations. A meta-analysis, of small study size (n = 786), demonstrated a significant risk ratio [relative risk (RR) 1.78, 95% confidence interval (CI) 1.07–2.94] of increased anomalies in infants exposed to first-trimester ACEIs and ARBs compared to the general population.[21] However, when the group exposed to ACEI/ARB was compared to a group of women who were exposed to other antihypertensive drugs, used in pregnancies, there was no statistically significant difference in congenital malformations. Although, fetal exposure in the second and third trimesters is clearly associated with a fetal renin–angiotensin–aldosterone system blockade syndrome, which includes renal failure, oligohydramnios, hypotension, intrauterine growth restriction and death.[22] The decision to discontinue an ACEI or ARB prior to pregnancy should be discussed with the woman and may depend on the indication for use and availability of an effective alternative medication. However, ACE inhibitors and ARBs should be discontinued once pregnancy is diagnosed.

DOES PREGNANCY AFFECT THE CLINICAL COURSE AND MANIFESTATIONS OF DIABETIC NEUROPATHY?[23]

Autonomic neuropathy (AN) involving the GI system may be difficult to determine as nausea, vomiting, and constipation are common symptoms of normal pregnancy. Prevalence of diabetic neuropathy (DN) in pregnancy varies between 8.5 and 32%. Exacerbation of AN during pregnancy has been reported. AN is associated with an increased risk of severe hypoglycemia. The blunted counter-regulatory responses to hypoglycemia in women with DN appear to diminish even further during pregnancy. The presence of gastroparesis is associated with exacerbation of hyperemesis of pregnancy, which results in irregular absorption of nutrients, inadequate nutrition and aberrant glucose control. In summary, it seems that pregnancy does not alter the natural course of diabetic AN. Although a successful outcome of the pregnancy is possible in the presence of symptomatic DN, significant maternal and perinatal morbidity may occur.

Painful Peripheral Neuropathy Management

All medications used in pregnancy, benefits need to be weighed against risk of their use. In the relatively small number of reported pregnancies in which women were exposed to first trimester gabapentin monotherapy (n = 294), no increased risk of congenital malformations was found.[24] However, neonatal gabapentin withdrawal has been reported with maternal oral dose of 600 mg three times daily throughout pregnancy.[25]

WHAT ARE THE RISKS ASSOCIATED WITH PREGNANCY IN WOMEN WITH DIABETIC CORONARY ARTERY DISEASE?

Women with diabetes have three-fold risk of atherosclerosis and fatal myocardial infarction (MI). Although rare, cardiovascular disease (CVD) can occur in women of reproductive age with diabetes. Long-standing diabetes significantly increases the risk of coronary artery disease (CAD) among women in their reproductive years. MI in pregnancy is associated with poor maternal and fetal outcomes.[26] Apparently, hyperglycemia has a direct toxic influence on the arterial wall by increased accumulation of irreversible glycosylation end products; and secondly, it provokes endothelial dysfunction. In women with pre-existing CAD, the cardiovascular changes associated with pregnancy and delivery can result in inadequate myocardial oxygenation, leading to MI and heart failure. Increased cardiac output, decreased systemic vascular resistance with shunting of blood away from the coronaries, increased oxygen consumption during physical activity, increased vascular return during uterine contractions, and acute blood loss at delivery may all contribute to an absolute or relative decrease in the ability of the coronary blood flow to meet the demands of the myocardium. Additionally, these women are extremely vulnerable to myocardial damage and pulmonary edema in the immediate postpartum period. After a vaginal delivery, there is an immediate 60–80% increase in cardiac output[27] due to release of venocaval obstruction, autotransfusion of uteroplacental blood, and rapid mobilization of extravascular fluid, resulting in increased venous return and stroke volume. These fluid shifts are less pronounced after cesarean delivery using controlled analgesia.[23]

Recommendations

Women with known CVD should be evaluated and counseled about the significant risks associated with pregnancy. Also, statins and/or fibrates should be discontinued prior to pregnancy as they are not safe to use during pregnancy.[13]

HOW DOES HYPERTENSION AFFECT THE COURSE OF PREGNANCY IN WOMEN WITH DIABETES?

Women may have pre-existing HT or develop preeclampsia (pregnancy induced HT) during gestation. About 40–45% of women with T1DM and T2DM may have HT complicating pregnancy. A systematic review of risk factors for preeclampsia demonstrated a 3.7 risk (RR 3.1–4.3) for the development of preeclampsia in women with pre-existing diabetes.[28] Preeclampsia is more often associated with T1DM, whereas chronic HT is more often associated with T2DM. Other risk factors for HT which can be modifiable is poor glycemic control in early pregnancy. Some studies, but not all,[29] have found that increased urinary protein excretion in early pregnancy is associated with an increased risk of HT. The HT of any type and degree is associated with adverse outcomes. A large randomized controlled trial in pregnant women with nonproteinuric pre-existing or gestational HT (that included women with GDM) showed that targeting a diastolic BP of 85 mm Hg versus 100 mm Hg reduced neonatal respiratory complications, severe maternal HT (i.e. >160/110 mm Hg) and did not increase the incidence of small for gestational age.[30] Finally, a number of antihypertensive medications are safe and effective in pregnancy, including calcium channel blockers, labetalol and methyldopa.

Although there are no intervention trials for acetylsalicylic acid (ASA) prophylaxis for the prevention of preeclampsia specific to women with pre-existing diabetes, ASA prophylaxis started between 12 and 16 weeks of gestation is likely to be beneficial, given the evidence of benefit in other high-risk populations.[31]

Based on a meta-analysis and systematic review, calcium supplementation (of at least 1,000 mg/day) in high-risk populations, especially in those with low-dietary calcium intake, may reduce preeclampsia rates by up to 40%, although evidence is limited.[32]

SHOULD WOMEN WITH DIABETES EXPECT AN INCREASED INCIDENCE OF PREECLAMPSIA?

The rate of preeclampsia in women with DM is generally being higher than the 5–7% in the general population. Acute hypertensive complications occurred in 51.6% of pregnant women with diabetic microvascular disease, versus 32.9% of those without microvascular disease.[33] By reducing glycated hemoglobin (HbA1c) both before and during pregnancy results in significantly lower incidence of preeclampsia. Kovilam et al.[34] have shown that each increment of 1% in the HbA1c during pregnancy conveyed a 37% increase in the risk of preterm delivery.

Recommendation

In women with DM and chronic HT, aggressive control of HT should be initiated preconceptionally in order to decrease long-term macrovascular and microvascular complications, maintaining BP below 130/80 mm Hg. Aggressive control of maternal HT is of utmost importance to optimize pregnancy outcome. Use of ACEI/ARBs during pregnancy is contraindicated due to their potential adverse effects on the fetus. Preferred medications are methyldopa, nifedipine, labetalol, α-adrenergic blockers and diuretics (targeted BP <130/80 mm Hg).

CONCLUSION

To determine the risks of maternal T1DM and T2DM in pregnancy, it requires a full assessment of maternal vascular disease, including examination for nephropathy, retinopathy, neuropathy, dyslipidemia and HT. The presence of one or more of these factors should prompt a cautious appraisal of the risks of pregnancy. The level of glycemic control achieved during pregnancy seems to modify this risk downward. Younger women with fewer vascular complications and good glycemic control are, unsurprisingly, less likely to suffer an adverse outcome during pregnancy. T2DM is often perceived as a benign form of diabetes, but rates of perinatal mortality and congenital malformation are significantly greater than those in background populations and at least as poor as those in T1DM.

REFERENCES

1. International Diabetes Federation (IDF) Diabetes Atlas, 7th edition. 2015
2. Hod M, Kumar A, Sacks DA, et al. The International Federation of Gynecology and Obstetrics (FIGO) Initiative on gestational diabetes mellitus: A pragmatic guide for diagnosis, management, and care. Int J Gynecol Obstet. 2015;131(Suppl 3):S173-211.
3. Howarth C, Gazis A, James D. Associations of Type 1 diabetes mellitus, maternal vascular disease and complications of pregnancy. Diabet Med. 2007;24:1229-34.
4. Dunne F. Type 2 diabetes and pregnancy. Semin Fetal Neonatal Med. 2005;10:333-9.
5. Lykke JA, Langhoff-Roos J, Sibai BM, et al. Hypertensive pregnancy disorders and subsequent cardiovascular morbidity and type 2 diabetes mellitus in the mother. Hypertension. 2009;53(6):944-51.
6. Reichard P, Britz A, Carlsson P, et al. Metabolic control and complications over 3 years in patients with insulin dependent diabetes (IDDM): The Stockholm Diabetes Intervention Study (SDIS). J Intern Med. 1990;228:511-7.
7. The Diabetes Control and Complications Trial Research Group. The effect of intensive treatment of diabetes on the development and progression of long-term complications in insulin-dependent diabetes mellitus. N Engl J Med. 1993:329:977-86.
8. Dahl-Jorgensen K. Oslo Study. BMJ. 1985;290:811-53.
9. Kaaja R, Loukovaara S. Progression of retinopathy in type 1 diabetic women during pregnancy. Curr Diabetes Rev. 2007;3:85-93.
10. Feghali M, Khoury JC, Shveiky D, et al. Association of vaginal delivery efforts with retinal disease in women with type I diabetes. J Matern Fetal Neonatal Med. 2012;25:27-31.
11. Chew EY, Mills JL, Metzger BE, et al. Metabolic control and progression of retinopathy. The Diabetes in Early Pregnancy Study. National Institute of Child Health and Human Development Diabetes in Early Pregnancy Study. Diabetes Care. 1995;18:631-7.
12. Gordin D, Kaaja R, Forsblom C, et al. Pre-eclampsia and pregnancy-induced hypertension are associated with severe diabetic retinopathy in type 1 diabetes later in life. Acta Diabetol. 2013;50:781-7.
13. Feig DS, Berger H, Donovan L, et al. Diabetes and Pregnancy, Diabetes Canada Clinical Practice Guidelines Expert Committee, 2018 Clinical Practice Guidelines. Can J Diabetes. 2018;42:S255-S282.
14. Ekbom P, Damm P, Feldt-Rasmussen B, et al. Pregnancy outcome in type 1 diabetic women with microalbuminuria. Diabetes Care. 2001;24:1739-44.
15. Reece EA, Wan M, Hobbins JC, et al. Does pregnancy alter the rate of progression of diabetic nephropathy? Am J Perinatol. 1990;7:193-7.
16. Khoury JC, Özalkaya E, Topcuoglu S, et al. Efficacy of levetiracetam in premature infants: our experience and review of the literature. J Matern Fetal Neonatal Med. 2002;11:238-44.
17. Bar J, Ben-Rafael Z, Padoa A, et al. Prediction of pregnancy outcome in subgroups of women with renal disease. Clin Nephrol. 2000;53:437-44.
18. Klemetti MM, Laivuori H, Tikkanen M, et al. Obstetric and perinatal outcome in type 1 diabetes patients with diabetic nephropathy during 1988–2011. Diabetologia. 2015;58:678-86.
19. Bogaerts A, Van den Bergh BR, Ameye L, et al. Interpregnancy weight change and risk for adverse perinatal outcome. Obstet Gynecol. 2013;122:999-1009.
20. Nielsen LR, Damm P, Mathiesen ER. Improved pregnancy outcome in type 1 diabetic women with microalbuminuria or diabetic nephropathy: Effect of intensified antihypertensive therapy? Diabetes Care. 2009;32:38-44.
21. Walfisch A, Al-maawali A, Moretti ME, et al. Teratogenicity of angiotensin converting enzyme inhibitors or receptor blockers. J Obstet Gynaecol. 2011;31:465-72.
22. Bullo M, Tschumi S, Bucher BS, et al. Pregnancy outcome following exposure to angiotensin-converting enzyme inhibitors or angiotensin receptor antagonists: A systematic review. Hypertension. 2012;60:444-50.
23. Minodovnik M. Preconceptional counseling for women with diabetes. In: Langer OP (Ed). The Diabetes in Pregnancy Dilemma, Leading Change with Proven Solutions. Lanham, Maryland: University Press of America; 2006. pp. 501-30.
24. Guttuso T Jr, Shaman M, Thornburg LL. Potential maternal symptomatic benefit of gabapentin and review of its safety in pregnancy. Eur J Obstet Gynecol Reprod Biol. 2014;181:280-3.
25. Carrasco M, Rao SC, Bearer CF, et al. Neonatal gabapentin withdrawal syndrome. Pediatr Neurol. 2015;53:445-7.
26. Bagg W, Henley PG, Macpherson P, et al. Pregnancy in women with diabetes and ischaemic heart disease. Aust N Z J Obstet Gynaecol. 1999;39:99-102.
27. Ueland K, Metcalfe J. Circulatory changes in pregnancy. Clin Obstet Gynecol. 1975;18:41-50

28. Bartsch E, Medcalf KE, Park AL, et al. Clinical risk factors for pre-eclampsia determined in early pregnancy: Systematic review and meta-analysis of large cohort studies. BMJ. 2016;353:i1753.
29. How HY, Sibai B, Lindheimer M, et al. Is early-pregnancy proteinuria associated with an increased rate of preeclampsia in women with pregestational diabetes mellitus? Am J Obstet Gynecol. 2004;190: 775-8.
30. Magee LA, von Dadelszen P, Rey E, et al. Less-tight versus tight control of hypertension in pregnancy. N Engl J Med. 2015;372:407-17.
31. LeFevre ML. U.S. Preventive Services Task Force. Low-dose aspirin use for the prevention of morbidity and mortality from preeclampsia: U.S. Preventive Services Task Force recommendation statement. Ann Intern Med. 2014;161:819-26.
32. Tang R, Tang IC, Henry A, et al. Limited evidence for calcium supplementation in preeclampsia prevention: A meta-analysis and systematic review. Hypertens Pregnancy. 2015;34:181-203.
33. Reece EA, Sivan E, Francis G, et al. Pregnancy outcomes among women with and without diabetic microvascular disease (White's classes B to FR) versus non-diabetic controls. Am J Perinatol. 1998;15:549-55.
34. Kovilam O, Khoury J, Miodovnik M, et al. Use of antihistamine drugs in early pregnancy and delivery outcome. J Matern Fetal Neonatal Med. 2002;11:245-8.

Chapter 66

Female Gender is the Key to Noncommunicable Diseases Prevention

V Seshiah

INTRODUCTION

The prevalence of diabetes is increasing globally and India is no exception. The concern is that India would be having the highest population of diabetes by 2025. The increased prevalence is attributed to the aging population structure, urbanization, the obesity epidemic and physical inactivity.[1] While all these factors contribute to the epidemic of diabetes, early life exposures are emerging as potential risk factors. The "fetal origin of disease" hypothesis proposes that gestational programming may critically influence adult health and disease. Gestational programming is a process whereby stimuli or stresses that occur at critical or sensitive periods of development, permanently change structure, physiology and metabolism, which predispose individuals to disease in adult life. Traditionally and convincingly, lifestyle modifications and drug interventions have proved to delay or postpone the development of overt diabetes in persons diagnosed to have impaired glucose tolerance (IGT). This is a postprimary prevention strategy. The primary prevention of type 2 diabetes mellitus (T2DM) at best would mean to keep genetically or otherwise susceptible individuals normoglycemic and not only preventing T2DM from developing. The primary prevention is more important than postprimary prevention, as this effort is likely to reverse or halt the epidemic of disease. Women with gestational diabetes mellitus (GDM) are an ideal group for the primary prevention of diabetes as they are at increased risk of developing diabetes predominantly T2DM as are their children. GDM is defined as carbohydrate intolerance of variable severity with onset or first recognition during the present pregnancy. Women with GDM have an increased lifetime risk of developing diabetes, at over three times compared to the controls at 16 years after index pregnancy.[2] By 17 years of age, one-third of children born to GDM mothers have had evidence of IGT or T2DM.[3]

IMPACT OF MATERNAL HYPERGLYCEMIA

It has been now recognized that GDM may be playing an important role in increasing the prevalence of diabetes. Also, it may be causing insulin resistance, obesity, dyslipidemia, increased inflammatory markers, endothelial dysfunction, hypertension and ultimately leading to the increased risk of cardiovascular diseases (CVDs). Maternal hyperglycemia in pregnancy is an independent risk factor for putting the offspring at increased risk of IGT, obesity, hypertension at 7 years of age, while cardiovascular (CV) risk continues to increase from adolescent to adulthood. There is also effect on childhood adiposity which is only evident in girls and not boys.[4] (Published Data) There has been an association of maternal hyperglycemia with offspring's adiposity and insulin resistance. Intrauterine exposure to hyperglycemia has deleterious effects that are in addition to those related to genetic predisposition.[5] Also, in utero exposure to hyperinsulinemia is an independent predictor of abnormal glucose tolerance in later childhood. Maternal hyperglycemia in pregnancy predisposes both mother and child at future risk of developing diabetes and CVD (Flowchart 1).[6]

Glucose that normally acts as fuel for developing fetus, in hyperglycemic state, it becomes deleterious for growing fetus. That gave rise to hypothesis called "the fuel-mediated teratogenesis."[7,8] This concept was first

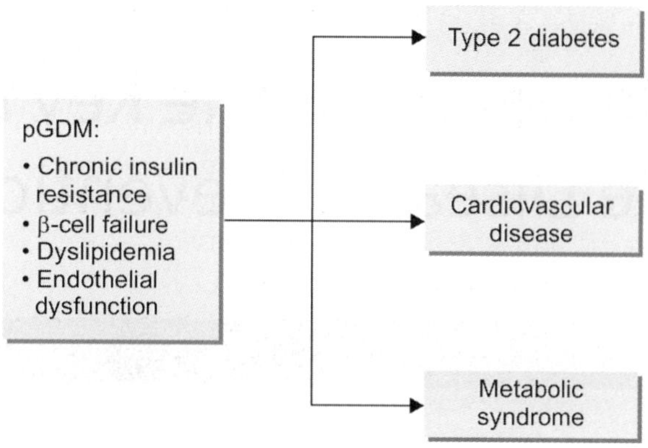

(pGDM: pregestational diabetes mellitus.)

Flowchart 1 Gestational diabetes mellitus and its consequences on adult offspring.

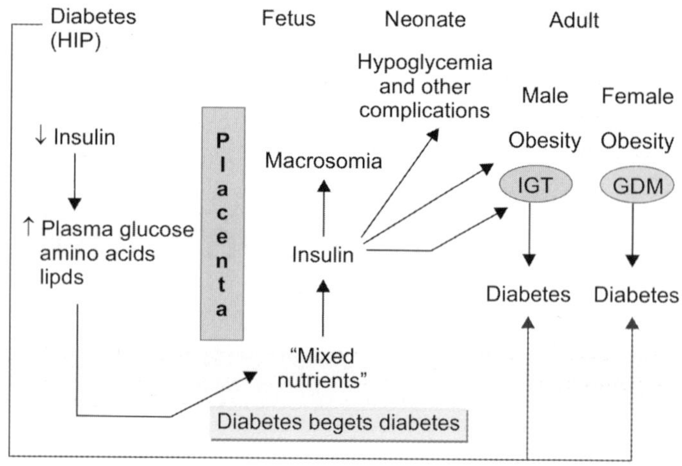

(IGT: impaired glucose tolerance; GDM: gestational diabetes mellitus.)

Flowchart 2 Effects of maternal fuels on fetal and offspring development.

proposed to explain the association of excessive growth of the fetus with maternal hyperglycemia. Maternal insulin does not cross placenta freely, while maternal glucose does, and in response to that, fetal pancreas tries to balance by producing more insulin. This in turn acts as fetal growth hormone and becomes responsible for promoting growth and adiposity (Flowchart 2). The male offspring develops IGT and ultimately diabetes. Whereas the female offspring develops GDM during pregnancy and in postpartum most of them develop diabetes.

ROLE OF ADIPOINSULAR AXIS

An endocrine feedback loop called adipoinsular axis connects the endocrine pancreas with adipose tissue and the brain. This axis regulates hunger and fat storage through the hormones named insulin and leptin. Insulin is responsible for promoting development of fat mass and leptin production. Leptin reduces energy intake and suppresses the insulin secretion via leptin receptors on pancreatic β cells. Abnormal functioning of this adipoinsular axis may lead to hyperphagia, dysregulation of the energy balance and excessive adiposity (Flowchart 3).[9]

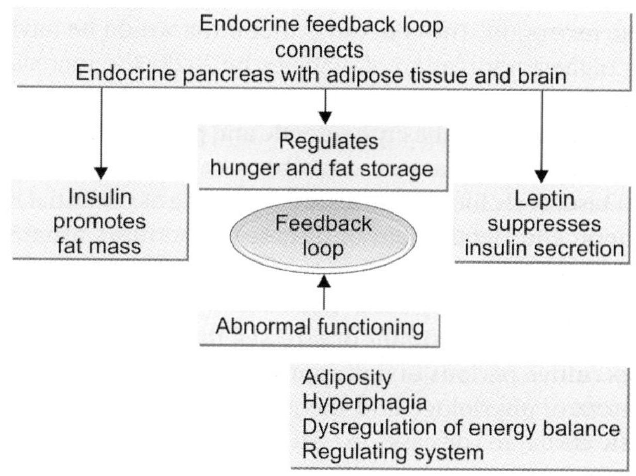

Flowchart 3 Role of adipoinsular axis.

MATERNAL OBESITY AND ITS INFLUENCE ON OFFSPRING AND CARDIOVASCULAR DISEASE

Exposure to maternal hyperglycemia in intrauterine life confers an additional risk of developing CVD in later part of life. This risk is independent of any genetic predisposition or adiposity. Studies are required to explain the mechanisms of maternal hyperglycemia conferring the CV risk. There is an increasing interest in another hypothesis on maternal obesity that leads to metabolic consequences in offsprings. This can add up to accelerate the obesity epidemic too, which is independent to genetic or environmental factors.[10] The glycemic index of diets also has an influence on birth weight of offsprings. Exposure to high glycemic index diets led to higher birth weight and skinfold thickness compared to exposure to a low glycemic diet.

It can be safely concluded that exposure to a hyperglycemic environment in the intrauterine life is associated with increased occurrence of IGT and a defective insulin secretory responses. Gestational diabetes mellitus GDM gives an opportunity wherein development of T2DM and CVD in young women can be prevented. Women with previous GDM (PGDM) are at increased risk of developing type 2 diabetes. Sometimes, GDM may represent an early stage in the natural history of type 2 diabetes. Also in subsequent years after the index pregnancy, these women with PGDM show deranged CV profile with an increased incidence of CVD.

DIAGNOSTIC TESTS PROCEDURE

Women of Asian origin and more so ethnic Indians are at a higher risk of developing GDM and subsequent type 2 diabetes. Universal screening for GDM is essential, and early screening should be done in population where there is a higher prevalence of T2DM. As per new recommendations, all women should be screened for GDM even if there are no symptoms. Compared to selective screening, universal screening of GDM detects more cases and ultimately improves maternal and neonatal outcomes.

Based on the Hyperglycemia and Adverse Pregnancy Outcome (HAPO) study, International Association of the Diabetes and Pregnancy Study Groups (IADPSG) has suggested the guidelines.[11] Predominantly, HAPO study was performed in Caucasian population, and population from India, China, South Asian countries (except the city of Bangkok and Hong Kong), Middle East, and Sub-Saharan countries were not included. The IADPSG recommendations include that the diagnosis of GDM is made when any of the following plasma glucose (PG) values meet or exceed—fasting - 92 mg/dL, (≥5.1 mmol/L), 1-h - 180 mg/dL (≥10.0 mmol/L), 2-h - 153 mg/dL (≥8.5 mmol/L) with 75 g oral glucose tolerance test. The IADPSG also suggests - fasting PG (FPG) 126 mg/dL (>7.0 mmol/L), and A1c >6.5% in the early weeks of pregnancy is diagnostic of overt diabetes. Fasting >92 mg/dL and <126 mg/dL is diagnosed as GDM.

Disadvantages of the IADPSG recommendations are:

- Most of the time pregnant women do not come in the fasting state because of the belief that they should not fast for long hours. The dropout rate is very high if they are asked to come back for repeat test for glucose tolerance. In many situations, attending the first prenatal visit in the fasting state is almost impractical
- The hallmark of GDM is that in all cases FPG values do not reflect the 2-h post glucose with 75 g oral glucose (2-h PG). Two-hour PG values are much higher in ethnically Asian Indians compared to Caucasians as they have high insulin resistance.[12] The insulin resistance during pregnancy is further increased; hence, FPG is not an appropriate option to diagnose GDM in Asian Indian women. About 76% of pregnant women would have missed the diagnosis of GDM made by WHO criterion by following FPG >5.1 mmol/L as cut-off value, in this population.[13,14]

Diabetes in Pregnancy Study Group India (DIPSI) has recommended single-step procedure for diagnosing GDM in community.[15] DIPSI diagnostic criteria of 2-h PG ≥140 mg/dL is similar to WHO criteria 2-h PG ≥140 mg/dL. This was developed due to the practical difficulty in performing glucose tolerance test in the fasting state, challenge of women revisiting the prenatal clinic and that too in fasting state. Hence, it was important to have a test that detects the glucose intolerance at first visit itself, irrespective of fasting or fed state.

Procedure in the antenatal clinic should include, after completing preliminary clinical examination of pregnant women, she should be given 75 g oral glucose load, irrespective of her fasting/nonfasting status and without regard to the time from the last meal. A venous blood sample is to be collected at 2 h for estimating PG by the glucose oxidase–peroxidase method. GDM is diagnosed if 2-h PG is ≥140 mg/dL (7.8 mmol/L). In case 75 g glucose packet is not available, remove and discard five level teaspoons (not heaped) of glucose from a 100 g packet which is freely available. In hospitals where glucose is supplied in bulk, a cup or container of 75 g may be used. The marketed glucose is available in anhydrous form.

As glucose concentrations are affected little by the time since the last meal in a normal glucose-tolerant woman, it makes it a rationale to perform this test in the nonfasting state. After a meal, a normal glucose-tolerant woman would be able to maintain euglycemia due to brisk insulin response against glucose challenge. Whereas, a woman with GDM would not be able to do so due to impaired insulin secretion that leads to increase in her glycemic levels with glucose challenge and the glycemic excursion may exaggerate further. There are several advantages of the DIPSI procedure, such as pregnant women need not be fasting, it causes least disturbance in routine activities of a pregnant woman, and it serves as both screening and diagnostic procedure. This single-step procedure has been approved by Ministry of Health, Government

Box 1: National guidelines for diagnosis and management of gestational diabetes mellitus (GDM).

Methodology: Test for diagnosis

- Single step testing using 75 g oral glucose and measuring plasma glucose 2-h after ingestion
- 75 g glucose is to be given orally after dissolving in approximately 300 mL water whether the PW (pregnant woman) comes in fasting or nonfasting state, irrespective of the last meal. The intake of the solution has to be completed within 5 min
- A plasma standardized glucometer should be used to evaluate blood glucose 2-h after the oral glucose load
- If vomiting occurs within 30 min of oral glucose intake, the test has to be repeated the next day, if vomiting occurs after 30 minutes, the test continues
- The threshold plasma glucose level of ≥140 mg/dL (≥140) is taken as cut-off for diagnosis of GDM

of India (Box 1).[16] It is also recommended by WHO,[17] International Federation of Gynecology and Obstetrics,[18] and International Federation of Diabetes.[19]

The chances of detecting unrecognized type 2 diabetes before pregnancy (pre-GDM) are likely to be missed if usual recommendation for screening between 24 weeks and 28 weeks of gestation is followed. In case 2-hour PG is >200 mg/dL in the early weeks of pregnancy, she may be a pre-GDM, and in this case, A1c of ≥6.5 becomes confirmatory.[20] A pregnant woman found to have normal glucose tolerance, in the first trimester, should be tested again for GDM around 24–28th weeks and finally around 32nd–34th weeks.

CONCLUSION

Female gender: The key to noncommunicable diseases (NCDs) prevention (Fig. 1) and thus maternal health is the link to the NCD epidemic. GDM is the mother of NCD. Hence, preventive measures against T2DM should start right from intrauterine period and continue throughout life from early childhood.[21] GDM offers an important opportunity for the development, testing and implementation of clinical strategies for diabetes prevention and NCD.[22] Public health priority is to initiate the action in screening all pregnant women for glucose intolerance, achieving euglycemia in them and ensuring adequate nutrition, as both low birth weight offsprings and large for gestational age birth weight offsprings are prone to develop NCD in the adulthood. This, in turn in all probability, will help in preventing the epidemic of diabetes and CVD. During postpartum period, women

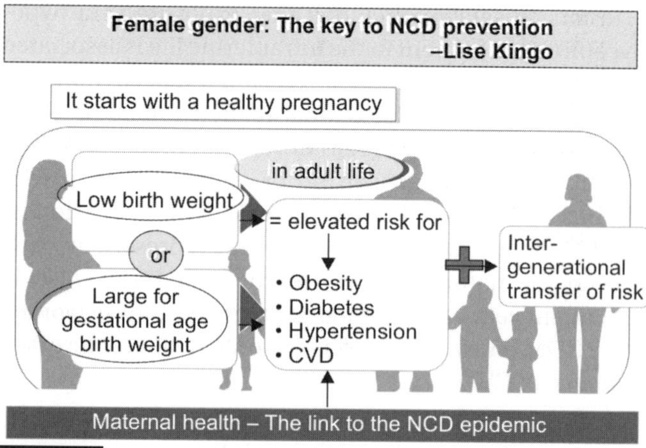

Figure 1 Maternal health is the key link to the NCD epidemic.

should be screened periodically for glucose intolerance and advised proper diet plan and physical activities. Their offsprings should also be advised to follow the healthy diet and healthy lifestyle.

REFERENCES

1. Hunt KJ, Schuller KL. The increasing prevalence of diabetes in pregnancy. Obstet Gynecol Clin North Am. 2007;34:173-99.
2. Henry OA, Beischer NA. Long-term implications of gestational diabetes for the mother. Baillieres Clin Obstet Gynaecol. 1991;5:461-83.
3. Silvermen BL, Rizzo TA, Cho NH, et al. Long-term effects of the intrauterine environment. The Northwestern University Diabetes in Pregnancy Center. Diabetes Care. 1998;21(Suppl 2):B142-9.
4. Tam WH, Ma RCW, Ozaki R, et al. In utero exposure to maternal hyperglycemia increases childhood cardiometabolic risk in offspring. Diabetes Care. 2017;40:679-86.
5. Krishnaveni GV, Hill JC, Leary SD, et al. Intrauterine exposure to maternal diabetes is associated with higher adiposity and insulin resistance and clustering of cardiovascular risk markers in Indian children. Diabetes Care. 2010;33:402-4.
6. McIntyre HD, Oats JJ, Zeck W, et al. Matching diagnosis and management of diabetes in pregnancy to local priorities and resources: an international approach. Int J Gynecol Obstet. 2011;115(Suppl 1):S26-9.
7. Dabelea D, Crume T. Maternal environment and the transgenerational cycle of obesity and diabetes. Diabetes. 2011;60:1849-55.
8. Macfarlane CM, Tsakalakos N. The extended pedersen hypothesis. Clin Physiol Biochem. 1988;6(2):68-73.
9. McMillen IC, Edwards LJ, Duffield J, et al. Regulation of leptin synthesis and secretion before birth: implications for the early programming of adult obesity. Reproduction. 2006;131:415-27.
10. Catalano PM. Obesity and pregnancy—the propagation of a vicious cycle? J Clin Endocrinol Metab. 2003;88:3505-6.
11. International Association of Diabetes and Pregnancy Study Groups Consensus Panel. International association of diabetes and pregnancy study groups recommendations on the diagnosis and classification of hyperglycemia in pregnancy. Diabetes Care. 2010;33(3):676-82.
12. Das S, Behera MK, Misra S, et al. Beta-cell function and insulin resistance in pregnancy and their relation to fetal development. Metab Syndr Relat Disord. 2010;8(1):25-32.

13. Balaji V, Balaji M, Anjalakshi C, et al. Inadequacy of fasting plasma glucose to diagnose gestational diabetes mellitus in Asian Indian women. Diabetes Res Clin Pract. 2011;94(1):e21-3.
14. Sacks DA, Hadden DR, Maresh M, et al. Frequency of gestational diabetes mellitus at collaborating centers based on IADPSG consensus panel-recommended criteria: the Hyperglycemia and Adverse Pregnancy Outcome (HAPO) Study. Diabetes Care. 2012;35(3):526-8.
15. Anjalakshi C, Balaji V, Balaji M, et al. A single test procedure to diagnose gestational diabetes mellitus. Acta Diabetol. 2009;46(1):51-4.
16. <www.mohfw.gov.in> & <www.nhm.gov.in>.
17. Colagiuri S, Falavigna M, Agarwal MM, et al. Strategies for implementing the WHO diagnostic criteria and classification of hyperglycaemia first detected in pregnancy. Diabetes Res Clin Pract. 2014;103(3):364-72.
18. Hod M, Kapur A, Sacks D, et al. The International Federation of Gynecology and Obstetrics (FIGO) initiative on gestational diabetes mellitus: a pragmatic guide for diagnosis, management, and care. Int J Gynaecol Obstet. 2015;131(Suppl 3):S173-211.
19. Purandare CN, Sadikot S, Cho NH. FIGO-IDF joint statement and declaration on hyperglycemia in pregnancy. Diabetes Res Clin Pract. 2018;pii: S0168-8227(18):30293-6.
20. Balaji V, Madhuri BS, Ashalatha S, et al. A1C in gestational diabetes mellitus in Asian Indian women. Diabetes Care. 2007;30(7):1865-7.
21. Tuomilehto J. Prevention of Diabetes Mellitus. A paradigm shift is needed in the primary prevention of type 2 DM, 1st edition. New York, NY: John Wiley & Sons Limited; 2005. pp. 153-65.
22. Buchanan TA, Xiang A, Kjos SL, et al. What is gestational diabetes? Diabetes Care. 2007;30(2):S105-11.

Chapter 67

Gestational Diabetes Mellitus to Diabetes Mellitus—A Window of Opportunity

Minal Mohit

INTRODUCTION

Gestational diabetes mellitus (GDM)—a transitory form of diabetes first recognized during pregnancy complicates between <1% and 28% of all pregnancies worldwide. GDM has important short and long-term health consequences for both the mother and her offspring. GDM predisposes the woman to diabetes mellitus type 2, as was made evident by the definition of GDM given by O'Sullivan and Mahan way back in 1964.[1] They defined GDM if a pregnant woman under-going a 3-hour 100-g oral glucose tolerance test (OGTT) had glucose values exceeding two standard deviations above the mean on two of the four values. [2]

Multiple studies worldwide thereafter have demonstrated a broad ethnic and geographic distribution of GDM, but all studies share the increased risk of subsequent diabetes after delivery.[3] GDM is a perfect window of opportunity for the prevention of DM in not two generations, but three as is understood now. The incidence of GDM is increasing in our country and so is the incidence of type 2 diabetes mellitus in women. To prevent adverse pregnancy outcomes and to prevent or delay future onset of type 2 diabetes in mother and offspring, timely detection, optimum treatment and preventive postpartum care and follow-up is necessary. Awareness of the condition among antenatal women and timely diagnosis of the disease will translate into prevention. However, the area remains grossly under-prioritized.

PREVALENCE OF DIABETES AFTER GESTATIONAL DIABETES MELLITUS

Pregnancy is a diabetogenic state. It creates a state of metabolic stress that unmasks a compensated type 1 or type 2 diabetic woman and brings to surface an uncompensated hyperglycemic state, which in the background of pregnancy is coined GDM. Diagnosing diabetes in the first trimester of pregnancy probably reflects the already existing but undiagnosed and asymptomatic diabetes. Diabetes risk assessment postpartum is influenced by:

- The criteria used to define GDM
- The testing undertaken postpartum
- The length of follow-up.

Oral glucose tolerance test is recommended at 4–6 weeks postpartum. Some recommend following the fasting plasma glucose alone. The studies have shown that fasting plasma glucose above 90 mg/dL doubles the risk of diabetes within 4 months postpartum, whereas fasting plasma glucose more than 120 mg/dL increases the risk 21-fold. [4] Reliance on fasting glucose screens alone and failing to perform OGTT reduces the sensitivity of identifying subsequent diabetes.[5] Kitzmiller et al. re-emphasized the limitations of the fasting glucose as a screen, drawing data from a multiethnic cohort. They demonstrated only 34% of impaired glucose tolerance or diabetes being picked up. [6]

There is no temporal window for postpartum diabetes development, but rather the risk persists, requiring lifelong evaluation to completely capture the risk of diabetes. A meta-analysis of 28 studies was done, and together they demonstrate a consistent pattern of diabetes occurrence over time. Differences among studies were explained by differential follow-up, ethnicity and retesting rates. When cumulative incidence of diabetes is plotted against follow-up after delivery rapid conversion to diabetes is seen over the first 5 years, with a slower progression subsequently. The Diabetes Prevention Program (DPP) involved women with a history of GDM and impaired glucose tolerance to participate in a long-term diabetes prevention study. [7] A total of 350 women (of 1,810 parous women randomized) provided a history of GDM with a mean of 12 years since the index GDM pregnancy. Women who rapidly transitioned from GDM to type 2 diabetes before entry into the DPP were excluded from entry, yielding a survival cohort of high-risk women who had impaired glucose tolerance. The results showed women with a history of GDM were 8 years younger than the non-GDM cohort, but were otherwise well matched for ethnicity, parity, BMI, level of glucose intolerance or insulin resistance. Even after adjusting for age, the women with a history of GDM in the placebo group had a 74% increased hazard for developing diabetes than their non-GDM control subjects. [8] This is to say that even when temporally removed from the index pregnancy, GDM confers a markedly increases the risk for developing diabetes, even when compared with a comparably glucose-intolerant population.

PREDICTORS OF TYPE 2 DIABETES AFTER GESTATIONAL DIABETES MELLITUS

- Fasting plasma glucose—It is the strongest predictor of early postpartum development of diabetes.[4] It is also the strongest independent predictor of long-term development of type 2 diabetes in the mother[9]
- Area under the OGTT curve—In the open-label observational study, Pioglitazone in Prevention of Diabetes (PIPOD), it was seen that during an intravenous glucose tolerance test, lower glucose levels and higher acute insulin responses were present in women remaining diabetes free. [10] Thus the lack of change in insulin area after the intravenous glucose tolerance tests in the first year of follow-up and the higher the baseline OGTT glucose areas are independent predictors of diabetes development
- One-hour and 2-hour glucose levels—The absolute plasma glucose values post-OGTT typically correlate with diabetes risk
- Maternal body mass index (BMI)—Once the glycemic parameters are controlled for in multivariate analysis, mother's BMI, either before or during pregnancy, correlated with diabetes risk
- Insulin therapy during pregnancy-The total daily insulin dose requirement (TDD) frequently predicts subsequent maternal diabetes, [11] but may simply be a reflection of the degree of fasting hyperglycemia
- Serum insulin levels—Assessment of insulin secretion, both during and after pregnancy, provides the strongest independent predictors of diabetes in the mother.[12,13]

LESS SIGNIFICANT CONTRIBUTORS[9,14,15]

- Gestational weight gain
- Postpartum BMI
- Maternal age
- Parity
- Prior GDM
- Family history of diabetes
- Fetal outcomes have not been predictive of maternal risk of diabetes.

HALTING THE JOURNEY FROM GESTATIONAL DIABETES MELLITUS TO DIABETES MELLITUS

Reduction in cell workload may preserve subsequent cell function. Protection from conversion to type 2 diabetes can be conferred by a reduction in insulin resistance, resulting in large reductions in insulin output. This can be achieved by therapeutic life style, which includes medical nutrition therapy (MNT), and regular physical activity. Drugs that reduce insulin resistance like metformin and glitazones may also be used to as preventive strategy.

CURRENT RECOMMENDATIONS FOR POSTPARTUM FOLLOW-UP

The American Diabetes Association (ADA) recommends, "women with gestational diabetes should be screened for diabetes 4–6 weeks postpartum and should be followed up with subsequent screening for the development of diabetes or prediabetes".[16] The American College of Obstetrics and Gynecology (ACOG) makes no specific recommendation on follow-up other than to suggest that postpartum testing may be performed.[17] Survey data suggest that 75% of practicing obstetricians who are ACOG fellows routinely test patients with GDM in the postpartum state[18]; however, a more detailed chart review revealed far fewer women with GDM actually receive any glucose follow-up.[19] Two-thirds of women with GDM history underwent some form of glycemia assessment at a mean of 136 days postpartum. Only 37% underwent either a fasting glucose or OGTT at a median of 14 months after delivery.

Recommendations for actual intervention to prevent progression to diabetes are even less clear. Without clearly specifying GDM as a risk factor, the ADA[16] recommends the following:

- Individuals at high risk for developing diabetes need to become aware of the benefits of modest weight loss and participating in regular physical activity, and
- Monitoring for the development of diabetes should be performed every 1–2 years. The ACOG suggests, "individuals at increased risk should be counseled regarding diet, exercise, and weight reduction or maintenance to forestall or prevent the onset of type 2 diabetes".[17] The National Diabetes Education Program (NDEP) is currently promoting a GDM Diabetes Prevention Initiative, targeting both providers and women with a GDM history.[20] Key messages are illustrated in Box 1. The rationale for such recommendations is now being developed from a variety of clinical trials; however, these are based on clinical expert committee recommendations.

Box 1: Gestational diabetes mellitus diabetes prevention initiative from the National Diabetes Education Program.

- GDM imparts lifelong risk for diabetes, mostly type 2
- Modest weight loss and physical activity can delay or prevent type 2 diabetes
- Offspring can lower risk by eating healthy foods, being active and not becoming overweight

Conservative recommendations to patients include:

- Let healthcare practitioners know of any history of GDM
- Get tested 6–12 weeks postpartum, then every 1–2 years
- Reach pre-pregnancy weight 6–12 months postpartum
- If still overweight, lose at least 5–7% of weight slowly, over time and keep it off

Adapted from the National Diabetes Education Program.[20]
(GDM: gestational diabetes mellitus.)

CONCLUSION

It is clear that GDM confers a lifelong increased risk for the development of diabetes, and in most cases, this turns out to be type 2 diabetes. Progression from GDM to type 2 diabetes correlates with progressive cell failure to compensate for the ongoing insulin resistance. Postpartum follow-up of at-risk women is inadequate, and the recommendations for screening from ACOG and the ADA are at variance. Consistent recommendations, together with a professional and public health campaign to raise the awareness of GDM as a diabetes predictor, will be necessary to improve postpartum care of women at highest risk. Recommendations for follow-up of GDM stemming from the Fifth International Workshop-Conference are summarized in Table 1.[6] Clinical trials now provide level A evidence for the impact of multiple interventions to prevent the progression to type 2 diabetes in women with a history of GDM. Both lifestyle modification and pharmacological therapies (metformin and pioglitazone) have been shown to reduce diabetes development by 50% or more. The diagnosis of GDM should initiate a long-term intervention and diagnostic process to minimize the risk of developing diabetes or to diagnose it as early in the course of disease as possible.

TABLE 1: Metabolic assessments recommended after gestational diabetes mellitus.

Time	Test	Purpose
After delivery (1–3 days)	Fasting or random plasma glucose	Detect persistent, overt diabetes
Early postpartum (around the time of postpartum visit)	75 g 2-h OGTT	Postpartum classification of glucose metabolism*
1-year postpartum	75 g 2-h OGTT	Assess glucose metabolism
Annually	Fasting plasma glucose	Assess glucose metabolism
Triannually	75 g 2-h OGTT	Assess glucose metabolism
Pre-pregnancy	75 g 2-h OGTT	Classify glucose metabolism*

*Classification of glucose metabolism by criteria recommended by the American Diabetes Association.17
(OGTT: oral glucose tolerance test.)
Reproduced from the Summary and Recommendations of the Fifth International Workshop-Conference on Gestational Diabetes Mellitus.[6]

REFERENCES

1. O'Sullivan JB, Mahan CM. Criteria for the oral glucose tolerance test in pregnancy. Diabetes. 1964;13:278-85.
2. O'Sullivan JB. Diabetes mellitus after GDM. Diabetes. 1991;40 (Suppl. 2): 131-5.
3. Buchanan TA, Xiang AH. Gestational diabetes mellitus. J Clin Invest. 2005; 115:485-91.
4. Schaefer-Graf UM, Buchanan TA, Xiang AH, et al. Clinical predictors for high risk for the development of diabetes mellitus in the early puerperium in women with recent gestational diabetes mellitus. Am J Obstet Gynecol 2002;186:751-6.
5. Woerle HJ, Pimenta WP, Meyer C, et al. Diagnostic and therapeutic implications of relationships between fasting, 2- hour postchallenge plasma glucose and hemoglobin a1c values. Arch Intern Med. 2004;164: 1627-32.
6. Metzger BE, Buchanan TA, Coustan DR, et al. Summary and recommendations of the Fifth International Workshop-Conference on Gestational Diabetes Mellitus. Diabetes Care. 2007;30(Suppl. 2):S251-60.
7. Diabetes Prevention Program Research Group: The Diabetes Prevention Program: Design and methods for a clinical trial in the prevention of type 2 diabetes mellitus. Diabetes Care. 1999;22:623-34.
8. Diabetes Prevention Program Research Group: Prevention of diabetes in women with a history of gestational diabetes. J Clin Endocrinol Metab. In press.
9. Kim C, Newton KM, Knopp RH. Gestational diabetes and the incidence of type 2 diabetes. Diabetes Care. 2002;25:1862-8.
10. Xiang A, Peters R, Kjos S, et al. Effect of pioglitazone on pancreatic beta cell function and diabetes risk in Hispanic women with prior gestational diabetes. Diabetes. 2006;55:517-22.
11. Catalano P, Vargo K, Bernstein I, et al. Incidence and risk factors associated with abnormal postpartum glucose tolerance in women with gestational diabetes. Am J Obstet Gynecol. 1991;165:914-9.
12. Metzger B, Cho N, Roston S, et al. Prepregnancy weight and antepartum insulin secretion predict glucose tolerance five years after gestational diabetes mellitus. Diabetes Care. 1993;16:1598-1605.
13. Buchanan T, Xiang A, Kjos S, et al. Antepartum predictors of the development of type 2 diabetes in Latino women 11–26 months after pregnancies complicated by gestational diabetes. Diabetes. 1999;48:2430-36.
14. Seghieri G, DeBellis A, Anichin R, et al. Does parity increase insulin resistance during pregnancy? Diabet Med. 2005;22:1574-80.
15. Lobner K, Knopff A, Baumgartner A, et al. Predictors of postpartum diabetes in women with GDM. Diabetes. 2006;55:792-7.
16. American Diabetes Association. Standards of medical care in diabetes (Position Statement). 2005;28(Suppl. 1):S4-36.
17. American Association of Obstetricians and Gynecologists. Gestational Diabetes, ACOG Practice Bulletin No. 30. Obstet Gynecol. 2001;98:525-38.
18. Gabbe SC, Gregory RP, Powers ML, et al. Management of diabetes mellitus by obstetricians-gynecologists. Obstet Gynecol. 2004;103:1229-34.
19. Smirnakis KV, Chasen-Taber L, Wolf M, et al. Postpartum diabetes screening in women with a history of gestational diabetes. Obstet Gynecol. 2005;106:1297-1303.
20. National Diabetes Education Program: http://www.ndep.nih.gov/diabetes/ pubs/ NeverTooEarly_Tipsheet.pdf [Accessed 1 June 2006].

Chapter 68

Gestational Diabetes Mellitus—Diagnosis and Management: A Diabetologist's Perspective

Shalini Jaggi

INTRODUCTION

The explosive rise in diabetes and obesity gripping the world today has resulted in a parallel rise in the number of cases of gestational diabetes mellitus (GDM), affecting about 15% women worldwide, with almost 4 million women having GDM in India alone.[1] It is associated with serious implications both for the mother and the fetus, not only during pregnancy but also after delivery. GDM significantly increases the future risk of development of type 2 diabetes (T2D) in the mother, and also makes the baby more prone to develop obesity as well as glucose intolerance as it grows, thus affecting two generations. An early diagnosis and adequate management of GDM provides us with a golden window of opportunity for intervention which has beneficial effects both on the present pregnancy and the future risk for both mother and baby.

WHAT IS GESTATIONAL DIABETES MELLITUS AND WHY IS IT IMPORTANT?

Gestational diabetes mellitus is defined as "glucose intolerance of any degree with the onset or first recognition during pregnancy" (in the second or third trimester), which may or may not resolve after delivery; Women with previously unknown diabetes who have a glycated hemoglobin (HbA1c) ≥6.5% in the first trimester, type 1 diabetes, and monogenic diabetes can sometimes present for the first time in pregnancy; and are all said to have overt diabetes and have to be differentiated from true GDM.[2,3] The prevalence of GDM varies from 3.8% to 21% in different parts of India, with an increased prevalence in urban than rural areas.[4,5]

Gestational diabetes mellitus is associated with an increase in maternal as well as fetal morbidity and mortality (Box 1).[6,7] Though it may revert after delivery in a majority of women, it has far-reaching consequences

Box 1: Hyperglycemia-related maternal and fetal complications.[7]

Maternal complications:
- Miscarriages in early pregnancy
- Higher incidence of infections
- Pre-eclampsia
- Preterm labor
- Birth trauma
- Assisted delivery and cesarean sections
- Hypoglycemia
- Acute metabolic complications such as DKA
- Worsening of pre-existing microvascular complications

Fetal complications:
- Congenital malformations, particularly cardiac and neural tube defects but sacral agenesis is the most pathognomonic
- Higher incidence of stillbirths
- Polyhydramnios
- Macrosomia
- Shoulder dystocia
- Prolonged labor
- Birth trauma and Erb palsy
- Neonatal asphyxia
- Neonatal hypoglycemia

(DKA: diabetic ketoacidosis.)

translating into an increased risk of future development of T2D in the mother, as well as obesity and metabolic syndrome in the offspring. Thus, prompt and early diagnosis and management ensures a safe pregnancy and improved maternal and fetal outcomes.

PATHOPHYSIOLOGY OF GESTATIONAL DIABETES MELLITUS

Pregnancy involves a major alteration in the mother's hormonal milieu, characterized by an increase in estrogen, progesterone, prolactin, cortisol, human chorionic gonadotropin (hCG), prolactin as well as placental hormones. These hormones alter the maternal insulin resistance to enable adequate supply of nutrients to the fetoplacental unit for growth. These metabolic changes promote adipose tissue deposition in early pregnancy, followed by increasing insulin resistance and facilitated lipolysis in late pregnancy.

The hallmark of late second and third trimesters is increasing insulin resistance, caused by alterations in adipocytokines such as lower levels of adiponectin, and increase in leptin, tumor necrosis factor-alpha (TNF-α), interleukin-6, and resistin, etc. as well as marked increase in counter-regulatory hormones. These include human placental lactogen (30-fold rise), human placental growth hormone (6–8 fold rise), prolactin (7–10 fold rise) and cortisol. As a consequence, insulin-mediated glucose disposal is reduced by almost 50% and there is a compensatory 200–250% increase in insulin secretion in late pregnancy.[8,9]

The increased insulin resistance and diabetogenic stress due to placental hormone surge in the second half of pregnancy place a huge demand for compensatory increase in insulin secretion. If this demand for massive increase in insulin secretion is not adequately fulfilled, it leads to dysglycemia and a clinical presentation of GDM.

RISK FACTORS FOR DEVELOPMENT OF GESTATIONAL DIABETES MELLITUS

- Obesity [Body Mass Index (BMI) ≥30 kg/m^2]
- Family history of diabetes (first-degree relative with diabetes)
- Bad obstetric history
- Previous macrosomic baby weighing ≥4.5 kg
- Previous history of GDM
- Elderly primigravida
- Hydramnios
- Multiparity or twin gestation
- Previous or current pregnancy-induced hypertension (PIH)
- *High risk ethnicity:* South Asian, Black Caribbean and Middle Eastern.

DIAGNOSIS OF GESTATIONAL DIABETES MELLITUS

The screening strategy for GDM has been controversial and has been changed from time to time. Many international diabetes associations and organizations recommend screening only the high-risk pregnancies for GDM, but universal screening is recommended for all high-risk ethnicities such as Asian Indians, Hispanics, Pacific Islanders, and Afro-Americans, etc. Indian pregnant women, being part of the high-risk ethnic group, need to be screened for diabetes at their first antenatal visit itself. Those found to be normal should be screened again at 24–28 weeks for GDM.

Current American Diabetes Association/ European Association for the Study of Diabetes 2018 Recommendations[10]

As per the American Diabetes Association (ADA), diagnosis of GDM can be made by either one-step or a two-step screening approach as shown in Box 2.

- *One-step approach:* 2-hour 75-g oral glucose tolerance test (OGTT) [the International Association of Diabetes and Pregnancy Study Groups (IADPSG) Consensus]
- *Two-step approach:* with a 1-hour 50 g (nonfasting) screen followed by a 3-hour 100-g OGTT for those who screen positive, i.e. 1 hour more than or equal to 140 mg/dL [National Institutes of Health (NIH) Consensus].

*Different diagnostic criteria will identify different magnitudes of maternal hyperglycemia and maternal/ fetal risk.

The Diabetes In Pregnancy Study Group India Criteria for Gestational Diabetes Mellitus Diagnosis in India

A developing country like India has an ethnic population highly predisposed to T2D as well as high prevalence of GDM which often goes undiagnosed, especially in rural areas. Some of the challenges for GDM screening in our country include lack of trained phlebotomists as well as

Box 2: Current screening and diagnosis of gestational diabetes mellitus as per American Diabetes Association.[10]

"One-step" (IADPSG consensus)

Perform a 75-g OGTT, with plasma glucose measurement fasting and at 1 h and 2 h, at 24–28 weeks of gestation in women not previously diagnosed with overt diabetes.

The OGTT should be performed in the morning after an overnight fast of at least 8 h.

The diagnosis of GDM is made when any of the following plasma glucose values are exceeded:

- Fasting: ≥92 mg/dL (5.1 mmol/L)
- 1 h: ≥180 mg/dL (10.0 mmol/L)
- 2 h: ≥153 mg/dL (8.5 mmol/L)

"Two-step" (NIH consensus)

Perform a 50-g GLT (nonfasting), with plasma glucose measurement at 1 h (step 1), at 24–28 weeks of gestation in women not previously diagnosed with overt diabetes.

If the plasma glucose level measured 1 h after the load is ≥140 mg/dL* (7.8 mmol/L), proceed to 100-g OGTT (step 2). The 100-g OGTT should be performed when the patient is fasting.

The diagnosis of GDM is made when at least two of the following four plasma glucose levels (measured fasting, 1 h, 2 h, 3 h, after the OGTT) are met or exceeded:

	Carpenter/Coustan	or NDDG
• Fasting	95 mg/dL (5.3 mmol/L)	105 mg/dL (5.8 mmol/L)
• 1 h	180 mg/dL (10.0 mmol/L)	190 mg/dL (10.6 mmol/L)
• 2 h	155 mg/dL (8.6 mmol/L)	165 mg/dL (9.2 mmol/L)
• 3 h	140 mg/dL (7.8 mmol/L)	145 mg/dL (8.0 mmol/L)

*The American Collage of Obstetricans and Gynecologists (ACOG) recommends a lower threshold of 135 mg/dL (7.5 mmol/L) in high-risk ethnic minorities with higher prevalence of GDM; some experts also recommend 130 mg/dL (7.2 mmol/L).

(IADPSG: The International Association of Diabetes and Pregnancy Study Groups; GDM: gestational diabetes mellitus; GLT: glucose loading test; NDDG: National Diabetes Data Group; NIH: National Institutes of Health; OGTT: oral glucose tolerance test.)

standardized laboratory facilities for blood glucose (BG) estimation, as well as the difficulty of getting all pregnant women to come fasting for an OGTT. To circumvent these challenges, the Diabetes In Pregnancy Study group India (DIPSI) recommends doing a single point nonfasting 75 g oral glucose test for all pregnant Indian women coming to the antenatal clinic in first trimester and again repeating it at 24–28 weeks as well as 32–34 weeks, if negative at prior visit.[11] The test involves giving 75 g oral glucose to the pregnant woman irrespective of fasting/nonfasting status and collecting a 2 hours postglucose sample. A value of 140 mg/dL or more establishes the diagnosis of GDM and calls for putting in place all lifestyle and diet measures followed by pharmacotherapy as per the need.

Though it is a simple, economical, and feasible test, and has been included in the guidelines issued by the Ministry of Health and Family Welfare, Government of India,[12] concerns have been raised by many studies as this single point nonfasting test when compared to a fasting IADPSG recommended or World Health Organization (WHO) recommended 75-g OGTT has much lower sensitivity, thus missing out a significant number of true GDM women as well as those with fasting hyperglycemia. There has been a justifiable call for more studies and a relook into the viability of following these criteria nationwide.[13,14]

SELF-MONITORING OF BLOOD GLUCOSE

Self-monitoring of blood glucose (SMBG) is essential during pregnancy. Factors such as type of treatment (diet or insulin), risk of hypoglycemia, as well as type and time of physical activity can help determine the number of daily tests required.

Ideally, 7-point capillary glucose testing at home which includes all three premeal as well as 1-hour or 2-hour postmeal blood sugars should be checked along with a bedtime glucose value, especially in patients on insulin. Many studies have demonstrated that postprandial hyperglycemia is the main predictor of fetal macrosomia. Hence, strict monitoring of postprandial glucose is of extreme importance during pregnancy. As peak plasma glucose excursions in pregnancy occur between 60 and 90 minutes after eating, 1-hour or 2-hour postmeal testing is generally recommended in pregnancy except in cases of women with delayed gastric emptying, those on high-fat meal, or those using regular insulin instead of analogs for prandial bolus, where a 2-hour value may be checked. Continuous glucose monitoring system (CGMS) or ambulatory glucose profiling is also being used currently especially in detecting missed postmeal peaks or unrecognized hyper- as well as hypoglycemia, though data on their use in pregnancy is yet insufficient.

Due to the increased risk of nocturnal hypoglycemia during pregnancy, testing during the night is often necessary in patients receiving insulin. Because starvation ketosis is common in pregnancy and may have detrimental effects on the fetus, urine and/or blood monitoring of ketones is also warranted to confirm that the diet is adequate.

TARGETS OF GLYCEMIC CONTROL IN GESTATIONAL DIABETES MELLITUS

The goals for glycemic control in GDM pregnancy recommended both by the *American College of Obstetricians and Gynecologists* (ACOG) as well as the ADA are:

- Fasting BG ≤95 mg/dL (5.3 mmol/L)
- One-hour postmeal BG ≤140 mg/dL (7.8 mmol/L)
- Two-hour postmeal BG ≤120 mg/dL (6.7 mmol/L).

In women who experience significant hypoglycemia in achieving these targets, ADA recommends less stringent targets based on clinical experience and individualization of care.

ROLE OF DIET: MEDICAL NUTRITION THERAPY

Lifestyle modification and medical nutrition therapy (MNT) is an integral part of management of GDM. Lifestyle therapy in terms of increased physical activity along with an optimal dietary prescription should provide optimum caloric and nutrient needs to sustain pregnancy and fetal growth without causing detrimental postprandial hyperglycemia. As postmeal peaks are linked to diabetic fetopathy and macrosomia, these excursions can be blunted with adequate restriction of simple carbohydrates. Carbohydrate intake should be restricted to 35–45% of total calories,[15] i.e. about 175 g/day. Saturated fats should also be limited (less than 10% of total calories) as they increase insulin resistance, and further increase triglycerides and free fatty acids for fetal growth. Monounsaturated fats are preferred. High fiber and low glycemic index carbohydrates are recommended to delay food absorption and prevent postmeal surges.

Approximately, 30–40 kcal/kg ideal body weight or an increment of about 300 kcal/day above the basal requirement is needed in pregnancy. The ADA recommends an intake of 2,000–2,500 kcal/day based on 35 kcal/kg of present pregnancy weight, but these need to be adjusted for each individual patient depending on her weight gain and glycemic control. Calorie restriction of about 30–33% benefits women with BMI of 30 kg/m^2 or above. Pregnancy is not the ideal time for obesity correction. Higher baseline BMI of the mother and gestational weight gain are shown to independently increase the risk of a large-for-date infant.

Physical activity complements diet therapy and unless contraindicated or forbidden by the obstetrician, all pregnant women should exercise/walk regularly as advised.

PHARMACOLOGICAL MANAGEMENT OF GESTATIONAL DIABETES MELLITUS

Insulin Treatment

Insulin is essential when MNT fails to achieve euglycemia in a GDM pregnancy even after 2 weeks of strict discipline. As insulin does not cross placenta, it is the safest and recommended first-line pharmacological agent for management of hyperglycemia in pregnancy.[10] Regular insulins being nonimmunogenic are safe and even analog insulins—rapid-acting insulin aspart and lispro as well as basal analog insulin detemir—are considered safe and given category B approval by the United States Food and Drug Administration (USFDA) for use in pregnancy.

For women with only postmeal rise in BG, premeal rapid-acting insulins/regular insulins can be given and doses titrated to achieve targets of control. In women whose fasting BG levels are also high, a basal insulin can be added at bedtime, as per the basal-bolus insulin regime to achieve euglycemia. NPH (neutral protamine Hagedorn) insulin can also be used as basal insulin, though chances of hypoglycemia with basal analog insulin are lower because of its flatter profile and no peak action.

Use of insulin pumps [continuous subcutaneous insulin infusion (CSII)], if affordable, is also indicated being the most physiological, flexible and fastest way to better regulate the blood sugars, especially in conjunction with CGMS.

Role of Oral Drugs in Pregnancy

The USFDA as well as ADA[10] do not recommend any oral drug in pregnancy as first-line therapy for GDM or diabetes in pregnancy.

- *Glyburide:* Glyburide crosses the placenta much less than all other sulfonylureas and has been shown to affect fetal insulin levels minimally. It has been shown to be associated with a higher rate of neonatal hypoglycemia and macrosomia than patients treated with insulin or metformin
- *Metformin:* Though metformin may be associated with a lower risk of neonatal hypoglycemia and less maternal weight gain compared to insulin, it has been shown to slightly increase the risk of prematurity. Also, quite a large proportion of GDM women treated with metformin eventually need insulin as pregnancy progresses to achieve adequate glycemic control.

Hence, patients unwilling for insulin and treated with oral agents should be informed that they cross placenta, and though various short-term studies have shown no adverse effects on the fetus, long-term data on their safety is still lacking. Current ADA/European Association for the Study of Diabetes 2018 guidelines recommend insulin as the first-line pharmacotherapy due to its established safety in pregnancy. It also opines against continuing metformin in polycystic ovary syndrome (PCOS) women due to lack of any evidence-based need to for its continuation in the background of no demonstrable benefits of metformin in preventing spontaneous abortion or GDM in these patients.

LONG-TERM MATERNAL RISKS: "DIABETES BEGETS DIABETES"

Gestational diabetes mellitus confers a lifelong increased risk for the development of diabetes, and in most cases this is T2D. Progression from GDM to T2D correlates with progressive β-cell failure to compensate for the ongoing insulin resistance. Postpartum follow-up of at-risk women needs to be emphasized. The presence of GDM doubles the risk of diabetes within 4 months postpartum, whereas fasting plasma glucose more than 121 mg/dL during the pregnancy increased the risk 21-fold.[16] A 75-g OGTT should be performed within 4–12 weeks postpartum to establish their glucose status and repeated every 1–3 years thereafter.[10] Women with previous GDM should plan future pregnancies in consultation with their health care providers.

All women with GDM should be counseled on a healthy lifestyle as well dietary discipline and the importance of losing excess weight as important measures to prevent progression to diabetes.

LONG-TERM RISKS IN OFFSPRING

Many studies have demonstrated that offspring exposed to GDM are at increased risk of obesity, impaired glucose tolerance (IGT), and frank diabetes especially if large for gestational age and born to obese mothers. In a Canadian cohort of children exposed to GDM, 7% had IGT at age 7–11 years.[17] In the Pima Indian population, as many as 70% of offspring exposed to diabetes in utero had T2D at age 25–35 years.[18] Breastfeeding may lower the risk.[19] The need for increased surveillance of these children requires further study.

CONCLUSION

Gestational diabetes affects almost 15–18% pregnancies in India today and the number is fast increasing along with a rise in number of cases of obesity and diabetes. An early diagnosis and prompt management has benefits seen across not one but two generations, i.e. both the mother and her offspring. Though there have been conflicting guidelines and treatment protocols, recent studies have all demonstrated improved maternal and neonatal outcomes with tight glycemic control. Diagnosis can be made using IADPSG criteria with 75-g 2-hour OGTT. Management is multifaceted and involves glucose monitoring, diet, and lifestyle measures as well as pharmacotherapy when needed to maintain adequate glycemic control. As oral drugs are still not approved for use in pregnancy, insulin therapy forms the mainstay of treatment. Delivery should be as close to term as possible. Breastfeeding must be encouraged owing to its beneficial effects in reducing insulin resistance and improving glycemia. Keeping in mind the future risks to both mother and her offspring, lifestyle modification must be impressed and need for regular screening for diabetes must be explained.

REFERENCES

1. International Diabetes Federation. Gestational diabetes. [online] Available from: https://www.idf.org/our-activities/care-prevention/gdm [Accessed October 2018].
2. American Diabetes Association. Diagnosis and classification of diabetes mellitus. Diabetes Care. 2011;34(Suppl 1):S62-9.
3. Barbour LA. Diabetes and pregnancy. In: McDermott MT (Ed). Endocrine Secrets, 6th edition. Philadelphia: Elsevier Saunders; 2013. p. 45.
4. Seshiah V, Balaji V, Balaji MS, et al. Prevalence of gestational diabetes mellitus in South India (Tamil Nadu): a community based study. J Assoc Physicians India. 2008;56:329-33.
5. Seshiah V, Balaji V, Balaji MS, et al. Pregnancy and diabetes scenario around the world: India. Int J Gynaecol Obstet. 2009;104(Suppl 1):S35-8.
6. Macintosh MC, Fleming KM, Bailey JA, et al. Perinatal mortality and congenital anomalies in babies of women with type 1 and type 2 diabetes in England, Wales, and Northern Ireland: population based study. BMJ. 2006;333(7560):177.
7. Lambert K, Germain S. Pre-existing type 1 and type 2 diabetes in pregnancy. Obstet Gynaecol Reprod Med. 2010;20(10):353-8.
8. Barbour LA, McCurdy CE, Hernandez TL, et al. Cellular mechanisms for insulin resistance in normal pregnancy and gestational diabetes. Diabetes Care. 2007;30(Suppl 2):S112-9.
9. Catalano PM, Huston L, Amini SB, et al. Longitudinal changes in glucose metabolism during pregnancy in obese women with normal glucose tolerance and gestational diabetes mellitus. Am J Obstet Gynecol. 1999;180(4):903-916.
10. American Diabetes Association. Management of diabetes in pregnancy-Standards of Medical Care in Diabetes 2018. Diabetes Care. 2018;41 (Suppl 1):S114-9.
11. Seshiah V, Das AK, Balaji V, et al. Diabetes in Pregnancy Study Group. Gestational diabetes mellitus – Guidelines. J Assoc Physicians India. 2006;54:622-8.
12. Maternal Health Division, Ministry of Health & Family Welfare. National Guidelines for Diagnosis and Management of Gestational Diabetes Mellitus, 2015.
13. Tripathi R, Verma D, Gupta VK, et al. Evaluation of 75 g glucose load in non-fasting state [Diabetes in Pregnancy Study group of India (DIPSI)

criteria] as a diagnostic test for gestational diabetes mellitus. Indian J Med Res. 2017;145(2):209-214.
14. Mohan V, Mahalakshmi MM, Bhavadharini B, et al. Comparison of screening for gestational diabetes mellitus by oral glucose tolerance tests done in the non-fasting (random) and fasting states. Acta Diabetol. 2014;51:1007-1013.
15. Reader DM. Medical nutrition therapy and lifestyle interventions. Diabetes Care. 2007;30 (Suppl 2):S188-93.
16. Schaefer-Graf UM, Buchanan TA, Xiang AH, et al. Clinical predictors for a high risk for the development of diabetes mellitus in the early puerperium in women with recent gestational diabetes mellitus. Am J Obstet Gynecol. 2002;186(4):751-6.
17. Malcolm JC, Lawson ML, Gaboury I, et al. Glucose tolerance of offspring of mother with gestational diabetes mellitus in a low-risk population. Diabet Med. 2006;23(5):565-70.
18. Dabelea D, Knowler WC, Pettitt DJ. Effect of diabetes in pregnancy on offspring: follow-up research in the Pima Indians. J Matern Fetal Med. 2000;9(1):83-8.
19. Plagemann A, Harder T, Franke K, et al. Long-term impact of neonatal breastfeeding on body weight and glucose tolerance in children of diabetic mothers. Diabetes Care. 2002;25(1):16-22.

Chapter 69

Diabesity: The Recent Concern

Anil Kumar Virmani

INTRODUCTION

The twin epidemics of obesity and diabetes are threatening the health of society and have recently become a matter of great concern. "Diabesity" is a term coined by the former US Surgeon General, Everett Koop, and is the registered trademark of "Shape Up America". However, its prevalence is also rising in Asians, with an enormous impact on health and economics.

Diabesity is a constellation of signs including abdominal obesity, hypertension, systemic inflammation, dyslipidemia, diabetes and a tendency to form clots. It has an enormous health impact leading to long-term chronic complications of diabetes, reduced quality of life and health-related functioning, and reduced life expectancy. Unfortunately, not only obesity increases the prevalence of diabetes, but it also becomes challenging to treat.

PREVALENCE

The Nurses' Health Study showed that body mass index (BMI) is the most important risk factor for developing diabetes. The relative risk of developing diabetes is 38.8% in women with a BMI of 35 kg/m^2 or higher, and 20.1% for women with BMI of 30–34.9 kg/m^2 as compared to women with BMI of <23 kg/m^2.[1]

As per the National Family Health Survey 3, the obesity (>25 kg/m^2) prevalence in India, in men, is 15.9% and 5.6% in urban and rural areas, and in women, it is 23.5% and 7.2% in urban and rural areas, respectively. It also directly correlates with a higher socioeconomic status.[2]

The Indian Council of Medical Research–India Diabetes study also showed a higher prevalence of both generalized and abdominal obesity in urban areas, especially in Chandigarh, Tamil Nadu, Maharashtra and Jharkhand.[3]

As per the World Health Organization website, in 2016, more than 1.9 billion adults more than 18 years were considered overweight, and of these, more than 600 million were classified as obese.

The rising prevalence of diabetes is parallel to the rising trend of obesity.

DEFINITION OF OBESITY

Obesity is defined as a chronic, relapsing, multifactorial, neurobehavioral disease, wherein an increase in body fat promotes adipose tissue dysfunction and abnormal fat mass physical forces, resulting in adverse metabolic, biomechanical and psychosocial health consequences.[4]

It is basically excessive fat accumulation that poses a risk to health and can be measured by BMI, waist circumference, and body fat distribution. The waist-to-height ratio (cut-off of >0.5) is a better indicator of cardiovascular risk, regardless of age or ethnicity.[5]

Excessive body fat is multifactorial in origin and may be due to genetic or development errors, various infections, endocrinal diseases including hypothalamic injury, drugs, improper nutrition, unfavorable environmental factors, etc. leading to oxidative stress.

Obesity is considered to be an imbalance of energy regulation, resulting from a failure of normal weight and energy regulatory mechanisms leading to an elevated body fat set point.

PATHOPHYSIOLOGY OF OBESITY AND TYPE 2 DIABETES MELLITUS

Obesity has a complex relationship with the insulin resistance leading to hypothalamic inflammation and leptin resistance in the brain, increased lipolysis and macrophage accumulation in the adipose tissue, increased glucose and triacylglyceride production in the liver, decreased efficiency of glucose uptake in the muscle, and decreased β-cell function in the pancreatic cells.

The proatherogenic, prothrombotic, and proinflammatory profile of obesity leads to insulin resistance and increased cardiovascular risk and mortality, thus hindering the management of diabetes.

MANAGEMENT OF DIABESITY

- Goals of management are to improve patients' health, quality of life and body weight and composition along with good glycemic, hypertension and dyslipidemia control
- Detailed history with psychological evaluation is a must
- Evaluation of BMI, waist circumference, glycemic status and related comorbidities and complications and patients' hunger pattern and eating habits
- Routine investigations, endocrinal tests, sleep study
- A structured behavioral change leading to weight loss. A 10% weight loss can lead to the reduction in diabetes-related mortality by 30–40%, glycosylated hemoglobin by 15%, fasting glucose by 30–50%, and total cholesterol by 10%
- Weight loss should be the "Gold Standard" in outcomes of diabesity. In addition to weight loss, maintenance of optimal weight is most challenging
- A healthy, balanced diet with small frequent meals, restriction of total calories and avoidance of unappreciated sources of excessive calories, such as soft drinks and fruit juices. Since, it is often difficult to change lifetime dietary habits, a sympathetic and individualized approach is warranted
- A structured, individualized exercise is recommended with the encouragement of small changes in overall lifestyle
- Avoidance or change of drugs that cause weight gain, especially antidepressants, antipsychotics, anticonvulsants, and antidiabetic drugs, such as insulin, sulfonylureas and glitazones
- Drugs to reduce weight are recommended with BMI >30 kg/m^2 or with BMI >27 kg/m^2 associated with comorbidities. Drugs used are Orlistat, lorcaserin, phentermine/topiramate, naltrexone/bupropion, liraglutide and semaglutide. Lorcaserin, which works by high-affinity binding to 5-hydroxytryptamine 2C receptors in the hypothalamic proopiomelanocortin pathway, has recently shown to be cardio safe, but with a higher rate of hypoglycemia in the CAMELLIA-TIMI 61 trial[6]
- Antidiabetic drugs of choice in diabesity are (1) weight neutral—metformin/dipeptidyl peptidase-4 inhibitors and α-glucosidase inhibitors; (2) weight loss—glucagon-like peptide 1 receptor agonist and sodium-glucose cotransporter 2 inhibitors; and (3) basal insulins preferred to premixed insulins
- Metabolic surgery, such as gastric binding, gastric sleeve, gastric bypass or Roux-en-Y, may be needed and are very effective in altering the "set-point" with systemic physiological changes affecting glucose homeostasis, lipids, hormones, gastrointestinal factors and energy balance
- Obesity treatment success rates are (1) lifestyle modification—1–5% on average; (2) lifestyle + pharmacotherapy—5–15% on average; and (3) lifestyle + surgery—20–40% on average.[7,8]

CONCLUSION

- Diabesity is a rapidly growing epidemic of great concern with enormous impact on morbidity and mortality
- The presence of obesity in a patient with diabetes can hinder both control of diabetes and the obesity management
- Weight reduction through dietary interventions, exercise and pharmacologic therapy is the first and long-lasting step in the management of diabesity
- Bariatric/metabolic surgery may be indicated in selected cases
- Counseling, education and behavioral therapy remain the cornerstone of successful management
- Multidisciplinary approach is the most successful way to manage both conditions.

REFERENCES

1. Hu FB, Manson JE, Stampfer MJ, et al. Diet, lifestyle, and the risk of type 2 diabetes mellitus in women. N Engl J Med. 2001;345(11):790-7.
2. International Institute for Population Sciences (IIPS) and Macro International. National Family Health Survey (NFHS-3), 2005-06, India, vol. I. Mumbai: IIPS; 2007. [online] Available from https://dhsprogram.com/pubs/pdf/frind3/frind3-vol1andvol2.pdf [Accessed September, 2018].
3. Pradeepa R, Anjana RM, Joshi SR, et al.; The ICMR-INDIAB Collaborative Study Group. Prevalence of generalized & abdominal obesity in urban & rural India—the ICMR—INDIAB Study (Phase-I) [ICMR—INDIAB-3]. Indian J Med Res. 2015; 142(2):139-50.
4. Bays HE, Seger JC, Primack C, et al. (2017). Obesity Algorithm 2017. Presented by the American Society of Bariatric Physicians; 2016-2017. [online] Availble from www.obesityalgorithm.org. [Accessed September, 2018].
5. Ashwell M, Gunn P, Gibson S. Waist-to-height ratio is a better screening tool than waist circumference and BMI for adult cardiometabolic risk factors: systematic review and meta-analysis. Obes Rev. 2012;13:275-86.
6. Bohula EA, Wiviott SD, McGuire DK, et al. Cardiovascular safety of lorcaserin in overweight or obese patients. N Engl J Med. 2018;379:1107-17.
7. Mechanic JI, Youdim A, Jones DB, et al. Clinical practice guidelines for the perioperative nutritional, metabolic, and nonsurgical support of the bariatric surgery patient—2013 update: cosponsored by American Association of Clinical Endocrinologists, the Obesity Society, and American Society for Metabolic & Bariatric Surgery. Surg Obes Relat Dis. 2013;9:159-91.
8. Yanovski SZ, Yanovski JA. Long-term drug treatment for obesity: a systematic and clinical review. JAMA. 2014;311:74-86.

Chapter 70

Novel Antiobesity Drugs

Manoj Saluja

INTRODUCTION

Obesity is a multifactorial chronic disease, defined as excessive fat accumulation caused by an imbalance between energy intake and expenditure. Its pathogenesis involves the interaction of genetic, environmental, and behavioral factors. Prevalence of obesity is increasingly globally affecting almost every 10th adult. As per World Health Organization (WHO) report, developing countries exhibit rapidly rising rates of obesity and obesity-related mortality.[1]

According to the latest guidelines, the mainstay of the treatment of obesity is a comprehensive lifestyle intervention consisting of hypocaloric diet, exercise, and behavioral strategies.[2] In individuals with a body mass index (BMI) >30 or those with a BMI ≥27 and at least one obesity-related comorbidity, pharmacotherapy can be considered as an adjunct to achieve the target of at least 5% weight loss and consequent health benefits. The pharmacotherapy of obesity is a field of continuous, strenuous research. Over past decades, a number of antiobesity drugs have been developed with demonstrable efficacy in cell lines, animal models, and humans, but only a few of them could stand the test of time. Currently, marketed pharmacological options for weight loss include orlistat, phentermine/topiramate, bupropion/naltrexone, lorcaserin, and liraglutide in the United States, whereas orlistat, bupropion/naltrexone, and liraglutide are approved for prescription in Europe.

PATHOPHYSIOLOGY OF OBESITY

Before discussing various antiobesity drugs, it is important to have a basic understanding of the pathophysiology of obesity. The arcuate nucleus (ArcN) of the hypothalamus is the key regulatory center of hunger and satiety, receiving signals by several hormones and peptides synthesized mainly by the adipose tissue and gut as shown in Figures 1 and 2.

PROMISING ANTIOBESITY AGENTS WITH FUTURE PERSPECTIVES

Various molecules involved at multiple levels of the brain-gut axis with their specific mode of action offer the potential of generating new drugs. Gut hormones are critical mediators of energy balance resetting and the consequent weight loss after bariatric surgery [particularly the Roux-en-Y gastric bypass (RYGB) and vertical sleeve gastrectomy (VSG)]. These procedures have been shown to enhance meal-stimulated secretion of anorexigenic insulin, peptide tyrosine tyrosine (PYY), and glucagon-like peptide-1 (GLP-1), an effect that is sustained for at least 10 years.[3] Developing drugs mimicking the hormonal–humoral–enteroendocrine milieu induced by the bariatric surgery have been under exploration. A bariatric pharmacotherapy is going to be a reality in future. Antiobesity drugs target different molecules of the energy balance cascade and match the patients' metabolic

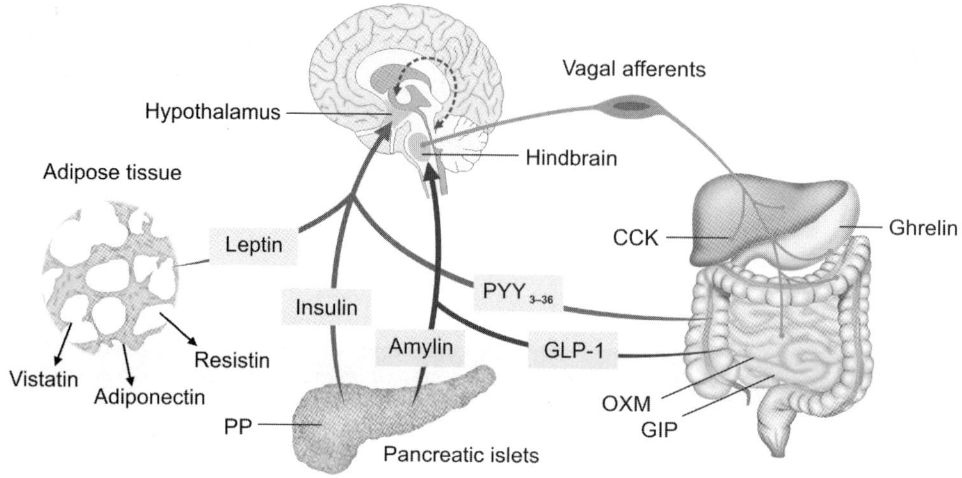

(CCK: cholecystokinin; GI: gastrointestinal; GLP: glucagon-like peptide; OXM: oxyntomodulin; PYY: peptide tyrosine tyrosine; PP: pancreatic polypeptide)

Figure 1 Brain–gut axis in obesity.

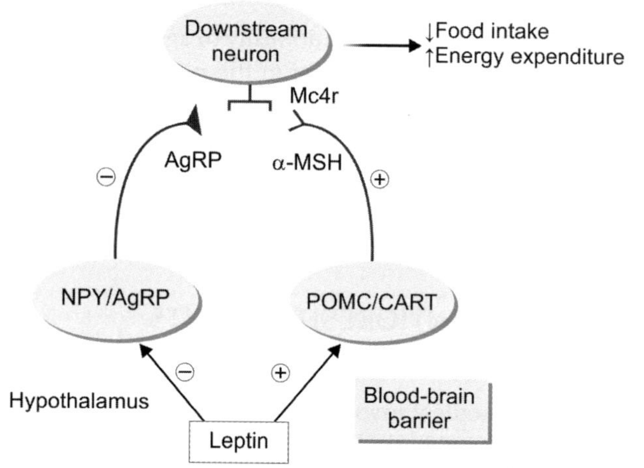

(AgRP: agouti-related peptide; CART: cocaine- and amphetamine-regulated transcript; NPY: neuropeptide Y; POMC: pro-opiomelanocortin).

Figure 2 Hypothalamic control.

needs, thus resulting in a beneficial metabolic profile. The present review covers the current pharmaceutical weight-loss remedies based on data of ongoing clinical trials and experimental studies (Table 1).

TABLE 1: Novel antiobesity agents.

Drug description	Drug
Leptin analog	Metreleptin
Amylin analog	Pramlintide
Amylin analog/amphetamine derivative	Pramlintide/phentermine
GABA inhibitor	Topiramate
Y5 receptor antagonist	Velneperit
Y2/Y4 receptor agonist	Obinepitide
GLP-1 receptor agonist	Lixisenatide
GLP-1 receptor agonist	Albiglutide
GLP-1 receptor agonist	Taspoglutide
GLP-1 receptor agonist/ recombinant human albumin	CJC-1134-PC
GLP-1 analog/PYY$_{3-36}$	NA
Y2 receptor agonist	PYY$_{3-36}$
GLP-1 receptor agonist	Oxyntomodulin
Antighrelin vaccine	NOX-B11

(GABA: gamma-aminobutyric acid; GLP: glucagon-like peptide; PYY: peptide tyrosine tyrosine).

CENTRALLY ACTING ANTIOBESITY DRUGS

Leptin, Leptin Analogs and Leptin Sensitizers

The protein leptin is secreted primarily from the adipose tissue. It stimulates the anorexigenic pro-opiomelanocortin (POMC) neurons and inhibits the orexigenic neuropeptide Y (NPY) neurons in the ArcN. Thus, it promotes satiety and weight loss. Metreleptin, a leptin analog has been under evaluation in various trials. Combined treatment with pramlintide (an amylin analog) and metreleptin has shown significant weight reduction of 12.7% ± 0.9% (11.5 kg ± 0.9 kg) without plateau in obese patients significantly more than treatment with pramlintide alone (8.4%) and this effect was dose- and initial BMI-dependent and sustained throughout.[4]

Subtype-selective Serotonin Receptor Agonists: Lorcaserin

Serotonin [5-hydroxytryptamine (5-HT)] participates in feeding behavior and energy balance modulation. The 5-HT system modulates directly the hypothalamic POMC and NPY networks and thus enhances satiety and causes hypophagia. These effects are mediated by 5-HT2C and 5-HT1B receptors located on hypothalamic POMC and NPY neurons, respectively. Thus, by increasing α-MSH (α-melanocyte-stimulating hormone) and decreasing agouti-related peptide (AgRP) release—it promotes satiety. Activation of the 5-HT1B receptor has been implicated in both primary pulmonary hypertension and valvulopathy,[5] so 5-HT2C receptor subtype has been targeted for therapeutic intervention. The BLOSSOM (Behavioral Modification and Lorcaserin Second Study for Obesity Management), BLOOM (Behavioral Modification and Lorcaserin for Overweight and Obesity Management), and BLOOM-DM (Diabetes Management) showed that 47.2% of patients treated with 10 mg lorcaserin twice daily lost at least 5% of their body weight, compared to 2.5% for placebo. It is to be used with caution in patients with congestive heart failure. It was approved as an addition to diet and exercise chronic management.

Naltrexone-bupropion Combination

An oral, sustained-release combination of dopamine and norepinephrine reuptake antagonist bupropion and the opioid antagonist naltrexone leading to complementary stimulation of central melanocortin pathways, results in increased energy expenditure and reduced appetite.[6] In a double-blind, placebo-controlled study of 1,496 obese or overweight subjects with dyslipidemia, hypertension, or both, weight loss was greater in the combination group than in the placebo at week 28 (6.5% vs. 1.9%, respectively) and week 56 (6.4% vs. 1.2%, respectively) and they showed greater improvements in various cardiometabolic risk markers, quality of life, and eating behavior.

Topiramate

Topiramate is an anticonvulsant/antimigraine agent associated with weight loss. It acts on the orexigenic gamma-aminobutyric acid (GABA) systems, causing appetite suppression. Studies employing different doses of topiramate reported clinically significant weight loss (losses of 7.0%, 9.1%, and 9.7% of patients' baseline body weight for doses of 96, 192, and 256 mg/day, respectively, compared to 1.7% body weight loss in the placebo group), along with improvements in blood pressure and glucose tolerance.[7] Binge eating and bulimia have been successfully treated with topiramate. Higher doses (192 mg/day or more) of topiramate were associated with suicidality, metabolic acidosis, acute myopia, and secondary angle closure glaucoma.

Topiramate-Phentermine Combination

Phentermine is an amphetamine derivative with central anorectic effects. The CONQUER trial has demonstrated the weight-loss efficacy of the new, orally administered controlled release formulation of topiramate/phentermine combination for appetite suppression.[8] The average weight losses were 14.4%, 6.7%, and 2.1% with the higher dose (phentermine 15.0 mg plus topiramate 92.0 mg), lower dose (phentermine 7.5 mg plus topiramate 46.0 mg), and placebo, respectively. The EQUATE study (756 obese subjects) and the EQUIP study (1,267 morbidly obese subjects) have demonstrated that higher doses were associated with depression, anxiety, and sleep disorders, increase in heart rate, amnesia and accentuated disturbances in attention and memory. The combination was approved by Food and Drug Administration (FDA).

Neuropeptide Y Inhibitors

The ArcN NPY neurons inhibit the anorexigenic POMC neurons (via NPY Y1 and Y5 receptors) and promote the release of the orexigenic neuropeptides orexin and melanin-concentrating hormone in the lateral hypothalamic area, promoting food intake.[9] Thus, NPY blockage could be a promising option for obesity management. NPY Y5 receptor antagonists show limited efficacy in weight loss. The combined NPY Y1/Y5 receptor antagonism may be more efficient. The Y2 and Y4 receptors are the targets of the satiety hormones PYY and pancreatic polypeptide (PP), respectively. Two drugs—a Y2/Y4 receptor agonist (obinepitide) and a selective PP Y4 receptor agonist (TM30339)—are under clinical trials with initial promising results.

GASTROINTESTINAL AND PANCREATIC PEPTIDES THAT REGULATE FOOD INTAKE

Lower Intestinal Peptides

The gut-brain axis plays an important role in appetite regulation. Anorexigenic peptides such as gastrin-releasing peptide, cholecystokinin (CCK), PYY, GLP-1, PP, glucagon, and amylin are secreted during feeding, whereas orexigenic peptide ghrelin is secreted before meals and acts to increase hunger and meal initiation. Some of them act directly on brain and other peptides act indirectly by modulating the activity of neurons such as the vagal nerve.

Glucagon-like Peptide-1 Analogs

The GLP-1 is produced primarily by L cells in the distal small intestine and colon. GLP-1 analogs are used in the treatment of diabetes. Currently, Exenatide, lixisenatide, dulaglutide, and liraglutide are in use. These agents contribute to appetite control, leading to weight loss, through vagal and possibly direct central pathways.[10] The GLP-1 receptor R (GLP-1R) is expressed by the gut, pancreas, brainstem, hypothalamus, and vagal-afferent nerves, and is the principle mediator of the anorectic effects of GLP-1.[11] In a randomized, double-blind, placebo-controlled study, liraglutide has shown significant weight loss ($p = 0.003$ for the 1.2-mg liraglutide dose and $p < 0.0001$ for 1.8–3.0-mg liraglutide doses). Mean weight losses with the 1.2-, 1.8-, 2.4-, or 3.0-mg liraglutide doses were 4.8, 5.5, 6.3, and 7.2 kg, respectively. It was approved by FDA for treatment of obesity. The SCALE study demonstrated the efficacy of liraglutide in maintaining weight loss.[12] Some other GLP-1 analogs such as lixisenatide, albiglutide, and taspoglutide are currently under investigation for weight loss. The most common adverse effects are related to gastrointestinal physiology (e.g. nausea, vomiting), occur early in therapy, and usually resolve after 4–8 weeks. With the help of sodium *N*-[8-(2-hydroxybenzoyl) amino]caprylate carrier, an orally administered combination of PYY_{3-36} and GLP-1 has been developed and being evaluated as a novel therapeutic option.[13]

Peptide Tyrosine Tyrosine

It is produced in response and proportionally to caloric load by the distal intestinal L cells. The Bioactive product, PYY_{3-36}, delays gastric emptying and promotes satiety. Short-term intravenous administration of PYY_{3-36} has been shown to decrease caloric intake by approximately 30% in a dose-dependent manner (maximal inhibition, 35%; $p < 0.001$). Antiorexigenic effect of PYY is by Y2 receptor-mediated NPY inhibition thus maximum when injected in fasting state or in the early dark cycle times when NPY secretion is naturally enhanced.[14]

Oxyntomodulin

Produced in the L cells of the distal small intestine and colon, it modulates the energy homeostasis system partly via GLP-1R.[11] Oxyntomodulin (OXM) activates neurons in the hypothalamus. In human studies, intravenously infused OXM acts acutely as an endogenous satiety signal, reducing appetite and food intake as demonstrated in various studies. The combination of OXM and PYY has shown superior effects. The short half-life of OXM limits its clinical application. Analogs with altered pharmacological profile and longer duration of action have good safety profile, lead to body weight reduction, and act favorably on glucose metabolism.

Ghrelin Vaccines and Inhibitors

Ghrelin is the only known potent orexigenic hormone. It is produced by the stomach and proximal small intestine, and its secretion increases before meals and is suppressed by nutrients. Antighrelin vaccine (NOX-B11) has been evaluated in various trials. Antighrelin vaccine-induced antibodies block effect of ghrelin, but this did not show substantial weight loss. The discovery of the main receptor of ghrelin (ghrelin receptor 1a) has resulted in development of potent, selective, and orally bioavailable ghrelin antagonists. Inhibitors of ghrelin O-acyltransferase, the enzyme responsible for octanoylation and its biological activity may potentially prevent or treat obesity.[15]

Pancreatic Peptides

Pancreatic Polypeptide

The PP resembles PYY. PP acting on peripheral and central Y4 and Y5 receptors modulates biliary and exocrine pancreatic function, gastric acid secretion, and GI motility. Initial human studies have shown the anorexigenic effect of a lower infusion rate of PP (5 pmol/kg/min) in lean fasted volunteers. A synthetic analog (TM30338) (obinepitide) of both PYY_{3-36} and PP, an agonist of both the Y2 and Y4 receptors, and a selective Y4 agonist (TM303390) have shown promising results regarding early meal termination and weight loss.[16]

Amylin and Amylin Analogs

Cosecreted postprandially with insulin by pancreatic beta-cells has glucoregulatory and anorexigenic actions through its effect on area postrema in central nervous system (CNS). It inhibits gastric emptying and glucagon secretion and decreases meal size and caloric intake (fat specific) in a dose-dependent manner.[17] Pramlintide is a stable, soluble, nonaggregating, equipotent amylin analog with similar pharmacodynamic and pharmacokinetic profile. Adjunctive pramlintide treatment (120 μg) in patients with T1DM and T2DM shows sustained reductions in food intake and a mild progressive weight loss. Pramlintide is currently approved for the treatment of T1DM and T2DM. Well-designed randomized, double-blind, placebo-controlled studies of nondiabetic individuals showed significant weight loss from baseline (31% vs. 2%). Davalintide is another amylin-mimetic peptide under trials.

Neurohormone Combinations

Amylin treatment has been shown to enhance the hypothalamic anorexigenic signaling of leptin. Combination of amylin and leptin resulted in substantial, synergistic reductions in food intake (up to 45%), and fat-specific weight loss (up to 15%).[4] Their respective analogs, pramlintide and metreleptin, in combination have may hold promise for effective obesity treatment. Combination of amylin and PYY_{3-36} shows synergistic anorexigenic and additive weight-reducing effects.[18]

Prophylactic and Therapeutic Vaccine

Human adenovirus 36 (Ad36) has been found to be associated with higher body weight and fat content. It belongs to serotype D and it is antigenically distinct. High prevalence of anti-adenovirus antibodies has been observed among obese persons of various ethnicities across nations. Ultraviolet-inactivated Ad36 vaccine has been associated with reduced levels of inflammatory cytokines, immune cell in the fat deposits, thus preventing increase in body weight and fat. Anti-Ad36 can prove a prophylaxis against obesity.

CONCLUSION

In spite of decades of intensive research till date expectations of medical management of obesity remain unmet in terms of safety, efficacy, and long-term weight-loss maintenance. The physiology and pathophysiology of appetite regulation and energy balance is complex and reveals the intriguing interrelation of multiple mechanisms. This becomes a reason for limited success of monotherapies. Additionally, the heterogeneity of the obese population along with poor compliance due to unsatisfactory therapeutic goals, random follow-ups, and the unpleasant side effects are greatly responsible for the poor performance of antiobesity drugs.

Future antiobesity pharmacotherapeutics will comprise of molecules with maximal multilevel action (CNS-periphery) and minimal side effects. Further individualization is the cornerstone of appropriate management of obesity. Currently, research is directed toward the development of combinations based on gut hormones that mimic the changes following surgically induced weight loss. Interestingly, skepticism about the unacceptable health risks of bariatric surgery and the fact that the desired result is critically mediated by gut hormonal signals has changed the scenario in favor of medical antiobesity options. Future ideal antiobesity pharmacotherapy would be a much more advanced version of bariatric medicine, in which gut hormones would interact synergistically and in a complementary mode to induce lipolysis, enhance energy expenditure, and restore disruptions of the energy homeostasis system without affecting basic systemic functions (e.g., reproduction, neurobehavioral functions). Further the genetics of obesity is a new and exciting field of exploration. Genome-wide association studies (GWAS) has accelerated the progress of polygenic obesity research. A better understanding of these pathways will lead to novel drug targets and effective prevention strategies.

REFERENCES

1. Hamdy O, Uwaifo GI, Oral EA. (2011). Obesity. NewYork: Medscape Drugs Dis. [online] Available from http://emedicine.medscape.com/article/123702-overview. [Accessed October, 2018].
2. Jensen MD, Ryan DH, Apovian CM, et al. 2013 AHA/ACC/TOS guideline for the management of overweight and obesity in adults: a report of the American College of Cardiology/American Heart Association/Task Force on Practice Guidelines and The Obesity Society. Circulation. 2014;129(25 Suppl. 2):102-38.
3. Dar MS, Chapman WHIII, Pender JR, et al. GLP-1 response to amixed meal: What happens 10 years after Roux-en-Y gastric bypass (RYGB). Obes Surg. 2012;22(7):1077-83.
4. Roth JD, Roland BL, Cole RL, et al. Leptin responsiveness restored by amylin agonism in diet-induced obesity: evidence from nonclinical and clinical studies. Proc Natl Acad Sci USA. 2008;105(20):7257-62.
5. Launay JM, Herv'e P, Tournois C, et al. Function of the serotonin 5-hydroxytryptamine 2B receptor in pulmonary hypertension. Nat Med. 2002;8(10):1129-35.

6. Padwal R. Contrave, a bupropion and naltrexone combination therapy for the potential treatment of obesity. Curr Opin Investig Drugs. 2009;10(10):1117-25.
7. Wilding J, Van Gaal L, Rissanen A, et al. A randomized double-blind placebo-controlled study of the long-term efficacy and safety of topiramate in the treatment of obese subjects. Int J Obes. 2004;28:1399-410.
8. Gadde KM, Allison DB, Ryan DH, et al. Effects of low-dose, controlled release, phentermine plus topiramate combination on weight and associated comorbidities in overweight and obese adults (CONQUER): a randomized, placebo-controlled, phase 3 trial. Lancet. 2011;377:1341-52.
9. Broberger C, Landry M, Wong H, et al. Subtypes Y1 and Y2 of the neuropeptide Y receptor are respectively expressed in pro-opiomelanocortin and neuropeptide Y containing neurons of the rat hypothalamic arcuate nucleus. Neuroendocrinology. 1997;66:393-408.
10. Abbot CR, Monteiro M, Small CJ, et al. The inhibitory effects of peripheral administration of peptide YY3–36 and glucagon-like peptide-1 on food intake are attenuated by ablation of the vagal–brainstem–hypothalamic pathway. Brain Res. 2005;1044:127-31.
11. Baggio LL, Huang Q, Brown TJ, et al. Oxyntomodulin and glucagon-like peptide-1 differentially regulate murine food intake and energy expenditure. Gastroenterology. 2004;127:546-58.
12. Wadden TA, Hollander P, Klein S, et al. Weight maintenance and additional weight loss with liraglutide after low-calorie-diet-induced weight loss: the SCALE Maintenance randomized study. Int J Obes. 2013;37:1443-51.
13. Steinert RE, Poller B, Castelli MC, et al. Oral administration of glucagon-like peptide 1 or peptide YY 3–36 affects food intake in healthy male subjects. Am J Clin Nutr. 2010;92:810-7.
14. Batterham RL, Cowley MA, Small CJ, et al. Gut hormone PY3–36 physiologically inhibits food intake. Nature. 2002;418:650-4.
15. Yang J, Zhao TJ, Goldstein JL, et al. Inhibition of ghrelin O-acyltransferase (GOAT) by octanoylated pentapeptides. Proc Natl Acad Sci USA. 2008;105:10750-55.
16. 7TM Pharma. (2007). 7TM Pharma obtains patent protection for the use of both obinepitide and TM30339 in the treatment of obesity. [online] Available from http://www.patentdocs.org/2007/07/7tm-pharma-obta.html. [Accessed October, 2018].
17. Roth JD, Anderson C. Anti-obesity effects of the β-cell hormone amylin in diet-induced obese rats: effects on food intake, body weight, composition, energy expenditure and gene expression. Endocrinology. 2006;147:5855-64.
18. Roth JD, Coffey T, Jodka CM, et al. Combination therapy with amylin and peptide YY[3–36] in obese rodents: anorexigenic synergy and weight loss additivity. Endocrinology. 2007;148:6054-61.

Chapter 71

Obesity Management: Surgical Knife or Drugs and Lifestyle?

Neeta Deshpande

INTRODUCTION

The epidemic of obesity shows no signs of ebbing worldwide. On the contrary, there is an alarming increasing trend that threatens to explode into a pandemic of several related metabolic disorders. Diabetes and macrovascular complications, nonalcoholic fatty liver disease (NAFLD) and its consequences, malignancies, hormonal disorders such as polycystic ovarian disease are but a few conditions that have their roots in obesity. It is well known that the successful prevention/treatment of obesity is far more beneficial than the treatment of the individual disorders mentioned above.

Unfortunately, the management of obesity, whatever the clinical setting, has been far from successful, for a variety of reasons. Lifestyle modification (LSM), the backbone of obesity management, is ill understood by even healthcare professionals,[1] difficult to follow for long periods and mired in controversy as several stakeholders, not all of them qualified or knowledgeable enough have entered the fray of nutrition and dietetics. Historically, drugs for treatment of obesity have been more controversial than useful. Several agents that were introduced had to be withdrawn on account of unacceptable adverse events. Additionally, the weight loss is maintained only for as long as the agent is being administered, making the therapy practically lifelong, which is not feasible. The quantum of weight loss achieved with these agents has not been very impressive. Bariatric surgery, supposedly the final option, is being advocated nowadays, especially for morbid obesity. This is perhaps the only option that offers huge weight loss, relatively quickly and at the same time ameliorating most comorbid conditions. However, it comes with its attendant flaws such as operative complications, nutritional deficiency, weight regain, etc.

Lifestyle modification, pharmacotherapy and bariatric surgery all have an evidence base to support their use. It is imperative that healthcare professionals familiarize themselves with the various modalities available to treat obesity and to weigh the risks versus benefits of choosing one option over the other. Obviously, one size does not fit all. The therapy in any particular patient is dictated by several considerations such as the behavioral patterns, weight loss target, cost of therapy, adherence, compliance to follow-up, family support, etc.

LIFESTYLE MODIFICATION

Lifelong LSM is the key to achieve weight loss and its long-term maintenance. Regardless of other therapies chosen, LSM has to be practiced alongside. It basically comprises diet therapy, physical activity and behavioral therapy.

Diet Therapy

There are two aspects under consideration in diet therapy for obesity. The first is calorie restriction and second is the macronutrient composition of the diet. There is general consensus and sufficient evidence that caloric restriction results in varying degrees of weight loss. There is no mathematical equation of the quantum of weight loss that can be achieved with a specific caloric deficit, as several other factors such as metabolic rate, age, sex, skeletal muscle mass, etc. influence weight loss. Nevertheless, caloric restriction underlies almost all types of diets designed for weight loss. Low-calorie diets (LCD) and very low-calorie diets (VLCD) have been effective in causing substantial weight loss.

The concept of macronutrient composition for weight loss diets has undergone several paradigm shifts over the last few decades. Low-fat diets are slowly being contested in favor of low-carbohydrate diets. Low-carbohydrate diets, by default, are either high protein or high fat or both. Several meta-analyses show that all these diets have data in their favor, giving rise to varying degrees of weight loss. However, what distinguish the different diets are factors such as ease of use, acceptability, tolerability, costs, adherence, long-term effects, metabolic effects and durability of weight loss. Different diets such as Atkins, Mediterranean, Paleo, ketogenic diets, etc. have all got evidence in their favor. Each has its own merits and demerits. Therefore, customized diets work best.

Physical Activity

Although physical activity alone is never enough to result in weight loss, it has a pivotal role to play in the maintenance period after weight loss has been achieved. The other benefits of physical activity include a sense of well-being, motivation, improved stamina, cardiovascular (CV) fitness, better joint mobility and flexibility, improved metabolic parameters and a better quality of life. However, motivating patients to get physically active and engage in structured exercise programs on a long-term basis is a difficult task. There are several barriers including comorbid conditions and musculoskeletal restrictions imposed by obesity itself. An important form exercise, strength training, is often ignored.

PHARMACOTHERAPY

Pharmacotherapy can be a good supplementary therapy to diet and physical activity. Guidelines advocate use of pharmacotherapy when the BMI (body mass index) >30 or when it is >27 with at least one obesity-related comorbid state.[2] Pharmacotherapy of obesity has always shown less than satisfactory results when used without proper adjunctive LSM. In fact, the placebo-subtracted weight loss with the approved agents is not >5 kg.[3] Several agents in the past had to be withdrawn on account of various side effects. The few that are available now result in very modest weight loss and need to be administered on a long-term basis. Liraglutide, a glucagon-like peptide (GLP)-1 receptor agonist and an antidiabetic agent has now been approved in some countries for use as an antiobesity agent, at a dose of 3 mg/day.[4] The efficacy is proven and the cognitive and psychological adverse events seen with earlier drugs are not there. Additionally, in the obese diabetic, liraglutide reduces death from CV causes.[4] However, it is not yet approved for treatment of obesity in India. Currently, the only available antiobesity drug is the lipase inhibitor (Orlistat). The efficacy and tolerability are both very modest. Around the world, some other drugs have been approved. Most of these are centrally acting. Lorcaserin is a combination of topiramate and phentermine. But the long-term use of these drugs has to be under strict medical monitoring due to psychological and cognitive side effects. The same is true of another combination—that of bupropion and naltrexone. However, not all patients respond uniformly to these drugs. The response in the first 3–4 months is predictive. On account of the less than modest weight loss, costs, adverse events and the need for long-term use, antiobesity drugs are not used as much as would be expected as per what the guidelines suggest.

BARIATRIC SURGERY

Weight loss surgery is today used interchangeably with metabolic surgery owing to all the metabolic benefits that ensue. What started off as treatment for weight loss has today found its way into guidelines as a valid treatment for type 2 diabetes.[5] There is observational data that it reduces all-cause mortality.[6] Various studies have reported losses of 15–30% weight loss from baseline. There are several procedures that qualify as bariatric surgery. There are restrictive procedures and malabsorptive procedures and some combined. The gastric bypass (Roux-en-Y), vertical sleeve gastrectomy and gastric banding are the usual procedures practiced worldwide. The quantum of weight loss in all these procedures is huge.[7] Therefore, it is often used as the treatment of choice in severe obesity. There is still controversy over whether it should be the method of choice in lesser degrees of obesity. The procedures themselves, although very refined in today's time, are still not entirely without risk.[8] Besides, there is a need for lifelong supplements and vigilance, especially after malabsorptive procedures. There are other long-term complications after surgery that one has to be prepared for. The most distressing among them is weight regain. Approximately, there is a regain of 5–10% of weight at the end of 10 years postsurgery.

CHOICE OF THERAPY

Although guidelines are available,[9,10] the choice of therapy often needs to be individualized. Several factors need to be considered. The target weight loss, presence of comorbid conditions, cost of therapy, ease of administration, expected adherence, etc. In any case, LSM takes precedence, not only because any other modalities do not work without it, but also because it practically carries no risk.[11] Lifestyle measures have never really been given their due. Both physician and patient factors are responsible for this. There is robust evidence in recent times that certain diets can result in >10% weight loss. That being the case, LSM would certainly be the preference as first line and perhaps the only line of treatment. Supplementation with pharmacotherapy in selected cases may be required, especially to speed up weight loss and to treat minor relapses. Therefore, a judicious combination of LSM and appropriate pharmacotherapy may obviate the need for surgery in most cases. This approach, if administered by efficient healthcare personnel, followed-up carefully, would be the best approach. The Look AHEAD trial,[12] the DiRECT trial,[13] and the Diabetes Prevention Program (DPP)[14] have provided ample proof that structured advice for nutrition and physical activity can result in substantial weight loss. Although weight regain is common after a lifestyle program, there is evidence to show that it can be sustained, if there is regular contact and support from healthcare professionals.

On the other hand, bariatric surgery, although having impressive results in terms of weight loss and resolution of metabolic disorders, cannot yet be recommended as first-line therapy in any patient. Both short-term and long-term risks of surgery make it an option only after other attempts have failed. It does have a place, but in failed attempts at LSM that have been explored fully. It also seems to be imperative in cases of severe obesity, where LSM alone may not be able to reach the goal of weight loss. Severe comorbid conditions such as uncontrolled diabetes, obstructive sleep apnea and fatty liver disease will resolve very well with bariatric surgery.[15]

Whatever be the modality of treatment used, behavior counseling is of utmost importance to ensure adherence to the given therapy, which in turn ensures long-term weight maintenance.[11]

CONCLUSION

Obesity is a global pandemic. Healthcare professionals need to equip themselves with the current trends in scientific management of weight loss. While pharmacotherapy and bariatric surgery are options in specific indications, lifestyle change remains the cornerstone of therapy. There are several different diets to choose from. But the one that works best long term is the one that one adheres to. Pharmacotherapy is underused for a variety of reasons. It can be a useful adjunct to LSM. Appropriate nutrition, physical activity and healthful behaviors need to be practiced lifelong to maintain weight and prevent obesity. Bariatric surgery offers the largest weight loss. However, it is best reserved for specific indications, after appropriate attempts at LSM and pharmacotherapy. Behavioral counseling is an integral part of any obesity management plan.

REFERENCES

1. Antognoli EL, Seeholzer EL, Gullett H, et al. Primary care resident training for obesity, nutrition, and physical activity counseling: a mixed-methods study. Health Promot Pract. 2017;18(5):672-80.
2. Apovian CM, Aronne LJ, Bessesen DH, et al. Pharmacological management of obesity: an Endocrine Society clinical practice guideline. J Clin Endocrinol Metab. 2015;100:342-62.
3. Khera R, Murad MH, Chandar AK, et al. Association of pharmacological treatments for obesity with weight loss and adverse events: a systematic review and meta-analysis. JAMA. 2016;315:2424-34.
4. Pi-Sunyer X, Astrup A, Fujioka K, et al. A randomized, controlled trial of 3.0 mg of liraglutide in weight management. N Engl J Med. 2015;373(1):11-22.
5. Courcoulas AP, Belle SH, Neiberg RH, et al. Three-year outcomes of bariatric surgery vs. lifestyle intervention for type 2 diabetes mellitus treatment: a randomized clinical trial. JAMA Surg. 2015;150:931-40.
6. Sjöström L, Narbro K, Sjöström CD, et al. Effects of bariatric surgery on mortality in Swedish obese subjects. N Engl J Med. 2007;357:741-52.
7. Bray GA, Frühbeck G, Ryan DH, et al. Management of obesity. Lancet. 2016;387(10031):1947-56.
8. O'Brien P. Surgical treatment of obesity. In: De Groot LJ, Chrousos G, Dungan K et al. (Eds). Endotext. South Dartmouth, MA: MDText.com; 2016.
9. Garvey WT, Mechanick JI, Brett EM, et al. American Association of Clinical Endocrinologists and American College of Endocrinology comprehensive clinical practice guidelines for medical care of patients with obesity. Endocr Pract. 2016;22:Suppl 3:1-203.
10. Canadian Obesity Network. (2016). 5As Team project. [online] Available from https://obesitycanada.ca/5as-team/. [Accessed October, 2018].
11. American College of Cardiology/American Heart Association Task Force on Practice Guidelines, Obesity Expert Panel, 2013. Expert Panel Report: guidelines (2013) for the management of overweight and obesity in adults. Obesity (Silver Spring). 2014;22:Suppl 2:S41-410.
12. The Look AHEAD Research Group, Pi-Sunyer X, Blackburn G, et al. Reduction in weight and cardiovascular disease risk factors in individuals with type 2 diabetes: one-year results of the look AHEAD trial. Diabetes Care. 2007;30:1374-83.
13. Lean ME, Leslie WS, Barnes AC, et al. Primary care-led weight management for remission of type 2 diabetes (DiRECT): an open-label, cluster-randomised trial. Lancet. 391(10120):541-51.
14. Diabetes Prevention Program Research Group. Reduction in the incidence of type 2 diabetes with lifestyle intervention or metformin. N Engl J Med. 2002;346:393-403.
15. Ikramuddin S, Billington CJ, Lee WJ, et al. Roux-en-Y gastric bypass for diabetes (the Diabetes Surgery Study): 2-year outcomes of a 5-year, randomised, controlled trial. Lancet Diabetes Endocrinol. 2015;3:413-22.

Chapter 72

Use of Fibrates in the Metabolic Syndrome and Diabetics: Practical Tips

Sudarshan Ramachandran, Mithun Bhartia, Alan Jones, Richard Charles Strange

INTRODUCTION

Cardiovascular disease (CVD), a cause of mortality worldwide, accounted for 28% of the UK deaths in 2012.[1] Risk reduction is based on improving modifiable risk factors with lipid-lowering therapy being particularly useful.[2] Because of the importance of reducing serum low-density lipoprotein cholesterol (LDL-C), statins remain an effective way of reducing CVD risk.[2] However, despite statin use, there remains a high residual CVD risk, due perhaps to other risk-associated lipoproteins.[3] Fibrates may be useful in targeting these atherogenic lipoproteins, especially in type 2 diabetes mellitus (T2DM) and the metabolic syndrome (MetS).[4] We describe evidence of the usefulness of fibrates, identify patient groups who may benefit from their use, outline factors to be monitored during follow-up, and describe effective holistic treatment of an anonymized clinic case.

Fibrates activate the peroxisome proliferator-activated receptor (PPAR)-α which, by upregulating transcription of various proteins associated with lipid metabolism, influences fatty acid and lipoprotein metabolism in hepatic, muscle, and renal tissues.[5] This results in a variable increase in high-density lipoprotein cholesterol (HDL-C), a greater reduction in triglycerides (TGs) levels, and a modest decrease in LDL-C.[4,5]

MACROVASCULAR OUTCOMES: A SUMMARY OF CURRENT EVIDENCE FROM RANDOMIZED CONTROLLED TRIALS

A timeline of statin, ezetimibe and proprotein convertase subtilisin/kexin type 9 (PCSK9) inhibitor, and fibrate randomized controlled trials (RCTs) is interesting. Since 1994, successive statin, ezetimibe and PCSK9 inhibitors RCTs have given rise to the largely accepted LDL hypothesis.[6] In contrast, after significant CVD risk reduction with gemfibrozil treatment in the Helsinki Heart Study (HHS) and Veterans Affairs High-Density Lipoprotein Cholesterol Intervention Trial (VA-HIT), evidence for the usefulness of fibrate therapy has diminished;[4] three nongemfibrozil studies [Bezafibrate Infarction Prevention (BIP) study, Fenofibrate Intervention and Event Lowering in Diabetes (FIELD), and Action to Control Cardiovascular Risk in Diabetes (ACCORD-LIPID)] failed to achieve their primary outcomes.[4] Interestingly, the Diabetes Atherosclerosis Intervention Study, with atherosclerosis progression on angiogram as the primary outcome (not clinical end points) in individuals with T2DM, showed a slower rate of atherosclerosis progression.[7]

Thus, fibrate RCT outcomes vary, and doubts remain whether these agents are useful. However, the RCTs have used varying inclusion criteria, and it is possible that a subgroup of individuals may benefit from fibrate use.

MACROVASCULAR OUTCOMES: SUMMARY OF CURRENT EVIDENCE FROM SUBGROUP AND META-ANALYSES

Subgroup analysis of patients in the HHS with elevated TG and reduced HDL-C showed greater relative risk reduction than in the remaining cohort.[8] This suggests that fibrate therapy may benefit particularly patients with atherogenic dyslipidemia characterizing the MetS. Bruckert et al. analyzed individuals with HDL-C, and

TG values closest to those of atherogenic dyslipidemia; HDL-C <0.91 mmol/L (35 mg/dL) and TG >2.2 mmol/L (195 mg/dL) in the five major fibrate RCTs (HHS, VAHIT, BIP, FIELD, and ACCORD-LIPID).[9] These characteristics were found in 11–33% of the total cohorts, and a significant reduction in CVD of 28% was observed. Importantly, the complementary group demonstrated only a nonsignificant 6% reduction in risk.[4,9] A meta-analysis of fibrates trials carried out by Jun et al. included 18 RCTs comprising 45,058 individuals with outcomes including major CV events, coronary events, coronary revascularization, stroke, heart failure, CV deaths, new-onset albuminuria and adverse effects due to the drugs.[10] Significant decreases were observed in major CV events. No significant change in mortality was apparent. Subgroup analysis demonstrated a greater effect in trials with higher mean TG levels.[10] Clearly, there are limitations in interpreting the analysis of subgroup data, not least the lack of power to detect the heterogeneity of treatment effects, and a further RCT designed to include narrower inclusion criteria would be valuable.

MICROVASCULAR OUTCOMES: SUMMARY OF EVIDENCE

The first RCT demonstrating microvascular benefit from fibrates was the FIELD study; a significant reduction in the rate of progression of albuminuria was noted with albuminuria often improving in those on fenofibrate.[11] Following washout, the benefit was maintained 5 years later. Similarly, microalbuminuria/macroalbuminuria development was reduced by fenofibrate in the ACCORD-LIPID, the microvascular benefit also extending to retinopathy.[12] In the FIELD study, there was a decrease in laser therapy in those on fenofibrate.[13]

Who should be Treated with Fibrates?

The National Institute for Health and Care Excellence lipid modification guidelines issued in 2014 do not recommend fibrates for primary/secondary prevention, chronic kidney disease, and T2DM/type 1 diabetes.[2] It states that fibrates may be considered in mixed dyslipidemia/hypertriglyceridemia, especially in individuals with TG between 4.5 and 9.9 mmol/L, as statin trials usually recruited subjects with TG <4.5 mmol/L.

The role of HDL-C as a CVD risk predictor is not well established. The Framingham Heart Study showed an inverse relationship between HDL-C and CVD.[14] In contrast, the Dallas Heart Study demonstrated that cholesterol efflux, not HDL-C, was associated with CVD.[15] Further, RCTs with niacin and cholesteryl ester transfer protein (CETP) inhibitors, both HDL-C raising agents did not show CVD benefits.[16,17] In contrast, in the Investigation of Lipid Level Management to Understand its Impact in Atherosclerotic Events (ILLUMINATE) study, torcetrapib, a CETP inhibitor increased HDL-C by 72.1% but significantly increased CVD and mortality.[17] Anacetrapib, another CETP inhibitor, was associated with a small but significant effect on CVD events, but this appeared to be due to lowering of non-HDL-C rather than doubling of HDL-C.[18]

Thus, in our view, fibrates should be considered solely as TG-reducing agents. Fibrate therapy in patients with TG >4.5 mmol/L after lifestyle advice can be justified, though a lowering of this threshold to 2.2 mmol/L could be accepted.

What can We Expect Following Fibrate Therapy?

We now consider observations made in our outpatient setting (Table 1). The changes observed in total cholesterol (TC), TG, and non-HDL-C following fibrates were associated with baseline values (greater decrease in patients with higher baseline values) and statistically significant in all subgroups. Treatment duration was not associated with response. The greatest change was in TG levels, but as expected TC and non-HDL-C levels also did improve. We believe fibrates should not be used to raise HDL-C. As previously reported, HDL-C change was variable; statin treatment, T2DM, and smoking appeared to blunt any increase in HDL-C.[19] Fenofibrate was the commonest fibrate used (~75%) with bezafibrate used in the remaining patients barring one on ciprofibrate (we avoided gemfibrozil as it could not be used with a statin). We have previously reported improvements in the liver function tests suggesting that it may be due to improvements in nonalcoholic fatty liver disease.

CLINICAL MONITORING FOLLOWING FIBRATE THERAPY

The FIELD study confirmed an increase in creatinine levels [an estimated glomerular filtration rate (eGFR) decrease] that was reversible on fibrate discontinuation.[13] Clinically, this is important, as a lower eGFR could lead to withdrawal of metformin, incretins, and sodium glucose

TABLE 1: Pre- and postfibrate lipid values observed in our practice.

	Mean lipid values/SD							
	Prefibrate TC	Postfibrate TC	Prefibrate TG	Postfibrate TG	Prefibrate HDL-C	Postfibrate HDL-C	Prefibrate non HDL-C	Post fibrate non HDL-C
Total group	6.8/2.5 (n = 242)	5.5/1.4 (p <0.0001)	8.0/7.7 (n = 241)	3.8/4.0 (p <0.0001)	1.1/0.4 (n = 204)	1.2/0.4 (p = 0.03)	5.5/2.0 (n = 204)	4.3/1.3 (p <0.0001)
Males	6.8/2. 7 (n = 176)	5.6/1.5 (p <0.0001)	8.8/8.7 (n = 175)	4.1/4.6 (p <0.0001)	1.1/0.3 (n = 149)	1.1/0.3 (p = 0.16)	5.4/2.0 (n = 149)	4.4/1.3 (p <0.0001)
Females	7.0/2.1 (n = 66)	5.5/1.2 (p <0.0001)	5.9/3.8 (n = 66)	2.9/1.6 (p <0.0001)	1.3/0.41 (n = 55)	1.3/0.5 (p = 0.07)	6.0/4.0 (n = 55)	4.0/1.3 (p <0.0001)
T2DM	6.7/2.6 (n = 79)	5.5/1.8 (p <0.0001)	8.9/8.8 (n = 78)	4.7/5.7 (p <0.0001)	1.1/0.4 (n = 64)	1.0 I 0.3 (p = 0.19)	5.2/1.6 (n = 64)	4.2/1.5 (p <0 0001)
No T2DM	6.9/2.5 (n = 162)	5.6/1.2 (p <00001)	7.6/7.3 (n = 162)	33/2 8 (p<00001)	1.1/0.4 (n = 139)	1.2/0.4 (p = 0.0002)	57/2.1 (n = 139)	4.3/1.2 (p <0 0001)
On statins	6.4/2.5 (n = 127)	5.4/1.4 (p <0.0001)	7.9/8.3 (n = 126)	3.7/4.2 (p <0.0001)	1.1/0.4 (n = 100)	1.1 I 0.4 (p = 0.63)	5.1/1 6 (n = 100)	4.1/1.2 (p <0 0001)
Not on statins	7.3/5.7 (n = 115)	5.7/1.4 (p <0.0001)	8.3/7.2 (n = 115)	3.8/3.8 (p <0.0001)	1.1/0.3 (n = 104)	1.2/0.3 (p = 0.017)	6.0/2.3 (n = 104)	4.4/1.3 (p <0.0001)
Current smokers	6.1/1.7 (n = 47)	5.5/1.4 (p = 0.037)	7.5/5.4 (n = 47)	4.3/4.6 (p = 0.0006)	1.0/0.3 (n = 41)	1.0 I 0.3 (p = 0.57)	5.1/1.6 (n = 41)	4.5/4.5 (p = 0.034)
Ex-/ nonsmoker	7.0/2.7 (n = 179)	5.6/1.4 (p <0.0001)	8.3/8.5 (n = 178)	3.7/4.0 (p <0.0001)	1.1/0.3 (n = 149)	1.2/0.4 (p = 0.023)	5.6/2.0 (n = 149)	4.3/1.3 (p <0.0001)
Alcohol: 0 units/week	6.8/2.5 (n = 57)	5.2/1.4 (p <0.0001)	8.0/6. 7 (n = 57)	3.4/2. 7 (p <0.0001)	1.0/0.4 (n = 49)	1.1/0.3 (p = 0.56)	5.3/1. 7 (n = 49)	3.9/1.15 (p <0.0001)
Alcohol: 1-28 units/week	6.8/2.4 (n = 115)	5.6/1.4 (p <0.0001)	7.4/6.3 (n = 11 4)	3.7/4.2 (p <0.0001)	1.1/0.4 (n = 97)	1.2/0.4 (n = 0.11)	5.8/2.4 (n = 97)	4.4/1.4 (p <0.0001)
Alcohol: >28 units/week	7.3/3.2 (n = 46)	5.7/1.1 (p = 0.0028)	10.2/11.2 (n = 46)	3.8/2.7 (p = 0.0005)	1.1/0.3 (n = 37)	1.2/0.4 (p = 0.42)	5.5/1.4 (n = 37)	4.5/1.0 (p <0.0001)

(HDL-C: high-density lipoprotein cholesterol; T2DM: type 2 diabetes mellitus; TG: triglyceride; TC: total cholesterol.)

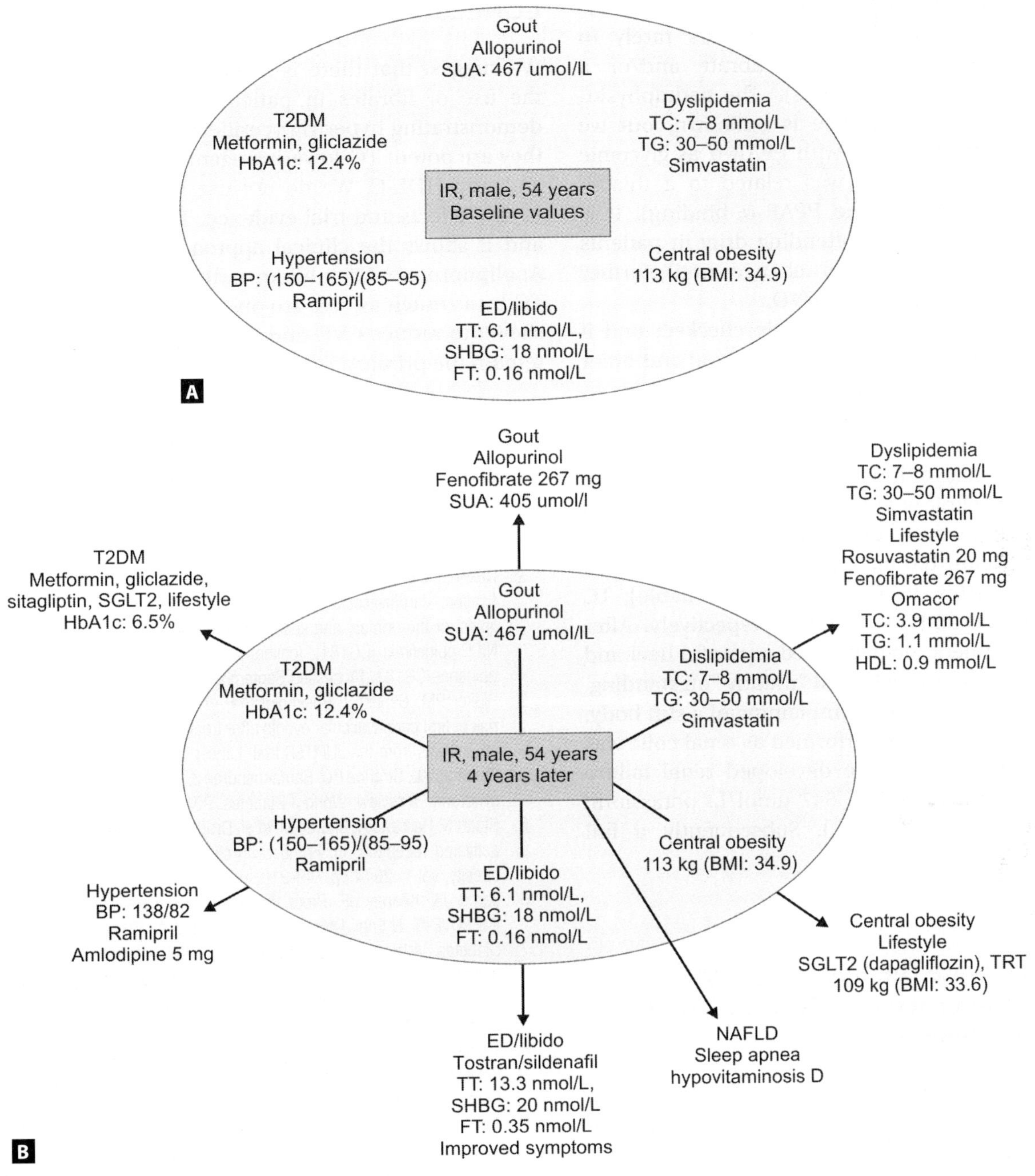

(ED: Erectile dysfunction, NAFLD: Nonalcoholic fatty liver disease; T2DM: type 2 diabetes mellitus; TG: triglyceride; TC: total cholesterol; BP: blood pressure; SGLT2: sodium-glucose cotransporter-2; SHBG: sex hormone binding globulin; IR: insulin resistance.).

Figure 1 (A) Details of patient IR when referred to the metabolic/diabetes clinic. (B) Details of patient IR 3 postreferral (~4 years). Treatment and metabolic parameters after 4 years of holistic care is presented together with details at initial consultation.

transporter 2 inhibitors in T2DM. We identified patients where hypercreatininemia was more likely male gender, lower baseline creatinine concentrations, nondiabetics, and greater decrease in TG levels. In our experience, it is worth commencing a lower dose of the fibrate after 2–3 months of washout or switching to a different fibrate.

A phenomenon termed paradoxical HDL-C decrease (defined by us as >50% decrease) occurs rarely in individuals treated with either a fibrate and/or a thiazolidinedione (PPAR-γ agonists).[4] The pathophysiology of this unusual occurrence is unknown, but we suggested that it is associated with PPAR-α as glycemic control improved when this was related to a thiazolidinedione (which have some PPAR-α binding). It is advisable to discontinue the offending drug in patients demonstrating this paradoxical change until further clarity is available on HDL-C and CVD.

Creatinine kinase (CK) is routinely checked; and if the value is 5 times the upper limit of normal and other causes (strenuous activity, muscular causes, and hypothyroidism) discounted, we would consider stopping the fibrate. The following case demonstrates the need for vigilance.[20] A 29-year-old man with type 3 dyslipidemia attended the lipid clinic with TC and TG values of 14.8 and 6.86 mmol/L, respectively. Following lifestyle advice, he received ciprofibrate 100 mg daily which was increased to 200 mg daily (this dose is no longer available); TC and TG fell to 6.6 and 1.9 mmol/L, respectively. After 6 months of treatment, he developed a painful heel and started ibuprofen; his urine turned "muddy" on standing, and he presented to hospital complaining of a stiff body. Intravenous urography was performed as renal colic was suspected. Two days later, he developed renal failure (urea: 23 mmol/L, creatinine: 647 μmol/L, potassium: 6.2 mmol/L, CK: 13,740 IU/L). Subsequently a full recovery was made.

CASE REPORT

Where does Fibrate Therapy Fit in with Clustering of Risk Factors in Type 2 Diabetes and Metabolic Syndrome?

We end by illustrating that fibrates in T2DM/MetS must be considered in combination with other treatments due to the clustering of CVD risk factors in these states. Mr IR, who had become increasingly demotivated, was referred to the diabetes clinic. He had issues with virtually all factors associated with the MetS (Fig. 1A). We decided that we needed to improve motivation and compliance; hence, lifestyle advice and fenofibrate were the first line of action. Improvement was noted within 3 months (TG decrease: 50–12 mmol/L), and then all other areas were addressed. The improvement is clear (Fig. 1B) and illustrates the importance of a holistic approach.

CONCLUSION

We suggest that there is sufficient evidence to support the use of fibrates in patients with T2DM and MetS demonstrating hypertriglyceridemia. Our data show that they are potent TG-lowering agents, which also lower TC and non-HDL-C. We do not use nicotinic acid in view of side effects and trial evidence. The case in Figures 1A and B shows the clinical approach should be holistic. Apolipoprotein C3 inhibitors that promise to decrease TG by as much as 75% are on the horizon. Until they are shown to reduce CVD and be cost-effective, fibrates will remain the primary TG-reducing agents.

REFERENCES

1. British Heart Foundation. Cardiovascular disease statistics 2014. Oxford, United Kingdom: British Heart Foundation Centre on Population Approaches for Non-Communicable Disease Prevention, Nuffield Department of Population Health, University of Oxford; 2014.
2. National Institute for Health and Care Excellence. (2014). Lipid modification: cardiovascular risk assessment and the modification of blood lipids for the primary and secondary prevention of cardiovascular disease. NICE guidelines [CG181]. [online] Available from http://www.nice.org.uk/guidance/CG181. [Accessed September, 2018].
3. Ridker PM, Genest J, Boekholdt SM, et al. HDL cholesterol and residual risk of first cardiovascular events after treatment with potent statin therapy: an analysis from the JUPITER trial. Lancet. 2010;376(9738):333-9.
4. Shipman KE, Strange RC, Ramachandran S. Use of fibrates in the metabolic syndrome: a review. World J Diabetes. 2016;7(5):74-88.
5. Stuart K, Hartland A, Bhartia M, et al. Drugs and the peroxisome proliferator activated receptors. In: Frontiers in clinical drug research: diabetes and obesity, vol 1. 2014.pp.149-210.
6. Jarco JA, Keaney JF. Proof that lower is better—LDL cholesterol and IMPROVE-IT. N Engl J Med. 2015;372(25):2248-50.
7. Diabetes Atherosclerosis Intervention Study Investigators. Effect of fenofibrate on progression of coronary-artery disease in type 2 diabetes: the Diabetes Atherosclerosis Intervention Study, a randomised study. Lancet. 2001;357(9260):905-10.
8. Tenkanen L, Manttari M, Manninen V. Some coronary risk factors related to the insulin resistance syndrome and treatment with gemfibrozil. experience from the Helsinki Heart Study. Circulation. 1995;92(7):1779-85.
9. Bruckert E, Labreuche J, Deplanque D, et al. Fibrates effect on cardiovascular risk is greater in patients with high triglyceride levels or atherogenicdyslipidemia profile: a systematic review and meta-analysis. J Cardiovasc Pharmacol. 2011;57(2):267-72.
10. Jun M, Foote C, Lv J, et al. Effects of fibrates on cardiovascular outcomes: a systematic review and meta-analysis. Lancet. 2010;375(9729):1875-84.
11. Davis TM, Ting R, Best JD, et al. Effects of fenofibrate on renal function in patients with type 2 diabetes mellitus: the Fenofibrate Intervention and Event Lowering in Diabetes (FIELD) Study. Diabetologia. 2011;54(2): 280-90.
12. Chew EY, Ambrosius WT, Davis MD, Danis RP, et al.; ACCORD Study Group, ACCORD Eye Study Group. Effects of medical therapies on retinopathy progression in type 2 diabetes. N Engl J Med. 2010;363(3):233-44.

13. Keech AC, Mitchell P, Summanen PA, et al. Effect of fenofibrate on the need for laser treatment for diabetic retinopathy (FIELD study): a randomised controlled trial. Lancet. 2007;370(9600):1687-97.
14. Mendis S. The contribution of the Framingham Heart Study to the prevention of cardiovascular disease: a global perspective. Prog Cardiovasc Dis. 2010;53(1):10-4.
15. Rohatgi A, Khera A, Berry JD, et al. HDL cholesterol efflux capacity and incident cardiovascular events. N Engl J Med. 2014;371(25):2383-93.
16. Boden WE, Probstfield JL, Anderson T, et al.; AIM-HIGH Investigators. Niacin in patients with low HDL cholesterol levels receiving intensive statin therapy. N Engl J Med. 2011;365(24):2255-67.
17. Barter PJ, Caulfield M, Eriksson M, et al. Effects of torcetrapib in patients at high risk for coronary events. N Engl J Med. 2007;357(21):2109-22.
18. Bowman L, Hopewell JC, Chen F, et al. HPS3/TIMI55–REVEAL Collaborative Group. Effects of anacetrapib in patients with atherosclerotic vascular disease. N Engl J Med. 2017;377(13):1217-27.
19. Ramachandran S, Abbas A, Saraf S, et al. Significant increase in high-density lipoprotein cholesterol with fibrates is associated with low pretreatment high-density lipoprotein cholesterol: findings from an outpatient clinic setting. Metab Syndr Relat Disord. 2012;10(3):189-94.
20. Ramachandran S, Giles PD, Hartland A. Acute renal failure due to rhabdomyolysis in the presence of concurrent ciprofibrate and ibuprofen treatment. BMJ. 1997;314(7094):1593.

Chapter 73

Lipid Disorders: Looking beyond Statins in Diabetes

Satinath Mukhopadhyay, Deep Dutta

INTRODUCTION

Statins form the cornerstone of managing dyslipidemia. Apart from its strong cholesterol reducing properties, improving cardiovascular (CV) morbidity and mortality, a lot of pleotrophic benefits have been attributed to statins.[1] However, it has also been realized hat a significant amount of CV risk remains in patients who have been treated with full dose of statins.[1] Statins reduce atherosclerotic cardiovascular disease (ASCVD) risk by 15–37%.[1] The residual CV risk contributes to major vascular event in about 20% of patients with coronary heart disease even under the optimal statin treatment.[1] Also statins many not be the best agents in managing hypertriglyceridemia. This chapter reviews the current literature on the role of different anti-lipid medications beyond statins in the holistic management of dyslipidemia in 2018.

NON STATIN LIPID MEDICATIONS

Fibrates, bile acid binding agents, ezetimibe, niacin, PCSK9 inhibitors and saroglitazar are some of the major non statin lipid medications. Each of these drugs has a unique and differential effect on lipid profile. However, CV risks reduction with them has not been equivocally documented as with statins.

SCOPE FOR NON STATIN MEDICATIONS

Statins are the primary treatment agents for hypercholesterolemia. Non statin agents are needed in case of statin intolerance, inability to reach low-density lipoprotein (LDL)-C targets with statins alone in patients with very high cholesterol levels like in patients with familial hypercholesterolemia, and in patients with mixed dyslipidemia. Statins are not the primary agents for managing hypertriglyceridemia. Also statins have minimal to no role in raising high-density lipoprotein (HDL)-C levels. Bile acid resins (BABR) and ezetimibe can be used with or without statins to reduce LDL-cholesterol levels. BABR are less potent agents. They are mainly used as adjunctive therapy. Data is ezetimibe is much stronger and its co-use with statins leads to additional reduction in LDL-C levels.

Hypertriglyceridemia

As per the ICMR-INDIAB study, the most common dyslipidemia in India is low HDL-C seen in 70–74% of the population, followed by hypertriglyceridemia (33%).[2] Elevated LDL-C was observed only in 10% people. This is the pattern of dyslipidemia, which is seen in Asian Indian, which is also known as atherogenic dyslipidemia.[2] Insulin resistance and thrifty phenotype are primarily responsible for atherogenic dyslipidemia in Indians. This is in stark contrast to Caucasians, where the predominant dyslipidemia is hypercholesterolemia. Niacin and fibrates help correct lipid abnormalities in patients with a low HDL-cholesterol level, high triglyceride levels, or both.

Niacin

Niacin (or nicotinic acid) is vitamin B used for treating dyslipidemia for over five decade now. Niacin decreases triglyceride hydrolysis and the transport of free fatty acids from adipose tissue to the liver, resulting in decreased substrate for the hepatic production of triglyceride and very low density lipoprotein (VLDL) cholesterol. Niacin increased HDL-cholesterol by 10–30%, decrease triglyceride by 20–50%, reduce LDL-cholesterol by up to 25%, and lower levels of lipoprotein (a) by 10–30%. The extended-release formulation can be used in combination with statins or BABR. Aspirin can also reduce niacin-induced flushing, which occurs through activation of GPR109A on dermal Langerhans cells leading to increased prostaglandin D2 and E2. Co-administration of niacin with the DP1 antagonist laropiprant reduces flushing. Studies from well-designed clinical trials showed that additional treatment with niacin in statin-treated patients with raised LDL-cholesterol levels is not associated with additional CV clinical benefit (AIM HIGH study, HPS2 THRIVE study).[1] In 2018, the practical use of niacin has significantly reduced in clinical practice. Concerns of worsening dysglycemia, bleeding and infections along with poor tolerability have limited the use of niacin laropiprant formulation. Niacin remains perhaps the only agent in clinical practice, which also has a HDL-C elevating property along with lipoprotein (a) reducing property. Use of niacin in today's world is limited to managing refractory hypercholesterolemia not managed with stains alone or with ezetimibe.

Fibrates

Fibrates have the strongest CV safety data among all the triglyceride reducing medications. Fibrates are commonly used with statins in India to tackle the dual problem of raised triglycerides and raised LDL-C in Indians living with diabetes. The Helsinki heart study and VA-HIT study showed for the first time the CV risk reducing properties with fibrates (gemfibrozil). However, similar results were not generated with fenofibrate in FIELD study and ACCORD studies. Criticisms for these studies include the allowed co-use of other lipid medications in the study groups like statins (simvastatin) making it difficult to document the independent effect of fenofibrate. However, the subgroup analysis of the ACCORD trial and FIELD trial suggested that patients with the combination of high triglyceride and low HDL-cholesterol levels would be likely to experience the greatest clinical and CV risk reduction benefit with fenofibrate treatment.[1] This is the very specific pattern of dyslipidemia, which we seen in Indians (Indian atherogenic dyslipidemia).

Saroglitazar

Saroglitazar is a pan Peroxisome proliferator-activated receptor (PPAR)-α and PPAR-γ agonist, which is approved by Drug Control General of India (DCGI) for use in India for the management of hypertriglyceridemia. Saroglitazar is a potent triglyceride reducing agent, with lesser impact on LDL-C levels. Literature is available on the beneficial effects of saroglitazar in fatty liver disease. A very mild HbA1c reducing property has been attributed to saroglitazar. Saroglitazar is a molecule belonging to the glitazar family. Previous molecules in this family (muraglitazar, tesaglitazar) did not see the light of the day due to serious side effects (soft tissue tumors) seen in animal models of dyslipidemia and insulin resistance. However, saroglitazar is significantly different from those molecules and has not been reported to be associated with similar side effects in animal models as well as from whatever data are available from human studies. In contrast to the previous glitazars, saroglitazar is a predominantly PPAR-α agonistic agent with some PPAR-γ agonstic properties also.

HYPERCHOLESTEROLEMIA

Familial Hypercholesterolemia

Familial hypercholesterolemia (FH), especially the homozygous version, is a difficult to treat condition. Patients with homozygous familial hypercholesterolemia might benefit from lomitapide, a microsomal triglyceride transfer protein inhibitor, and mipomersen, an antisense inhibitor of apolipoprotein B synthesis.

Apolipoprotein B Synthesis Inhibitors

Mipomersen is a second-generation, 20-nucleotide antisense oligonucleotide that targets the coding region of apolipoprotein B–100 mRNA. It has a very potent LDL-C reducing property, much greater than what observed with statins. This molecule was approved in the USA in early 2013 as an orphan drug for the treatment of homozygous FH. Administered by weekly subcutaneous injection, mipomersen has demonstrated substantial additional reductions in LDL-cholesterol levels in patients already receiving maximal lipid-lowering (statin with or without fibrates) therapy without LDL apheresis in four phase III clinical trials. Hence, this drug can be said to have an LDL apheresis sparing effect. However, in all four of these phase

III trials, patients receiving mipomersen had a higher rate of adverse events leading to study discontinuation than those receiving placebo (pooled data: 18.0% vs. 2.3%).

PCSK9 Inhibitors

Proprotein convertase subtilisin/kexin type 9 (PCSK9) is a serine protease, which is expressed in hepatocytes, kidney mesenchymal cells, intestine as well as in embryonic brain telencephalon neurons.[3] The fully humanized monoclonal antibody SAR236553/ REGN727 (Sanofi/ Regeneron, Alirocumab) has been shown to reduce effectively LDL-C in healthy individuals as well as in patients with heterozygous familial hypercholesterolemia (HeFH) and individuals with polygenic hypercholesterolemia in conjunction with statins. The net LDL-C reduction is an additional 50–60% above that achieved by statins alone. Currently there are five ongoing phase III trials for bococizumab in familial heterogenous hypercholesterolemia (SPIRE-HF), patients with high CV risk (SPIRE-LDL), among others. Food and Drug Administration (FDA) has approved PCSK9 inhibitors for clinical use in patients with severe hypercholesterolemia not controlled with statins. These include patients with FH and patients with residual CV risk in patients with high-risk ASCVD. There is an FDA warning about possible cognitive adverse effects with PCSK9 inhibitors. Hence, FDA has recommended neurocognitive testing to be included in all phase III clinical trials involving PCSK9 inhibitors. Injection site irritation is a common minor side effect.[3]

HDL-C Elevating Agents

Cholesteryl ester transfer protein (CETP) inhibitors are the primary agents for raising HDL-C levels. Torcetrapib and dalcetrapib are the two main molecules of this class. However, none of them have been approved for clinical use due to the unfavorable side effects in phase III clinical trials (ILLUMINATE and dal-OUTCOME trials), which include elevation of blood pressure and concerns for raised CV risk.[4]

Newer molecules in this class like anacetrapib and evacetrapib have been found to be safer and free of the side effects seen with previous molecules. Large-scale CV outcomes trials in patients with atherosclerotic vascular disease are currently on with anacetrapib (Reveal Trial) and evacetrapib (Accelerate Trial) and their results which determine the future of this class of drugs.[4]

FUTURE DIRECTIONS

A vaccine, that targets PCSK9 in under advanced phase of development. This vaccine uses virus like particle to carry the PCSK9 antigenic peptide. This leads to in vivo generation of high titers of IgG antibodies which bind to and inhibit circulating PCSK9 in the patients. Berberine has been found to have some PCSK9 inhibiting properties.

CONCLUSION

Statins remain the primary agent for managing hypercholesterolemia. PCSK9 inhibitors are novel and very potent agents for managing resistant hypercholesterolemia. PCSK9 inhibitors are very good for managing difficult hypercholesterolemia of FH. They have probable additional CV risk reducing properties over statin. There use in patients with ASCVD is increasingly being studies. Fibrates and saroglitazar are the best agents when the primary target is to control hypertriglyceridemia. They perhaps have more relevance in Indian atherogenic dyslipidemia. There is an urgent need for generating CV safety data for these medications from India.

REFERENCES

1. Dutta D, Mukhopadhyay S. Intervening at prediabetes stage is critical to controlling the diabetes epidemic among Asian Indians. Indian J Med Res. 2016;143:23-26.
2. Noto D, Cefalu AB, Averna MR. Beyond statins: new lipid lowering strategies to reduce cardiovascular risk. Curr Atheroscler Rep. 2014;16:414.
3. Rosenson RS, Hegele RA, Fazio S, et al. The evolving future of PCSK9 inhibitors. Journal of the American College of Cardiology. 2018;72(3):314-329.
4. Lüscher TF, Taddei S, Kaski JC, et al. Vascular effects and safety of dalcetrapib in patients with or at risk of coronary heart disease: the dal-VESSEL randomized clinical trial. Eur Heart J. 2012;33(7):857-65.

Chapter 74

Obesity and Diabetes—Common Soil Hypothesis

Sunil Kumar Kota, Sambit Das, Lalit Kumar Meher

INTRODUCTION

Cardiovascular disorders (CVD) are the major cause of morbidity and mortality in type 2 diabetes patients. Diabesity too is burgeoning in prevalence. In fact obesity, diabetes and cardiovascular diseases are described as a compendium.[1] Patients with metabolic syndrome (MetS) have increased risk of both diabetes (5-fold) and CVD (2-fold) over the next 5–10 years. The microvascular complications in type 2 diabetes are overtly related to preceding hyperglycemia. But large vessel atherosclerosis which is the harbinger of macrovascular complications can precede the development of diabetes. This suggests that atherosclerosis and diabetes, rather than one being the complication of the other, both disorders have common genetic and environmental antecedents. Therefore, it is suggested that both of them spring from a "common soil".[2] It all started with the publication by Jarrett in 1984 titled "Type 2 (non-insulin-dependent) diabetes mellitus and coronary heart disease: chicken, egg or neither?"[3]

The concept was further strengthened by publications of Barker et al. hypothesizing early environment theory for both diabetes and coronary disease.[4] They demonstrated greater prevalence of diabetes and incidence of coronary disease in the regions of United Kingdom, which had high rates of infant mortality 50 years earlier. Inadequate nutritional intake during the perinatal period (manifesting in the form of low birth weight and low rates of weight gain in the first year of life) coupled with a subsequent situation with an excess calorie were associated with increased incidence of diabetes, hypertension and coronary disease.[5] It was hypothesized that fetal malnutrition could give rise to fewer adipocytes and also lead to pancreatic beta cells misregulation. Probably there is hypertrophy of visceral adipocytes, more readily than adipocytes from other fat depots, thereby becoming the preferable storage sites. During subsequent state of abundance with excess calorie ingestion, there would be hypertrophy of these cells, with undesired metabolic consequences.[4,5]

The basis for all these is MetS, which arises out of a combination of excess calorie intake and relatively deficient physical activity. It is a proinflammatory and prothrombotic state in the back drop constellation of abdominal obesity, dyslipidemia, glucose intolerance and hypertension arising because of insulin resistance.

INSULIN RESISTANCE AS THE ANTECEDENT OF DIABETES AND CARDIOVASCULAR DISEASE

Insulin resistance is a direct risk factor for type 2 diabetes. The impending hyperinsulinemia ensues as a compensatory response to insulin resistance and is a risk factor for diabetes. In due course of time, the ongoing demand for insulin hypersecretion for maintenance of glucose homeostasis ultimately leads to islet cell exhaustion resulting in over hyperglycemia. The elevated proinsulin in states of insulin resistance is sometimes depicted as a stronger risk factor for future diabetes.

Insulin resistance contributes to atherogenic dyslipidemia by increasing free fatty acid (FFA) flux to the liver. It gives rise to increased hepatic secretion of very low-density lipoprotein (VLDL) and other apolipoprotein (apo) B containing lipoproteins. Additionally the suppressive effect of insulin on apoB secretion is blunted giving rise to either decreased degradation of apoB or inhibition of microsomal triglycerides (TGs) transfer protein activity. It results in elevated TG levels in blood. Cholesteryl ester transfer protein (CETP) transfers TG from VLDL to high-density lipoprotein (HDL) creating TG-rich HDL particles, which are avidly hydrolyzed by hepatic lipase leading to rapid clearance from plasma. CETP mediated transfer of TGs from VLDL to low-density lipoprotein (LDL) contributes to the formation of small dense LDL particles. The combination of low HDL and increased small dense LDL is a strong risk factor of CVD.[6]

Insulin itself is atherogenic.[2] The elevated level of plasminogen activator inhibitor 1 (PAI-1) is associated with almost all of the features of the MetS.[2] The elevated PAI-1, by inhibition of fibrinolysis aids the prothrombotic state.

OXIDATIVE STRESS AS THE PATHOGENETIC MECHANISM

Oxidative stress is common in overnutrition, insulin resistance, impaired glucose tolerance (IGT), diabetes, and CVD. Overnutrition and decreased physical activity lead to increased glucose and FFA loads in cells. This is accompanied by increased free radicals generation (oxidative stress) (Flowchart 1). There are several mechanisms by which oxidative damage results in insulin resistance, beta-cell and endothelial cell dysfunction, IGT, diabetes and CVD. The individual causative mechanisms are elaborated below.

Role of Oxidative Stress in Development of Insulin Resistance from Overfeeding

When energy expenditure is surpassed by excess caloric intake, there is an excess flux of substrates (glucose/FFA) into muscle and adipose tissues. The glucose through pyruvate or FFA by beta-oxidation produce mitochondrial acetyl coenzyme A. This enters citric acid cycle which produces an excess of mitochondrial nicotinamide adenine dinucleotide reduced (mNADH) and reactive oxygen species (ROS). In order to protect themselves against harmful effects of ROS, cells either reduce the formation of ROS and/or enhance their removal. ROS formation is reduced by preventing the build-up of mNADH by inhibiting insulin stimulated nutrient uptake

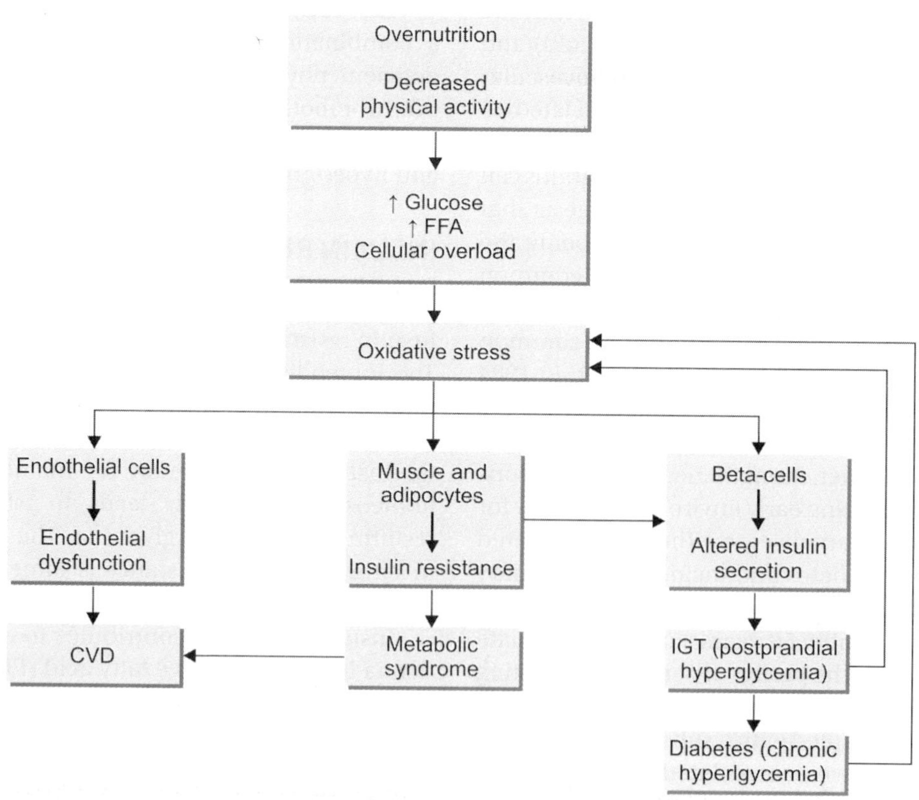

(CVD: cardiovascular disease; FFA: free fatty acid; IGT: impaired glucose tolerance.)

Flowchart 1 Overnutrition and decreased physical activity induced oxidative stress.

and preventing the entrance of substrates (pyruvate, FFA) into the mitochondria. An increase in intracellular FFA leads to reduced glucose transporter type 4 (GLUT-4) translocation to the plasma membrane, resulting in resistance to insulin mediated glucose uptake in both muscle and adipose tissue.[7]

Oxidative Stress Resulting In Beta-cell and Endothelial Cell Dysfunction (Flowchart 2)

High glucose or FFA levels alone or in combination give rise to beta-cell dysfunction. Because of lesser content of antioxidant enzymes like catalase, superoxide dismutase and glutathione peroxidase, the pancreatic beta-cells are very sensitive to ROS. The oxidative stress leads to increased levels of p21 (a regulator of cell cycle progression at G_1 and S phase) and decreased levels of insulin mRNA, cytosolic adenosine triphosphate (ATP), and calcium flux in cytosol and mitochondria. Mitochondrial ROS inhibits the key glycolytic enzyme glyceraldehyde 3-phosphate dehydrogenase (GAPDH), thereby suppressing the first phase of insulin secretion.[7] Additionally both FFA and glucose activate uncoupling of protein 2 leading to impaired beta-cell insulin secretion.[8]

Similarly glucose and FFA overload induced oxidative stress mediates endothelial cell dysfunction. There is

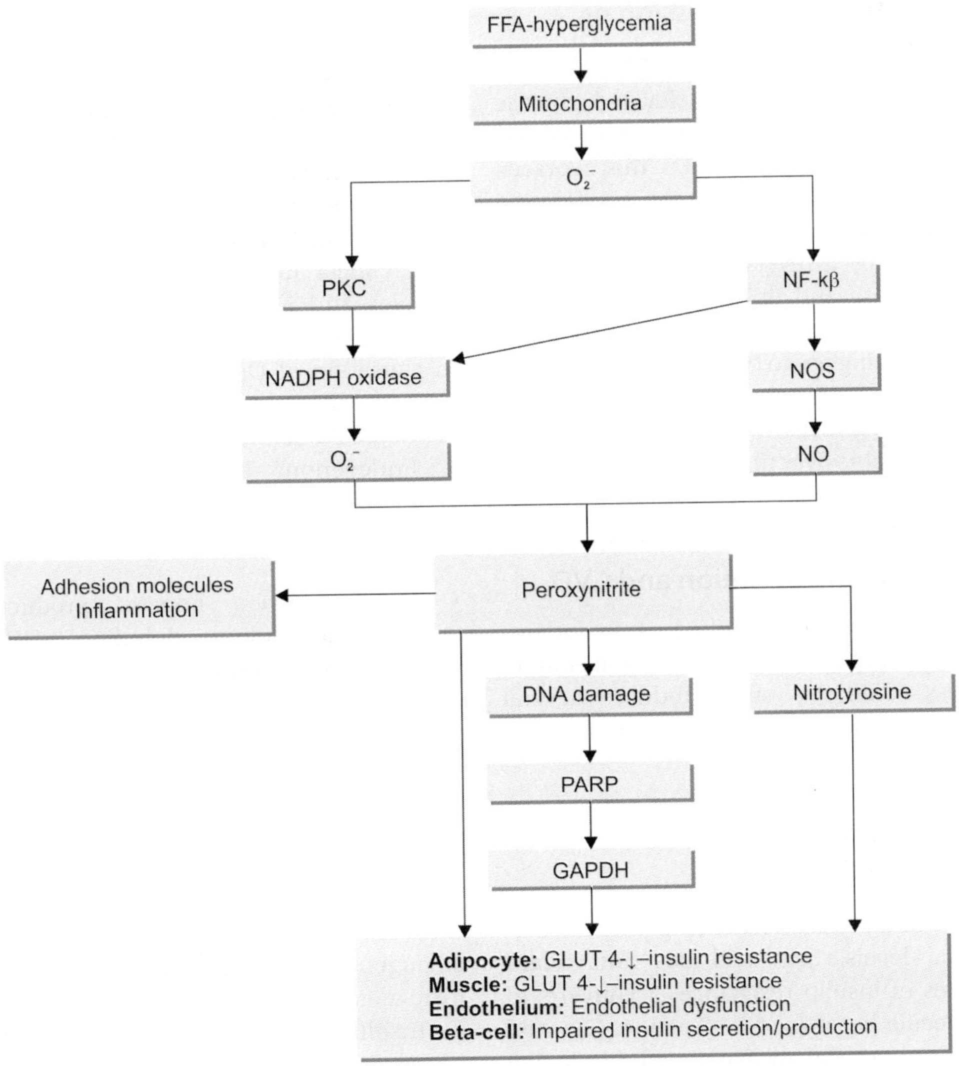

(ADP: adenosine diphosphate; DNA: deoxyribonucleic acid; FFA: free fatty acid; GAPDH: glyceraldehyde 3-phosphate dehydrogenase; GLUT-4: glucose transporter type 4; NADPH: nicotinamide adenine dinucleotide phosphate; NF-kβ: nuclear factor-kappa beta; NO: nitric oxide; NOS: NO synthase; PARP: poly (ADP-ribose) polymerase; PKC: protein kinase C.)

Flowchart 2 Hyperglycemia and free fatty acid-induced dysfunction.

superoxide over production by mitochondrial electron transport chain machinery. The endothelial nitric oxide synthase (NOS) and inducible NOS increase nitric oxide generation, which leads to formation of peroxynitrite, a strong oxidant. This damages the DNA, leading to activation of the nuclear enzyme poly [adenosine diphosphate (ADP)-ribose] polymerase, giving rise to depletion of the intracellular concentration of its substrate nicotinamide adenine dinucleotide (NAD). The reduced NAD in turn slows the rate of electron transport, and ATP formation, and produces an ADP-ribosylation of the GAPDH. This inactivated GADPH deters glycolysis. All these steps finally lead to acute endothelial dysfunction.[9]

Role of Oxidative Stress in Progression of Insulin Resistance to IGT and Diabetes

Hyperinsulinemia in association with elevated glucose and/or FFA increase ROS production (oxidative stress) and activate stress-sensitive pathways.[7] This worsens both insulin action and secretion, thereby accelerating the progression to overt type 2 diabetes. Initially, this damage is manifested by a reversible defective insulin gene expression. Glucose and lipid toxicity induce the gradual, time-dependent damage of cellular components of insulin production giving rise to blunted insulin content and secretion. Repeated onslaught of hyperglycemia and increased FFA levels can give rise to beta-cell dysfunction, which becomes irreversible over time.[10]

Link between Insulin Resistance-induced Oxidative Stress and Inflammation and CVD

Atherosclerosis has long been described as an inflammatory process. And inflammation is a manifestation of oxidative stress. Oxidative stress induces several mediators of inflammation like adhesion molecules, interleukins etc.[11]

URIC ACID: FUELING THE COMMON SOIL HYPOTHESIS

Uric acid is produced by oxidation during purine catabolism. At normal levels, uric acid has antioxidant properties. In states of insulin resistance, it converts to a pro-oxidant molecule because of ROS action. Elevated uric acid leads to endothelial dysfunction by inducing antiproliferative effects on endothelium and impairing nitric oxide production and inflammation by means of increased C-reactive protein expression.[12] Uric acid additionally gives rise to immune activation with increased chemokine and cytokine expression. Uric acid has some renal effects like increased glomerular pressure and sodium reabsorption, which are enhanced by high plasma insulin, further deteriorating glucose tolerance. Two prospective studies have demonstrated significant association between increased plasma concentrations of uric acid and incidence of type 2 diabetes and increased mortality from coronary heart disease, congestive heart failure and stroke.[12]

COMMON SOIL HYPOTHESIS: DIABETES AND CANCER IN PATIENTS WITH METABOLIC SYNDROME

Some authors consider MetS to increase cancer risk and mortality. Both MetS and cancer have common modifiable and nonmodifiable risk factors, including age, genetic factors, physical inactivity, unhealthy diet, obesity, smoking, alcohol, circadian rhythm disturbances and air pollution. MetS is associated with increased risk of colorectal cancers in both sexes; increased liver cancer in males; increased pancreatic cancer in females and increased breast, endometrial cancers in postmenopausal women.[13] The role of insulin resistance in causation of Diabetes is a well understood fact. The potential mechanisms implicated in causation of cancer are depicted below:

- Endogenous hyperinsulinemia and the resultant increased insulin like growth factor- 1(IGF-1) activate the carcinogenic Ras/Raf/MAPK and PI3K/Akt/mTOR pathways
- Insulin lowers hepatic production of steroid hormone-binding globulin (SHBG). Additionally insulin like growth factor-1 (IGF-1) increases the aromatase activity in adipose cells. Combined the higher free estradiol and androgens levels lead to the upregulation of both estrogen and androgen receptors in breast and prostate cancer cells.

Estrogens may contribute to both tumor development and growth directly, by stimulating cellular proliferation and inhibiting apoptosis and indirectly, by stimulating vascular endothelial growth factor (VEGF) mediated angiogenesis or inducing gene mutations induced by toxic metabolites.

- Insulin stimulates white adipose tissue (WAT) inflammation, which release FFAs into the bloodstream. These FFAs serve as the main energy substrates for cancer cells promoting their growth and sustenance. The FFA get accumulated in the bloodstream resulting in ectopic lipid storage in other organs (liver, pancreas, kidneys)

- Obesity induced high leptin to adiponectin ratio is involved in altered energetic metabolism and insulin action leading to inflammation, neoangiogenesis and cell growth, thereby potentiating cancer initiation and progression[13]
- Chronic subclinical inflammation in WAT in obese patients leads to infiltration by macrophages and lymphocytes, which produce proinflammatory factors [e.g. tumor necrosis factor-alpha (TNF-α) and interleukin-6]. In some organs closely associated with inflamed WAT (e.g. breast, pancreas, colon, kidneys,), this can play an important role in cancer development[13]
- There is increased expression of nuclear transcription factor such nuclear factor-kappa beta, which is a tumor promoter in inflammation-associated cancer and is helpful for tissue factor (TF) expression.[14] TF has important role in the activation of the clotting cascade and it also serves as a signalling mediator in cancer cell migration and angiogenesis[14]
- Disruption of circadian rhythm results in detrimental effects including metabolic disorders, uncontrolled cell growth and cancer. It is seen more in elderly and shift workers because of dyssynchrony in circadian rhythm.[13]

CONCLUSION

Considering the impact of obesity in causes of metabolic disorders, cardiovascular disorders and cancers in a long run, it is highly imperative to strike the right chord very early on in the life of a person. This can be done by achievement and maintenance of a healthy weight throughout life; adoption of a physically active lifestyle, consumption of a healthy diet with an emphasis on plant-based foods and mitigation of modifiable risk factors like alcohol, smoking, etc. Ongoing and future, target oriented research is essential to identify potential pathogens in causation of this dual dynamo, so that more specific pharmacological agents can be invented.

REFERENCES

1. Scherer PE, Hill JA. Obesity, diabetes, and cardiovascular diseases: A compendium Circ Res. 2016;118:1703-5.
2. Stern MP. Diabetes and cardiovascular disease. The "common soil" hypothesis. Diabetes. 1995;44:369-74.
3. Jarrett RJ. Type 2 (non-insulin-dependent) diabetes mellitus and coronary heart disease-chicken, egg or neither? Diabetologia. 1984;26:99-102.
4. Barker DJ, Osmond C. Infant mortality, childhood nutrition, and ischemic heart disease in England and Wales. Lancet. 1986;1:1077-814.
5. Barker DJ, Hales CN, Fall CH, et al. Type 2 (non-insulin-dependent) diabetes mellitus, hypertension, and hyperlipidaemia (syndrome X): Relation to reduced fetal growth. Diabetologia. 1993;36:62-75.
6. Bitzur R, Cohen H, Kamari Y, et al. Triglycerides and HDL cholesterol: Stars or second leads in diabetes? Diabetes Care. 2009;32(Suppl 2):S373-7.
7. Ceriello A, Motz E. Is oxidative stress the pathogenic mechanism underlying insulin resistance, diabetes, and cardiovascular disease? The Common Soil Hypothesis Revisited. Arterioscler Thromb Vasc Biol. 2004;24:816-23.
8. Krauss S, Zhang CY, Scorrano L, et al. Superoxide-mediated activation of uncoupling protein 2 causes pancreatic beta cell dysfunction. J Clin Invest. 2003;112:1831-42.
9. Garcia Soriano F, Virag L, Jagtap P, et al. Diabetic endothelial dysfunction: The role of poly(ADP-ribose) polymerase activation. Nature Med. 2001;7:108-13.
10. Poitout V, Robertson RP. Mini review: Secondary beta-cell failure in type diabetes—a convergence of glucotoxicity and lipotoxicity. Endocrinology. 2002;143:339-42.
11. Roebuck KA. Oxidant stress regulation of IL-8 and ICAM-1 gene expression: differential activation and binding of the transcription factors AP-1 and NF-kappaB. Int J Mol Med. 1999;4:223-30.
12. Koenig W, Meisinger C. Uric acid, type 2 diabetes, and cardiovascular diseases: Fueling the common soil hypothesis? Clinical Chemistry. 2008;54:231-3.
13. Bellastella G, Scappaticcio L, Esposito K, et al. Metabolic syndrome and cancer: The common soil hypothesis. Diabetes Res Clin Pract. 2018;143:389-97.
14. Donati MB. The "common soil hypothesis": Evidence from population studies? Thromb Res. 2010;125 Suppl 2:S92-5.

Chapter 75

Metabolic Karma—The Atherogenic Legacy of Diabetes

Subhash Kumar Wangnoo, Swati Tayal Goray

INTRODUCTION

It is well established that cardiovascular disease (CVD) is still the principal cause of mortality and morbidity among patients with diabetes mellitus. A lot has been achieved in the management of risk factors in diabetes including hyperglycemia, lowering of blood pressure and cholesterol levels. However the ability to retard and reverse cardiovascular (CV) events such as myocardial infarction, stroke and peripheral vascular disease in diabetics continues to elude us.

There has been some ambiguity with respect to CV outcomes in patients with diabetes especially those subjected to intensive glycemic control.The Steno-2 randomized trial demonstrated favorable effects with regard to vascular complications and CV mortality when at-risk patients with type 2 diabetes were subjected to intensive intervention with multiple drug combinations and behavior modification for 7.8 years.[1] In a further follow-up of the same study, it was revealed that intensified treatment was associated with a prolonged median lifespan over a period of 21.2 years follow-up. This was attributed to reduced risk of incident CVD and mortality.[2]

In a 2009 meta-analysis, which comprised data from four major trials, including Action to Control Cardiovascular Risk in Diabetes (ACCORD), Action in Diabetes and Vascular Disease: Preterax and Diamicron Modified Release Controlled Evaluation (ADVANCE), UK Prospective Diabetes Study (UKPDS) and Veterans Affairs Diabetes Trial (VADT), it was established that more intensive glycemic control can achieve only a modest CV benefit. It failed to show any effect on all cause and CV mortality with an added risk for increased hypoglycemic events.[3]

However, not all hope is lost as certain newglucose-lowering agents are showing improved effect on CV outcomes. Dipeptidyl peptidase-4 (DPP-4) inhibitors like saxagliptin, alogliptin and sitagliptin are seen to not alter the rates of major adverse CV events in diabetic patients.[4-6] On the other hand, Sodium-glucose cotransporter 2 (SGLT2) inhibitors were associated with improved CV outcomes in patients with type 2 diabetes as demonstrated in the Canagliflozin Cardiovascular Assessment Study (CANVAS) and EMPA-REG OUTCOME trials.[7,8] In addition to this, encouraging results with decreased CV mortality have also been reported from use of liraglutide and semaglutide in patients with type 2 diabetes.[9,10] Despite this, the burden of CVD in diabetics is still significant and several mechanisms for elevated atherosclerotic CV risk have been mentioned including presence of inflammation, reactive oxygen species (ROS), endothelial dysfunction, hypercoagulability and vascular calcification.[11]

To illuminate on the molecular and cellular mechanisms responsible for the diabetic macrovascular complications, there has been the lack of a suitable animal model. To study atherosclerosis in murine models has not been an easy task, as rodents are inherently resistant to development of macrovascular disease. However, it has been observed that mice deficient in apolipoprotein E (apo $E^{-}/^{-}$) mouse are highly susceptible to atherosclerosis. Thus, to determine the pathways in which diabetes accelerates the incidence and progression of vascular lesions, (apo $E^{-}/^{-}$) mice were made diabetic using streptozotocin.[12] Based on these models, studies have shown the importance of renin-angiotensin system in the pathogenesis of atherosclerosis in diabetes and its diminution with angiotensin-converting enzyme (ACE) inhibitor treatment.[13,14] In a similar murine model, activation of the receptor for advanced glycation end products (RAGE) was found to play a key role in the mediation of atherogenesis in diabetes and highlighted the potential for targeting RAGE activation in the prevention and treatment of diabetic macrovascular complications.[15]The diabetic (apo $E^{-}/^{-}$) mouse remains one of the preferred models by the JDRF/National Institutes of Health-sponsored Animal Models of Diabetic Complications Consortium (AMDCC) for the study of diabetes-associated CVD.[16]

ADVANCED GLYCATION PATHWAY

In diabetes, non-enzymatic glycation and oxidation of proteins and lipids results in a build-up of permanently formed advanced glycation end products (AGEs). These AGEs occupy their receptor in cells of vessel wall leading to a cascade of reactions responsible for development of vascular lesions. In a first of a kind study in diabetic mice deficient for apolipoprotein E (apo $E^{-}/^{-}$), soluble receptor for advanced glycation end products (sRAGE) were administered. This pivotal study revealed complete suppression of diabetic atherosclerosis in a glycemia- and lipid-independent manner and identified the importance of receptor as a new therapeutic target in diabetic macrovascular disease.[12] Following this few more studies have endorsed the significance of RAGE in development of endothelial dysfunction and atherosclerotic plaque development in a mouse model of atherosclerosis in diabetes.[15,17]

There are several ways in which AGE-RAGE interaction accelerate vascular injury and plaque development. Activation of RAGE by AGEs is responsible for the up regulation of the transcription factor nuclear factor κ-B and its target genes simultaneously increasing the endothelial permeability. The soluble AGEs are responsible for activation of monocytes and AGEs in the basement membrane inhibit monocyte migration. In view of the rising evidence of adverse effects of AGEs on the vasculature of patients with diabetes, a number of differenttherapies to inhibit AGEs are under investigation.[18]

Furthermore, the AGE-RAGE interaction also triggers the release of ROS, thereby altering gene expression. In a recent study, the role of NADPH oxidase (Nox) was delineated in the generation of ROS which provides a mechanism for altered gene expression in AGE-related disorders.[19]

Few studies have been undertaken investigating treatment strategies targeting AGE. In a mouse model with established atherosclerosis and diabetes, delayed treatment with alagebrium chloride and pyridoxamine dihydrochloride was studied in comparison with quinapril. The blockade of AGE accumulation was associated with significant reduction the development of atherosclerosis in diabetes, further underscoring the role of AGE-mediated pathways.[20]

In a similar model with streptozotocin induced diabetes in (apo $E^{-}/^{-}$) mice, the role of AGE cross-link breaker ALT-711, or the inhibitor of AGE formation amino guanidine (AG) in atherosclerosis was evaluated. Both the molecules demonstrated substantial decrease in vascular AGE accumulation in addition to lessening atherosclerosis in these diabetic mice.[21]

More recently, role of toxic metabolites comprising of reactive dicarbonyls like methylglyoxal (MG) is also being recognized for the harmful effects of hyperglycemia especially on the vessel wall. The abnormal build-up of dicarbonyls which is metabolized by glyoxalase 1, accounts for the protein and DNA alteration causing cellular dysfunction in aging and disease. This dicarbonyl stress exists thereby promotes the metabolic and vascular complications in not only diabetes but also obesity and renal failure.[22] The insight into these mechanisms has led to studies evaluating novel drugs such as the role of glyoxalase 1 inducer in obesity. In a recent study glyoxalase 1 inducers were found to be showing significant improvement in glucose control, insulin sensitivity and vascular function[23] identifying their potential to prevent and treat diabetes.

In another study, increasing plasma MG was seen to enhance atherogenesis in euglycemic apolipoprotein E knockout mice to a similar magnitude as that observed in mice with diabetes. The RAGE partly contributes to the vessel damage and inflammation together with oxidative stress triggered by dicarbonyls. This would suggest that a synergistic combination of RAGE antagonism and antioxidants may present a unique opportunity in the management of vascular complications in diabetes.[24]

OXIDATIVE STRESS

Oxidative stress significantly contributes to the pathogenesis of atherosclerosis and diabetes mellitus. To its aid comes the superoxide-generating enzyme Nox, which plays a fundamental role in the release of ROS.

There exist multiple isoforms of Nox enzyme which are currently under investigation. Of these isoforms, Nox1 is known to play a vital part in the progression of accelerated atherosclerosis in diabetes. It has been observed that Nox1 deletion leads to marked reduction of ROS and inflammatory markers serving as a prospective candidate in the treatment of diabetic vascular complications. Moreover, treatment with GKT137831 (a specific Nox inhibitor) demonstrated significant decrease in progression of atherosclerosis.[25]

However, appearance of ROS in atherosclerosis is apparently not always a undesirable oxidative stress, but can also have protective effects. It has been also recognized that Nox4 offers protection in diabetes-associated atherosclerosis by acting as a negative modulator of inflammation and remodeling thus providing vascular protection. These results have implications on how to judge ROS formation in CVD and need to be considered in the development of Nox inhibitory drugs.[26]

A study was undertaken to establish the importance of combined Nox1/4 inhibition using GKT137831 in the presence of already recognized diabetic complications. Consistent with previous studies, Nox1/4 inhibition with GKT137831 did demonstrate renoprotective effects; however, with regards to reducing atherosclerosis, a dose dependent phenomenon was observed.[27]

The role of Nox5-derived ROS has also been identified in the development of renal dysfunction in few studies. These studies have helped in underlining the importance of Nox5 isoform in the development of nephropathy and Nox5 may emerge as an innovative pharmacological target for decreasing chronic kidney disease progression.[28,29]

EPIGENETIC PATHWAYS AND METABOLIC MEMORY

A crucial discovery in patients with type 1 and 2 diabeties with intensive blood glucose control has been the presence of sustained benefits after termination of the randomized intervention. This 'legacy effect' or 'metabolic memory' demonstrates continued reduction in microvascular risk, CV events and mortality on follow-up, despite the presence of similarities in glycated hemoglobin levels between the intensive- therapy and the conventional-therapy group. The UKPDS categorically proved the advantages of better glycemic control in decreasing the microvascular complications; however, the risk reductions in CV events and death were noted only on extended post-trial follow-up.[30]

The results of the Diabetes Control and Complications Trial (DCCT) suggested that patients with type 1 diabetes assigned to intensive glycemic control had a decreased risk of progression to complications like nephropathy and neuropathy in comparison to those in conventional therapy. In the following Epidemiology of Diabetes Interventions and Complications (EDIC) study phase, both groups were placed on intensive therapy and underwent long-term follow-up. It was observed that, despite achieving similar levels of glycated hemoglobin in both groups during the EDIC study, patients in the initial DCCT intensive treatment group had substantially lower risks of developing microvascular and macrovascular complications compared with original conventional treatment group. [31,32]

Additionally, based on the results of a meta-analysis, greater reduction in CV risk was observed in with type 1 diabetes than among those with type 2 diabetes with regards to improved glycemic control.[33]

The underlying explanation at a molecular and/ or cellular level for this phenomenon remains to be determined. Several groups have hypothesized the role of epigenetic mechanisms in elucidation of the metabolic memory.[34-36]

Epigenetic mechanisms cause altered gene expression by DNA methylation, histone modifications in chromatin, rather than the alteration in DNA sequence. The significance of epigenetic mechanisms in macrovascular disease in diabetes has been highlighted in a recent review article. It is further explained that in diabetes, presence of hyperglycemia, growth factors, oxidant stress and inflammatory factors leads to disruption of these epigenetic mechanisms. This ultimately causes modified expression of pathological genes in target cells such as endothelial, vascular smooth muscle, retinal and cardiac cells. Thus, persistence of epigenetic alterations initiated by diabetic stimuli could be one of theessential mechanisms fundamental to metabolic memory.[35]

In another study, it was shown that transient hyperglycemia was responsible for continued atherogenic effects following normoglycemia. This was triggered by long-term alterations in chromatin remodeling, recruitment of the histone methyltransferase Set7 and increased H3K4 monomethylation in the proximal NF-κB promoter, leading to increased expression of p65, MCP-1 and VCAM-1.[37]

A recent study presented the positive effects of exercise on epigenetic marks linked to diabetes.[38] Because epigenetic changes are potentially reversible in nature, combination therapies with epigenetic drugs (epidrugs)[39] and antagomirs (miRNA inhibitors)[40] could be considered to complement the current treatments for complications.

On the whole, ongoing research in the subject of epigenetics could identify much required new biomarkers and drug targets for the early detection and treatment of the debilitating vascular complications of diabetes.[35]

REFERENCES

1. Gæde P, Lund-Andersen H, Parving HH, et al. Effect of a multifactorial intervention on mortality in type 2 diabetes. N Engl J Med. 2008;358(6): 580-91.
2. Gæde P, Oellgaard J, Carstensen B, et al. Years of life gained by multifactorial intervention in patients with type 2 diabetes mellitus and microalbuminuria: 21 years follow-up on the Steno-2 randomised trial. Diabetologia. 2016;59(11):2298-307.
3. Control Group, Turnbull FM, Abraira C, et al. Intensive glucose control and macrovascular outcomes in type 2 diabetes. Diabetologia. 2009;52(11): 2288-98.
4. Scirica BM, Bhatt DL, Braunwald E, et al. Saxagliptin and cardiovascular outcomes in patients with type 2 diabetes mellitus. N Engl J Med. 2013;369(14):1317-26.
5. White WB, Cannon CP, Heller SR, et al. Alogliptin after acute coronary syndrome in patients with type 2 diabetes. N Engl J Med. 2013;369(14):1327-35.
6. Green JB, Bethel MA, Armstrong PW, et al. Effect of sitagliptin on cardiovascular outcomes in type 2 diabetes. N Engl J Med. 2015;373(3):232-42.
7. Neal B, Perkovic V, Mahaffey KW, et al. Canagliflozin and cardiovascular and renal events in type 2 diabetes. N Engl J Med. 2017;377(7):644-57.
8. Zinman B, Wanner C, Lachin JM, et al. Empagliflozin, cardiovascular outcomes, and mortality in type 2 diabetes. N Engl J Med. 2015;373(22):2117-28.
9. Marso SP, Daniels GH, Brown-Frandsen K, et al. liraglutide and cardiovascular outcomes in type 2 diabetes. N Engl J Med. 2016;375(4):311-22.
10. Marso SP, Bain SC, Consoli A, et al. Semaglutide and cardiovascular outcomes in patients with type 2 diabetes. N Engl J Med. 2016;375(19): 1834-44.
11. Low Wang CC, Hess CN, Hiatt WR, et al. Clinical update: cardiovascular disease in diabetes mellitus: Atherosclerotic cardiovascular disease and heart failure in type 2 diabetes mellitus - mechanisms, management, and clinical considerations. Circulation. 2016;133(24):2459-502.
12. Park L, Raman KG, Lee KJ, et al. Suppression of accelerated diabetic atherosclerosis by the soluble receptor for advanced glycation end products. Nat Med. 1998;4(9):1025-31.
13. Candido R, Allen TJ, Lassila M, et al. Irbesartan but not amlodipine suppresses diabetes-associated atherosclerosis. Circulation. 2004;109(12):1536-42.
14. Candido R, Jandeleit-Dahm KA, Cao Z, et al. Prevention of accelerated atherosclerosis by angiotensin-converting enzyme inhibition in diabetic apolipoprotein E-deficient mice. Circulation. 2002;106(2):246-53.
15. Soro-Paavonen A, Watson AMD, Li J, et al. Receptor for advanced glycation end products (RAGE) deficiency attenuates the development of atherosclerosis in diabetes. Diabetes. 2008;57(9):2461-9.
16. Hsueh W, Abel ED, Breslow JL, et al. Recipes for creating animal models of diabetic cardiovascular disease. Circ Res. 2007;100(10):1415-27.
17. Harja E, Bu D, Hudson BI, et al. Vascular and inflammatory stresses mediate atherosclerosis via RAGE and its ligands in apoE-/- mice. J Clin Invest. 2008;118(1):183-94.
18. Goldin A, Beckman JA, Schmidt AM, et al. Advanced glycation end products: Sparking the development of diabetic vascular injury. Circulation. 2006;114(6):597-605.
19. Wautier MP, Chappey O, Corda S, et al. Activation of NADPH oxidase by AGE links oxidant stress to altered gene expression via RAGE. Am J Physiol Endocrinol Metab. 2001;280(5):E685-94.
20. Watson AMD, Soro-Paavonen A, Sheehy K, et al. Delayed intervention with AGE inhibitors attenuates the progression of diabetes-accelerated atherosclerosis in diabetic apolipoprotein E knockout mice. Diabetologia. 2011;54(3):681-9.
21. Forbes JM, Yee LTL, Thallas V, et al. Advanced glycation end product interventions reduce diabetes-accelerated atherosclerosis. Diabetes. 2004;53(7):1813-23.
22. Rabbani N, Xue M, Thornalley PJ. Methylglyoxal-induced dicarbonyl stress in aging and disease: First steps towards glyoxalase 1-based treatments. Clin Sci (Lond). 2016;130(19):1677-96.
23. Xue M, Weickert MO, Qureshi S, et al. Improved glycemic control and vascular function in overweight and obese subjects by glyoxalase 1 inducer formulation. Diabetes. 2016;65(8):2282-94.
24. Tikellis C, Pickering RJ, Tsorotes D, et al. Dicarbonyl stress in the absence of hyperglycemia increases endothelial inflammation and atherogenesis similar to that observed in diabetes. Diabetes. 2014;63(11):3915-25.
25. Gray SP, Di Marco E, Okabe J, et al. NADPH oxidase 1 plays a key role in diabetes mellitus-accelerated atherosclerosis. Circulation. 2013;127(18): 1888-902.
26. Gray SP, Di Marco E, Kennedy K, et al. Reactive oxygen species can provide atheroprotection via NOX4-dependent inhibition of inflammation and vascular remodeling. Arterioscler ThrombVasc Biol. 2016;36(2):295-307.
27. Gray SP, Jha JC, Kennedy K, et al. Combined NOX1/4 inhibition with GKT137831 in mice provides dose-dependent reno- and atheroprotection even in established micro- and macrovascular disease. Diabetologia. 2017;60(5):927-37.
28. Holterman CE, Thibodeau JF, Towaij C, et al. Nephropathy and elevated BP in mice with podocyte-specific NADPH oxidase 5 expression. J Am SocNephrol. 2014;25(4):784-97.
29. Jha JC, Banal C, Okabe J, et al. NADPH Oxidase Nox5 accelerates renal injury in diabetic nephropathy. Diabetes. 2017;66(10):2691-703.
30. Holman RR, Paul SK, Bethel MA, et al. 10-year follow-up of intensive glucose control in type 2 diabetes. N Engl J Med. 2008;359(15):1577-89.
31. Diabetes Control and Complications Trial/Epidemiology of Diabetes Interventions and Complications Research Group, Lachin JM, Genuth S, Cleary P, et al. Retinopathy and nephropathy in patients with type 1 diabetes four years after a trial of intensive therapy. N Engl J Med. 2000;342(6):381-9.
32. Writing Team for the Diabetes Control and Complications Trial/Epidemiology of Diabetes Interventions and Complications Research Group. Sustained effect of intensive treatment of type 1 diabetes mellitus on development and progression of diabetic nephropathy: The Epidemiology of Diabetes Interventions and Complications (EDIC) study. JAMA. 2003;290(16): 2159-67.
33. Stettler C, Allemann S, Jüni P, et al. Glycemic control and macrovascular disease in types 1 and 2 diabetes mellitus: Meta-analysis of randomized trials. Am Heart J. 2006;152(1):27-38.
34. Keating ST, El-Osta A. Epigenetics and metabolism. Circ Res. 2015;116(4): 715-36.
35. Reddy MA, Zhang E, Natarajan R. Epigenetic mechanisms in diabetic complications and metabolic memory. Diabetologia. 2015;58(3):443-55.
36. Keating ST, Plutzky J, El-Osta A. Epigenetic changes in diabetes and cardiovascular risk. Circ Res. 2016;118(11):1706-22.
37. El-Osta A, Brasacchio D, Yao D, et al. Transient high glucose causes persistent epigenetic changes and altered gene expression during subsequent normoglycemia. J Exp Med. 2008;205(10):2409-17.
38. Hodgin JB, Nair V, Zhang H, et al. Identification of cross-species shared transcriptional networks of diabetic nephropathy in human and mouse glomeruli. Diabetes. 2013;62(1):299-308.
39. Baylin SB, Jones PA. A decade of exploring the cancer epigenome - biological and translational implications. Nat Rev Cancer. 2011;11(10):726-34.
40. Kato M, Natarajan R. Diabetic nephropathy--emerging epigenetic mechanisms. Nat Rev Nephrol. 2014;10(9):517-30.

Chapter 76

PCSK9 Inhibitors in Diabetic Dyslipidemia

Sudarshan Ramachandran, Mithun Bhartia, Alan Jones, Richard Charles Strange

INTRODUCTION

The association between cardiovascular disease (CVD) risk and raised serum total cholesterol and low-density lipoprotein cholesterol (LDL-C) has been demonstrated in epidemiology and intervention trials showing significant decreases in CVD following use of LDL-C-reducing agents, such as statins and ezetimibe, and has given rise to the low-density lipoprotein (LDL) hypothesis.[1,2] However, even with statin/ezetimibe combination treatment, many patients fail to achieve LDL-C targets. The proprotein convertase subtilisin/kexin type 9 (PCSK9) inhibitors are monoclonal antibodies that bind and inactivate PCSK9, leading to decreased LDL receptor degradation, and hence enhanced LDL receptor recycling back to the liver surface (up to 150 times) and increased LDL uptake.[3] The PCSK9 inhibition was identified as a potential modifier of CVD risk, as loss of function mutations in the *PCSK9* gene were associated with low LDL-C and reduced CVD.[4] We will explore efficacy (trials and outpatient data) and outcome evidence with emphasis on patients with diabetes mellitus (DM), especially type 2 DM (T2DM).

PROPROTEIN CONVERTASE SUBTILISIN/KEXIN TYPE 9 INHIBITOR EFFICACY

Alirocumab and evolocumab were licensed in 2015 and given as monotherapy or in combination with statins/ezetimibe leading to LDL-C reductions of 45–70%.[5] Tables 1 to 4 provide details of LDL-C reductions seen with alirocumab and evolocumab in some trials evaluating efficacy. The LDL-C reductions were similar in the total cohort and patient subgroups; DM, without DM, T2DM, type 1 diabetes, metabolic syndrome, mixed dyslipidemia and impaired fasting glucose. Further, treatment-related mortality, adverse events, and treatment discontinuation were similar in the PCSK 9 inhibitor and control groups in all the studies described (Tables 1 to 4). Nasopharyngitis, upper respiratory tract infections and injection site reactions (generally mild) were the commonest adverse effects.[5] None of the above phenomena were more common in individuals with DM; in fact, lower local injection site reactions were observed.[5]

Local Efficacy Data

Proprotein convertase subtilisin/kexin type 9 inhibitors were approved for use in the National Health Service (NHS) by the National Institute for Health and Care Excellence (NICE) in 2016 in secondary prevention and heterozygous familial hypercholesterolemia (FH) (https://www.nice.org.uk/guidance/ta393, https://www.nice.org.uk/guidance/ta394) when LDL-C remained above specific threshold levels after the use of statins (maximally tolerated dose) and ezetimibe. In secondary prevention, LDL-C treatment thresholds of 4.0 and 3.5 mmol/L are recommended in patients considered high risk (history of acute coronary syndrome, coronary or other arterial revascularization procedures, chronic heart disease, ischemic stroke, peripheral arterial disease) and very high risk (recurrent cardiovascular events or cardiovascular events in more than one vascular bed) of CVD, respectively. In contrast, an LDL-C threshold >5.0 mmol/L was recommended in FH after maximal statin/ezetimibe treatment. We evaluated the LDL-C reductions in 42 patients commenced on fortnightly alirocumab 150 mg (n = 30) and evolocumab 140 mg (n = 12) after the first 6 months of use (Table 5, Fig. 1).

TABLE 1: Allirocumab efficacy data (alirocumab vs. control groups) with subgroup analysis based on diabetes.

	Total cohort		Diabetes		No Diabetes	
	Alrocumab	Control	Alrocumab	Control	Alrocumab	Control
Alirocumab trials	% Mean LDL-C change (n)					
ODYSSEY LONG TERM (150 mg vs. placebo) + max tolerated lipid lowering (24 weeks)	−61.0 (1530)	+0.8 (780)	−60.0 (545)	−1.0 (273)	−61.6 (985)	+1.8 (507)
ODYSSEY FH1 and FH2 (pooled analysis) (75 mg/150 mg vs. placebo) + max tolerated lipid lowering (24 weeks)	−48.8 (488)	+7.1 (244)	−51.4 (37)	+2.4 (29)	−48.5 (451)	+7.6 (215)
ODYSSEY COMBO I (75 mg/150 mg vs. placebo) + max tolerated lipid lowering (24 weeks)	−48.2 (205)	−2.3 (106)	−42.2 (94)	−2.6 (41)	−53.2 (111)	−2.0 (65)
ODYSSEY COMBO II (75 mg/150 mg vs. ezetimibe) + max tolerated lipid lowering (24 weeks)	−50.6 (479)	−20.7 (241)	−49.1 (148)	−18.4 (77)	−51.2 (331)	−21.8 (164)

(LDL-C: low-density lipoprotein cholesterol)

TABLE 2: Allirocumab efficacy data (alirocumab vs. control groups) in type 1 diabetes mellitus and type 2 diabetes mellitus.

	T2DM		T2DM	
	Alrocumab	Control	Alrocumab	Control
Alirocuma b trials	% Mean LDL-C change (n)			
ODYSSEY DM-INSULIN (75 mg/150 mg vs. placebo) + max tolerated lipid lowering (24 weeks)	−48.2 (287)	+0.8 (142)	−51.8 (49)	−3.9 (25)

(LDL-C: low-density lipoprotein cholesterol; T1DM: type 1 diabetes mellitus; T2DM: type 2 diabetes mellitus.)

Interestingly, baseline LDL-C (5.0 mmol/L) and LDL-C reductions were nearly identical for both treatments (https://www.atherosclerosis-journal.com/article/S0021-9150(17)31051-1/pdf). The LDL-C change was associated with baseline levels, but not treatment duration (>2 months). We noted a wider variation in LDL-C reduction: 21–83% (Fig. 2) than some of the phase 3 PCSK9 inhibitor trials reviewed above.[5] We speculated that baseline PCSK9 activity, etiology of the hypercholesterolemia, and concurrent use of other lipid-lowering agents may have led to this variation. Unfortunately, low patient numbers prevented stratification of the group by DM. It was reassuring that the efficacy was in accordance with that observed in published phase 3 trials (Tables 1 to 4).

OUTCOME TRIALS WITH PROPROTEIN CONVERTASE SUBTILISIN/KEXIN TYPE 9 INHIBITORS

Several randomized controlled trials have demonstrated the effectiveness of statins in primary and secondary prevention.[6] The Collaborative Atorvastatin Diabetes Study trial compared the effect of atorvastatin (10 mg) against placebo in primary prevention patients with T2DM and an LDL-C ≤4.14 mmol/L together with one of the following conditions, retinopathy, albuminuria, history of current smoking and hypertension as inclusion criteria.[7] The trial was discontinued 2 years early due to the end point (CVD reduction) being met prematurely; a 37% relative risk reduction of CVD was seen. The individual components of CVD also showed significant event reductions; coronary heart disease: 36%, coronary revascularizations: 31%, strokes: 48%. Total mortality decreased by 27% albeit not significantly.

Cardiovascular disease reduction with PCSK9 inhibitors was hinted at by post hoc analyses of the OSLER[8] and ODYSSEY LONG TERM[9] efficacy trials. The GLAGOV study investigated 970 patients with angiographic coronary artery disease (LDL-C ≥2.07 mmol/L or between 1.55 and and 2.07mmol/L with one major or 3 minor cardiovascular risk factors) over 78 weeks of treatment.[10] The evolocumab was associated with reduction in

TABLE 3: Allirocumab efficacy data (alirocumab vs. control groups) in patients with type 2 diabetes mellitus and mixed dyslipidemia.

	T2DM + mixed dyslipidemia	
	Alrocumab	Control
Alirocumab trials	% Mean LDL-C change (n)	
ODYSSEY DM-DYSLIPIDEMIA (75 mg/150 mg vs. placebo) + max statin therapy (12 weeks)	−43.3 (273)	−0.3 (136)
TG change	alirocumab −15.4%	fenofibrate −24.4%
	alirocumab −12.4%	omega-3 fatty acids −9.6%
Lp(a) change	alirocumab −23.7%	standard care +3.7%
	alirocumab −26.2%	ezetimibe +3.2%
	alirocumab −18.9%	fenofibrate +3.9%
	alirocumab −18.3%	omega-3 fatty acids +5.7%

(LDL-C: low-density lipoprotein cholesterol; T2DM: type 2 diabetes mellitus.)

atheroma volume (primary outcome) on angiography with more individuals demonstrating plaque regression (64.3% vs. 47.3%) and fewer developing major adverse cardiac events (12.2% vs. 15.3%) compared to controls (secondary outcomes).

The FOURIER was the first clinical outcome trial comparing evolocumab against placebo in 27,564 patients with atherosclerotic CVD, LDL-C ≥1.8 mmol/L or non-high-density lipoprotein cholesterol (HDL-C) ≥2.6 mmol/L and receiving moderate-to-high-intensity statin therapy.[11] During a median 2.2 years follow-up, a statistically significant reduction [hazard ratio (HR): 0.85, 95% confidence interval (CI): 0.79–0.92, p <0.001] in a composite major adverse cardiac events end point (primary outcome) of cardiovascular death, myocardial infarction, stroke, hospital admission with unstable angina or coronary revascularization was observed (evolocumab: 9.8%, placebo: 11.3%).[11] Relative risk reduction in the FOURIER trial was in accordance with benefit seen in statin trials when follow-up was taken into account. Patients with (n = 11,031) and without (n = 16,533) DM showed similar reduction in the primary outcome, with DM (HR: 0.83, 95% CI: 0.75–0.93, p = 0.0008) and without DM (HR: 0.87, 95% CI: 0.79–0.96, p = 0.0052).[12] No difference in adverse events was observed between DM patients at baseline (evolocumab: 78.5%, placebo: 78.3%) and those without DM (evolocumab: 76.8%, placebo: 76.8%).

TABLE 4: Evolocumab efficacy data (evolocumab vs. control groups) in patients with type 2 diabetes mellitus, metabolic syndrome and impaired fasting glucose.

	T2DM			No DM		
Evolocumab trials	Evolocumab	Controls	% LDL-C difference	Evolocumab	Controls	% LDL-C difference
LAPLACE-2 and RUTHERFORD-2 (140 mg/2 weeks or 420 mg/4 weeks) vs. placebo + max tolerated lipid lowering (24 weeks)	210	94	−60.0%	1127	573	−66.0%
DESCARTES (r 420 mg/4 weeks vs. placebo) + max tolerated lipid lowering (52 weeks)	Total cohort			T2DM		
	599	302	−57.0%	77	43	−50.8%
	Impaired fasting glucose			Mets		
	194	99	−59.40%	182	107	−55.0%
	No impaired fasting glucose or MetS			–		
	294	119	−58.1%	–	–	–
FOURIER (140 mg/2 weeks or 420 mg/4 weeks vs. placebo) + max tolerated lipid lowering (48 weeks)	Total cohort			DM		
	13,784	13,779	−59.0%	5,515	5,516	−57.0%
	No DM			–		
	8,269	8,264	−60.0%	–	–	–

(DM: diabetes mellitus; LDL-C: low-density lipoprotein cholesterol; MetS: metabolic syndrome; T2DM: type 2 diabetes mellitus.)

TABLE 5: Low-density lipoprotein cholesterol values before and after proprotein convertase subtilisin/kexin type 9 inhibitors in an outpatient setting.

	n	Pre-PCSK91 LDL-C Mean (SD)	Post-PCSK91 LDL-C Mean (SD)	LDL-C change Mean (SD)	% LDL-C change Mean (SD)
Alirocumab	30	5.0 (1.3) mmol/L	2.3 (1.3) mmol/L	2.7 (0.9) mmol/L	55.7 (17.0)
Evolocumab	12	5.0 (1.3) mmol/L	2.3 (1.3) mmol/L	2.7 (1.2) mmol/L	5 4 .2 (20.4)

(LDL-C: low-density lipoprotein cholesterol; PCSK91: proprotein convertase subtilisin/kexin type 91; SD: standard deviation.)

Source: Data from the clinics at Good Hope and Birmingham Heartlands Hospitals, now part of University Hospitals Birmingham.

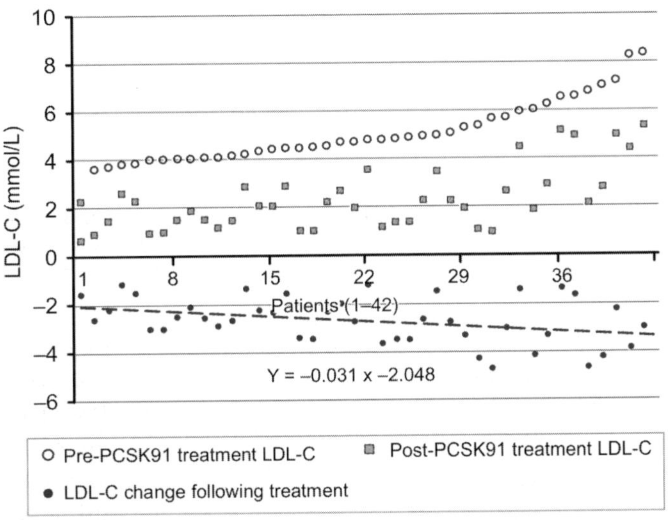

(LDL-C: low-density lipoprotein cholesterol; PCSK91: proprotein convertase subtilisin/kexin type 91.)

Figure 1 Low-density lipoprotein cholesterol (LDL-C): Pre- and post-treatment values in an outpatient setting. Greater decrease in LDL-C was associated with higher baseline LDL-C (multiple regression analysis): c = 0.26, 95% CI: 0.03–0.50, p = 0.026. No difference between the 2 PCSK9 inhibitors or duration of treatment was observed.

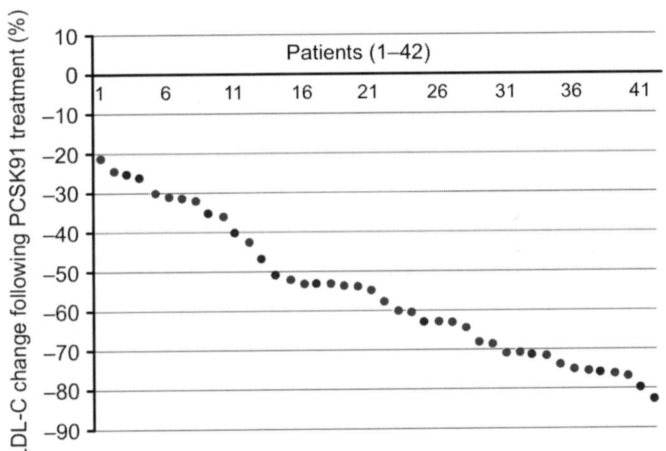

(LDL-C: low-density lipoprotein cholesterol; PCSK91: proprotein convertase subtilisin/kexin type 91; Pink dots: alirocumab; black dots: evolocumab.)

Figure 2 Low-density lipoprotein cholesterol: Percentage change following proprotein convertase subtilisin/kexin type 9 inhibitors in an outpatient setting.

The as yet unpublished, ODYSSEY OUTCOMES trial, presented at the American College of Cardiology Annual Scientific Sessions in March 2018, evaluated as primary outcome over 48 months, a composite of mortality associated with coronary heart disease, nonfatal myocardial infarction, fatal or nonfatal stroke or hospitalization due to unstable angina in 18,924 patients (http://www.clinicaltrialresults.org/Slides/ACC2018/ODYSSEY_Steg.pdf) following alirocumab treatment (75 mg, titrated up to 150 mg depending on whether target LDL-C was achieved). Inclusion criteria consisted of age ≥40 years, occurrence of acute coronary syndrome 1–12 months prior to randomization, being on high-intensity statins and elevated lipids (LDL-C ≥1.8 mmol/L, non-HDL-C ≥2.6 mmol/L, or apolipoprotein B ≥80 mg/dL). The LDL-C reductions seen with alirocumab, compared with placebo, were 62.7%, 61.0% and 54.7% after 4, 12 and 48 months, respectively. The alirocumab (9.5%) was associated with fewer events (primary outcome) (HR: 0.85, 95% CI: 0.78–0.93, p = 0.0003) compared to placebo (11.1%). Analysis of specified groups suggested that maximum benefit was in 5,629 individuals with a baseline LDL-C ≥2.59 mmol/L (HR: 0.76, 95% CI: 0.65–0.87, p = 0.0003). We await analyses of data from the 5,444 DM patients.

DO PROPROTEIN CONVERTASE SUBTILISIN/KEXIN TYPE-9 INHIBITORS INCREASE THE RISK OF DIABETES?

Following conflicting results on new-onset diabetes associated with statin therapy,[13] Sattar et al. carried out a meta-analysis of 13 trials between 1994 and 2009 comparing statin therapy with placebo of 91,140 individuals without DM.[14] The statin therapy was associated with an increase in new-onset diabetes [4.89%, odds ratio (OR): 1.09, 95% CI: 1.02–1.17] compared with placebo (4.5%).

So far, PCSK9 inhibitors have not been associated with new-onset diabetes. In the FOURIER trial, evolocumab treatment did not increase the risk of new-onset DM in individuals without DM (HR: 1.05, 95% CI: 0.94–1.17) and with prediabetes (HR: 1.00, 95% CI: 0.89–1.13) at recruitment.[12] Further, HbA1c and fasting plasma glucose concentrations were similar between evolocumab and placebo groups during follow-up in patients classified as having DM, prediabetes or normoglycemia at baseline.[12]

Data from the ODYSSEY OUTCOMES trial showed alirocumab was not associated with new-onset DM during follow-up; alirocumab: 9.6%, placebo: 10.1% (http://www.clinicaltrialresults.org/Slides/ACC2018/ODYSSEY_Steg.pdf). Further, patients on alirocumab did not experience worsening glycemic control or development of DM-related complications; alirocumab: 18.8%, placebo: 21.2%. Despite the above outcome trials suggesting that new-onset DM was not associated with PCSK9 inhibitors, further study over a longer follow-up is needed.

CONCLUSION

The PCSK9 inhibitor studies have added confirmatory evidence to the LDL-C hypothesis. Statins will be frontline treatment for the foreseeable future because of safety data spanning three decades, cost, and wealth of evidence. Although the efficacy of ezetimibe is not similarly substantiated, it will remain as add-on to statin treatment due to cost and outcome evidence. PCSK9 inhibitors have proven efficacy and with the FOURIER and ODYSSEY OUTCOMES trials have clinical outcome evidence. Efficacy and outcomes are similar in patients with and without DM. They do not appear to be related to new-onset T2DM, though studies with longer follow-up are required. Clinical outcomes in patients with elevated lipoprotein (a) levels need assessing in view of reduced levels after PCSK9 inhibitor treatment.

At present, the PCSK9 inhibitors will remain as third in line because of cost. Our clinical experience shows that they are very useful in high-risk patients unable to tolerate statins. We estimated that following an initial high uptake because of an accumulated cohort of patients not meeting LDL-C targets, PCSK9 inhibitors in the United Kingdom will be used in relatively small numbers of patients referred to dyslipidemia/metabolic clinics (5.2%, 2.2%, 1.5% and 0.4% in patients with LDL-C >3.0, 3.5, 4.0 and 5.0 mmol/L, respectively).[15] In healthcare systems funded by general taxation such as the NHS in the United Kingdom, cost benefit has led to NICE guidelines with LDL-C thresholds of 3.5, 4.0 and 5.0 mmol/L in high-risk patients. Other healthcare systems will have to build these agents into their own guidelines based on outcome evidence, cost and high tolerability.

REFERENCES

1. Mendis S. The contribution of the Framingham Heart Study to the prevention of cardiovascular disease: a global perspective. Prog Cardiovasc Dis. 2010;53(1):10-4.
2. Jarco JA, Keaney JF. Proof that lower is better—LDL cholesterol and IMPROVE-IT. N Engl J Med. 2015;372(25):2248-50.
3. Brown MS, Anderson RG, Goldstein JL. Recycling receptors: the round-trip itinerary of migrant membrane proteins. Cell. 1983;32(3):663-7.
4. Horton JD, Cohen JC, Hobbs HH. PCSK9: a convertase that coordinates LDL catabolism. J. Lipid Res. 2009;50(Suppl.):S172-7.
5. Handelsman Y, Lepor NE. PCSK9 inhibitors in lipid management of patients with diabetes and high cardiovascular risk: a review. J Am Heart Assoc. 2018;7(13):e008953.
6. Abbas A, Milles J, Ramachandran S. Rosuvastatin and atorvastatin: comparative effects on glucose metabolism in non-diabetic patients with dyslipidaemia. Clin Med Insights Endocrinol Diabetes. 2012;5:13-30.
7. Colhoun HM, Betteridge DJ, Durrington PN, et al. Primary prevention of cardiovascular disease with atorvastatin in type 2 diabetes in the Collaborative Atorvastatin Diabetes Study (CARDS): multicentre randomised placebo-controlled trial. Lancet. 2004;364(9435):685-96.
8. Sabatine MS, Giugliano RP, Wiviott SD, et al. Open-Label Study of Long-Term Evaluation against LDL Cholesterol Investigators. Efficacy and safety of evolocumab in reducing lipids and cardiovascular events. N Engl J Med. 2015; 372(16):1500-9.
9. Robinson JG, Farnier M, Krempf M, et al. Efficacy and safety of alirocumab in reducing lipids and cardiovascular events. N Engl J Med. 2015;372(16):1489-99.
10. Nicholls SJ, Puri R, Anderson T, et al. Effect of evolocumab on progression of coronary disease in statin-treated patients: the GLAGOV randomized clinical trial. JAMA. 2016;316(22):2373-84.
11. Sabatine MS, Giugliano RP, Keech AC, et al. Evolocumab and clinical outcomes in patients with cardiovascular disease. N Engl J Med. 2017; 376(18):1713-22.
12. Sabatine MS, Leiter LA, Wiviott SD, et al. Cardiovascular safety and efficacy of the PCSK9 inhibitor evolocumab in patients with and without diabetes and the effect of evolocumab on glycaemia and risk of new-onset diabetes: a prespecified analysis of the FOURIER randomised controlled trial. Lancet Diabetes Endocrinol. 2017;5(12):941-50.
13. Belalcazar LM, Raghavan VA, Ballantyne CM. Statin-induced diabetes: will it change clinical practice? Diabetes Care. 2009;32(10):1941-3.
14. Sattar N, Preiss D, Murray HM, et al. Statins and risk of incident diabetes: a collaborative meta-analysis of randomised statin trials. Lancet. 2010;375(9716):735-42.
15. Groves C, Shetty C, Strange RC, et al. A study in high risk, maximally pretreated patients to determine the potential use of PCSK9 inhibitors at various thresholds of total and LDL cholesterol levels. Postgrad Med J. 2017;93(1098):205-8.

Chapter 77

Current Technologies in Diabetes Management

Jothydev Kesavadev

INTRODUCTION

With the advancements in technology during the past two decades, many of the shortcomings of conventional diabetes care practices have started to resolve in an appreciable manner. Blood glucose monitors integrated with mobile apps and web apps available today, makes diabetes management much simpler and easier. Likewise, continuous glucose monitoring systems (CGMS) can provide constant insight into changing glucose levels enabling users to manage their diabetes better.[1,2] Insulin pump therapy though originally meant for type 1 diabetes (T1D), currently it is approved for use in any type of diabetes as an advanced gadget for delivering insulin replacing the conventional syringes and pens. The Indian insulin pump guidelines advocate the use of pumps in eligible and affordable patients as an alternative drug delivery device with proven benefits.[3,4] Open loop technologies are gradually being replaced with partially closed loop and hybrid closed-loop systems. Artificial pancreas (AP) systems with multiple glucoregulatory hormones have successfully completed clinical trials. These new generation devices and upcoming technologies are all supposed to be cost-effective and path-breaking which could address and overcome the major challenges in diabetes management. Some of the recently introduced technologies for diabetes care are discussed here.

ONETOUCH VERIO FLEX™ METER AND THE ONETOUCH REVEAL™ APP

The OneTouch Verio Flex® meter with Color Sure™ technology (Fig. 1) instantly shows the users if their blood glucose levels are in or out of range. The range indicator arrow points to the corresponding blue, green or red color bar below the meter display.

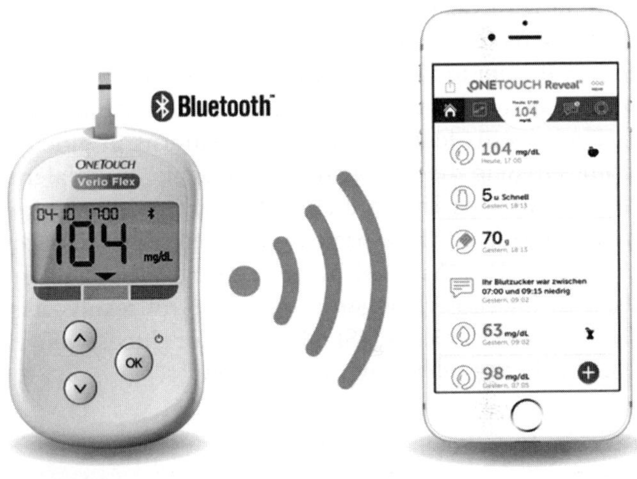

Figure 1 OneTouch Verio Flex™ Meter and the OneTouch Reveal™ app. ***(For color version, see Plate 6)***

The OneTouch Verio Flex® meter also connects wirelessly with the OneTouch Reveal® mobile app and syncs data directly to the patient's smartphone or tablet. The electronic visual logbook in the mobile app automatically logs and organizes blood glucose results and transforms data into quick visual snapshots. Color Sure™ technology highlights patterns and can motivate patients to perform structured self-monitoring of blood glucose (SMBG). The data can be shared with the healthcare provider. The app also facilitates the entry of data on medications, insulin dosages, carbs and physical activity. For the healthcare team, the OneTouch Reveal

Web App facilitates setting of individualized short-term and long-term treatment goals, quick subgroup analysis of the patients and generate ready to publish data.[5]

CONTOUR® NEXT ONE BLOOD GLUCOSE MONITORING SYSTEM

The CONTOUR® NEXT ONE smart meter and CONTOUR® DIABETES app (Fig. 2) seamlessly connect to capture the blood glucose readings via Bluetooth, which can be accessed on a smartphone, tablet or computer. The captured readings will be automatically synced and logged and over time, helps create meaningful insights. The CONTOUR® NEXT ONE smart meter system has many salient features such as the 1) Smartlight® feature (an instant indicator of the blood glucose levels, i.e. green for within target, amber for above target and red for below target), Second-Chance® sampling (allows users to reapply blood to the same test strip if the first sample was insufficient to take a reading), options to add events like diet, activity, medication, photos and voice memos etc. my patterns feature detects the patterns in glucose readings to help the user gain more insights, smart alerts when glucose readings are critically out of range, share reports with healthcare professionals, etc. The smallest error range demonstrated by the glucose meter system was that, for subject fingertip tests, 95% of results met ±8.4 mg/dL or ±8.4% (vs. YSI reference) for glucose values <100 mg/dL or ≥100 mg/dL, respectively.[6]

iPro®2 CONTINUOUS GLUCOSE MONITORING SYSTEM

The iPro®2 (Medtronic, Inc. Diabetes) professional CGMS procures interstitial fluid (ISF) glucose profile (Fig. 3) and consists of Enlite Sensor, iPro2 recorder and the Enlite serter. The iPro2 recorder collects (up to 7 days of data) and stores data from the glucose sensor and is intended for multiple patient use (can be used up to 60 times). The data can be uploaded into CareLinki Pro® Therapy Management Software for Diabetes, to generate reports and store the data. The reports provide a quick visualization of the patient's glucose excursions as well as possible explanations/suggestions based on the glucose trends, allowing the healthcare provider to take optimal treatment decisions.[7]

FREESTYLE LIBRE™ PRO CONTINUOUS GLUCOSE MONITORING SYSTEM

Abbott's FreeStyle Libre™ Flash Glucose Monitoring system (FGM) comes in two versions FreeStyle Libre (real time) and FreeStyle Libre Pro (professional version). Only the professional version, FreeStyle Libre Pro (Fig. 4), is marketed in India. The system consists of a small, round sensor that can be worn on the back of the upper arm, which measures ISF glucose every minute. The sensor comes in a factory-calibrated mode and has a recommended sensor wear-time of 14 days. The system

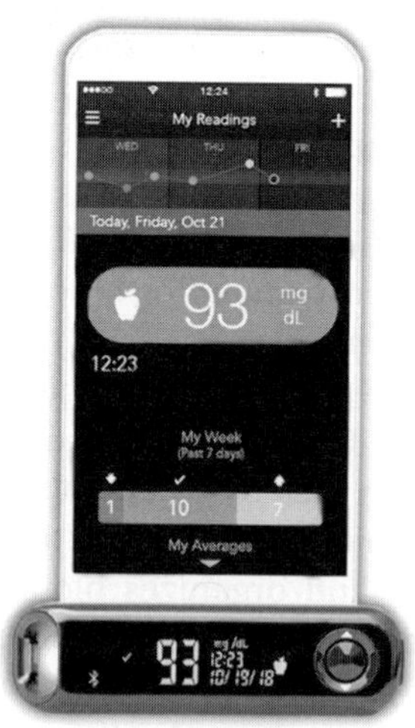

Figure 2 CONTOUR® NEXT ONE blood glucose monitoring system. ***(For color version, see Plate 6)***

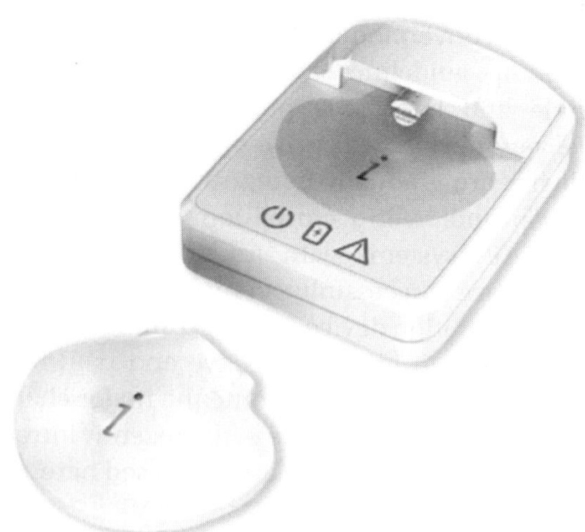

Figure 3 iPro®2 professional continuous glucose monitoring system. ***(For color version, see Plate 6)***

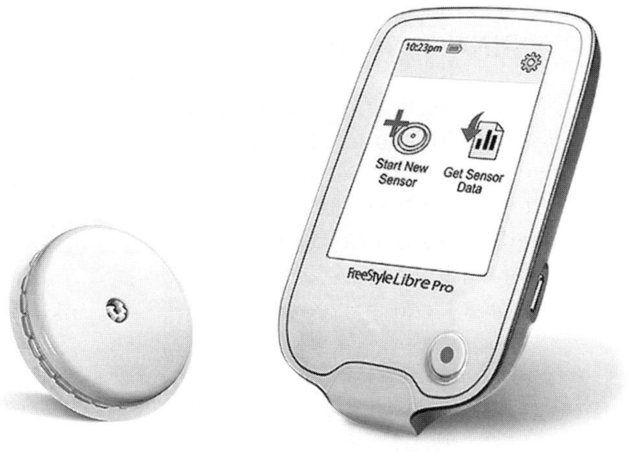

Figure 4 FreeStyle Libre™ Pro continuous glucose monitoring system. ***(For color version, see Plate 7)***

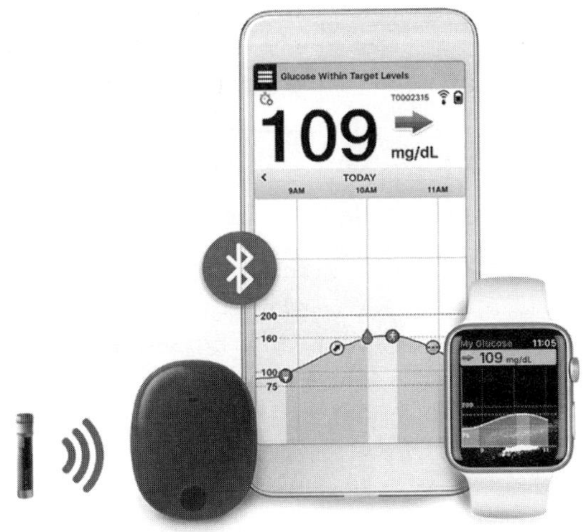

Figure 5 Eversense® 90-day implantable continuous glucose monitoring system. ***(For color version, see Plate 7)***

captures as many as 1340 glucose values which can be procured by the healthcare provider's FreeStyle Libre Pro reader in as little as 5 seconds (a single reader can be used to scan Freestyle Libre Pro sensors of multiple patients). The comprehensive glucose report generated, 'Ambulatory Glucose Profile (AGP)' provides a visual snapshot of glucose levels and is found to be an effective basis for education and increasing involvement in diabetes self-management.[8,9]

EVERSENSE® 90-DAY IMPLANTABLE CONTINUOUS GLUCOSE MONITORING SYSTEM

Eversense® CGMS (Fig. 5) is the first and only CGMS to feature an implantable glucose sensor and provides long-term continuous monitoring for up to 90 days. The system includes a pill-sized sensor implanted in the upper arm, an on-body transmitter and a mobile app that displays glucose data and issues alert to high and low blood glucose values. Eversense's 90-day wear thus eliminates the need for frequent sensor insertions required by other CGMS. This is also the first CGMS to provide on-body vibration alerts and thus notifies the user in the event of highs and lows.[10]

GUARDIAN™ CONNECT CONTINUOUS GLUCOSE MONITORING SYSTEM

Guardian™ Connect CGMS (Fig. 6) works with three elements: a thin sensor (Guardian Sensor 3 which is FDA approved to be used to control the AP system, MiniMed™

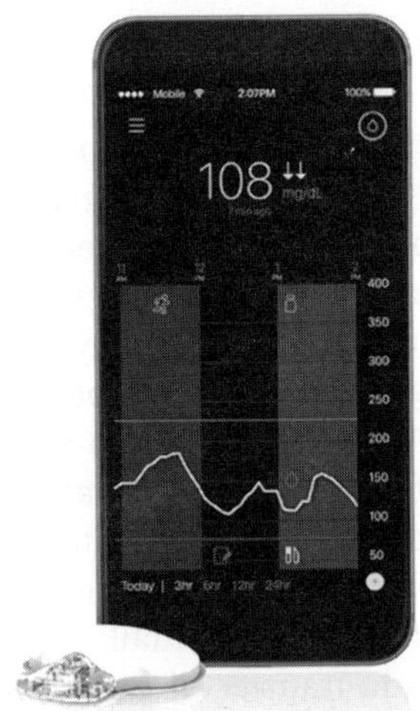

Figure 6 Guardian™ Connect continuous glucose monitoring system. ***(For color version, see Plate 7)***

670G), a small transmitter attached to the sensor and the Guardian Connect app on a compatible iOS device. It is thus the first smart standalone CGMS that does not require a receiver and directly sends the continuous sensor glucose data from the sensor transmitter to a smartphone. The Sugar.IQ™ smart diabetes assistant app continually analyzes how an individual's glucose levels respond to food intake, insulin dosages, daily routines and other factors. The system has customizable alerts that can notify the users about future high and low glucose events up to 60 minutes in advance, and also allows the caregivers to track the user's glycemic status remotely.[11]

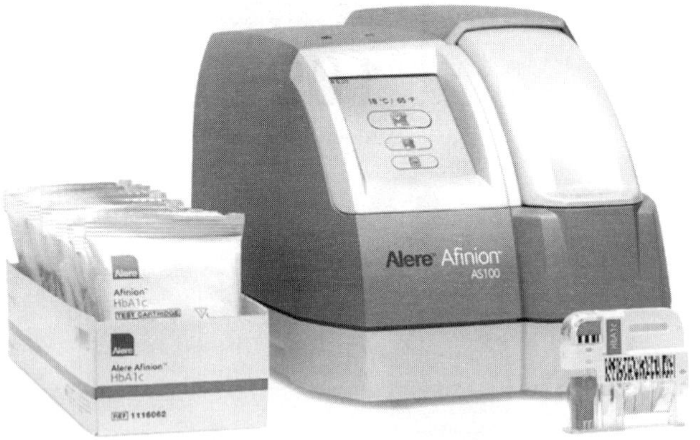

Figure 7 Point-of-Care HbA1c testing device alere Afinion™ HbA1c Dx. ***(For color version, see Plate 7)***

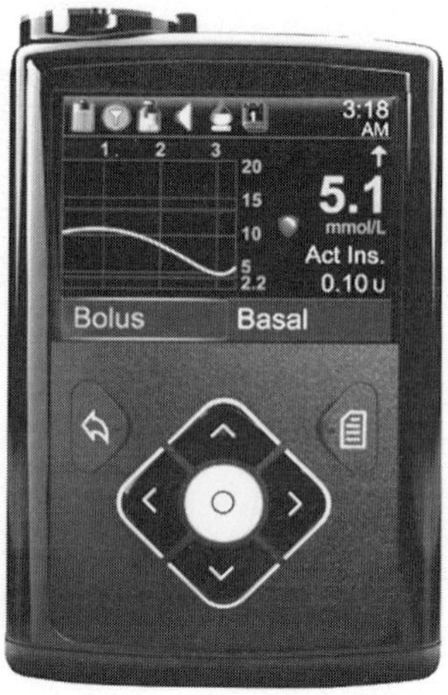

Figure 8 MiniMed™ 640G Insulin Pump. ***(For color version, see Plate 7)***

ALERE AFINION™ HbA1c

Alere Afinion™ HbA1c (Fig. 7) is a point-of-care HbA1c testing device, a desktop-size analyzer designed for use in a physician's office, a treatment room or at a bedside. It uses a finger-prick capillary blood sample which when applied to a test cartridge, is analyzed within several minutes. The system has several potential advantages over laboratory A1c testing such as simple to perform, accurate (insignificant lot-to-lot variation and total error of <6%) and rapid test results expedite medical decision-making, more convenient for patients and can improve health system efficiency. A small connectivity device facilitates automatic transfer of data from the analyzer to a laboratory, information system or other electronic record systems.[12]

MINIMED™ 640G SENSOR-AUGMENTED INSULIN PUMP

The MiniMed™ 640G Insulin Pump (Fig. 8) is a sensor-augmented pump (SAP) and has built-in intelligent features including the SmartGuard technology, active insulin tracking, bolus progress bar and predictive battery life. The SmartGuard technology predicts when a patient is approaching low glucose levels 30 minutes in advance and automatically stops insulin delivery. When the glucose levels recover, SmartGuard will automatically resume insulin delivery. Multiple low limits can be set throughout the day to give increased protection.[13]

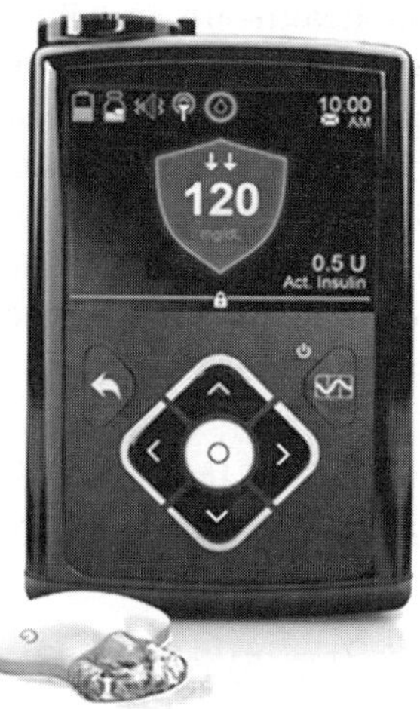

Figure 9 MiniMed™ 670G hybrid closed-loop insulin pump. ***(For color version, see Plate 7)***

MINIMED™ 670G INSULIN PUMP–THE WORLD'S FIRST HYBRID CLOSED-LOOP SYSTEM

The Medtronic's MiniMed™ 670G hybrid closed-loop insulin pump system (Fig. 9) consists of MiniMed 670G insulin pump, the Guardian Link 3 Transmitter, the Guardian Sensor 3, One-Press Serter, and the Contour NEXT Link 2.4 Glucose Meter. The MiniMed 670G system features an advanced algorithm, the SmartGuard HCL, which enables greater glucose control with reduced user input. The suspend on low feature stops insulin delivery for up to 2 hours when the sensor reaches a preset low

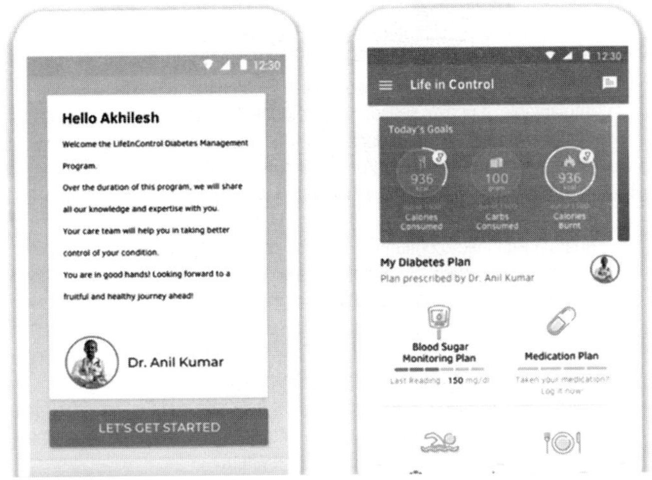

Figure 10 Life in Control™ Diabetes Coach. ***(For color version, see Plate 8)***

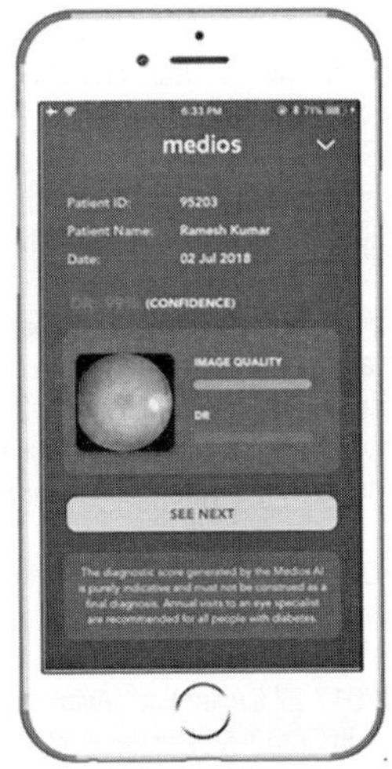

Figure 11 Medios Technologies AI assistant to detect diabetic retinopathy. ***(For color version, see Plate 8)***

and the suspend before low option stops insulin delivery up to 30 minutes before reaching the preset low limits and automatically resumes when the glucose levels recover. When in auto mode, the system automatically adjusts the user's basal insulin every 5 minutes based on the CGM readings. The 670G will thus reduce time at dangerous high and low blood sugar levels, improve time-in-range, reduce glucose variability, bring much greater night-time safety and target morning blood sugars.[14]

LIFE IN CONTROL™ DIABETES COACH—A MULTI-MODEL BOT ENABLED DIABETES CARE PLATFORM

The multi-model BOT enabled diabetes care platform Life in Control™ Diabetes Coach app (Fig. 10) is designed to keep doctors and patients connected. It allows integration with hospital electronic medical record and monitoring devices and thus guides and supports the users to set goals and daily tasks, improve their lifestyle, track calorie intake and physical activities, get glycemic rating, nutritional information and personalized diet plans etc. It also analyzes the user's medical history to predict secondary complications so as to prevent diabetes and promote wellness. It helps clinicians improve their overall productivity and is proven to be a highly cost-effective and time-saving option.[15,16]

MEDIOS TECHNOLOGIES AI ASSISTANT TO DETECT DIABETIC RETINOPATHY

Medios Technologies AI assistant (Fig. 11) uses deep learning to help doctors diagnose diabetic retinopathy (DR) during a typical diabetes check-up. It works by taking an image of the eye, running it through a software programme which then provides an almost-immediate diagnosis. Artificial intelligence automatically grades fundus images, detects all cases of referable DR including moderate NPDR, severe nonproliferative diabetic retinopathy (NPDR) and proliferative DR. The first model is capable of detecting if a retinal image needs a referral with 98% sensitivity.[17]

CONCLUSION

Conventional diabetes treatment and management processes were usually centered around hospitals and primary care physicians which had their own limitations such as enabling most of the times only a physician-centered one-way communication, unable to provide a systematic assistance via social support to address the psychological needs of the patients and unable to readily adopt advanced health information technologies that could otherwise facilitate effective healthcare. Newer technologies, while replacing the existing ones, are simpler, user-friendly, cost-effective and ensure successful short-term and long-term outcomes in the treatment of both T1D and type 2 diabetes. Physicians should adopt technologies in eligible and affordable candidates to successfully overcome the major barriers in treatment and help patients retain the quality of life while surviving longer with the disease.

REFERENCES

1. Kesavadev J, Vigersky R, Shin J, et al. Assessing the Therapeutic Utility of Professional Continuous Glucose Monitoring in Type 2 Diabetes Across Various Therapies: A Retrospective Evaluation. Adv Ther. 2017;34(8):1918-27.

2. Kesavadev J, Krishnan G, Saboo B, et al. Better Outcomes in Type 2 Diabetes Management with a User Friendly Flash Glucose Monitoring System: Freestyle Libre Pro. Diabetes Technol Ther. 2017;19(S1): A1-133.
3. Kesavadev J, Jain SM, Muruganathan A, et al. Consensus evidence-based guidelines for use of insulin pump therapy in the management of diabetes as per Indian clinical practice. J Assoc Physicians India. 2014;62(7 Suppl):34-41.
4. Kesavadev J, Das AK, Unnikrishnan R, Joshi SR, Ramachandran A, Shamsudeen J, et al. Use of insulin pumps in India: suggested guidelines based on experience and cultural differences. 2010;12(10):823-31.
5. OneTouch Reveal® mobile and web apps for patients [cited 2018 30 August]. Available from: https://professional.onetouch.com/software-and-apps/reveal-app.
6. CONTOUR®NEXT ONE blood glucose monitoring system [cited 2018 31 August]. Available from: https://www.contournextone.com/.
7. Medtronic MiniMed I. iPro™2 Professional Continuous Glucose Monitoring (CGM) 2017 [cited 2017 27 December]. Available from: http://professional.medtronicdiabetes.com/ipro2-professional-cgm.
8. Abbott. Real-World Data from Abbott's FreeStyle® Libre Show Association Between Higher Frequency of Glucose Monitoring and Improved Glucose Control for People with Diabetes: Cision PR Newswire; 2017 [cited 2017 27 December]. Available from: https://www.prnewswire.com/news-releases/real-world-data-from-abbotts-freestyle-libre-show-association-between-higher-frequency-of-glucose-monitoring-and-improved-glucose-control-for-people-with-diabetes-300407487.html
9. Kesavadev J, Shankar A, Ashok AD, et al. Our First 825 T2DM Patients on 14-Day Factory-Calibrated Glucose Monitoring System: Clinical Utility and Challenges. J Diabetes Sci Technol. 2018;12(1):230-1.
10. FDA approves first continuous glucose monitoring system with a fully implantable glucose sensor and compatible mobile app for adults with diabetes [press release]. June 21 2018. Available from: https://www.fda.gov/newsevents/newsroom/pressannouncements/ucm611454.htm
11. Medtronic MiniMed I. The Guardian™ Connect CGM 2018 [cited 2018 14 August]. Available from: https://www.medtronicdiabetes.com/products/guardian-connect-continuous-glucose-monitoring-system.
12. Foerster V, Severn M. Point-of-Care Glycated Hemoglobin Testing to Diagnose Type 2 Diabetes. 2017.
13. The MiniMed™ 640G insulin pump with SmartGuard [cited 2018 5 September]. Available from: https://www.medtronic-diabetes.co.uk/minimed-system/minimed-640g-insulin-pump.
14. Medtronic MiniMed I. MiniMed™ 670G Insulin Pump System 2018 [cited 2018 14 August]. Available from: https://www.medtronicdiabetes.com/products/minimed-670g-insulin-pump-system.
15. Life in Control Diabetes Coach [cited 2017 12th July]. Available from: http://www.lifeincontrol.com/mobile-app/.
16. Kesavadev J, Saboo B, Ramachandran L, et al. Utility of a multi-model bot enabled and doctor led intervention for diabetes management-clinician and patient perspectives. Diabetes Technol Ther. 2018;20:A39-40.
17. Medios Technologies [cited 17 Aug 2018]. Available from: https://mediostech.com/.

Chapter 78

Paradigm Shift in Diabetes

Sundeep Ruder

INTRODUCTION

The global burden of diabetes has increased massively and the number of new treatments continue to increase with little change in the trajectory of the epidemic and markers of treatment success. Current World Health Organization (WHO) figures suggest that globally over 420 million people are affected by type 2 diabetes (T2D). Africa and developing countries are facing the highest rates of increase in the epidemic. The number of people living with diabetes in Africa is predicted to increase by 140% by the year 2040. Developing countries also face the highest mortality rates from diabetes complications. The number of deaths globally from diabetes exceeded the combined mortality from HIV/AIDS, tuberculosis and malaria in 2015.[1]

A paradigm shift denotes a fundamental change in thinking or a change in approach to underlying assumptions. It is an important change that happens when the usual way of thinking about or doing something is replaced by a new and different way.

The principle of causality, so deeply embedded in humans' minds that it has been thought of as immediately evident, is the very foundation not only of all three monotheistic world religions but also of the first staggering steps of science [*de nihilo nihil* (*nothing can be born of nothing*); Lucretius 1951].[2]

The law of causality is fundamental in medicine. It simply states that every cause has an effect and every effect has a cause. Understanding the root cause of disease helps one to change the cause, which leads to the undesirable effect (the disease) being vanquished.

The solution to the diabetes epidemic lies in determining the root cause of this undesired effect. Causality cannot be understood simplistically (Box 1).

Box 1: On causality.[2]

- A cause is something that produces or creates an effect
- A cause is a condition without which the effect cannot occur. A cause is a condition with which the effect must occur
- A cause is made up of several components, no single one of which is sufficient of its own, which taken together must lead to the effect
- A cause is a condition that increases the probability of occurrence of the effect
- A cause is a condition that, if present, makes a difference in (the probability of) the outcome

Source: Adapted from Kundi M. Causality and the interpretation of epidemiologic evidence. Environ Health Perspect. 2006;114(7):969-74.

Pure examination of the peripheral factors of causality leads to treatments and interventions that only address such. Understanding risk factors and complications such as cardiovascular disease (CVD) and renal disease is essential as this leads to treatment, which alleviates suffering temporarily and may prolong life. Risk factor modification interventions are usually self-limiting and patients are often neutralized to diets and exercise regimens. Ultimately, these approaches are associated with great cost and burden to individuals and society and result in little or no change in the trajectory of the epidemic.[3] A paradigm shift appears necessary.

CURRENT APPROACH

Through science, many mechanisms have been described explaining the "causes" of diabetes. But one needs to be cautious in oversimplifying causality. Box 2 outlines the risk factors associated with diabetes. Genetic factors contribute

Box 2: Risk factors for type 2 diabetes.

- Older age
- Non white ancestry
- Family history of type 2 diabetes mellitus (T2DM)
- Low socioeconomic status
- Genetic factors (e.g. carrying risk alleles in the TCF7L2 gene)
- Components of the metabolic syndrome (increased waist circumference, increased blood pressure, increased plasma levels of triglycerides, low-plasma levels of HDL cholesterol and small, dense LDL cholesterol particles)
- Overweight or obese (BMI ≥25 kg/m^2)
- Abdominal or central obesity (independent of BMI)
- Cigarette smoking
- Sedentary lifestyle
- History of gestational diabetes mellitus or delivery of neonates >4 kg in weight
- Some medications, such as statins, thiazides and beta-blockers
- Psychosocial stress and depression

(BMI: body mass index; HDL: high-density lipoprotein; LDL: low-density lipoprotein.)

Source: Zheng Y, Ley SH, Hu FB. Global aetiology and epidemiology of type 2 diabetes mellitus and its complications. Nat Rev Endocrinol. 2018;14(2):88-98.

risk,[4,5] but there is consensus that lifestyle factors are have the greatest impact on disease expression and genetic risk can be subverted by changing lifestyle factors.[3]

Globalization is quoted as cause of diabetes. The "globalized" life, which is reflection of "Western living" involves many of the risk factors listed in the Box 2. With such a multitude of risk factors that contribute to causality in diabetes and an increasing disease burden, it places on individuals and society, it seems almost impossible to address every need individually.[6]

The modern medical or western approach is to find "pharmaceutical" treatments at the physiological level for the causes and complications of diabetes. This requires the necessary scientific approach of the current model of investigative and evidence-based medicine, which has led to excellent insights and treatments. Diabetic patients now have access to a multitude of treatment options beyond the traditional metformin and insulin. New classes of drug therapies such as glucagon-like peptide 1 (GLP-1) analogs and sodium-glucose cotransporter-2 (SGLT2) inhibitors address many unmet needs (weight, hypoglycemia risk and heart failure) and offer CV benefit. Together with antihypertensives and statin therapies, the risk of CV complications is reduced but not completely nullified. All new therapies, however, are associated with a host of new side effects, which require vigilance.

And many challenges remain. The reasons for this are multifold, incomplete knowledge on the mechanisms of CV risk, treatment non-adherence and non-compliance and physician factors such as physician apathy. Also, real world behavior differs from trial behavior and 75% of the loss of efficacy of medication in the real world is due to non-adherence.[7]

Medication burden is high among individuals with established T2D. Results from a systematic review indicate that patients with diabetes take in the range of four to ten medications a day. Evidence also suggests high levels of prescription of other drug classes for example, treatment for neuropathy, depression and gastric and rheumatological symptoms.[8]

It may appear that the current approach is unsustainable in the long term.

THE WAY FORWARD

In addressing the root cause of diabetes, one has to cognize that all human behavior is driven by desire. The globalized way of life is driven my materialistic acquisition and enjoyment at the center of which is economic success.[9] While economic success is necessary for survival needs, today's utilitarian version of acquisition of luxury by a few, marginalizes others to the fringes of society. Thus creating, a wide socioeconomic gap and class consciousness. Mill defines utilitarianism as a theory based on the principle that "actions are right in proportion as they tend to promote happiness, wrong as they tend to produce the reverse of happiness". Yet, both classes (low- and high-socioeconomic groups) now suffer increasingly high-diabetes rates. It would be pertinent thus to deeply understand the drivers of human desire to understand better the behaviour patterns associated a higher risk of diabetes and non - adherence for those on treatment already.

Aristotle once said *"All human beings by nature desire to understand."* One needs to understand the complex socioeconomic play, and drivers of human desire and behavior behind this epidemic.

Science deals with the particularized and concrete characteristics of the world. It is theoretical, knowledge based and is partitive and analytical in nature.

Philosophy, on the other hand, deals with the essential, universal and abstract nature of things. It is an attempt to study the essence of truth and knowledge itself. Through "wisdom" rather than knowledge, philosophy plays a unitive and synthetic role in medicine.

It becomes clear that for the truth-seeking human, philosophy is essential.

The philosophical approach to understanding the root cause of human suffering was practiced in the eastern cultures (India, Japan and China) and the some cultures of the middle East. Even the Greek philosopher physicians, Hippocrates and Epicurus approached medicine with a philosophical perspective.[10]

The Islamic philosopher physician, Avicenna once quoted *"The knowledge of anything, since all things have causes, is not acquired or complete unless it is known by its causes".*

In India, Ayurvedic practitioners called *vaidya*, meaning a person of profound knowledge, primarily made use of what is called rational therapy. He examined the individual as a whole and not just the disease. *Vaidyas* laid equal emphasis on the cure of disease as well as health promotion and prevention. They prescribed a daily and seasonal routine as well as attention to nutrition for maintenance of a balanced state of health. They advocated harmony of body and mind, and a harmonious interaction between man and universe for a healthy life.[11]

The philosophical approach requires an examination of the essence of human behavior and purpose, which is driven by desires. Learning to govern unregulated human desire seems crucial in combating diabetes.[12]

Volumes have been written by great Indian sages on the nature of human desire (*vasanas*) and volumes more have been written on how to understand and regulate them through self-effort (yogas).

They described the human being as having three equipments—(1) the body, (2) the mind and (3) the intellect.[9]

The body comprises the organs of perception, which are the senses that sense the sense-objects of the world and the organs of actions (limbs and speech) through which we act in the world. The eyes see color and form, skin feels touch and the tongue tastes food. The organs of action execute the action, which are influenced by the mind.[9]

Philosophically speaking the mind is composed of feelings, emotions, likes and dislikes. Through it, we experience joy, sorrow, love hatred, anger and jealousy. This is the emotional personality.[9,13]

It is the logical centre of reason which if developed well can assist decision making and curb the vascillations of the desire driven mind, which influences diabetes patients behaviour.

The subtle intellect, however, crosses the limit of the terrestrial world to consider something beyond the transcendental purpose of life. It distinguishes the eternal from the ephemeral. This is the contemplator in us—the spiritual personality.[13]

A powerful intellect can govern the child mind and thus direct desires into purposeful action.

The intellect is developed through questioning and not accepting anything at face value. The paradigm shift proposed here is to restructure diabetes education that encourages critical thinking together with traditional health literacy tools.

Thus, diabetes education must be geared toward developing critical thinking, which develops the intellect. A powerful intellect supports patients in becoming self-sufficient in decision making. For example, soft drinks companies advertise happiness and well-being. A person with a strong intellect will question this claim investigate and come to their own conclusions that this is not the case and choose not to partake of it.

The Indian mathematician and sage Swami Rama Tirtha once said that *"Heredity reigns supreme in the lower animal kingdoms. Man also owes his physical powers and organs to the principles of heredity. But man arises to his fullest most refined, full blown and perfect state more especially through adaptation and education".*

Along with education that is aimed at developing critical thinking, public health policies and advocacy should to be escalated to support education projects. The word advocacy is derived from the Latin word "advocare", which means "a summons or call to aid". Policy change through advocacy helps create con-ducive environments for human well being. This would be in keeping with the Indian concept of 'satsang' or 'environment or company of the good', which propels the intellect forward. Physicians should take on this role more strongly and restore the trust of the public as being the greatest advocates for health and purpose-driven life.[14]

Public health intervention such as a sugary drinks tax, banning of soft drinks to children, sin tax on smoking, banning advertising of junk food to children must be emphasized and every country should consider implementing such. Physician led advocacy should drive the process through policy pressures on government. Media should be used to increase public awareness of such policies to counter the propaganda of junk food industry.

"The purpose of advertising is to convince people to purchase things they do not need."

Commercial appeals did not become commonplace until the advent and widespread adoption of television and grew exponentially with the advent of cable television, which allowed programmers to develop entire channels of child-oriented programming and advertising. Opportunities to advertise to children further expanded with the explosive growth of the Internet, and thousands of child-oriented websites with advertising content have appeared in the past few years.[15]

Current approaches to eating are often hedonistic and not purpose driven.

Ancient philosophies and religions tried to inculcate sensible eating through observance of one's nature. The idea was to eat to maintain the body to do purposeful work in the world, which contributed to collective good. In the Vedic sciences sattvika food is described. These are fleshy vegetables, oleaginous nuts and fruit. Modern studies such as the recent PURE studies confirm the benefits of such.[16] Protein in the form of meat was not taboo but eaten considerately for a need. Diets were not prescriptive, but functional and purpose driven. So, critical thinking around eating habits needs to be inculcated.

Current diabetes education interventions show inconsistent results. Some show improvement in metabolic and psychological parameters and other do not show significant effects.[17]

CONCLUSION

There is clearly a need for diabetes education models to be re-evaluated. The author's proposal is that in the traditional knowledge systems of India such as the Vedas, there is wealth of knowledge on how to develop critical thinking, not only as pertains to health but all spheres of human life. This knowledge ought to be conveyed in a contemporary way and used to reassess our modern approach in the management of the diabetes epidemic. It is beyond the scope of this manuscript to go into the details of such an endeavor. The purpose of this manuscript is to invite the reader to consider this concept and critically think around it.

To quote Swami Rama Tirtha:

> *"Is it not laziness to keep floundering in the quagmire of conventionality and let oneself flow down the current of custom and fashion, and sink like a dead weight in a well of appearances and be caught in the pond of possession and spend the time, which should be God's, in making gold and call it 'doing good'?"*

REFERENCES

1. The Society for Endocrinology; Metabolism and Diabetes of South Africa Type 2 Diabetes Guidelines Expert Committee. The 2017 SEMDSA Guideline for the Management of Type 2 Diabetes Guideline Committee. JEMDSA. 2017;21(1)(Supplement 1):S1-S196.
2. Kundi M. Causality and the interpretation of epidemiologic evidence. Environ Health Perspect. 2006;114:969-74.
3. Zheng Y, Ley SH, Hu FB. Global aetiology and epidemiology of type 2 diabetes mellitus and its complications. Nat Rev Endocrinol. 2018;14(2):88-98.
4. Franks PW, Pearson E, Florez JC. Gene-Environment and Gene-Treatment Interactions in Type 2 Diabetes. Diabetes Care. 2013;36:1413-21.
5. Hu FB. Globalization of Diabetes: The role of diet, lifestyle, and genes. Diabetes Care. 2011;34(6):1249-57.
6. Edelman SV. Type 2 Diabetes in the Real World: The Elusive Nature of Glycemic Control. Diabetes Care. 2017;40(11):1425-32.
7. Odegard PS, Capoccia K. Medication taking and diabetes: a systematic review of the literature. Diabetes Educ. 2007;33:1014-29.
8. Manderbacka K, Sund R, Koski S, et al. Diabetes and depression? Secular trends in the use of antidepressants among persons with diabetes in Finland in 1997–2007. Pharmacoepidemiol Drug Saf. 2011;20:338-43.
9. Parthsarathy A. The Fall of the Human Intellect, 3rd edition. India: Springer; 2008.
10. Yapijakis C. Hippocrates of Kos, the Father of Clinical Medicine, and Asclepiades of Bithynia, the Father of Molecular Medicine. In Vivo. 2009;23:507-14.
11. Saini A. Physicians of ancient India. J Family Med Prim Care. 2016;5(2):254-8.
12. Parthasarathy A. Vedanta Treatise, 17th edition. 2015. Published by A. Parthsarathy, 1A Landsend, Mumbai, 400006, India
13. Parthasarathy A. Governing Business and Relationships, 1st edition. 2010. Published by A. Parthsarathy, 1A Landsend, Mumbai, 400006, India
14. Nutbeam D. Health literacy as a public health goal: a challenge for contemporary health education and communication strategies into the 21st century, Health Promotion International, Volume 15, Issue 3. UK: Oxford University Press; 2000. pp. 259-67.
15. Wilcox BL, Kunkel D, Cantor J, et al. (2004). Report of the APA Task Force on Advertising and Children. [online] Available from http://www.apa.org/pi/families/resources/advertising-children.pdf. [Accessed October, 2018].
16. Dehghan M, Mente A, Zhang X, et al.; on behalf of the Prospective Urban Rural Epidemiology (PURE) study investigators. Associations of fats and carbohydrate intake with cardiovascular disease and mortality in 18 countries from five continents (PURE): a prospective cohort study. Lancet. 2017;390(10107):2050-62.
17. Norris SL, Engelgau MM, Venkat Narayan KM. Effectiveness of Self-Management Training in Type 2 Diabetes. Diabetes Care. 2001;24(3):561-87.

Chapter 79

Camel Milk and Type 1 Diabetes Link

RP Agrawal

INTRODUCTION

No doubt the primary treatment of diabetes is insulin replacement. However, at present, complete physiological insulin replacement cannot be achieved, as required. Prevention and early treatment is important because diabetes interrupts normal development and growth in children and carries the threat of severe complication in more active period of life.

Composition of camel milk is different from other ruminant milk: having low cholesterol, low sugar, high minerals (sodium, potassium, iron, copper, zinc, magnesium and free calcium),[1] high vitamin C (Table 1).[2] These may act as antioxidant, thereby removing free radicals, which may provide a stress free situation. High concentrations of antioxidants and removal of fat from the body may enable the insulin receptors to respond better to available insulin. The milk protein lactoferrin, which is present in large quantities in camel milk, does have some antiviral and anti-bacterial properties.

Radioimmunoassay of camel milk has revealed high concentration of insulin (45–128 units/L) as compared to other milks. As is evident from the literature that one of the camel milk proteins has many characteristics similar to insulin and it does not form coagulum in acidic environment.[3] The lack of coagulum formation allows the camel milk to pass rapidly through the stomach together with the specific insulin like protein/insulin and remains available for absorption in intestine. Even if some insulin is destroyed, enough amount remains available for absorption in intestine.

HYPOGLYCEMIC EFFECT OF CAMEL MILK

The efficacy of raw camel milk on glycemic control risk factors and diabetes quality of life in patients of type 1 diabetes has been proved by several studies in different corners of the world.

EFFECT OF CAMEL MILK ON BLOOD GLUCOSE LEVEL

Various researches have advocated glucose lowering effect of camel milk. Twenty-four randomly selected patients with type 1 diabetes were enrolled in a study. These patients were divided into two groups. Group 1 ($n = 12$) received usual care (diet, exercise and insulin) and group 2 ($n = 12$) received 500 mL camel milk, two times daily (250 mL in morning and 250 mL in evening) in addition to usual care for 3 months. Frequent blood sugar monitoring was done to maintain euglycemia by titrating the doses of insulin. HbA1c, lipid profile, plasma insulin and C-peptide estimation were done at the beginning and after 3 months. After 3 months of treatment there was a significant improvement in fasting blood sugar.[4]

Similar results were found in a controlled cross over study. The requirement of insulin was 40.83 ± 7.12 at the beginning. It reduced to 26.83 ± 8.44, ($p < 0.05$) after camel milk supplementation. Improvement in mean blood glucose (7.11 ± 0.32 to 5.96 ± 0.31, $p < 0.05$) was observed in group 1. In the same group HbA1c reduced from 9.48 ± 2.17 to 8.19 ± 1.84. Statistically significant improvement was seen in DQL score. It is concluded that moderate

TABLE 1: Composition of camel milk and cow milk.

Components	Camel milk	Cow milk
Water	86–91%	88%
Lactose	4.2–5.0 g%	5.0 g%
Fat	2.49–3.1 g%	3.7 g%
Protein	3.78–3.9 g%	3.3 g%
Casein : albumin ratio	2.85	3.1
Sodium	38–68 mg/100 mL	35–60 mg/100 mL
Potassium	50–90 mg/100 mL	135–155 mg/100 mL
Magnesium	11.88–13.59 mg/100 mL	10–15 mg/100 mL
Phosphorus	41.72–47.21 mg/100 mL	75–110 mg/100 mL
Calcium	94.1–97.43 mg/100 mL	100–140 mg/100 mL
Iron	0.32–0.36 mg/100 mL	0.30–0.65 mg/100 mL
Zinc	1.2–6.3 mg/100 mL	1.0–3.0 mg/100 mL
Manganese	0.02–2.0 mg/100 mL	0.01–0.03 mg/100 mL
Copper	0.09–0.5 mg/100 mL	0.03–0.17 mg/100 mL
Vitamin A	0.03 mg%	0.34 mg%
Vitamin C	4–5 mg/100 g	1.6 mg/100 g
Vitamin E	0.27 mg%	0.1 mg%
Niacin	0.46 mg%	0.08 mg%
Vitamin-B1	0.03 mg%	0.42 mg%
Vitamin-B2	0.04 mg%	1.57 mg%

Immunoglobulins: IgM, IgG, IgA and even IgD were detected in camel milk.

intake of camel milk will reduce the insulin requirement with better glycemic control and diabetes quality of life without affecting lipid profile.[5]

In another, 52 weeks randomized controlled study after 1 year of treatment there was significant increase in body mass index (17 ± 4.4 to 19.7 ± 2.97 kg/m^2, $p < 0.001$), improvement in fasting blood sugar (119±19 to 95.42 ± 15.70 mg/dL, $p < 0.003$) and HbA1c (7.8 ± 1.38 to 6 ± 0.96%, $p < 0.001$). In group 2 there was a significant reduction in the mean doses. No significant treatment emerged adverse events were reported in either group.[6]

There is a traditional belief in the middle East that regular consumption of camel milk may aid in prevention and control of diabetes. This 16-week randomized study enrolled 54 type 1 diabetic patients. Subjects were randomly divided into two groups of 27 patients: one received usual management (diet, exercise and insulin), whereas the other received 500 mL of camel milk daily in addition to standard management. After 16 weeks of camel milk treatment fasting blood sugar (227.2 ± 17.7 vs. 98.9 ± 16.2 mg/dL), HbA1c [9.59 ± 2.05(%) vs. 7.16 ± 1.84(%)], serum anti-insulin antibodies (26.20 ± 7.96 vs. 20.92 ± 5.45 mIU/mL), urinary albumin excretion (25.17 ± 5.43 vs. 14.54 ± 5.62 mg/dL/24 h), daily insulin dose (48.1 ± 6.95 vs. 23 ± 4.05 units), and body mass index (18.43 ± 3.59 vs. 24.3 ± 2.95 kg/m^2). These results suggest that, as an adjunct to standard management, daily ingestion of camel milk can aid metabolic control in young type 1 diabetics.[7]

EFFECT OF CAMEL MILK ON INSULIN DOSE

There was a significant reduction in the mean doses of insulin (41.16 ± 10.32 to 30 ± 12.6 u, $p < 0.002$) in patient's receiving camel milk.[8] In further study a significant reduction in the mean doses of insulin (32 ± 12 to 17.83 ± 12.40, $p < 0.005$) was observed again.[5]

The important observation of the randomized controlled trial was a significant reduction in insulin requirement (46.15%) at the end of 2 years in patients

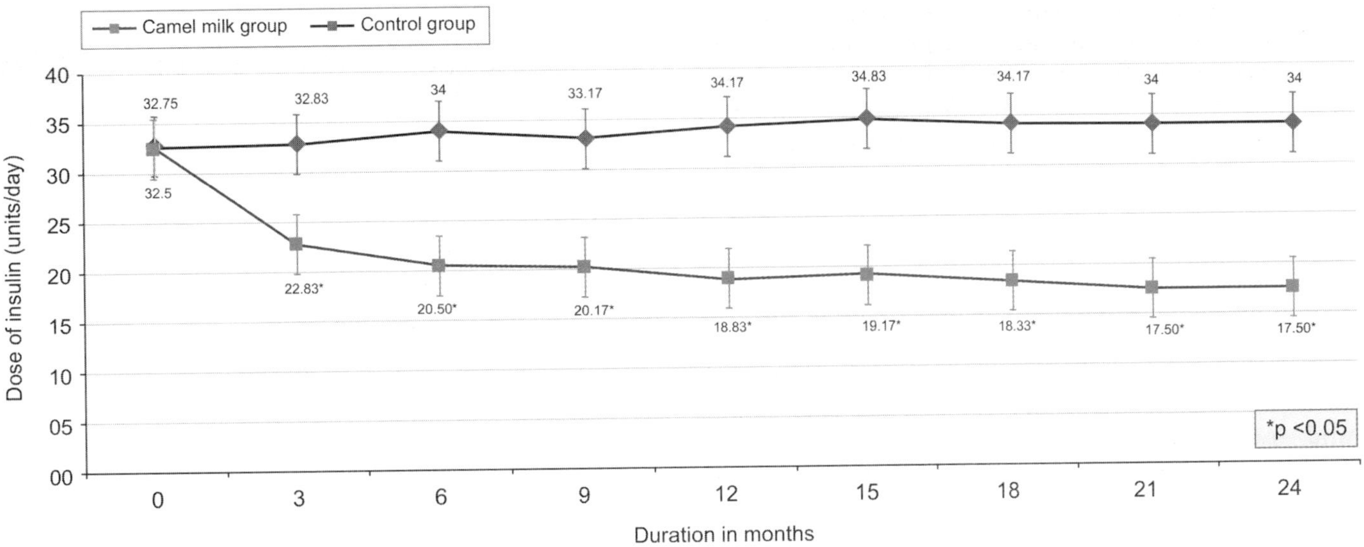

Figure 1 Mean dose of insulin of control and camel milk group.

Source: Agrawal RP., European Journal of Clinical Nutrition, 2011;65:1048-52.

taking camel milk. Amongst the twelve subjects in camel milk consuming group, the remarkable observation was gradual reduction upto zero in three subjects. These three subjects reached to this level on 12th, 18th and 21st month of the study and returned to this "no insulin requirement status" upto the end of study with some intermittent deviations. Two out of these three subjects maintained this zero level continuously from 18th and 21st month till the end of study (Fig. 1).[9]

EFFECT ON BETA-CELL FUNCTION

To understand how the camel milk is helping in type 1 diabetes and the effect of camel milk on residual β-cell function in recent onset type 1 diabetes a study was carried out and concluded that the mean basal C-peptide gradually increased in camel milk group from 0.14 ± 0.10 to 0.16 ± 0.10. The improvement in β-cell may be due to: (a) Euglycemia possibly reduces β-cell work, leading to β-cell rest, and thereby, preserving β-cell function; (b) Tolerance induction in the body due to high concentration of circulating insulin (antigen) leading to preservation of β-cell function; (c) Camel milk immunoglobulins are of relatively smaller size and weight due to only Y-shaped main chain which might offer an interplay with host cell protein thereby leading to an induction or activation of regulatory cells and finally leading to a downward regulation of immune system and β-cell salvage; (d) Protective effect of β-cell function may be due to presence of half cystine, lactoferrin or insulin like factor in camel milk.[10]

BENEFICIAL EFFECT OF CAMEL MILK IN DIABETIC NEPHROPATHY

A study was performed to observe the role of camel milk in controlling microalbuminuria level of type 1 diabetic patients. Twenty four patients were randomly recruited and then these patients were given camel milk in addition with usual care for 6 months. It was found that after adding camel milk to the usual regimen there was improvement in microalbuminuria (119.48 ± 1.68 to 22.52 ± 2.68; p 0.001). It may be due to good glycemic control or due to direct effect of camel milk.[11]

Possible Mechanisms Involved

The exact cause of hypoglycemic effect of camel milk is not known. It is possibly due to insulin like activity, regulatory and immunomodulatory function of β-cells.[12] Agamy found good amount of lysozyme, lactoferrin, lactoperoxidase, immunoglobulin G and secretory immunoglobulin A in camel milk.[13] The lack of coagulum formation of camel milk may also be helpful in taking the insulin present in it unchanged to intestine, where it can be absorbed even if some amount is destroyed in the passage. Beg has found that amino acid sequence of some of the camel milk protein is rich in half cystine, which has superficial similarity with insulin family of peptides.[14] Low prevalence of diabetes in camel breeder community (Raica) paves path to novel approaches lying behind the glycemic control attributed to camel milk.

CONCLUSION

For reducing insulin requirement in type 1 diabetes camel milk has played a potent therapeutic alternative. The most prompt and effective method for treatment of type 1 diabetes is insulin, but is somewhat painful and inconvenient for many individuals. Nowadays many alternative methods are being tested for insulin replacement which includes noninvasive techniques.[15] The alternatives ways for insulin delivery in diabetic patients include oral administration. It has been studied that oral insulin mimics the effect of pancreas secreted insulin after undergoing hepatic pass and inhibits hepatic gluconeogenesis.[16] Camel milk is one such alternative for oral insulin as it has protein similar to insulin like characteristics which does not form coagulum in stomach. It is not destroyed in acid environment and is available for absorption in intestine.[17] A number of studies have proved that camel milk as an adjunct to insulin therapy appears to be safe and efficacious in improving long-term glycemic control and helps in reduction of insulin requirement in type 1 diabetic patients. Camel milk is considered as the 'white gold' of the desert. Camel milk is already marketed as a health food and beauty product in the Gulf and several African countries and the global market potential for camel milk could be billions of dollars, according to estimates by the Food and Agriculture Organization (FAO) of the United Nations.

Hence, food industry could design and construct functional foods with probiotics. These food products could be positioned between conventional foods and medicines, with their uses targeting semi-healthy state of the body as a preventive measure against disease. This concept is consistent with the historic belief that natural substances play an important role in prevention and treatment of diseases.

REFERENCES

1. Gorban Ali MS, Omar IM. Mineral Content of Camel Milk and Colostrums. J. Dairy Res. 1997;64:471-4.
2. Knoess KH. Milk production of the dromedary. In: Camels. IFS Symposium, Sudan. 1979;201-14p.
3. Wangoh J. What steps towards camel milk technology? Int Jr of Anim Sci. 1993;8:9-11.
4. Agrawal RP, Swami SC, Beniwal R, et al. Effect of Camel Milk on Glycemic Control, Risk Factors and Diabetes Quality of Life in Type-1 Diabetes: A Randomised Prospective Controlled Study. Int Jour of Diab in Dev Countries. 2002;22:70-4.
5. Agrawal RP, Swami SC, Beniwal R, et al. Effect of camel milk on glycemic control lipid profile and diabetes quality of life in type-1 diabetes: a randomised prospective controlled cross over study. Indian Jr of Animal Sci. 2003;73(10):1105-10.
6. Agrawal RP, Sharma S, Beniwal R, et al. Camel milk as an adjunct to insulin therapy improves long-term glycemic control and reduction in doses of insulin in patients with type-1 diabetes A 1 year randomized controlled trial. Diab Res Clin Pract. 2005;68(2):176-7.
7. Mohamad RH, Zekry ZK, Al-Mehdar HA, et al. Camel milk as an adjuvant therapy for the treatment of type 1 diabetes: verification of a traditional ethnomedical practice. J Med Food. 2009;12(2):461-5.
8. Agrawal RP, Singh G, Nayak KC, et al. Prevalence of Diabetes in Camel Milk Consuming 'RAICA' Rural Community of North West Rajasthan. Int. J. Diab. Dev. Countries. 2004;24:109-14.
9. Agrawal RP, Jain S, Shah S, et al. Effect of camel milk on glycemic control and insulin requirement in patients with type 1 diabetes: 2-years randomized controlled trial. Euro. Jr of Clin Nutri. 2011;65:1048-52.
10. Agrawal RP, Saran S, Sharma P, et al. Effect of camel milk on residual b-cell function in recent onset type 1 diabetes. Diab Res and Clin Prac. 2007;77:494-5.
11. Agrawal RP, Dogra R, Mohta N, et al. Beneficial effect of camel milk in diabetic nephropathy. Acta Bio. 2009;80:131-4.
12. Lutz B. Insulin and antidiabetic activity of camel milk. Jr of Camel Res and Prac. 2002;9:43-5.
13. El-Agamy El, Ruppanner R, Ismail A, et al. Antibacterial and antiviral activity of camel milk protective proteins. J Dairy Res. 1992;59(2):169-75.
14. Beg OU, Bahr V, Lindrom H, et al. A camel milk protein rich in half cystine. Primary structure assessment of variations, internal repeat patterns and relationship with neurophysin and other active polypeptides. Euro Jr of Biochem. 1986;15:195-201.
15. Owens DR. New horizons-alternative routes for insulin therapy. Nature Rev Drug Discov. 2002;1:529-40.
16. Clement S, Still G, Kosutic G, et al. Oral insulin product hexyl-insulin monoconjugate 2 (HIM2) in type 1 diabetes mellitus: the glucose stabilization effects of HIM2. Diab Tech and Therap. 2002;4:459-66.
17. Abu-Lehia IHIS, Al-Mohizea, M.El-Behary. Studies on the production of ice cream from camel milk products. Aust. J. Dairy Technol. 1989;44:31-4.
18. Sahani MS, Mal G, Kumar R, et al. Annual Report on Camel milk and its role in tuberculosis. NRCC, Bikaner. 1989;7-8.
19. Ganong WF. Ganong's Review of Medical Physiology. 23 Edition. 1999;19:431.

Chapter 80

Can High Protein Content of Diet Prevent Diabetes?

Shilpa S Joshi

Asia accounts for 60% of the world's population with diabetes. In recent decades, many developing countries in Asia have undergone rapid economic development and urbanization leading to the nutritional transition.[1] These changes are believed to have led to an explosive increase in metabolic diseases more specifically diabetes prevalence within a relatively short time.

Prevalence of diabetes in India is about 8.8% (72 million individuals) of diabetes and it has been predicted to rise to 151 million by year 2045. Lifestyle modifications are shown to be corner stone of management of diabetes. Lifestyle modification which includes nutritional changes, exercise have shown to help control blood glucoses. Interestingly, research has shown that lifestyle modification is also most powerful tool to prevent diabetes.

OBESITY AND DIABETES

Obesity and/or overweight are the major driving forces of epidemic of diabetes across the globe. Interestingly, in case of Asian Indians lower body mass index (BMI) is associated with higher prevalence of diabetes as compared to Caucasians.[2] Computer-based tomography has shown that Asians have more visceral fat than Caucasians with the same waist circumference.[3] Hence, in case of Asian Indians, even a small amount of weight gain during adulthood increases the risk of diabetes. Indians also have a greater tendency to gain weight around abdomen. They also have less muscle mass compared to Caucasians which leads to increased predisposition to insulin resistance. Therefore, although they look thin, they are "metabolically obese". This "metabolically obese" phenotype among individuals with normal BMI may explain the increased propensity for diabetes.

THRIFTY GENOTYPE AND THRIFTY PHENOTYPE

The thrifty genotype hypothesis postulates that obesity and type 2 diabetes (T2D) are caused by positive selection of genotypes for efficiency of metabolism and energy and fat storage, thereby conferring advantage in times of nutrient scarcity.[4,5] It has been suggested that the populations having this genotype may have an enhanced predisposition to obesity and hence diabetes. This thrifty genotype, results from evolutionary selection by repeated feast and famine cycles. In contrast, Europeans are less likely to possess thrifty genotypes as they evolved in environments that were least affected by the feast and famine cycles. So, the thrify genotype shows that there is distinct mismatch our ancestral genes which evolved in nutritional scarcity and today's environment of nutrient excess.

The thrifty phenotype hypothesis postulates a mismatch between intrauterine and adult life environments. This hypothesis also has been widely used to explain the role of nutrition transition in the development of chronic diseases. This hypothesis postulates that there are adaptations in response to under nutrition in fetal stage. These lead to metabolic and structural changes (e.g. decreased β-cell mass and function and increased insulin resistance) that are necessary for early survival. These changes which are lifesaving in fetal life, may increase the risk of chronic diseases, such as T2D, in adulthood.[6,7] This hypothesis was validated from studies, consistently showing associations between low birth weight (LBW) and increased risk of T2D. LBW promotes a thrifty phenotype during intrauterine and early life. Catch up growth in early years and weight gain in later years, induces an insulin resistant state and low β-cell function.

Both these hypotheses show that there a deep link between nutrition and diabetes. Under nutrition in fetal stage and over nutrition/improper nutrition in later years of life leads to high risk of T2D. Hence, for treatment, prevention or delay of diabetes, right selection of food or right nutrition is important at all stages of life.

DIET

Excessive caloric intake is a major driving force behind increasing rates of obesity and T2D epidemics worldwide. Along with excessive caloric intake, diet quality or type of calories also has its independent effects. In the Nurses' Health Study (NHS), it was found that the quality of fats and carbohydrates play an important role in the development of diabetes. This association was independent of BMI and other risk factors.[8] It showed that diets that were higher dietary glycemic load (GL) and trans-fat were associated with increased diabetes risk. It was also found that greater consumption of cereal fibre and polyunsaturated fat is associated with decreased risk of diabetes. Evidence also shows that higher consumption of sugar-sweetened beverages (SSBs) increases the risk of T2D even after considering the effects of body weight. Meta-analysis[9] found that individuals in the highest amount of SSB intake (most often 1–2 servings/day) had a 26% greater risk of developing the disease than those in the lowest intake. This effect is due to large quantities of rapidly absorbable carbohydrates (e.g., sucrose) in SSBs. This large amount of sucrose result in a high dietary GL which leads to quick increases in blood glucose and insulin levels. A continuous consumption of high GL diet increases the insulin demand. This may lead to pancreatic β-cell exhaustion in the long run, which has been implicated in increased risk of T2D and cardiovascular disease.[10] Even fructose from high fructose corn syrup has also shown to play a role. Fructose is preferentially metabolized to lipid in the liver, leading to increased hepatic de novo lipogenesis, dyslipidemia, and insulin resistance.[11] It may also promote visceral adiposity predisposing to diabetes.

CAN NUTRITIONAL MODIFICATION PREVENT TYPE 2 DIABETES?

Excess adiposity reflected by higher BMI is the strongest risk factor for diabetes across the globe, and more specifically Asians tend to develop diabetes at a much lower BMI than those of European ancestry.[12] A meta-analysis of prospective cohort studies suggests that the risk associated with a higher waist circumference is slightly stronger than the risk associated with a higher BMI.[13] Lifestyle intervention, as demonstrated in the Diabetes Prevention Program (DPP), involving calorie-restriction and exercise, significantly reduced conversion to diabetes among high-risk patients with impaired glucose tolerance by 58%.[14] These effects were seen in all DPP studies involving individuals of multiple ethnicities like Finnish, Chinese, Americans and Indians.[14-17] In DPP studies this goal was 5–7% of weight loss achieved by lower fat, high fibre diet and restricting simple carbohydrates. Although, Indian DPP did not see much weight loss, lifestyle modification did reduce conversion to T2D.

CAN HIGH PROTEIN DIETS PREVENT DIABETES?

The DPP trials clearly indicated that life style interventions are important in prevention of diabetes. Most of the prevention trials actually focused on the modification of fat and carbohydrates in diet. In these studies there was more emphasis on decreasing the fat content to prevent insulin resistance or carbohydrate type. Most of these studies were done in Western world where protein intakes of individuals is liberal as compared to India. Pan Indian diet study, STARCH study has shown that diets in India of both individuals with or without diabetes is high in carbohydrates and very poor in proteins.[18] Chennai Rural and Urban Epidemiological study (CURES) also shows that diets in Southern part of India are high in refined carbohydrates like white rice and are poor in proteins.[19] Based on this evidence, international bodies such as the European Association for the Study of Diabetes, American Diabetes Association recommend a lower-fat and moderate (45–60% of energy)—carbohydrate diet for the prevention of T2D. These carbohydrates should be based on vegetables, legumes, fruit, and whole grain cereals which provide dietary fibre and are also low in glycemic index (GI). Recommended protein intake is 10–20% of energy (0.8–1.2 g/kg). In real world, a diet containing 0.8–1 g/kg body weight of protein is in itself a higher protein diet in India. Therefore, increasing protein content from baseline traditional low protein diets to diets containing recommended amount of protein would go a long way in preventing diabetes in India. For people on energy-reduced diets for weight-loss, which is recommended for prevention of diabetes, it is important to maintain or increase protein intake because using a fixed percentage of total calories to estimate a protein requirement may result in inadequate protein intake and lean muscle loss.[20]

To date, the evidence base has been insufficient to support specific recommendations for a higher-protein diet (>20% of energy) for T2D prevention.[21] There is, however, a growing body of research that shows that high protein diets may provide a useful aid for short-term weight loss. There is evidence building in support of low-fat (25–30% of energy), moderate carbohydrate (40–50% of energy), high protein (20–25% of energy) diets for longer-term maintenance of weight loss and, hence, for T2D prevention.[22-29] Higher dietary protein appears to promote and aid weight management.[22-26] A meta-analysis[29] of 32 trials assessing high protein diets selected on the basis of >12 month follow-up concluded that benefits observed in the short term persist to a smaller degree in the long term, with greater benefits associated with better compliance to the diet. A second meta-analysis of nine studies lasting for 6 months also confirmed a beneficial effect of high protein diets on weight loss in T2D cohorts.[30] In low carbohydrate, moderate energy diets substitution of carbohydrates for proteins leads to a greater benefit and a greater sustained weight loss. As gram-to-gram fat has more than double calories as one would get from carbohydrates and protein, substitution of carbohydrates for proteins is more achievable. Unravelling this issue, however, is complex. A recent review reported that weight loss and weight-maintenance depends on the high protein content of diet, but not on the "low carbohydrate" component of the diet.[31]Although this has not been a universal conclusion. Some studies have shown that low-carbohydrate diets promote weight loss, even when protein content remains little[32] or entirely unchanged.[33] Irrespective of the causative nutrient, decreasing the carbohydrate content of the diet has long been shown to have a positive effect on aspects of metabolic health, including serum lipids and lipoproteins, Very-low-density lipoprotein-triglycerides, and high-density lipoprotein cholesterol, with some evidence of improved blood pressure.[34]

To have an impact on T2D prevention, high protein diets must prevent the gradual weight gain and long-term weight regain which is associated with most weight-loss regimens. The Pan-European DioGenes (Diet, Obesity and Genes) study high protein diet group had the lowest dropout rate and least weight regain.[25] The DioGenes study has sparked renewed interest in high protein diets for longer-term weight maintenance and, in turn, amelioration of T2D risk.

MECHANISM OF ACTION OF HIGH PROTEIN DIETS

A number of well-established mechanisms acting on energy intake, expenditure, and utilization may contribute to the success of high protein diets for weight loss and the prevention of weight rebound.[71] Satiety is the most important mechanism. Dietary protein has long been shown to have favorable effects on hunger and satiety.[35-40]The mechanisms proposed is that dietary protein induced promotion of gluconeogenesis,[41] with increased intestinal glucose detected via sensing cells within the portal vein wall[42] and/or promotion of ketosis and secretion of β-hydroxybutyrate (BHB), all these promote satiety. When there is decreased portal glucose concentration, it has been shown to activate vagal afferent activity in animal models, triggering increased food intake.[43] The dietary protein, conversely promotes increased glucose concentrations via gluconeogenesis, there is little clinical evidence that appetite is directly suppressed through this mechanism.[41] However, increased concentrations of BHB and increased dietary fat oxidation, both clear markers of a ketogenic state, do appear to contribute to the appetite suppressive effect of HP diets.[41]

Protein may also differentially stimulate diet-induced thermogenesis. Another advantage is the anabolic effect of dietary protein on lean mass, such that branch chain amino acids enhance muscle protein synthesis and may protect against loss of lean mass during weight loss.[44] Maintenance of LM, as a metabolically active tissue, may in turn contribute to long-term weight maintenance. High protein diets may also improve glycemia,independent of body weight.[25,45,46,47,48]

TYPES OF PROTEINS IN HIGH PROTEIN DIETS FOR PREVENTION OF TYPE 2 DIABETES

Types of dietary protein to be included in diet for high protein diet are as important as amount of protein or percentage calories from protein. Study's have consistently shown that proteins from vegetarian sources such as dairy and soya have a greater advantage over proteins from animal sources.[48,49] Even proteins from marine sources have shown advantage over protein from animal sources.[50] The European Prospective Investigation into Cancer and Nutrition (EPIC) study showed a positive association between the consumption of animal-origin protein, e.g. red meat, processed meat, and chicken, but not fish and dairy, and greater weight gain over 6.5 years.[51,52] Pan et al. showed a strong correlation between red (particularly processed) meat consumption and T2D, with a 50% increased risk. Data from three Harvard Cohorts, the Health Professionals Follow-Up Study, the Nurses' Health Study, and the Nurses' Health Study 2, have shown that an additional 0.5 servings/day (42 g/day) of processed red meat over 4 years also is associated with up to a 50% increased risk of T2D.[53-55] Processed red meat is high in saturated fats, nitrate, sodium, and hemeiron, and is hypothesized to affect glucose metabolism, insulin resistance, endothelial function, glycoxidation and oxidative stress.[54]

CONCLUSION

Lifestyle modification is the key strategy to prevent T2D. The key component of lifestyle modification are diet and physical activity. In current Indian scenario, we are seeing increased imbalance diet and reduction of physical activity. Imbalanced diets in India include excessive amounts of energy coming in from refined carbohydrates and saturated or trans fats. This has led to having a pandemic of T2D in this country. High protein diets have shown consistently to cause weight loss and prevent glycemia. Hence, it is important that emphasis should be laid on protein content of diet. Besides improving glycemia and weight loss, they also prevent muscle loss which is critical in managing blood glucose and improving frailty in aging T2D patients. In Indian context, compliance to diets high in protein is an issue. Indians, essentially consume vegetarian diets, which have lower protein content. Also vegetarian proteins in form of legumes, pulses and diary are expensive and also difficult to consume in large quantities as they cause gastric discomfort. Therefore although, high protein diets have shown beneficial effects consuming them as part of natural food options is difficult. Due to this reason, use of protein supplements is gaining popularity. These are usually based of whey or casein. In case of vegan population there are options like soya protein and pea protein. These can be used just to normalize the protein content of diet to normalcy—0.8 g/kg body weight. This change can itself lead to increased satiety, weight loss and normalization of blood glucose.

REFERENCES

1. Chan JC, Malik V, Jia W, et al. Diabetes in Asia: epidemiology, risk factors, and pathophysiology. JAMA. 2009; 301:2129-40.
2. Yoon KH, Lee JH, Kim JW, et al. Epidemic obesity and type 2 diabetes in Asia.Lancet 2006;368:1681-8.
3. Lear SA, Humphries KH, Kohli S, et al. Visceral adipose tissue accumulation differs according to ethnic background: results of the Multicultural Community Health Assessment Trial (M-CHAT). Am J Clin Nutr. 2007;86:353-9.
4. Neel JV. Diabetes mellitus: a "thrifty" genotype rendered detrimental by "pr ogress"?AmJHumGenet.1962;14:353-62.
5. Neel JV. Diabetes mellitus: a "thrifty" genotype rendered detrimental by "progress"? 1962. Bull World Health Organ. 1999;77:694-703.
6. Hales CN, Barker DJ. The thrifty phenotype hypothesis. Br Med Bull. 2001;60:5-20.
7. Gluckman PD, Hanson MA, Bateson P, et al. Towards a new developmental synthesis: adaptive developmental plasticity and human disease. Lancet. 2009;373:1654-7.
8. Hu FB, Manson JE, Stampfer MJ, et al. Diet, lifestyle, and the risk of type 2 diabetes mellitus in women. N Engl J Med. 2001;345:790-7.
9. Malik VS, Popkin BM, Bray GA, et al. Sugar-sweetened beverages and risk of metabolic syndrome and type 2 diabetes: a meta-analysis. Diabetes Care. 2010;33:2477-83
10. Hu FB, Willett WC. Optimal diets for prevention of coronary heart disease. JAMA 2002;288:2569-78.
11. Stanhope KL, Havel PJ. Fructose consumption: recent results and their potential implications. Ann N Y Acad Sci. 2010;1190:15-24.
12. Hu FB. Metabolic consequences of obesity. Obesity epidemiology. New York: Oxford University Press; 2008. p. 149-73.
13. Vazquez G, Duval S, Jacobs DR Jr, et al. Comparison of body mass index, waist circumference, and waist/hip ratio in predicting incident diabetes: a meta-analysis. Epidemiol Rev. 2007;29:115–28.
14. Knowler WC, Barrett-Connor E, Fowler SE, et al. Reduction in the Incidence of Type 2 Diabetes with Lifestyle Intervention or Metformin. N Engl J Med. 2002;346(6):393-403.
15. Tuomilehto J, Lindström J, Eriksson JG, et al. Prevention of type 2 diabetes mellitus by changes in lifestyle among subjects with impaired glucose tolerance. N Engl J Med. 2001;344(18):1343-50.
16. Pan XR, Li GW, Hu YH, et al. Effects of diet and exercise in preventing NIDDM in people with impaired glucose tolerance. The Da Qing IGT and Diabetes Study. Diabetes Care. 1997;20(4):537–44.
17. Ramachandran A, Snehalatha C, Mary S, et al. The Indian Diabetes Prevention Programme shows that lifestyle modification and metformin prevent type 2 diabetes in Asian Indian subjects with impaired glucose tolerance (IDPP-1). Diabetologia. 2006;49(2):289-7.
18. Joshi SR, Bhansali A, Bajaj S, et al. Results from a dietary survey in an Indian T2DM population: a STARCH study. BMJ Open. 2014;4(10): e005138.
19. Mohan V, Radhika G, Sathya RM, et al. Dietary carbohydrates, glycaemic load, food groups and newly detected type 2 diabetes among urban Asian Indian population in Chennai, India (Chennai Urban Rural Epidemiology Study 59). Br J Nutr. 2009;102:1498-506.
20. Canadian Diabetes Assocaition Clinical Practice Guidelines Expert Committee. Clinical Practice Guidelines: Nutrition Therapy. Can J Diabetes. 2013;37:S45-55.
21. Amy Y Liu, Marta P Silvestre, et al. Prevention of Type 2 Diabetes through Lifestyle Modification: Is There a Role for Higher-Protein Diets? Adv Nutr. 2015;6:665-73.
22. Noakes M. The role of protein in weight management. Asia Pac J Clin Nutr. 2008;17:(Suppl 1):169-71.
23. Paddon-Jones D, Westman E, Mattes RD, et al. Protein, weight management, and satiety. Am J Clin Nutr 2008;87:1558S-61S.
24. Gilbert JA, Bendsen NT, Tremblay A, et al. Effect of proteins from different sources on body composition. Nutr Metab Cardiovasc Dis. 2011;21: (Suppl 2):B16-31.
25. Larsen TM, Dalskov SM, van Baak M, et al. Diets with high or low protein content and glycemic index for weight-loss maintenance. N Engl J Med. 2010;363:2102-113.

26. Morenga LT, Williams S, Brown R, et al. Effect of a relatively high protein, high-fiber diet on body composition and metabolic risk factors in overweight women. Eur J Clin Nutr. 2010;64:1323-31.
27. Johnstone AM, Horgan GW, Murison SD, et al. Effects of a high-protein ketogenic diet on hunger, appetite, and weight loss in obese men feeding ad libitum. Am J Clin Nutr. 2008;87:44-55.
28. Johnstone AM, Lobley GE, Horgan GW, et al. Effects of a high-protein, low-carbohydrate v. high-protein, moderate-carbohydrate weight-loss diet on antioxidant status, endothelial markers and plasma indices of the cardiometabolic profile. Br J Nutr. 2011;106:282-91.
29. Clifton PM, Condo D, Keogh JB. Long term weight maintenance after advice to consume low carbohydrate, higher protein diets–a systematic review and meta-analysis. Nutr Metab Cardiovasc Dis. 2014;24:224-35.
30. Dong JY, Zhang ZL, Wang PY, et al. Effects of high-protein diets on body weight, glycaemic control, blood lipids and blood pressure in type 2 diabetes: Meta-analysis of randomised controlled trials. Br J Nutr. 2013;110:781-9.
31. Soenen S, Bonomi AG, Lemmens SG, et al. Relatively high-protein or 'low-carb'energy-restricted diets for body weight loss and body weight maintenance? Physiol Behav 2012;107:374-80.
32. Feinman RD, Pogozelski WK, Astrup A, et al. Dietary carbohydrate restriction as the first approach in diabetes management: Critical review and evidence base. Nutrition. 2015;31:1-13.
33. Samaha FF, Iqbal N, Seshadri P, et al. A low-carbohydrate as compared with a low-fat diet in severe obesity. N Engl J Med. 2003; 348:2074-81.
34. Liebman M. When and why carbohydrate restriction can be a viable option. Nutrition. 2014;30:748-54.
35. Bowen J, Noakes M, Trenerry C, et al. Energy intake, ghrelin, and cholecystokinin after different carbohydrate and protein preloads in overweight men. J Clin Endocrinol Metab. 2006;91:1477-83.
36. Barkeling B, Rössner S, Björvell H. Effects of a high-protein meal (meat) and a high-carbohydrate meal (vegetarian) on satiety measured by automated computerized monitoring of subsequent food intake, motivation to eat and food preferences. Int J Obes. 1990;14:743-51.
37. Porrini M, Crovetti R, Testolin G, et al. Evaluation of satiety sensations and food intake after different preloads. Appetite. 1995;25:17-30.
38. Anderson GH, Moore SE. Dietary proteins in the regulation of food intake and body weight in humans. J Nutr. 2004;134:974S-9S.
39. Halton TL, Hu FB. The effects of high protein diets on thermogenesis, satiety and weight loss: A critical review. J Am Coll Nutr. 2004;23:373-85.
40. Poppitt SD, McCormack D, Buffenstein R. Short-term effects of macronutrient preloads on appetite and energy intake in lean women. Physiol Behav. 1998;64:279-85.
41. Veldhorst MA, Westerterp KR, Westerterp-Plantenga MS. Gluconeogenesis and protein-induced satiety. Br J Nutr 2012;107:595-600.
42. Penhoat A, Mutel E, Amigo-Correig M, et al. Protein-induced satiety is abolished in the absence of intestinal gluconeogenesis. Physiol Behav. 2011;105:89-93.
43. Jensen KJ, Alpini G, Glaser S. Hepatic nervous system and neurobiology of the liver. Compr Physiol. 2013;3:655-65
44. Josse AR, Atkinson SA, Tarnopolsky MA, et al. Increased consumption of dairy foods and protein during diet- and exercise-induced weight loss promotes fat mass loss and lean mass gain in overweight and obese premenopausal women. J Nutr. 2011;141:1626-34.
45. Kushner RF, Doerfler B. Low-carbohydrate, high-protein diets revisited. Curr Opin Gastroenterol 2008;24:198-203.
46. Layman DK, Baum JI. Dietary protein impact on glycemic control during weight loss. J Nutr. 2004;134:968S-73S.
47. Baum JI, Layman DK, Freund GG, et al. A reduced carbohydrate, increased protein diet stabilizes glycemic control and minimizes adipose tissue glucose disposal in rats. J Nutr. 2006;136:1855-61.
48. McGregor RA, Poppitt SD. Milk protein for improved metabolic health: A review of the evidence. Nutr Metab (Lond). 2013;10:46-59.
49. Cope MB, Erdman JJ, Allison DB. The potential role of soyfoods in weight and adiposity reduction: An evidence-based review. Obes Rev. 2008;9:219-35.
50. Sofi F, Macchi C, Abbate R, et al. Mediterranean diet and health. Biofactors. 2013;39:335-42.
51. Du H, van der A DL, van Bakel M, et al. Dietary glycaemic index, glycaemic load and subsequent changes of weight and waist circumference in European men and women. Int J Obes (Lond). 2009;33:1280-8.
52. Halkjær J, Olsen A, Overvad K, et al. Intake of total, animal and plant protein and subsequent changes in weight or waist circumference in European men and women: The Diogenes project. Int J Obes (Lond). 2011;35:1104-113.
53. Pan A, Sun Q, Bernstein AM, et al. Red meat consumption and risk of type 2 diabetes: 3 cohorts of US adults and an updated meta-analysis. Am J Clin Nutr. 2011;94:1088-96.
54. Pan A, Hu FB. Can eating red meat increase the risk of developing type 2 diabetes? Diabetes Management 2014;4:1-4.
55. Pan A, Sun Q, Bernstein AM, et al. Red meat consumption and mortality: Results from 2 prospective cohort studies. Arch Intern Med. 2012;172: 555-63.

Chapter 81

Hepatic 11-beta HSD-1 Enzyme in Pathophysiology of Type 2 Diabetes and Steroid-induced Diabetes

Vijay Negalur

INTRODUCTION

Glucocorticoids are steroid hormones, which are primary hormone to regulating a wide range of biological reactions, including the control of immune and stress responses, and modulating energy metabolism. Glucocorticoids, cortisol in man and corticosterone in mice and rats, stimulate glucose production in the liver and antagonize insulin-mediated glucose uptake in peripheral tissues such as adipose and muscle. They also increase lipolysis and fatty acid mobilization. Individuals with systemic glucocorticoid excess, or Cushing's syndrome, develop visceral obesity, insulin resistance, glucose intolerance, dyslipidemia, hypertension and increased cardiovascular risk. The phenotypic similarities between Cushing's syndrome and obesity/metabolic syndrome have led to the provocative hypothesis that the cardiometabolic consequences of obesity may be driven by glucocorticoid action. Paradoxically, while elevated circulating cortisol levels cause the phenotypic changes observed in Cushing's syndrome, blood cortisol levels are generally normal in patients with metabolic syndrome and simple obesity.[1]

Recent studies have shown that nonadrenal and tissue-specific metabolism of glucocorticoids occurs and is catalyzed by two enzymes, 11β-hydroxysteroid dehydrogenases type-1 (11β-HSD1) and type-2 (11β-HSD2). These two enzymes carry out the interconversion of nonreceptor-binding cortisone and the receptor-binding active form, cortisol. The 11β-HSD2, an NAD-dependent dehydrogenase, is expressed primarily in mineralocorticoid target tissues, such as kidney and colon, and inactivates cortisol to cortisone. The other isoform, 11β-HSD1, a nicotinamide adenine dinucleotide phosphate (NADPH)-dependent enzyme, acts primarily as an 11-keto reductase in vivo, converting inactive cortisone to active cortisol in metabolically important tissues including liver, adipose, vasculature, brain and macrophages. Therefore, 11β-HSD1 activity provides a mechanism for specific cell types to utilize circulating cortisone for intracellular, nonadrenal cortisol production. This local conversion of cortisone to cortisol in metabolically important tissues can drive glucocorticoid-mediated functional antagonism of insulin action in a manner that is independent of circulating cortisol levels.[2]

The cortisol-producing capacity of 11β-HSD1 within liver and adipose tissue is significant. Studies estimate that ~25% of circulating cortisol is derived from the splanchnic reactivation of cortisone. While this productive capacity underlies the attractiveness of pharmacological inhibition of 11β-HSD1 activity to modulate local glucocorticoid action, it also reinforces the need to examine carefully the endocrinologic effects of reducing this nonadrenal source of cortisol.[3]

PRECLINICAL EVIDENCE SUPPORTING 11-β-HSD1 AS A TARGET FOR METABOLIC DISEASE

Transgenic mice generated to mimic this modest overexpression of 11β-HSD1 under the control of the adipose tissue-specific adipocyte protein 2 (aP2) promoter possess elevated corticosterone levels in adipose tissue but normal plasma corticosterone concentrations.[4] These mice exhibit a phenotype closely resembling that of human metabolic syndrome including visceral obesity, insulin resistance, hyperlipidemia, hyperphagia and hypertension. Transgenic mice engineered to overexpress 11β-HSD1 specifically in liver utilizing the apolipoprotein E (ApoE) promoter develop mild-insulin resistance, fatty liver and dyslipidemia. Because splanchnic 11β-HSD1 reactivation of cortisol accounts for ~25% of circulating cortisol levels.[3] This increased adrenal corticosterone biosynthesis maintains normal daily corticosterone levels and rhythmicity. The preclinical evidence presented above supports the hypothesis that small molecule inhibition of 11β-HSD1 in key metabolic tissues, such as liver and adipose, will result in the suppression of intracellular glucocorticoid reactivation, leading to an improvement in hepatic and peripheral insulin sensitivity and overall glycemic control.

CLINICAL EVIDENCE SUPPORTING 11-β-HSD1 INHIBITION AS A TREATMENT FOR METABOLIC DISEASE

Carbenoxolone (CBX) is a steroidal, synthetic analog of glycyrrhetinic acid, itself a derivative of glycyrrhizin, the sweet-tasting compound from the licorice root. CBX is a nonselective inhibitor of 11β-HSD1 and 11β-HSD2 and exhibits only weak 11β-HSD1 pharmacodynamic activity in adipose and liver after oral administration. 100 mg of CBX administered q8h for 7 days in healthy and nondiabetic individuals has been shown to result in modest improvements in insulin sensitivity,[5] and more notably, in patients with type 2 diabetes mellitus (T2DM), the same regimen and treatment duration decreased glucose production rates via attenuation of glycogenolysis.[6] Most recently, Rosenstock et al.[7] have published the results of a 12-week efficacy study evaluating INCB13739 (Incyte Corporation, Wilmington, DE, USA) in patients with T2DM who are failing metformin monotherapy. INCB13739 is a potent (1.1 nM), small molecule, 11β-HSD1-selective inhibitor, which has been shown in previous clinical studies to achieve complete inhibition of both adipose tissue and liver 11β-HSD1 activity after oral administration, and improve clamp-based insulin sensitivity when administered for 4 weeks as monotherapy in patients with T2DM.[8] In this placebo-controlled, dose-ranging study evaluating 5, 15, 50, 100 and 200 mg once daily INCB13739 administered orally with failing metformin monotherapy (mean dose 1,500 mg daily; mean A1c at entry 8.2–8.3%; 66–67 mmol/mol), the 100- and 200-mg dose levels showed statistically significant ($p < 0.01$) reductions in hemoglobin A1c (HbA1c) relative to placebo of –0.5% (–5 mmol/mol) and –0.6% (–7 mmol/mol), respectively. The 200-mg dose group also achieved significant reductions relative to placebo in fasting plasma glucose (FPG) (–24 mg/dL) and homeostatic model assessment of insulin resistance (HOMA-IR) (–24%). While the patient population with T2DM studied by Rosenstock et al.[7] was both unselected and generally well controlled in terms of plasma lipids, a substantial proportion did exhibit ATP III-defined hyperlipidemia at baseline [total cholesterol >200 mg/dL, 38% of the baseline population; low-density lipoprotein (LDL)-cholesterol >130 mg/dL, 20%] or hypertriglyceridemia (>200 mg/dL, 31%). In these subjects, the 100-mg subgroup achieved significant ($p < 0.05$) reductions from baseline in total cholesterol (–6% or –16 mg/dL), LDL-cholesterol (–10% or –17 mg/dL) and triglycerides (–16% or –74 mg/dL). These data must be viewed cautiously, however, as changes in cardiovascular risk factors have not always translated into cardiovascular benefit. Nonetheless, such a profile could address a significant unmet medical need in this disease, as currently available antihyperglycemic agents have thus far failed to reduce the residual cardiovascular risk that is present in even well-controlled patients.

ENDOCRINE RESPONSE TO 11-β-HSD1 INHIBITION

The 11β-HSD1 is not involved in adrenal cortisol biosynthesis, but the enzyme's substantial activity within the splanchnic bed contributes approximately 25% of total cortisol production.[3] It follows, therefore, that significant inhibition of this activity is likely to require an adaptive HPA (hypothalamic, pituitary, adrenal) axis activation to ensure that basal cortisol homoeostasis is maintained. Adrenocorticotropic hormone (ACTH) is produced and secreted by the anterior pituitary and functions as a critical component of the HPA axis controlling the production and release of cortisol from the adrenal gland. Morning, fasting ACTH increased in a dose- and time-dependent manner following INCB13739 treatment of patients with T2DM. After 4 weeks of treatment, maximal ACTH concentrations were achieved in the 50-mg dose group ($p < 0.01$ from placebo), and neither longer durations of treatment (12 weeks) nor increased INCB13739 dose levels (100 and 200 mg) resulted in a further increase in ACTH concentrations. Mean ACTH concentrations in all treatment groups at all time points remained within normal reference ranges.

CONCLUSION

These data also presented a unique therapeutic proposition: inhibition of 11β-HSD1 in patients with T2DM may enable anti-hyperglycemic benefit through improved insulin sensitivity in a manner that concomitantly reduces macrovascular risk. In 2010, the results of a long-awaited clinical evaluation of a potent and selective 11β-HSD1 inhibitor, INCB13739, in patients with T2DM were published. These data not only showed that 11β-HSD1 inhibition can significantly reduce HbA1c and fasting glucose but they also provided provocative evidence that cholesterol and triglyceride levels can be improved in patients with hyperlipidemia and/or hypertriglyceridemia. Thorough endocrinologic assessments showed nothing other than the expected adaptive and compensatory HPA axis response to therapy that functions to maintain normal cortisol homoeostasis. Perhaps, most interesting is the observation that patients classified as obese benefited the greatest from INCB13739 therapy, possibly underscoring the importance of 11β-HSD1-mediated splanchnic cortisol reactivation to the metabolic sequelae of obesity. These data mark the beginning of a new chapter in the 11β-HSD1 evolution, one that will be devoted to the further characterization of cardiometabolic benefit and endocrine adaptation that arise from long-term therapy.

REFERENCES

1. Kraus-Friedmann N. Hormonal regulation of hepatic gluconeogenesis. Physiol Rev. 1984;64:170-259.
2. Smas CM, Chen L, Zhao L, et al. Transcriptional repression of pref-1 by glucocorticoids promotes 3T3-L1 adipocyte differentiation. J Biol Chem. 1999;274:12632-41.
3. Basu R, Singh RJ, Basu A, et al. Obesity and type 2 diabetes do not alter splanchnic cortisol production in humans. J Clin Endocrinol Metab. 2005;90:3919-26.
4. Kershaw EE, Morton NM, Dhillon H, et al. Adipocytespecific glucocorticoid inactivation protects against diet-induced obesity. Diabetes. 2005;54:1023-31.
5. Walker BR, Connacher AA, Lindsay RM, et al. Carbenoxolone increases hepatic insulin sensitivity in man: a novel role for 11-oxosteroid reductase in enhancing glucocorticoid receptor activation. J Clin Endocrinol Metab. 1995;80:3155-9.
6. Andrews RC, Rooyackers O, Walker BR. Effects of the 11 beta-hydroxysteroid dehydrogenase inhibitor carbenoxolone on insulin sensitivity inmen with type 2 diabetes. J Clin Endocrinol Metab. 2003;88:285-91.
7. Rosenstock J, Banarer S, Fonseca VA, et al. The 11-beta-hydroxysteroid dehydrogenase type 1 inhibitor INCB13739 improves hyperglycemia in patients with type 2 diabetes inadequately controlled by metformin monotherapy. Diabetes Care. 2010;33:1516-22.
8. Williams W, Huber R, Levy R, et al. Endocrine homeostasis with inhibition of tissue-specific cortisone reductase in healthy volunteers and obese insulin resistant subjects following oral INCB013739 inhibitor therapy [abstract]. In: 67th Scientific Sessions of the American Diabetes Association; 2007 June 22–26; Chicago, IL: Diabetes; p. A572. Abstract 2255, 2007.

Chapter 82

Restoring Insulin Secretion in Type 2 Diabetes Mellitus: Concept to Reality

Diksha Shirodkar, Shaila Shamanur Bhattacharyya, Arpandev Bhattacharyya

INTRODUCTION

Type 2 diabetes mellitus (T2DM) affects 1 in 11 adults aged 20–79 years. Diabetes is a global burden and threat—415 million adults had T2DM in 2015 and this number is predicted to rise to 592 million by 2035.[1] Low- and middle-income countries will experience the greatest increase in cases of diabetes. Glycemic control in T2DM not only improves symptoms and quality of life but also prevents/postpones micro- and macrovascular complications. From a number of studies, particularly from United Kingdom Prospective Diabetes Study (UKPDS), we know clearly that T2DM progresses with time. Whether β-cell dysfunction in the form of glucolipotoxicity or oxidative stress are similar and what are the best points at which we can resurrect the β-cell and help it get back to its normalcy to a large extent is the question. Here, in this chapter, we shall discuss interventions on T2DM (especially at its bud stage) to improve β-cell function based on a comprehension of previous and new data, practical experience and rational speculation.

β-CELL: NORMAL FUNCTION

β-cells synthesize, store and release insulin. To maintain euglycemia in a normal healthy individual, the body has a complex mechanism which includes interplay of insulin from pancreas, glucose from liver and insulin- and noninsulin-mediated glucose uptake in the tissues. Normally, insulin is secreted in the form of a basal output and after a meal. The two-phase insulin secretion is as follows:

1. *A fast phase which is adenosine triphosphate (ATP) dependent and requires release of Ca^{2+}:* Here, the insulin granules are already in the cytoplasm which is the "readily released pool" and these are "docked" and "energized" followed by release from the β-cell. About 5% of the total insulin released comes from this phase. This helps in priming the target tissues to maintain euglycemic homeostasis
2. The slow-phase (ATP dependent), wherein the insulin granules are moved from the "reserve pool" to the "readily released" pool of insulin granules. This accounts for the maximum levels of insulin (60 minutes postmeal).

In addition, it has been demonstrated that there is oscillatory release of insulin, with stable rapid pulses (occurring every 8–10 minutes) which are superimposed on low pulses.

The amplitude of these insulin oscillations is 100 times higher in the portal vein than in the systemic circulation (hepatic extraction of insulin pulses). Bergman and Cobelli[2] have found that this relationship between insulin secretion and insulin sensitivity is well extrapolated as a hyperbolic curve and the product of insulin sensitivity and insulin secretion is constant as long as normoglycemia is maintained. This product is called disposition index, which refers to insulin secretion adjusted by insulin sensitivity and depicts the true β-cell function in vivo. Abnormal glucose tolerance develops when the insulin secretion cannot increase to fight back the declining insulin sensitivity. The disposition index is, therefore, decreased and poor functioning of the β-cell has already commenced.

Biphasic Insulin Secretion

Figure 1 defines biphasic insulin secretion.

β-CELL: ABNORMALITY IN TYPE 2 DIABETES MELLITUS

Type 2 diabetes mellitus is an outcome of insulin resistance with failing β-cells, each one worsening itself and the other and causing the progression of T2DM (Flowchart 1).

The earliest abnormality of β-cell in T2DM is the loss of the first-phase of insulin release in response to a meal. Fasting plasma glucose level rising to 115–120 mg/dL denotes the first phase abnormality.

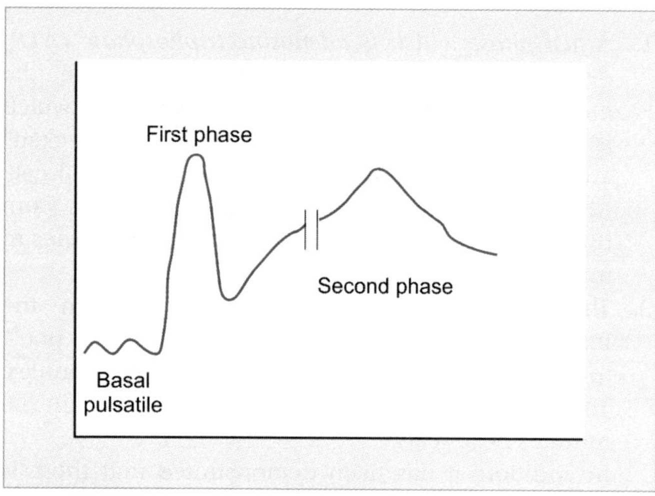

Figure 1 Biphasic insulin secretion.

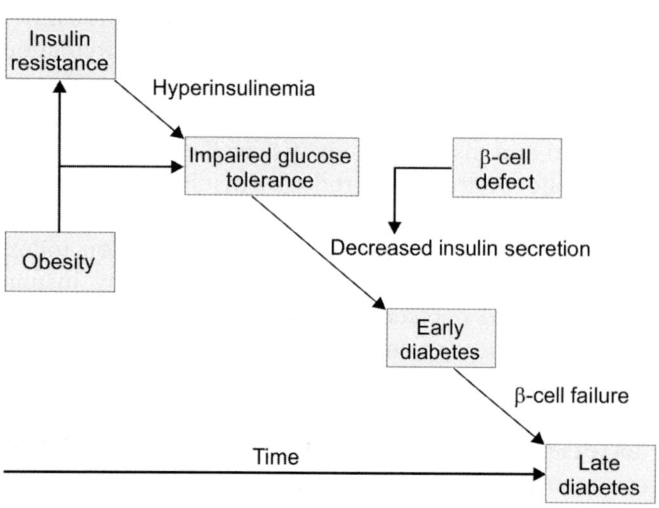

Flowchart 1 Stages of type 2 diabetes.

PHASES OF DETERIORATION OF β-CELL FUNCTION

- Phase 1: Successful adaptation to increased demand
- Phase 2: Mild decompensation
- Phase 3: Severe decompensation
- Phase 4: Decompensation with structural damage.

Hyperglycemia exerts a direct toxic effect on the β-cells 24-hour period of hyperglycemia decreasing the β-cell response by 20%. This is due to downregulation of receptors and appearance of postreceptor defects. Thus, hyperglycemia is not just a manifestation of diabetes but also a self-perpetuating etiological factor. The molecular mechanism of insulin resistance includes postreceptor defects since reduced insulin receptor levels are thought to be secondary to hyperinsulinemia which in turn cause defects in internalization and recycling of receptors. The postreceptor defects include reduced activation of insulin receptor substrate-1 and phosphatidylinositol-3 kinase and impaired translocation of GLUT-4 (insulin-regulated glucose transporter-4).

TYPE 2 DIABETES MELLITUS—A PROGRESSIVE DISORDER

In the UKPDS, β-cell function assessed by Homeostasis Model Assessment (HOMA) in patients with T2DM was already decreased by 50% at the time of diagnosis and progressively declined by 5% annually. β-cell function starts to decline 10 years prior to the onset of the disease.[3] There was decline in glycemic control with conventional treatment and with intensive treatment associated with declining β-cell function (Figs. 2 and 3).

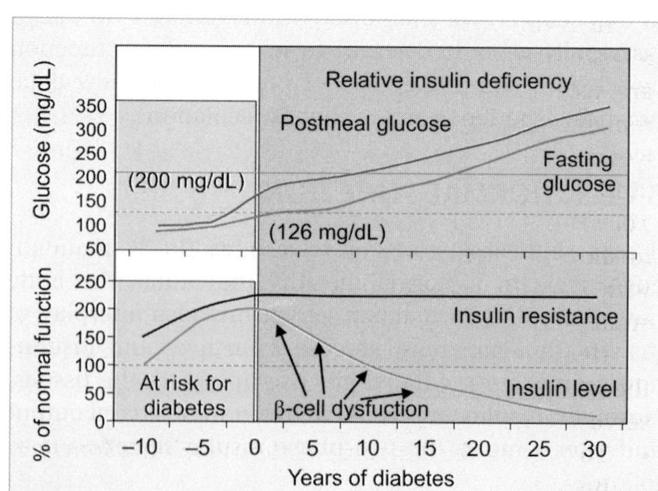

Figure 2 Natural history of type 2 diabetes.

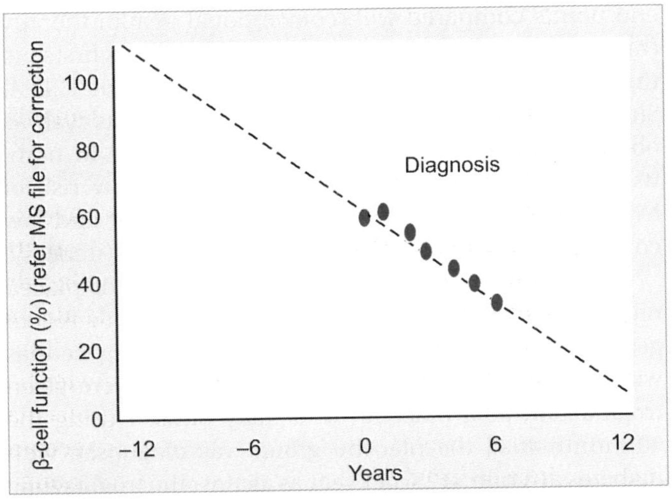

Figure 3 Progressive β-cell failure in type 2 diabetes mellitus.

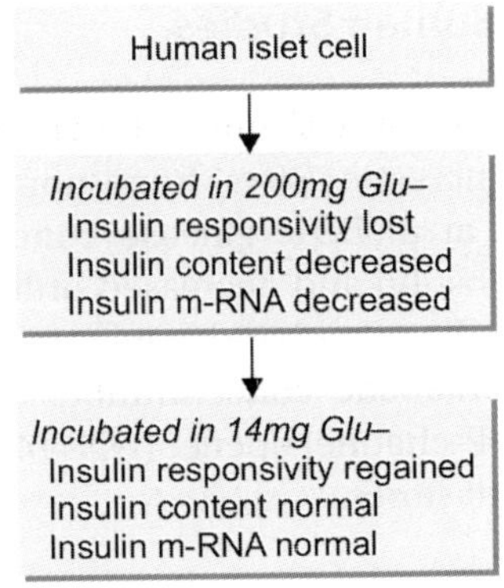

(Glu: glucose; mRNA: messenger ribonucleic acid.)

Flowchart 2 Improved insulin response in lower concentration of glucose as seen in study by Rasmussen et al.[4]

This rate of decline depends on the genetic, metabolic and environmental influences. The lifestyle modifications like regular exercise, eating healthy food, maintaining ideal body weight, waist hip ratio and moderating alcohol have a great role.

THE CONCEPT OF β-CELL REST/PROTECTION

This idea of β-cell rest causing rejuvenation and possibly return of function of the β-cell came about when researchers (Jackson et al. in 1940) began to notice a progressive decline in the need of exogenous insulin in type 1 diabetes children following recovery after the initial months of treatment—"The Honey Moon Phase". Here, there was a partial remission period and the endogenous secretion of insulin improved.

In T2DM with fasting plasma glucose of >140 mg/dL, >75% of the β-cell function is lost. Now, if sulfonylureas are used at this stage, it would mean whipping the remaining 25% to compensate for the loss—in other words working them to death! Just like the NAVIGATOR trial in 2010 (Nateglinide And Valsartan in Impaired Glucose Tolerance Outcomes Research) where nateglinide failed to show a reduction in progression to T2DM in patients with impaired glucose tolerance (IGT) suggesting that strategies to increase β-cell workload may not be effective.

Here is where we need to understand the concept and the basis behind giving the β-cells some form of rest to serve a couple of purposes, i.e.:

- To protect the function of the remaining functional β-cells
- To postpone the complications secondary to T2DM.

Firstly, there is a threshold that the pancreas can handle. When insulin resistance strikes, the β-cells overwork to produce more insulin for the necessary compensation. Over time, this high workload causes the β-cells to die. In addition, hyperglycemia per se also worsens β-cell function by the mechanism of glucotoxicity.

IN VITRO STUDIES

Patients with established T2DM have mainly a defect in insulin pulse mass. In a study done in Hagedorn Research Institute, it was proven that through intensive insulin treatment and potassium channel openers, β-cell mass is improved, in acutely diabetic BB rats. Here, when the β-cells were cultured in a medium with increased glucose concentration (200 mg/dL), there was lesser insulin secretion compared to when they were transferred to a normoglycemic culture (Flowchart 2).[4]

IN VIVO STUDIES

Animal Studies

In a study at Denmark,[5] NN414 an orally active SUR1/Kir6.2 selective potassium channel blocker was used in comparison with vehicle (V), on diabetic adult male Zucker obese rats. NN414- and V-treated rats had fasting blood sugars of 118 mg/dL and 154 mg/dL, respectively, at the end of the treatment. Fasting insulin levels were also significantly lower in NN414 rats compared to V. Basal insulin was significantly lower and first-phase insulin sensitivity significantly higher in NN414-treated rats.

Cadaveric Human Studies

Ritzel et al.[6] in 2004 demonstrated that incubation of cadaveric pancreatic islets from nondiabetic humans for 96 hours at diabetic glucose concentration caused depletion of insulin and decreased orderliness of insulin secretion. On the other hand, concurrent culture of islets at the same diabetic concentrations with a new cell-selective KATP-channel opener (NN414, KCO) prevented loss of islet cell stores.

Human Studies

Twelve-hour intravenous insulin infusion was used in nonobese uncontrolled T2DM patients to check whether there was any improvement in sulphonylurea sensitivity postinfusion. The results were positive and the insulin infusion showed significant improvement in β-cell function which was seen from the 2nd day and lasted for >6 months (Table 1).[7]

This proves that the 12-hour insulin infusion provided restoration of the blood glucose levels and caused β-cell resensitization to sulphonylureas resulting in normoglycemia for longer periods. So, in the same vein, there was an important conclusion made by Weng et al. in 2008[8] demonstrating early intensive insulin therapy (multiple daily injections and continuous insulin infusion) in patients with newly diagnosed T2DM having favorable outcomes on recovery, maintenance of β-cell function and early glycemic remission compared to oral hypoglycemic agents. In the ORIGIN (Outcome Reduction with Initial Glargine Intervention) trial, adding basal insulin was also shown to suppress progression from IGT to T2DM[9] through inducing β-cell rest.

The Kumamoto study involved a smaller number of T2DM patients who were nonobese with mild insulin resistance, requiring <30 units of insulin per day for intensive therapy. Over a 6-year period, it was shown that intensive insulin therapy [mean glycated hemoglobin (HbA1c) = 7.1%] significantly reduced microvascular end points compared with conventional insulin therapy (mean HbA1c = 9.4%).[10] Metformin is ranked as first-line therapy in most guidelines for the treatment of T2DM. Since metformin is effective in lean patients as well as obese patients with T2DM, it should be used in both. Its efficacy in reducing HbA1c (by -1.5%), low risk of hypoglycemia, favorable effect on body weight and low cost make it apt to use it to break the insulin resistance.[11]

Buchanan et al. tested whether the demands placed on β-cells could prevent T2DM in people with recent gestational diabetes.[12] In this study, 235 young Latinas with gestational diabetes in the recent past were given troglitazone or a placebo on a daily basis. During the 30-month trial, the placebo group was diagnosed with diabetes at a rate >12% per year as against the troglitazone group (5% per year). The woman whose β-cells worked most at the start of the study benefitted the most from the drug; this was because of "β-cell rest".

Fehse et al.[13] showed that exenatide-treated subjects had an insulin secretory pattern similar to healthy subjects in both first (0–10 min) and second (10–180 min) phases after glucose challenge in contrast to saline-treated T2DM subjects, thus proving that exenatide (incretin) brought about near-normal insulin secretion phases in T2DM. This is possible because of the biology of glucose-dependent insulinotropic peptide-1 (GLP-1) molecule which promotes β-cell proliferation and inhibits apoptosis. It also inhibits gastric emptying and glucagon causing the feeling of satiety-inducing β-cell rest (Fig. 4).

Bunck et al.[14] conducted a study on 69 metformin-treated patients with T2DM who were randomly assigned to exenatide or glargine. Treatment-induced change in combined glucose- and arginine-stimulated C-peptide secretion was 2.46-fold greater after a 52-week exenatide treatment compared with glargine treatment.

DeFronzo et al.[15] showed reduced risk of conversion of IGT to T2DM by 72% in the pioglitazone group compared to placebo. There were other advantages too—being reduction in diastolic blood pressure, increased

TABLE 1: Effect of 12-hour insulin infusion.

	Basal	2 days	7 days	2 months	4 months	6 months
FBG	201	167	135	146	136	145
C-pep (f) ng/mL	0.56	0.83	–	0.6	0.7	0.46
C-pep (pp)	1	1.46	–	0.86	0.96	0.96
HbA1c	8.3	–	–	6.4	6.5	6.7

N = 15, Age at diagnosis >35 years, nonobese, failed to diet and 15 mg Glib.
(c-PEP: C-peptide; FBG: fasting blood glucose; HbA1c: glycated hemoglobin.)
Source: Sinagra D, Greco D, Amanto M, et al. A 12-h intravenous insulin infusion restores the b-cell response to sulfonylureas in patients affected by type 2 diabetes. Diab Care. 2000;23:1857-8.

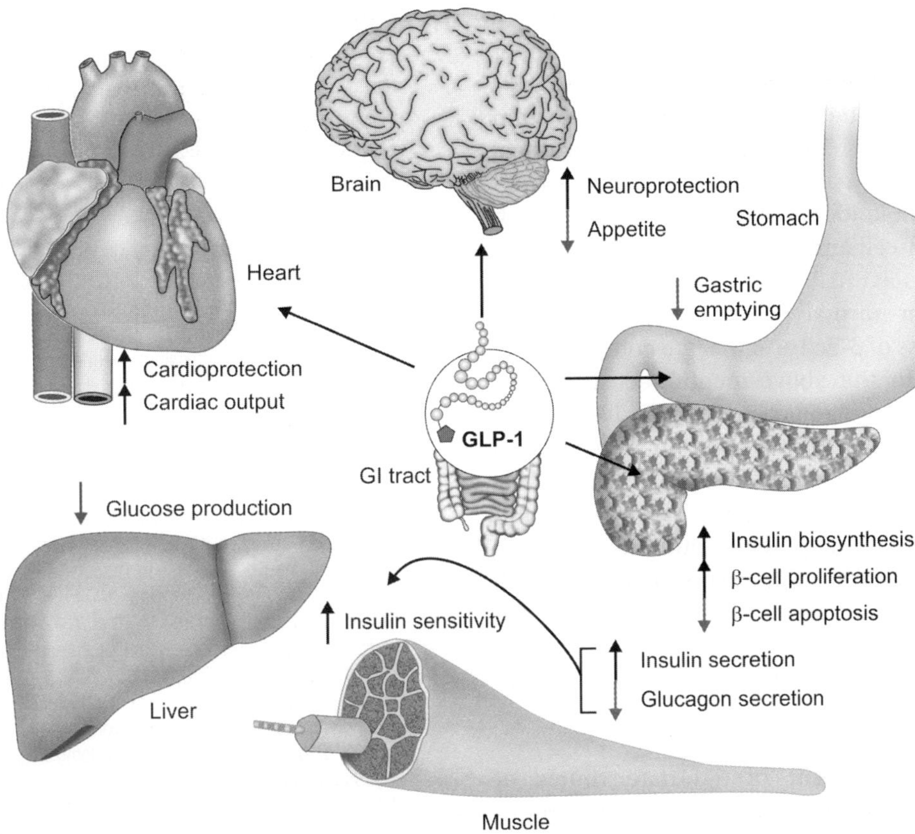

(GI: gastrointestinal; GLP-1: glucose-dependent insulinotropic peptide-1.)

Figure 4 Mechanism of action of incretin hormones.

Source: Drucker DJ. The biology of incretin hormones. Cell Metab. 2006;3(3):153-65.

high-density lipoprotein (HDL) cholesterol and reduced risk of cardiovascular disease. On the same strain in TODAY-2013 trial (Treatment Options for type 2 Diabetes in Adolescents and Youth), the combination of metformin with rosiglitazone proved to show lesser failure rates and better glycemic control thus improving β-cell function compared to metformin alone or metformin plus lifestyle modification.

A new concept has taken light in the midst of using only drugs to improve insulin sensitivity and provide β-cell protection. We all know pulsatile insulin secretion is governed by islet oscillations such as bursting electrical activity and periodic Ca^{2+} entry in β-cells and these are lost by fixing the glucose stimulus at a high concentration, but can be recovered by converting the glucose stimulus to a sinusoidal wave using microfluidics. Hence, Mc Kenna et al.[16] in his research put forward the hypothesis of a dual oscillator model in 2016. Here, oscillatory blood glucose levels recruit nonoscillating islets to enhance pulsatile insulin secretion from the pancreas.

In case of bariatric surgery, most of the surgeries do not affect the early phase of insulin secretion except laparoscopic sleeve surgery and biliopancreatic diversion. In the latter, early insulin secretion is not altered in nondiabetics but is increased in T2DM with an associated increase in insulin secretion for the second phase too.[17]

Earlier sodium-glucose cotransporter 2 (SGLT2) inhibitor was thought to be independent of β-cell function and the reduction of HbA1c was purely secondary to increased glucose excretion via the renal SGLT2 transporters. However, Cheng et al. showed[18] empagliflozin to be reported to improve glycemic control, by increasing β-cell mass along with its traditional function, in streptozotocin-induced type 1 diabetic rats. These effects are attributed to a reduction in apoptosis and reactive oxygen species in the β-cells.

Recently, "RISE (Restoring Insulin Secretion) Consortium 2014"[19] has commenced a study to preserve β-cell function in adults, children and adolescents with early diabetes or prediabetes. This study has three protocols.

The adult protocol randomizes patients to 12 months of placebo, metformin alone, liraglutide plus metformin, or insulin followed by metformin (9 months). The pediatric protocol randomizes patients to metformin or insulin followed by metformin. The adult surgical protocol randomizes patients to gastric banding or metformin (24 months). The whole idea is to devise ways by which we can salvage the β-cell and the results of this study are awaited.

Maintaining near-normal glycemia should at least reduce the rate of loss of β-cell and the late complications of central obesity. In the above-mentioned studies, it has been proved that early initiation of intensive therapy with insulin at least for a short duration is helpful to preserve and improve the β-cell function in T2DM. It is also evident that usage of metformin to break the insulin resistance, GLP-1 and dipeptidyl-peptidase inhibitors cause glucose-mediated insulin response and SGLT2 inhibitors (empagliflozin) could also help restore the β-cell mass.

CONCLUSION

In view of the development of alternate routes of insulin administration, possible theories with respect to mechanism of action of SGLT2 inhibitors, GLP-1 analogs, and dipeptidyl peptidase 4 (DPP-4) inhibitors—having β-cell protective mechanisms, it looks certain that the concept of β-cell preservation would become practical and acceptable. So, early insulin therapy may become an option soon as first-line therapy for those newly diagnosed with T2DM. Indeed, acceptance should come about by patients and the physicians. This does ring a bell in us that the earlier we diagnose the better is the outcome with respect to saving the islet function. Recommendation of early insulin therapy in T2DM will happen only when we have immense data and intervention trials which will put forward the guidelines, clearly delineating the basis on which β-cell protection strategies are used. Karvestedt et al. had shown that early insulin therapy for the preservation of β-cell function works well, but the initial effect does not last on continuous insulin use in T2DM.[20] So, can early intermittent therapy with insulin in T2DM be used? We cannot say for sure. Unfortunately, currently no universally accepted treatment strategies to improve β-cell functional mass have been established, we still have a hope ahead. Considering all the aspects, restoring the β-cell function is the way forward. Future advances in the area of β-cell failure mechanism and modulators may lead to the identification of possible novel therapeutic strategies.

REFERENCES

1. Guariguata L, Whiting DR, Hambleton I, et al. Global estimates of diabetes prevalence for 2013 and projections for 2035. Diab Res Clin Pract. 2014;103(2):137-49.
2. Bergman RN, Phillips LS, Cobelli C. Physiologic evaluation of factors controlling glucose tolerance in man: measurement of insulin sensitivity and beta-cell glucose sensitivity from the response to intravenous glucose. J Clin Invest. 1981;68:1456-67.
3. U.K. Prospective Diabetes Study 16: Overview of 6 Years' Therapy of Type II Diabetes: A Progressive Disease; U.K. Prospective Diabetes Study Group. Diabetes. 1995;44(11):1249-58.
4. Rasmussen SB, Sorensen TS, Hansen JB, et al. Functional rest through intensive insulin and potassium channel openers preserves residual beta-cell function and mass in acutely diabetic BB rats. Horm Metab Res. 2000;32:294-300.
5. Aizawa T, Taguchi N, Sato Y, et al. Prophylaxis of genetically determined diabetes by diazoxide: a study in a rat model of naturally occurring obese diabetes. J Pharmacol Exp Ther. 1995;275:194-9.
6. Ritzel RA, Hansen JB, Veldhuis JD, et al. Induction of beta-cell rest by a Kir6.2/SUR1-selective K(ATP)-channel opener preserves beta-cell insulin stores and insulin secretion in human islets cultured at high (11 mM) glucose. J Clin Endocrinol Metab. 2004;89(2):795-805.
7. Sinagra D, Greco D, Amanto M, et al. A 12-h intravenous insulin infusion restores the b-cell response to sulfonylureas in patients affected by type 2 diabetes. Diab Care. 2000;23:1857-8.
8. Weng J, Li Y, Xu W, et al. Effect of intensive insulin therapy on beta-cell function and glycemic control in patients with newly diagnosed type 2 diabetes: a multicentre randomized parallel-group trial. Lancet. 2008;371:1753-60.
9. Trial Investigators. Basal insulin and cardiovascular and other outcomes in dysglycemia. N Engl J Med. 2012;367(4):319-28.
10. Wake N, Hisashige A, Katayama T, et al. Cost-effectiveness of intensive insulin therapy for type 2 diabetes: a 10-year follow up of the Kumamoto study. Diab Res Clin Pract. 2000;48:201-10.
11. DeFronzo R, Barzilai N, Simonson DC. Mechanism of metformin action in obese and lean noninsulin-dependent diabetic subjects. J Clin Endocrinol Metabol. 1991;73(6):1294-301.
12. Buchanan TA, Xiang AH, Peters RK, et al. Preservation of pancreatic beta-cell function and prevention of resistance in high-risk Hispanic women. Diabetes. 2002;51:796-803.
13. Fehse F, Trautmann M, Holst JJ, et al. Exenatide augments first- and second-phase insulin secretion in response to intravenous glucose in subjects with type 2 diabetes. J Clin Endocrinol Metabol. 2005;90(11):5991-7.
14. Bunck MC, Diamant M, Cornér A, et al. One-year treatment with exenatide improves β-cell function, compared with insulin glargine, in metformin-treated type 2 diabetic patients: A randomized, controlled trial. Diab Care. 2009;32(5):762-8.
15. DeFronzo RA, Tripathy D, Schwenke DC, et al. Pioglitazone for diabetes prevention in impaired glucose tolerance. N Engl J Med. 2011;364:1104-15.
16. McKenna JP, Dhumpa R, Mukhitov N, et al. Glucose oscillations can activate an endogenous oscillator in pancreatic islets. In: Voit EO (Ed). PLoS Computational Biology. 2016;12(10):e1005143.
17. Bradley D, Magkos F, Klein S. Effects of bariatric surgery on glucose homeostasis and type 2 diabetes. Gastroenterology. 2012;143(4):897-912.
18. Cheng ST, Chen L, Li SY, et al. The effects of empagliflozin, an SGLT2 inhibitor, on pancreatic β-cell mass and glucose homeostasis in type 1 diabetes. PLoS ONE. 2016;11(1):e0147391.
19. The RISE Consortium. Restoring Insulin Secretion (RISE): Design of studies of β-cell preservation in prediabetes and early type 2 diabetes across the life span. Diab Care. 2014;37(3):780-8.
20. Karvestedt L, Anderson G, Efendic S, et al. A rapid increase in β-cell function by multiple insulin injections in type 2 diabetic patients is not further enhanced by prolonging treatment. J Intern Med. 2002;251:307-16.

Chapter 83

Adult Immunization in Diabetes—Current Recommendations

OP Sharma

INTRODUCTION

Demographic transition of population has modified the prevalence of many diseases.[1] This is a global phenomenon with reflections in India as well. With the rapid advances in medical field, there is a steady increase in average human longevity. This has led to an increased number of elderly people seeking medical attention for their age-related health problems. In addition, an improvement in socioeconomic status has also led to an increased prevalence of lifestyle diseases like diabetes mellitus (DM) in the elderly.[2] Most common type of diabetes in this age group is type 2 DM that is often associated with a state of diminished immunity.[3]

With the advancing age, the health decline in elderly is further compounded with comorbid conditions like obesity, hypertension, ischemic heart diseases, heart failure, chronic obstructive airway diseases, chronic kidney diseases, chronic liver diseases, etc. thereby increasing morbidity and mortality.[4] Additionally, the elderly have a higher incidence of infections (bacterial as well as viral). Unfortunately, repeated and injudicious use of antimicrobials often leads to the emergence of resistant strains, side effects of medication and longer stays in hospitals adding to cost[5] as multiple problems make management more difficult.[6]

Mortality[7] from various infections due to emerging drug resistance and mutations in bugs continues to rise.[8] This is despite the use of broad spectrum antibiotics and other support systems in intensive care units. There comes the role of preventions in which immunization/vaccination is of prime importance.[8]

Immunization is a means of providing specific protection against damaging pathogens. Specific immunity can be acquired naturally or artificially by either passive or active immunization. Vaccines greatly reduce the risk of infection by working with the body's natural defenses to safely develop immunity to disease. Vaccination thereby becomes a novel approach to boost immunity.

PASSIVE IMMUNITY

- Natural passive immunity is acquired without challenging the immune system with an antigen. It involves transfer of serum or gamma globulins from an immune donor to a nonimmune individual. For example, naturally acquired passive immunity is transferred from mother to fetus through placental transfer of IgG or colostral IgA
- Artificially acquired passive immunity is by transfusing with immune globulins or gamma globulins; this property is used in many acute infection situations like diphtheria, tetanus, measles, rabies and poisoning with insects, reptiles, botulism and as a prophylactic measure in hypogammaglobulinemia.[4]

ACTIVE IMMUNITY

- Active immunity is produced by the body following exposure to antigens
- Naturally acquired active immunity is produced after exposure to a pathogen leading to subclinical or clinical infection and results in a protective immune response against exposure to the pathogens

- *Artificially acquired active immunity* is transferred via administration of vaccines containing live or dead pathogens or their antigenic components.[8]

IMMUNIZATION IN DIABETICS

Based upon the observation that the diabetics have lowered immunity and are more prone to infections; the role of vaccines in them in preventable diseases is paramount. This is more common in the elderly as the advancing age reduces the body response to previous vaccination because of immunosenescence, a term coined by Roy Walford in 1969.

The American Diabetes Association, Advisory Committee on Immunization Practices, Center for Disease Control and Prevention, World Health Organization (WHO), United Kingdom Guidelines, Geriatric Society of India and Association of Physicians of India have given their recommendations for the use of vaccines in type 2 diabetes (T2D). These recommendations are for hepatitis B, influenza, pneumococcal, tetanus, diphtheria, pertussis and zoster vaccines.[9]

In addition, however, it advocates that people suffering from diabetes may also be given hemophilus influenza type B, hepatitis A, human papillomavirus, measles, mumps, rubella, meningococcal, typhoid, varicella and yellow fever vaccines under certain special circumstances.[10]

In this review, we shall be discussing hepatitis B, influenza, pneumococcal, tetanus, diphtheria, pertussis, hepatitis A, meningococcal, typhoid, zoster vaccines and yellow fever vaccine.

Hepatitis B Vaccine[11]

This is given to all unvaccinated people suffering from T2D. The case for vaccination becomes stronger in them if they have, in addition, a history of intravenous drug use, a household contacts of persons with chronic *hepatitis B virus* (HBV) infection, occupational exposure to HBV, human immunodeficiency virus (HIV) seropositivity, chronic liver disease (CLD), chronic kidney disease, use of blood products or multiple blood transfusions, or sexual exposure with patients having sexually transmitted disease. It is also indicated in medico-social workers and partners having hepatitis B surface antigen positive status. Post-exposure prophylaxis includes full course of vaccination and in addition to it, single intramuscular (IM) dose of hepatitis B Ig 0.06 mL/kg is also given.

Influenza Vaccine

First available in the 1940s, there are now two formulations per year: One for each hemisphere (Northern and Southern) are made available. WHO recommends the viral composition of each formulation, based on the predominant circulating viral strains grown in embryonated chicken eggs in the relevant geographical area based on surveillance and epidemiology.

There are two types of vaccines: killed and live attenuated vaccine.

The killed "trivalent inactivated influenza vaccine and the live attenuated influenza vaccine (LAIV)" are efficacious and recommended for use by the Advisory Committee on Immune Practice for prevention of influenza.

The seasonal influenza vaccine (LAIV)[12] is a trivalent vaccine containing two influenza A strains: One H_1N_1 type and another H_3N_2[12] strains and one influenza type B strain (each 15 mg) decided by the WHO on the epidemiologic and antigenic analysis of the currently circulating strains.

The annual influenza vaccination (LAIV) is advised to cover any mutation, which the circulating virus may undergo over the timescale. Seasonal influenza vaccine is prepared annually to include the most likely strain for the season. Over 100 countries in the world use influenza vaccines.

If an antigenic shift in the virus takes place, pandemic results. There is no pandemic virus vaccine available. Post-vaccination, antibodies develop in about 2 weeks' time, which gives protection against influenza virus infection.

Influenza in India

As India being a tropical country is geographically located in the Northern hemisphere, the vaccination should be done by October, if possible. Vaccination should continue as long as influenza viruses are circulating. However, being a tropical country, WHO places India in the Southern hemisphere for epidemiological purposes. As a matter of fact, because of different climatic variations in different parts of country, India has two peaks of influenza—first during the months of September to November and then during January to March. As the virus is circulating all the 12 months of the year—365 days of the year, the vaccine could be given any time, if available. The WHO also recommends that the latest vaccine formulation available should be given to the vulnerable population instead of waiting for the availability of vaccines, based on geographic discrimination.

Annual vaccination against influenza is recommended for all adult diabetics who want to reduce the risk of becoming ill with influenza. Vaccination is also recommended in diabetic women who are or will be pregnant during the influenza season. Stronger recommendations are for diabetics who additionally suffer from chronic pulmonary conditions [asthma, chronic obstructive pulmonary disease (COPD) and interstitial lung disease], cardiovascular diseases (except hypertension), CLDs, chronic kidney diseases, hematological diseases, metabolic disorders, persons who are on immune suppression, residents of nursing homes, chronic care facilities workers and contacts of caregivers with comorbid medical conditions.

Schedule of Vaccination[13]

Trivalent inactivated influenza vaccine is given only once as a single dose to elderly persons. It is available as 0.5-mL liquid in prefilled syringe. This is given as IM injection in the deltoid muscle or as intranasal. Yearly flu vaccination should begin in September, or as soon as vaccine is available.

Revaccination: Influenza vaccine is recommended to be administered annually.

Pneumococcal Vaccines

There are two types of vaccines, namely, pneumococcal polysaccharide vaccine [(PPSV)23] and pneumococcal conjugate vaccine [(PCV)13].

1. Pneumococcal polysaccharide vaccine 23:[14] In the year 1945, for the first time, a tetravalent PPSV was introduced in 1945. It was derived from a capsular polysaccharide of killed *Streptococcus pneumoniae.* The polysaccharide antigen was capable of inducing type-specific antibodies that enhanced opsonization, phagocytosis and killing of pneumococci by phagocytic cells

   After years of continuous research and development, by the year 1983, it gave way for the production of a 23-valent formulation of a PPSV23 containing long chains of polysaccharide molecules that make up the surface capsule of 23 types of pneumococci, which include 1, 2, 3, 4, 5, 6b, 7f, 8, 9v, 10a, 11a, 12f, 14, 15b, 17f, 18c, 19f, 19a, 20, 22f, 23f and 33f serotypes. It is particularly beneficial in invasive pneumococcal disease and has shown significant reduction in diseases caused by invasive serotypes
2. Pneumococcal conjugate vaccine 13:[15] In the year 2000, a new PCV7 was introduced to increase efficacy of existing vaccine. In the process of conjugation, bacterial polysaccharides are covalently conjugated to an immunogenic carrier protein containing nontoxic variety of diphtheria toxin. The conjugate vaccine acts by binding to polysaccharide-specific B-cells that communicate carrier protein antigen cross-reactive material 197 to T-cells. There is a T-cell-dependent immune response by the release of cytokines that facilitate B-cells to transform into plasma cells, which in turn release antibodies. Pneumococcal conjugate vaccine 7 over the years has been modified into a triskavalent vaccine (Prevnar13, PCV13) containing capsular polysaccharides from 13 serotypes of *pneumococcus* (1, 3, 4, 5, 6a, 6b, 7f, 9v, 14, 18c, 19a, 19f and 23f). This vaccine has caused significant reduction in the rates of pneumococcal disease in the United States

   Pneumococcal conjugate vaccine 13 has been approved by the US Food and Drug Administration in 2011 for use in adults 50 years of age or older to prevent pneumonia and invasive disease by S. pneumoniae (Table 1).

Schedule of Vaccination[15]

Pneumococcal polysaccharide vaccine 23 is given only once as a single dose to elderly persons. One dose of (0.5 mL) the vaccine contains 25 μg of each capsular polysaccharide antigen dissolved in isotonic saline solution with 0.25% phenol as a preservative. Revaccination is after 5 years have elapsed since getting the first dose of pneumococcal vaccine.

Pneumococcal conjugate vaccine 13 is administered once in lifetime, in a dose of 0.5 mL intramuscularly. The preferred site is the deltoid muscle of the upper arm.

Both the vaccines are indicated in type 2 DM, besides all adults above the age of 50 years and in some other conditions as described: persons with certain underlying medical conditions, such as coronary artery disease, congestive heart failure, cardiomyopathy, COPD, cirrhosis of liver and chronic renal failure—immunocompromised persons who are at high risk for pneumococcal infections, such as Ig deficiency, HIV infection, leukemia, lymphoma, multiple myeloma, Hodgkin's disease, non-Hodgkin's lymphoma, disseminated malignancy—persons receiving long-term therapy with corticosteroids and immunosuppressive agents—persons who have

TABLE 1: Advantages and disadvantages of pneumococcal polysaccharide vaccine (PPSV) and pneumococcal conjugate vaccine (PCV).

Vaccine	Advantages	Disadvantages
PPSV23	• Long experience (licensed in 1983) • Not expensive • At present, relatively high serotype coverage for IPD in elderly (60–70%) • Considerable efficacy proven against IPD (50–70%) in immunocompetent elderly • Cost-effective proven for elderly people even if it only prevents IPD	• T-cell-independent immune response (IgM antibody produced, response declines in 3–5 years and no anamnestic response at revaccination) • Decrease in memory B-cell frequency after PPV23 • Weak immunogenicity in some individuals • Unclear (null-to-small) efficacy against nonbacteremic pneumococcal pneumonia. No effect on nasopharyngeal carriage • No efficacy demonstrated in reducing nasopharyngeal carriage • No impact proven in reducing overall pneumococcal disease burden
PPSV23	• T-cell-dependent immune response (larger duration and boosting effect at revaccination) • High efficacy (80–90%) against vaccine type IPD proven in children • Significant efficacy against pneumococcal pneumonia (CAPiTA study) • Potential efficacy in reducing nasopharyngeal carriage • Considerable impact in reducing all pneumococcal disease burden shown by prior PCV7	• Short experience (approved in 2011) • Expensive • At present, relatively small serotype coverage for IPD in the elderly (30–40%) • Future reduction of vaccination impact in adults/elderly (because of probable indirect effects from PCV13 pediatric use)

(PPV: pneumovax IPD: invasive pneumococcal disease; CAPiTA: the community acquired pneumonia immunization trial in adults; IgM: mmunoglobulin M.)

undergone splenectomy, or exhibit anatomic asplenia, or sickle cell disease as they exhibit reduced clearance of encapsulated bacteria from the bloodstream. Additional indications are chronic smokers, persons suffering from sleep disorders and persons prone to nocturnal aspirations.

Tetanus, Diphtheria and Pertussis

Tetanus, diphtheria and pertussis (Tdap) is indicated in all type 2 diabetics who have not received Tdap in childhood or are in contact with infants, health-care personnel, during pertussis and in pregnant women. It is given 0.5-mL IM deltoid with booster dose once in every 10 years.[16,17]

Zoster Vaccine

Zoster vaccine is advised to diabetics aged 60 years and older regardless of whether they report a previous episode of herpes as a single 0.65-mL dose subcutaneous in the deltoid region. Contraindication to vaccines includes a history of immediate hypersensitivity reaction to gelatin or neomycin.[17]

Hepatitis A Vaccine

Hepatitis A vaccine is indicated in all type 2 diabetics specially if they are at high risks like illicit drug use, suffering from hemophilia, infected with other hepatitis viruses, having CLD and not immune to hepatitis A virus, received or awaiting liver transplant or are food handlers and methylsulfonylmethane.[18]

Measles, Mumps and Rubella

Measles, mumps and rubella (MMR) vaccine is indicated in all type 2 diabetics except those having suffered from all the three diseases or have received two doses of MMR vaccine in the childhood or if they are healthcare workers.

Meningitis Vaccine

Meningitis vaccine is advised to all type 2 diabetics during meningococcal outbreaks and if they are visiting fairs/mass religious congregations 10–14 days prior to their visits.[18]

Typhoid Vaccine

Typhoid vaccine is recommended as part of routine immunization in type 2 diabetics, like other adolescents or for travelers to areas where there is a moderate-to-high risk of exposure to Salmonella typhi. Either Ty21a or Vi vaccine may be used as both have comparable efficacy (51% vs. 55% at 3 years), and both are safe.[18]

Yellow Fever Vaccine

Yellow fever vaccine is advised to diabetics like any other person, if they are traveling to endemic zones of yellow fever.[18]

DRAWBACKS

There are many roadblocks and drawbacks in the path of proper immunization. These are due to apathy on the part of clinicians, diabetics taking immunization lightly, cost factors, nonreimbursement of vaccines, complicated regimens, etc. This is also a fact that all strains are not covered in the vaccine. Increasing immunosenescence with age sometimes leads to poor response and efficacy of vaccines to prevent disease. This also leads to some critics questioning the need for vaccination in elderly, although studies show the benefits far outweigh the failure rates.

CONCLUSION

Vaccination in children has yielded positive results, and based on the same logic, vaccinations in adults are also indicated to prevent serious diseases. Diabetes, a condition being equated to diminished immunity, leads to higher incidence of both bacterial as well as viral infections and thus all diabetics deserve protection from all vaccine preventable diseases. All strains in vaccines are not covered but still the protection offered is good enough to be lifesaving. Due to immunosenescence, the booster doses are required. Awareness on prevention needs to be made in medical community as well as in masses.[19] As the number of diabetics steadily increases, there is going to be a steady increase in morbid conditions and infections. Increased drug utilization and repeated hospitalization is a major dent on household economy. In a situation, like this, preventive vaccination will play a vital role in improving the health of diabetics and elderly.

REFERENCES

1. Sharma OP. Introduction. In: Principles & practice of geriatric medicine. New Delhi: Viva Books; 2015. pp. 1-6.
2. Whiting DR, Guariguata L, Weil C, et al. IDF diabetes atlas: global estimates of the prevalence of diabetes for 2011 and 2030. Diabetes Res Clin Pract. 2011;94:311-21.
3. Sengupta U. Immunology of ageing. In: Principles & practice of geriatric medicine. New Delhi: Viva Books; 2015. p. 23-34.
4. Sharma OP. Health promotion & preventive strategies. In: Principles & practice of geriatric medicine. New Delhi: Viva Books; 2015. p. 790-6.
5. Fradkin J, Rodgers GP. The economic imperative to conquer diabetes. Diabetes Care. 2008;31:624-5.
6. Sajith Kumar R. Infections. In: Principles & practice of geriatric medicine. New Delhi: Viva Books; 2015. pp. 52-9.
7. Mohan V, Shanthirani CS, Deepa M, et al. Mortality rates due to diabetes in a selected urban south Indian population—the Chennai Urban Population Study [CUPS-16]. J Assoc Physicians India. 2006;54:113-7.
8. Suresh Kumar D, Muruganathan A. Vaccination. In: Principles & practice of geriatric medicine. New Delhi: Viva Books; 2015. pp. 797-8.
9. Centres for Disease Control and Prevention. Recommended adult immunization schedule—United States. J Midwifery Women's Health. 2012;57:188-95.
10. Kesavadev J, Misra A, Das AK, et al. Suggested use of vaccines in diabetes. Indian J Endocrinol Metab. 2012;16(6):886-93.
11. Thompson ND, Perz JF. Eliminating the blood: ongoing outbreaks of hepatitis B virus infection and the need for innovative glucose monitoring technologies. J Diabetes Sci Technol. 2009;3:283-8.
12. Gupte S, Gupte N. ECAB clinical update. In: Seasonal influenza & pandemics: complete spectrum-1. Elsevier India; 2011. pp. 82-108.
13. Influenza Foundation of India News Letter. February 2008;2(Special Issue).
14. Macleod CM, Hodges RG, Heidelberger M, et al. Prevention of pneumococcal pneumonia by immunization with specific capsular polysaccharides. J Exp Med. 1945;82:44.
15. Sharma OP. Indian recommendations for vaccination in older adults—2015. In: Pneumococcal vaccination. New Delhi: Jaypee Brothers; 2015. pp. 28-35.
16. CDC. Possible side effects of vaccines and tetanus, diphtheria (TD), or tetanus, diphtheria, and pertussis (Tdap) vaccine. What you need to know.
17. Recommended adult immunization schedule—United States [Cited April 2012].
18. Sharma OP, Shankar PS, Sharma M. Hepatitis A vaccine. In: Vaccines at a glance. New Delhi: Geriatric Society of India; 2015. pp. 22-5.
19. Swenson CJ, Appel A, Sheehan M, et al. Using information technology to improve adult immunization delivery in an integrated urban health system. Jt Comm J Qual Patient Saf. 2012;38:15-23.

Chapter 84

— • Point–Counterpoint • —

Biosimilar Insulins—As Good as Gold

For the Motion

NK Soni, VB Jindal

INTRODUCTION

Biosimilars are generic versions of biopharmaceuticals which resemble the reference product, but cannot completely mimic it due to the variations and complexity in manufacture process. Biopharmaceuticals are the products containing the biotechnologically derived proteins as an active ingredient and include hormones like insulin. They are produced from the living organisms and are manufactured through complex processes and differ in many aspects from their chemically derived originator. There are various ways in which they differ from their conventional chemical originator. These differences include firstly their large size and complex structure compared to the small sized simple chemical molecules. Secondly, they differ in the nature of manufacturing process which decides the outcome i.e. even the minor change while manufacturing can lead to hazardous consequences. The other important difference is that their safety profile depends on the monitoring of quality aspects.[1] The patent production of many biopharmaceuticals like insulin and insulin analogs will be expired shortly, and hence many manufacturing companies are in the race to seek the approval in the market for introducing the generic versions of the biopharmaceutical insulin which are manufactured with modern biotechnological methods possessing the same amino acid structure and hence are known as Biosimilar insulins. They are also referred to as "follow-on-biologics" in US. These generics are the copies of the innovative molecules containing the exact active substance as in the reference medicine.

The first biosimilar insulin was approved in European Union in 2014.[2] Currently, the other biosimilars are entering the market. In order to make the place in the market, the manufacturing companies need to prove that the biosimilar insulins are equally efficacious and safe as that of the presently available insulins in the market. This warrants a careful approval process and stringent evaluation based on scientific and regulatory aspects as during manufacturing, modifications in the insulin molecule takes place leading to the production of insulin molecule which differs from the originator and hence these molecules are not exactly identical to their reference product. Apart from this, any manufacturing company cannot manufacture a precise replica of the product as the manufacturing process of the innovator products is never disclosed after its expiry.[3] According to the European Medicines Evaluation Agency (EMEA), biosimilar medicine is a medicine which contains the same active substance as present in the already authorized biopharmaceutical product i.e. the biological reference medicine. These should be similar in terms of quality, safety, efficacy and also the amino acid sequence in both is expected to be the same (Table 1).

The inherent variabilities, changes during the manufacturing process, presence of impurities, exposure to light and temperature may lead to production of a molecule which is not identical and hence these minor modifications if clinically relevant may even bring hazardous consequences in the biological effects while in use.[4] Due to the complexity of the issue, the regularity requirements before approval of these molecules are

TABLE 1: Shows the differences between generics and biosimilar medicines[2]

Generics	Biosimilars
Copies of small-molecule medicinal products derived from chemical manufacturing processes	Similar versions of biological medicinal products derived from biotechnological manufacturing processes
Identical chemical structures to those of already marketed products	Amino acid sequence to be identical to that of the reference product
Low molecular weight	Differences in biotechnological manufacturing processes between companies – biosimilar products cannot be described as identical
Known structure	Higher molecular weight
Stable at room temperature	Complex structure
Different routes of administration	Unstable, sensitive to heat and shear
Organic/chemical synthesis	Mostly parenteral administration
Homogeneous/high purity	Produced from living cells/ organisms
Rarely immunogenic	Heterogeneous/difficult to standardize
Not affected by slight changes in environment	Higher immunogenic risk
Simple purification and characterization	Affected by slight changes in environment
Simple detection and purification of contamination	Complex purification and characterization
	Difficult detection and purification of contamination
Reproducible	Reproducibility difficult

very essential. The European Medicines Agency (EMEA) became the first regularity body in UK followed by US. Accordingly, a company can apply for authorisation of the biosimilars only after the reference medicine has expired (Flowchart 1).

A consensus group of expert panel from Middle East discussed the currently available guidelines including the EMEA and concluded that due to the potential immunogenicity and complex nature of the biosimilar insulins, companies need to demonstrate their quality efficacy and efficacy in comparison with their original product along with post marketing pharmacovigilance monitoring for the adverse effects.[6]

There are other biosimilars available in India like monoclonal antibodies for treating malignancy, granulocyte colony stimulating factor, erythropoietin though dramatic increase in the number of cases of pure red cell aplasia occurring due to a minor change in packaging of erythropoietin raised an alarm and questioned the regulatory methods of these biosimilar products and warranted strict guidelines for their approval.[7] Another such incidence was of the "Marvel Insulin" where it was claimed that the marvel insulins were comparable to the reference insulins but the authorities discarded this fact by proving that the data was insufficient to prove the similarities,[8] despite the fact that biosimilars are cost effective, they can have short and long term safety issues if not vigilantly looked before approval. Immunogenicity is one safety concern to be looked for as development of antibodies may modify the dosage of insulin and blood sugar profile of the patients.

Marketing authorization to biosimilars can be given only after an evaluation of efficacy, safety and quality profile is conducted by a regulatory authority. Due to the difference in the size and manufacturing process, biosimilars cannot be introduced in the market following a standard approach.[9] This requires comparative data based on the quality, consistency, efficacy and safety profiles (Table 2).

In term of "Biosimilar Insulin as Good as Gold" we have to evaluate biosimilar insulin with gold standard on following parameters:

- Is biosimilar clinically comparable to reference insulin?
- How comparable is the bio similar to the reference insulin?
- Can a patent be switched from reference insulin to biosimilar?
- Can I change my practice seamlessly to use a cheaper biosimilar?
- How the side effect profile of biosimilar to established in practice if it is prescribed by generic name?

Recently, a large systematic review was conducted to compare the efficacy, pharmacokinetics and pharmacodynamics of the biosimilar insulins with the reference insulin products. Here 6945 articles were screened and 11 studies were included out of which 6 examined pharmacokinetics and pharmacodynamics while 5 examined clinical efficacy and immunogenicity. LY2963016, Basalin, Basalog and MK-1293 were compared to Lantus while SAR342434 was compared to Humalog. All studies showed parameters were within the specified margins.[10] The first biosimilar insulin Abasaglar

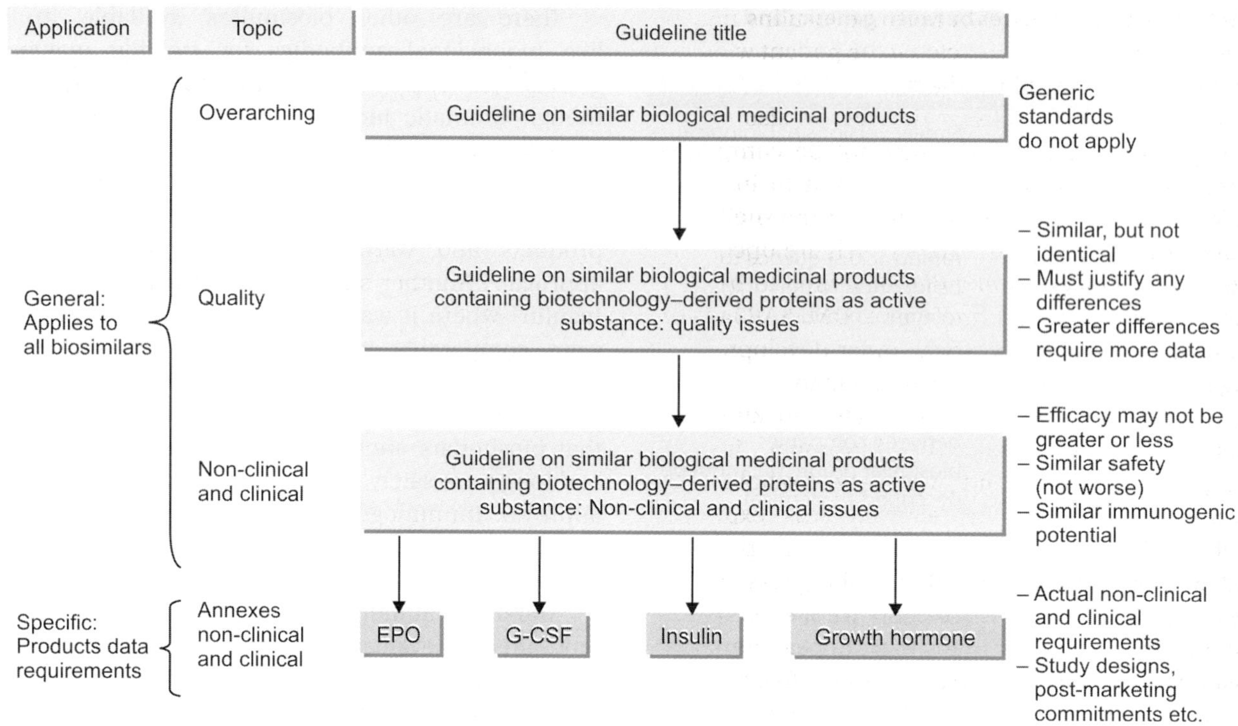

(EMEA: European medicines evaluation agency; EPO: Erythropoietin; G-CSF: granulocyte-colony stimulating factor.)

Flowchart 1 Shows the EMEA guidelines for the approval process of the biosimilars.

TABLE 2: **Current status of biosimilar insulin in india**[18]

Brand name	Company	Study
Biosulin	MJ Biopharma	NA
Lupisulin	Lupin	NA
Wosulin	Wockhardt	Phase I completed
Insugen	Biocon	Phase III to recruit
Glaritus	Wockhardt	Phase I and Phase III
Basalog	Biocon	Phase III

(LY2963016) is the biosimilar glargine insulin similar to its reference product Lantus. It was authorized by EMEA in 2014 and was launched in UK in 2015 September while in US it was approved in December 2015.

Studies demonstrated comparable pharmacokinetic, pharmacodynamics, bioavailability profiles of Abasaglar and Lantus before launch.[11,12] Randomized control phase III trials also demonstrated similar efficacy, immunogenicity and safety profiles in both the groups along with the similar change in HbA1c levels over 24 weeks.[13,14] The strength of both the insulins is same (100 Units/mL) with Abasaglar showing cost reduction of around 15%. Though these biosimilars are expensive than generics but they are cheaper than their reference product and hence the cost effectiveness of these biosimilar insulins is quite advantageous to the patients with the estimated cost around 20–30% lower than their originator drug. A recent estimate showed that US and UK health care systems can save upto $110 billion with biosimilars.

One of the important concerns while using biosimilar insulins is switching, substitution and interchangeability. Switching is when the physician decides to replace the reference product with biosimilars, while substitution is if the pharmacist substitutes the prescription with biosimilars without the physicians consent and is not permitted currently by any country. Interchange ability is when one medicine is switched with another known to produce the similar effects. Further evidence is required to demonstrate interchange ability while using biosimilar insulins.[15] In UK, change from an insulin to bioinsulin is not permitted unless clinically indicated. The indications of use of Abasaglar has been limited to the patients who are either newly initiated on insulin glargine or require a switching due to poor control of the blood sugars. Those patients who have stable blood sugar control should not be switched as the results with both the insulins may be variable and it cannot be predicted if the patient will have similar control with the biosimilars.

Importantly, insulin delivery devices are also unique to each type of insulin which may not be compatible for biosimilars, hence efforts are required to inculcate the patients for insulin delivery pens and the shelf lives. There are several other biosimilars which are upcoming. MK-1293 from Merck recently demonstrated to be non-inferior to Lantus in type 1 and type 2 DM. SAR34234 is insulin lispro biosimilar currently under development.[16] Basalog has recently been approved in Japan.

Interestingly a survey was conducted to know the patients perspective about the biosimilar insulins enrolling 3214 patients and were asked about their willingness to switch to a relatively less expensive biosimilar insulin approved by their healthcare provider. Around 665 patients showed their willingness for the same while 17% refused.[17] The acceptance was seen more in type 2 diabetes though their main concern remained the assurance of effectiveness, low side effects profile and delivery methods. Low cost might influence patients to use these biosimilar insulins, but assurance of quality remains the foremost concern.

CONCLUSION

The emergence of biosimilar insulins gives a broader choice available in clinical practice, enhances individualized treatment options and reduced costs. It is a better cost effective method compared to the reference product. Though due to the lack of experience to use and long term safety concerns, their use can be limited but can be used as gold with certain precaution and regulatory guidelines.[18]

- All new biological products unlike generic should be considered as new drugs
- Product levelling should be transparent and clear
- The prescription of biosimilar should not be based on their generic name, but on a unique name as proposed by World Health Organization to discourage automatic substitution and switching.

The use of these molecules is encouraged wherever indicated but unnecessary switching over in stable patients is not required. At the same time it is essential to remember that these are products manufactured through complex processes and hence cannot be considered identical to their reference molecule. Strict regulatory guidelines are essential for ensuring the safety, efficacy and quality of the new biosimilar insulins.

REFERENCES

1. Locatelli F, Roger S. Comparative testing and pharmacovigilance of biosimilars. Nephrology, dialysis, transplantation: official publication of the European Dialysis and Transplant Association - European Renal Association. 2006;21 Suppl 5:v13-6.
2. Davies M, Dahl D, Heise T, et al. Introduction of biosimilar insulins in Europe. Diabetic medicine : a journal of the British Diabetic Association. 2017;34(10):1340-53.
3. Mellstedt H, Niederwieser D, Ludwig H. The challenge of biosimilars. Annals of oncology : official journal of the European Society for Medical Oncology. 2008;19(3):411-9.
4. Declerck P, Farouk Rezk M. The road from development to approval: evaluating the body of evidence to confirm biosimilarity. Rheumatology. 2017;56(suppl_4):iv4-iv13.
5. Heinemann L, Hompesch M. Biosimilar insulins: how similar is similar? Journal of diabetes science and technology. 2011;5(3):741-54.
6. Bohlega S, Al-Shammri S, Al Sharoqi I, et al. Biosimilars: opinion of an expert panel in the Middle East. Current medical research and opinion. 2008;24(10):2897-903.
7. Locatelli F, Del Vecchio L, Pozzoni P. Pure red-cell aplasia "epidemic"--mystery completely revealed? Peritoneal dialysis international : journal of the International Society for Peritoneal Dialysis. 2007;27 Suppl 2:S303-7.
8. Owens DR, Landgraf W, Schmidt A, et al. The emergence of biosimilar insulin preparations--a cause for concern? Diabetes technology & therapeutics. 2012;14(11):989-96.
9. Nowicki M. Basic facts about biosimilars. Kidney & blood pressure research. 2007;30(5):267-72.
10. Tieu C, Lucas EJ, DePaola M, et al. Efficacy and safety of biosimilar insulins compared to their reference products: A systematic review. PloS one. 2018;13(4):e0195012.
11. Linnebjerg H, Lam EC, Seger ME, et al. Comparison of the Pharmacokinetics and Pharmacodynamics of LY2963016 Insulin Glargine and EU- and US-Approved Versions of Lantus Insulin Glargine in Healthy Subjects: Three Randomized Euglycemic Clamp Studies. Diabetes care. 2015;38(12):2226-33.
12. Zhang X, Lam ECQ, Seger ME, et al. LY2963016 Insulin Glargine and Insulin Glargine (Lantus) Produce Comparable Pharmacokinetics and Pharmacodynamics at Two Dose Levels. Clinical pharmacology in drug development. 2017;6(6):556-63.
13. Blevins TC, Dahl D, Rosenstock J, et al. Efficacy and safety of LY2963016 insulin glargine compared with insulin glargine (Lantus(R)) in patients with type 1 diabetes in a randomized controlled trial: the ELEMENT 1 study. Diabetes, obesity & metabolism. 2015;17(8):726-33.
14. Rosenstock J, Hollander P, Bhargava A, et al. Similar efficacy and safety of LY2963016 insulin glargine and insulin glargine (Lantus(R)) in patients with type 2 diabetes who were insulin-naive or previously treated with insulin glargine: a randomized, double-blind controlled trial (the ELEMENT 2 study). Diabetes, obesity & metabolism. 2015;17(8):734-41.
15. Dowlat HA, Kuhlmann MK, Khatami H, et al. Interchangeability among reference insulin analogues and their biosimilars: regulatory framework, study design and clinical implications. Diabetes, obesity & metabolism. 2016;18(8):737-46.
16. Garg SK, Wernicke-Panten K, Rojeski M, et al. Efficacy and Safety of Biosimilar SAR342434 Insulin Lispro in Adults with Type 1 Diabetes Also Using Insulin Glargine-SORELLA 1 Study. Diabetes technology & therapeutics. 2017;19(9):516-26.
17. Wilkins AR, Venkat MV, Brown AS, et al. Patient Perspectives on Biosimilar Insulin. Journal of diabetes science and technology. 2014;8(1):23-5.
18. Singh AK Boisimilar insulins. RSSDI UPDATE 2015;240-247.

Against the Motion

Rohit Kapoor, Shivam Kapoor, Rishabh Kapoor

INTRODUCTION

What are Biologics? What are originators? What are Biosimilars? The answer lies-biologics are substances consisting of sugars, nucleic acids, protens and or cells used to prevent, treat, or cure a condition or disease in human beings. The products listed include vaccines, allergenic products, blood components and recombinant therapeutic proteins. Originators or References are first biologics approved against which future related biologics are assessed. The biosimilars are biologic that is very much similar to a reference product (That is the originator) with no clinically meaningful differentiation in potency, purity and safety. Biosimilar insulins (BI) are accessible in several countries and will be made accessible in the United State in the near future.

The ground basis why BI are not considered generic products is because the term "generic" is restrained for copies of nonbiologics or small-molecule drugs because these copies contain the exact same active ingredient as their respective proprietary reference drugs. Generic manufacturing companies are able to identically replicate active ingredient of small-molecule drugs despite the fact that manufacturers do not divulge proprietary composition information or manufacturing protocols. In contrast, insulin is a large-protein, biological product that cannot be exactly replicated because of the greater complexity involved in manufacturing biologics. BI are manufactured in living organisms (e.g. yeast and bacteria) to produce large quantities of the desired large-protein product, which limits the ability to manufacture exact replicas of original biological medications.

Thus, the word "generic" I reserve red for exact replicas of the active ingredients of small-molecule drugs, and the term "biosimilar" was coined to address the fact that biological medications are not exact duplicates of their originator but are highly similar with no clinically meaningful difference in efficacy or safety. Nevertheless, there are concerns that these subtle differences may potentially alter the efficacy or safety of BI compared to its originator insulin.

NONCLINICAL STUDIES

In order to support biosimilarity, the European Medicines Agency (EMA) guideline of similar biological medical products states that relevant nonclinical studies should be performed before imitating clinical clinical trials. A stepwise approach is recommended for evaluation of the similarity of the biosimilar and the reference product. Analytical studies and in vitro pharmaco-toxicological studies should be conducted first and a decision than made as to the extent of what, if any, in vivo work in animal studies will be required.

It is important to note that, to design and appropriate nonclinical study programme, a clear understanding of the reference product characteristics is required. Results from the physicochemical and biological characterization studies (i.e. comparability of the biosimilar to the reference product) should be reviewed from the point-of-view of potential impact on efficacy and safety.

Step 1: In vitro Studies

In order to assess any potential difference in biological activity between the biosimilar and the reference medicinal product, data from a number of comparative in vitro studies, some of which may already be available from quality related assays, should normally be provided. These studies should include relevant assays on:

- Binding to target(s) (e.g. receptors, antigens and enzymes) know to be involved in pharmaco-toxicological effects and/or pharmacokinetics of the reference product
- Signal transduction and functional activity/viability of cells known to be of relevance for the pharmaco-toxicological effects of the reference product.

The studies should be comparative in nature and should not just assess the response per se. To obtain unambiguous results, the methods used should be scientifically valid and suitable for their purpose.

The studies should be sensitive, specific and sufficiently discriminatory to provide evidence that observed differences in quality attributes are clinically are clinically no relevant.

The studies should compare the concentration activity/binding relationship of the biosimilar and the reference medical product at the pharmacological target(s), covering a concentration range where potential differences are most sensitively detected. They should be performed with an appropriate number of batches of the reference product and of the biosimilar representative of the material intended for clinical use. Assay and batch-to-batch variability will affect the number needed. The number tested should be sufficient to draw meaningful conclusion on the variability of a given parameter for both the biosimilar and the reference product and on the similarity of both products.

Together, these assays should cover the whole spectrum of pharmacological/toxicological aspects known to be of clinical relevance for the reference product and for the product class. The applicant should discuss to what degree the in vitro assays used are representative/predictive for the clinical situation according to current scientific knowledge.

Step 2: Need for In-vivo Studies

It is acknowledged that biotechnology-derived proteins may medicate in vivo effects that cannot be fully elucidated by in vitro studies. Therefore, nonclinical evaluation in in vivo studies may be necessary to provide complementary information, provided that a relevant in-vivo model with regard to species or design is available.

Factors to be considered when the need for in vivo nonclinical studies is evaluated, include but are not restricted to:

- Presence of potentially relevant quality attributes that have not been detected in the reference product (e.g. new post-translation modification structures)
- Presence of potentially relevant quantitative difference in quality attributes between the biosimilar and the reference product
- Relevant difference in formulation, e.g. use of exception not widely used for biotechnology-derived proteins.

Although each of the factors mentioned above do not necessarily warrant in-vivo testing, these issue should be considered together to assess the level of concern and whether there is a need for in vivo testing.

Step 3: In vivo Studies

If an in vivo evaluation is deemed necessary, the focus of the study/studies (Pharmacokinetic (PK) and/or pharmacodynamic (PD) and/or safety) depends on the need for additional information. Animal studies should be designed to maximize the information obtained. The principles of the 3Rs (replacement, refinement and reduction) according to Article 4 of Directive 2010/63/EU should be considered when designing any in vivo study. Depending on the endpoints used, it may not be necessary to sacrifice the animals at the end of the study. The duration of the study (including observation period) should be justified, taking into consideration the PK behavior's of the reference medicinal product and its clinical use.

For Safety studies a flexible approach should be considered, in particular if nonhuman primates are the only relevant species. The conduct of standard repeated dose toxicity studies in nonhuman primates is usually not recommended. If appropriately justified, a repeated dose toxicity study with refined design (e.g. using just one dose level of biosimilar and reference product and/or just one gender and/or no recovery animals) or an in-life evaluation of safety parameters (such a clinical signs, body weight and vital functions.) may be considered. For repeated dose toxicity studies where only one dose is evaluated, this would usually be selected at the high and of the dosing range and should be justified on the basis of expected toxicity of the reference medicinal product.

The conduct of toxicity studies in nonrelevant species is not considered. Due to the different production processes used by the biosimilar and reference product manufacturers, qualitative difference of process related impurities can occur (e.g. host cell proteins). The level of such impurities should be kept to a minimum, which is the best strategy to minimize any associated risk.

Qualitative or quantitative difference (s) of product-related variants (e.g. glycosylation patterns, charge variants) may affect biological functions of the biotechnology-derived protein and are expected to be evaluated by appropriate in vitro assays. These difference and impurities may have an effect on immunogenic potential and the potential to cause hypersensitivity. It is acknowledged that these effects are difficult to predict from animal studies and should be further assessed in clinical studies. Although the immunogenicity assessment in animals is generally not predictive for immunogenicity in humans, it may be needed for interpretation of in vivo studies in animals. Therefore, blood samples should be taken and stored for future evaluations of pharmacokinetic/toxic kinetic data if then needed.

Studies regarding safety pharmacology, reproduction, toxicology and carcinogenicity are not required for nonclinical testing of biosimilar. Studies on local tolerance are usually not mandatory. However, if excipients are introduced for which there is no or slight experience with the proposed clinical route of administration, local tolerance may need to be estimated. If other in vivo studies are accomplished, estimation of local tolerance may be part of the design of that study instead of the presentation of separate local tolerance studies.

CLINICAL STUDIES

Also the EMA guideline has recognized that the manufacturing process of the biosimilar product will be augmented during development. However, it is suggested to generate the clinical data required for the biosimilar comparability implement with the biosimilar product derived from the commercial manufacturing process and therefore represent the quality profile of the batches to become commercialized. Any deviation from this reference should be accepted and supported by adequate additional bridging data.

The clinical biosimilar comparability exercise is normally a stepwise process that should begin with PKand, if possible, PD studies followed by clinical efficacy and safety trial or, in certain cases, confirmatory PK/PD studies for representing clinical biosimilar comparability.

Extrapolation of Efficacy and Safety from one Therapeutic Indication to Another

The reference medicinal product may have more than one beneficial indication. When biosimilar comparability has been established in one indication, extrapolation of clinical data to other indications of the reference product could be adequate, but needs to be scientifically warranted. In case, it is indistinct whether the safety and efficacy established in one indication would be relevant for another indication, extra information will be required. Extrapolation should be reflected in the light of the totality of data that is quality, nonclinical and clinical data. It is projected that the safety and efficacy can be extrapolated when biosimilar comparability has been confirmed by thorough physicochemical and structural analyses as well as by in vitro functional tests complemented with clinical information (efficacy and safety and/or PK/PD data) in one therapeutic indication. Additional information are required in certain circumstances, such as

- The active substance of the reference product interacts with several receptors that may have an altered impact in the tested and nontested therapeutic indications
- The studied therapeutic indication is not relevant for others in terms of efficacy or safety, that is, is not sensitive for differences in all applicable aspects of efficacy and safety
- The active substance itself has more than one active site and the sites may have an altered impact in different therapeutic indications.

Immunogenicity is associated to multiple factors including the route of administration, patient-related factors, dosing regimen and disease-related factors (e.g. co-medication, type of disease and immune status). Thus, immunogenicity could differ among indication. Extrapolation of immunogenicity from the studied indication/route of administration to other uses of the reference product should be justified.

PHARMACOVIGILANCE

Data from preauthorization clinical studies are usually insufficient to indentify rare adverse effects. Therefore, clinical safety of biosimilar must be monitored closely on an ongoing basis during the post approval phase including continued benefit-risk assessment.

Within the authorization procedure the applicant should present a description of the pharmacovigilance system and a risk management plan in accordance with current EU legislation and pharmacovigilance guidelines. The risk management plan should take into account indentified and potential risks associated with the use of the reference product and should detail how these issues will be addressed in postmarketing follow-up. Immunogenicity should specifically be addressed in postmarketing follow-up. Immunogenicity should specifically be addressed in this context. Any specific safety monitoring imposed on the reference medicinal product or product class should be adequately addressed in the pharmacovigilance plan of the biosimilar. Applicants are encouraged to participate in already existing pharmacoepidemiological, studies in place for the reference product. However, new studies might have to be initiated. Risk minimization activities in place for the reference medicinal product should, in principle, also be included into the risk management program of the biosimilar. Any deviation from this (e.g. when the risk minimization is linked to the device used with the reference product) should be justified.

For suspected adverse reactions relating to biological medicinal products, the definite identification of the concerned product with regard to its manufacturing is of particular importance. Therefore, all appropriate measures should be taken to indentify clearly any biological medicinal product which is the subject of a suspected adverse reaction report, with due regard to its brand name and batch number.

CONCLUSION

Biosimilars are anticipated to be an essential component in reducing health care costs and enhancing patient contact to important, often life saving medications. It is expected that the FDA will soon finalize these regulatory guidelines, clarify unreciprocated questions and establish a pathway for biosimilars that is based upon comprehensive scientific principles.

REFERENCES

1. U.S. Food and Drug Administration. Nonproprietary naming of biological products. Available from http://www.fda.gov/ downloads/Drugs/ GuidanceComplianceRegulatoryInformation/Guidances/ UCM459987.pdf.
2. Schellekens H. Biosimilar therapeutics – what do we need to consider? NDT Plus. 2009;2(Suppl 1):i27-i36.
3. U.S. Food and Drug Administration. FDA overview of biosimilar products: glossary. Available from http:// fdabiosimilars.e-paga.com/course/ framework/glossary.html#glossary_term_ Biological_product.
4. U.S. Food and Drug Administration. Drugs approvals and databases: Drugs@ FDA glossary of terms. Available from http://www.fda.gov/Drugs/ InformationOnDrugs/ucm079436.htm.
5. Owens DR, Landgraf W, Schmidt A, Bretzel RG, Kuhlmann MK. The emergenceof biosimilar insulin preparations – a cause for concern? Diabetes Technol Ther. 2012;14(11):989–96.
6. Kim AP, Bindler RJ. The Future of Biosimilar Insulins. Diabetes Spectrum. 2016;29(3):161-166.
7. DeVries JH, Gough SC, Kiljanski J, et al. Diabetes ObesMetab. 2015;17(5): 445-451.
8. Dolinar RO, Edelman S, Heinemann L, et al. Impact of biosimilar insulins on clinical practice: meeting report. J Diabetes Sci Technol. 2014;8:179-185.
9. U.S. Food and Drug Administration. Biosimilars: additional questions and answers regarding implementation of the Biologics Price Competition and Innovation Act of 2009. Available from http://www. fda.gov/downloads/ Drugs/Guidances/ UCM273001.pdf.
10. U.S. Food and Drug Administration. Quality considerations in demonstrating biosimilarity of a therapeutic protein product to a reference product. Available from http://www.fda.gov/downloads/Drugs/Guidance Compliance Regulatory Information/Guidances/UCM291134.pdf.
11. NHS England, Medical Directorate. What is a biosimilar medicine? 2015. Available from: https://www.england.nhs.uk/wp-content/uploads/2015/ 09/biosimilar-guide.pdf.
12. Heinemann L, Khatami H, McKinnon R, et al. An overview of current regulatory requirements for approval of biosimilar insulins. Diabetes TechnolTher.2015;17(7):510-26.
13. Weise M, Bielsky MC, De Smet K, et al. Biosimilars: what clinicians should know. Blood. 2012;120(26):5111-7.
14. Rovira J, Espin J, Garcia L, et al. The impact of biosimilars' entry in the EU market. 2011. Available from: http://ec.europa.eu/DocsRoom/ documents/7651/attachments/1/translations/en/renditions/pdf.

Chapter 85

Rationalizing Antidiabetic Therapy

Urman Dhruv, Banshi Saboo

INTRODUCTION

Type 2 diabetes is a progressively worsening metabolic disease which is assuming epidemic proportions. Globally, there are multiple guidelines directing physicians to manage the disease properly. However, it is also understood that the phenotype of patients vary across the country and across the globe. Even the genotype of the patients may vary similarly. This means that the guidelines created for one geographical area may not completely be applicable to the other. Adopting country-specific guidelines improves treatment outcomes in diabetes.

The Research Society for the Study of Diabetes in India (RSSDI) therefore published the clinical practice recommendations for the management of type 2 diabetes mellitus (T2DM) in 2015, which was adapted from the 2014 global guidelines for type 2 diabetes by International Diabetes Federation (IDF).[1,2] The recommendations were specifically designed considering the diverse socioeconomic and cultural background of Indians. The 2015 RSSDI guidelines were very well accepted by the healthcare practitioners across India and helped in decision-making. Every year, several publications are being added to the literature which can significantly impact holistic diabetes care. The consensus was updated in 2017, as diabetes research is evolving rapidly and continuously.

This chapter does not boast to discuss every part of guidelines laid down by RSSDI, but will emphasize the salient features of the same. It will also try to reveal the purpose of guidelines which has paved way ahead of "precision medicine" in diabetes by creating a RSSDI Wheel.

INDIAN PHENOTYPE

As per IDF, India has second largest population having diabetes and stands just next to China, the leader in this list.[1,2] Epidemiological studies in India have suggested that Indian patients with T2DM have distinctive clinical and biochemical characteristics, which makes them the so-called Asian Indian Phenotype.[3-6] These abnormalities include more insulin resistance (IR), elevated abdominal adiposity [i.e., higher visceral fat in spite of lower body mass index (BMI)], lower level of adiponectin, and a higher level of highly-sensitive C-reactive protein.[3-6] Moreover, they have greater propensity to develop cardiovascular (CV) complications such as coronary artery disease (CAD) and atherosclerosis at any age point. At the same BMI, more Asian Indians develop metabolic syndrome (MS) and diabetes compared to their Western counterparts. In spite of a relatively lower rate of obesity as defined by international BMI cut-off points, Indians tend to have larger waist circumference (WC) and waist-to-hip ratio (WHR), indicating a greater degree of central body obesity.

OBESE TYPE 2 DIABETES[7,8]

- Overweight and obese people with T2DM should be initiated on exercise therapy, prescribing a combination of aerobic and muscle strengthening activities
- Pharmacotherapy for obese patients with T2DM should be considered in addition to lifestyle changes in those with BMI >27 kg/m^2 without comorbidity or a BMI >25 kg/m^2 with comorbidity

    - Metformin should be first-line drug for all T2DM patients
    - Glucagon-like peptide (GLP)-1 analogs, dipeptidyl peptidase (DPP) 4 inhibitors, and sodium-glucose cotransporter (SGLT) 2 inhibitors may be preferred as add-ons to metformin in obese T2DM patients.
- Lipase inhibitors (orlistat) may be used for inducing weight loss
- Surgical treatment (bariatric surgery) is indicated in patients with BMI >32.5 kg/m^2 with comorbidity and BMI >37.5 kg/m^2 without comorbidity.

Prescribing a combination of aerobic and resistance training exercises in individuals with T2DM can improve metabolic control while reducing obesity and its related complications.

DIET IN DIABETES[9]

Management of diabetes requires proper understanding of diet and nutrition and is a team effort which requires the help of dietician and an enough time for education. Individualized nutrition plans are preferred and a blanket diet chart may not help the most. Individual's health needs, personal and cultural preferences, access to healthful choices, health literacy and numeracy must be kept in mind while discussing diet plans. The most beneficial metabolic profile is provided by a high-carbohydrate low-fat diet, and the worst metabolic profile results from low-carbohydrate high-fat diets.

EXERCISE[10]

- A total of 60 minute of physical activity is recommended every day for healthy Indians in view of the high predisposition to develop T2DM and CAD
    - At least 30 minutes of moderate-intensity aerobic activity
    - Fifteen minutes of work-related activity
    - Fifteen minutes of muscle-strengthening exercises (at least three times/week).
- In the absence of contraindications, encourage resistance training three times in a week
- Guidelines also makes mention of role of behavioural lifestyle intervention and yoga which bridge the gap between motivation and action.

CHALLENGES IN DIABETES MANAGEMENT IN INDIA[11]

The guideline nicely depicts the problems and barriers that are faced by health professionals while managing diabetes. Reduced awareness, lack of knowledge, delay in clinical practice, lack of time for education, lack of strong referral system, patients apathy to gather education, wrong perceptions and false beliefs are few of the lots of problems that is at the base of foundation of health system in India and also in Asia.

PHARMACOTHERAPY[12-15]

As per rest of other guidelines, oral glucose-lowering medications are to be initiated when life style interventions cannot keep glucose levels at a targets and metformin is the drug of first choice unless there is evidence of renal failure. The dose requires to be titrated over ensuing weeks to avoid gastrointestinal intolerance. If metformin is not tolerated, one can start with second line of agents.

There is no specific agent which requires to be selected as second or third line of agent. Rather than going by step wise approach, it is better to individualize drug treatment based on patient-centric approach.

The glucose-lowering effectiveness of oral antidiabetes drugs (OADs) is said to be high with metformin, sulfonylureas (SUs) and thiazolidinedione (expected A1c reduction ~1.0–1.5%) and comparatively lower for meglitinides, DPP-4 inhibitor, SGLT2 inhibitor, alpha-glucosidase inhibitors (AGIs), HYQ, colesevelam and bromocriptine.

RSSDI WHEEL

The RSSDI has created a RSSDI wheel which directs selection of different molecules based on eight different characteristics which is also known as ABCD (EFGH) approach for diabetes management for patient-centric management (see chapter 34 for RSSDI wheel):

- For patients who have been diagnosed with diabetes, consider a combination of metformin and one of the treatment options based on patients Age, BMI, CKD, Duration of diabetes Established CVD, Financial condition, Glycemic status and Hypoglycemia concern
- Drug choice should be based on patient preferences as well as presence of various comorbidities and complications and drug characteristics, with the goal of reducing blood glucose levels while minimizing side effects, especially hypoglycemia and weight gain.

A. **Age:** Estimated glomerular filtration rate adjusted doses of gliptins (linagliptin and teneligliptin do not require adjustment) or AGIs may be safer in elderly people. If cardiac ejection fraction is preserved, glitazones may be an alternative but should be avoided in postmenopausal females. Newer SUs like gliclazide modified release (MR) and glimepiride (due to low risk of hypoglycemia) and glinides (due to shorter half-life) can be safely used in elderly patients with T2DM. Use of SGLT2 inhibitors and GLP-1 receptor agonists may be safe under regular medical supervision only. Early initiation of insulin in older patients was found to be beneficial without increasing risk of hypoglycemia or greater total direct healthcare costs. Evidence suggests that basal insulin analogs like glargine and detemir were effective and safe without any risk of hypoglycemia and weight gain.

B. **BMI:** Metformin, AGIs, GLP-1 receptor agonists (GLP-1 RAs), and SGLT2 inhibitors are associated with weight loss characteristics, and DPP-4 inhibitors appear to be weight neutral and may be given preference in obese patients with diabetes, subject to the precautions needed. When used judicially, SGLT2 inhibitors and GLP-1 receptor agonists may work wonders. Use of newer SUs compared to older SUs and other OADs does not result in significant weight gain in patients with T2DM.

C. **Complications (chronic kidney disease):** Gliptins especially linagliptin or teneligliptin would be preferred drugs (rest of gliptins may require dose adjustments). Repaglinide is another agent which may be used across all stages of renal insufficiency.

Similarly, glitazones may be used in chronic kidney disease; however, one has to be careful about fluid retention. Short-acting SUs like glipizide can be preferred in patients with moderate/severe renal impairment. Furthermore, in mild/moderate renal impairment, gliclazide and glimepiride may also be used, preferably at lower doses. AGIs may be used in patients with mild to moderate renal disease. Insulin may be used in any stages of renal insufficiency and is the best agent for this purpose. Short-acting insulin analogs are preferred over conventional insulins.

D. **Duration of Diabetes:** Longer the duration of diabetes indicate reduced beta cell function. Contrary to this, shorter duration of diabetes (especially less than 5 years) require aggressive control as evidence suggest that early aggressive control reduce the chances of macro and microvascular complications later in life due to "legacy" or "metabolic memory" effect. It means that one should use the potent most agents in the early stages of diabetes. SU or glinide, as an add-on therapy to metformin, will be the best choices. Glitazones may also be helpful. Basal insulin analogs are often used in patients with long-standing diabetes to address insulinopenic states. GLP-1 RAs may be helpful as they are more potent than gliptins. SGLT2 inhibitors may also be useful as second add-on agent due to their insulin-independent action which is pathophysiologically different. AGIs are last choices due to their moderate efficacy.

E. **Established CVD:** Intensive glycemic control in the early stages of diabetes reduces cardiovascular disease (CVD). On the contrary, drugs potent enough to cause hypoglycemia are best avoided when there is established CVD with diabetes. DPP-4 inhibitors, GLP-1 analogs, and SGLT-2 inhibitors may be preferred in this scenario as they are less likely to cause hypoglycemia. Pioglitazone is better to avoid in patients with reduced ejection fraction as it may cause fluid retention and may aggravate heart failure. SGLT2 inhibitors and GLP-1 receptor agonists has proven benefits in such cases as depicted in LEADER, EMPA-REG and other trials. Glimepiride and gliclazide MR can be preferred over conventional SUs in patients at increased risk of CVD or with CVD.

F. **Financial Concern:** Newer drugs are quite safe, beneficial but costlier. So in a country with limited resources and poor economic conditions like we see in India, one needs to take in to account the cost factors of treatment as mostly this is a life-long treatment. SUs should be the first choice with metformin by considering their cost. Then after AGIs or glitazones should be used at next therapy level.

G. **Glycemic Status and Variability:** The order of glucose-lowering agents according to their efficacy of A1C reduction is insulin, SUs, GLP-1 RAs, pioglitazone, gliptins, SGLT2 inhibitors and AGIs. One should remember that better efficacy comes with a price tag omit either in the form of cost or safety. It is also necessary to understand that glycemic variability needs to be considered under this head as it directly affects the glycemic targets and there by rate of complications.

H. **Hypoglycemia Concern:** Hypoglycemia is the biggest hurdle that any medical fraternity is facing during treatment course of diabetes. In a set up where the elderly patient stays alone and cannot manage his hypoglycemia without assistance, situations with poor resources (no glucose meter available) severe retinopathy preventing management of hypoglycemia or cognitive impairment are conditions where one should use drugs which do not have higher potentials for hypoglycemia. In patients with history of hypoglycemia or for those at high risk of hypoglycemia, GLP-1 RA or gliptins should be considered as first choice with metformin. Other options include SGLT2 inhibitors, glitazones and AGIs. Last option for such patients should be glinides, SUs, or insulin since there are highchances of hypoglycemia with these agents. It must be understood that contrary to beliefs, glinides have high potency to cause hypoglycemia in all studies.

Patients in whom one should avoid hypoglycemia include:

- Those with established CVD
- Elderly patients
- Those suffering from retinopathy and cannot perform self-monitoring of blood glucose without help of others
- Those who stay alone, especially in remote areas
- Those who are having poor longevity
- Those who are having documented hypoglycemia unawareness
- Those who met with severe symptomatic hypoglycemia requiring hospitalization.

POSTPRANDIAL HYPERGLYCEMIA[16]

There are situations when fasting sugars are well controlled but there is a rapid rise in postprandial sugars. AGI glinides, gliptins and GLP-1 analogs may be helpful in these scenario.

INSULIN THERAPY[17-19]

Due to the progressive nature of diabetes and β-cell dysfunction, insulin replacement therapy is frequently required in T2DM patients.[5,7] Optimally, insulin aims to create a normal glycemic profile as possible without unacceptable weight gain or chances of hypoglycemia. A current National Insulin Summit (NIS) consensus from India reports that insulin therapy is the most effective antidiabetic agent and can reduce A1C by 1.5–3.5% from baseline when used as monotherapy in T2DM patients, whereas other antidiabetic agents can only reduce A1C to a range of 0.5–2.0%.

- Indications of insulin in T2DM in newly detected patients:
  - Those patients, who at the time of diagnosis are symptomatic, have one of the following:
    - A1c >9%
    - Fasting plasma glucose >250 mg/dL
    - Postprandial plasma glucose >300 mg/dL
    - Positive ketonuria
    - Catabolic status
    - Pregnant or planning pregnancy.
  - When patient presents with metabolic/CV/medical/surgical/obstetric crisis, insulin is safer as well as more effective
    - In these cases, insulin may be started as monotherapy or with metformin if the latter is not contraindicated and is well tolerated
    - As the patient's glucose toxicity resolves, the regimen can potentially be de-escalated, and a switch over to oral therapy may be considered.
- Indications of insulin in T2DM in patients with already established diagnosis:
  - If a trial of adequate doses of two to three non-insulin agents for 3–6 months fails to achieve A1c to target levels, or if organ dysfunction contra-indicates use of oral agents, addition of insulin may be justified as the landmark studies suggest that achieving intensive glycemic control (if not contraindicated) in initial few years of diagnosis is of profound benefit.

IMPORTANCE OF RSSDI WHEEL AND GUIDELINE

The RSSDI wheel was the first Asian step toward the thought process of "Precision Medicine". Although the guideline was based on ADA guideline emphasizing on patient-centric approach, it also seeded the idea of dividing patients in different classes based on eight different characteristics which could be easily defined and decide the therapy for each class. Thus from "one drug fits all" notion was terminated and an era of personalized medicine in type 2 diabetes was launched by RSSDI. This was the biggest achievement of this guideline. RSSDI wheel is one of the biggest gift of RSSDI to modern medicine.

REFERENCES

1. International Diabetes Federation. The International Federation (IDF) diabetes atlas, 7th Edn. 2015. Available from http://www.diabetesatlas.org/
2. IDF diabetes atlas—7th Edition 2015. Across the globe, available at http://www.diabetesatlas.org/across-the-globe.html
3. Mohan V, Sandeep S, Deepa R, et al. Epidemiology of type 2 diabetes: Indian scenario. Indian Journal of Medical Research. 2007;125(3):217.
4. Joshi SR, Anjana RM, Deepa M, et al. Prevalence of dyslipidemia in urban and rural India: the ICMR–INDIAB study. PLOS One. 2014;9(5):e96808.
5. Shah VN, Mohan V. Diabetes in India: what is different? Current opinion in endocrinology. Diabetes and Obesity. 2015;22(4):283-9.

6. Unnikrishnan R, Anjana RM, Mohan V. Diabetes in South Asians: is the phenotype different? Diabetes. 2014;63(1):53-5.
7. Haslam DW, James WP. Obesity. Lancet. 2005;366(9492):1197-209.
8. Gulati S, Misra A. Abdominal obesity and type 2 diabetes in Asian Indians: dietary strategies including edible oils, cooking practices and sugar intake. European Journal of Clinical Nutrition. 2017;71(7):850-7.
9. Evert AB, Boucher JL, Cypress M, et al. Nutrition therapy recommendations for the management of adults with diabetes. Diabetes Care. 2013;36(11):3821-42.
10. Madhu SV. World Diabetes Day 2015: healthy living & diabetes. The Indian journal of medical research. 2015;142(5):503.
11. Venkataraman K, Kannan AT, Mohan V. Challenges in diabetes management with particular reference to India. Int J Diabetes DevCtries. 2009;29(3):103-9.
12. Kalra S, Aamir AH, Raza A, et al. Place of sulfonylureas in the management of type 2 diabetes mellitus in South Asia: a consensus statement. Indian journal of endocrinology and metabolism. 2015;19(5):577.
13. Pai SA, Kshirsagar NA. Pioglitazone utilization, efficacy & safety in Indian type 2 diabetic patients: a systematic review & comparison with European Medicines Agency Assessment Report. The Indian Journal of Medical Research. 2016;144(5):672.
14. DeFronzo RA, Norton L, Abdul-Ghani M. Renal, metabolic and cardiovascular considerations of SGLT2 inhibition. Nature Reviews Nephrology. 2017;13(1):11-26.
15. John M, Gopinath D, Kalra S. Triple fixed drug combinations in type 2 diabetes. Indian Journal of Endocrinology and Metabolism. 2015;19(3):311.
16. Chawla A, Chawla R, Jaggi S. Microvasular and macrovascular complications in diabetes mellitus: distinct or continuum? Indian Journal of Endocrinology and Metabolism. 2016;20(4):546-51.
17. American Diabetes Association. Standards of medical care in diabetes. 2017. Available at: http://professional.diabetes.org/sites/ professional.diabetes.org/files/media/dc_40_s1_final.pdf
18. Shah S, Sharma SK, Singh P, et al. Consensus evidence-based guidelines for insulin initiation, optimization and continuation in type 2 diabetes mellitus. J Assoc Doctors India. 2014;62(7 Suppl):49-54.
19. Holman RR, Paul SK, Bethel MA, et al. 10-year follow-up of intensive glucose control in type 2 diabetes. New England Journal of Medicine. 2008;359(15):1577-89.

Chapter 86

Diabetes and Tuberculosis: Dual Epidemic

Vijay Viswanathan, TP Smina

INTRODUCTION

The incidence of diabetes is alarmingly increasing all over the world making it a major threat to the global public health. A greater proportion of the diabetes cases (80%) occur in low- and middle-income countries. Developing countries like India is facing a dual epidemic of diabetes and tuberculosis (TB). India carries the highest number of TB cases which is 23% of total global burden and hold second position in the number of diabetic people with an estimate of 65.1 million cases.[1] Diabetic people are considered to be at higher risk of contracting TB. Epidemiological studies carried out around the globe have established an increased prevalence of active TB among people with diabetes, highlighting the positive association between diabetes and TB.[2-4]

Studies conducted earlier in our hospital to screen TB patients for diabetes in India also indicated the higher incidence (25.3%) of TB patients with diabetes and pre-diabetes (24.5%).[4] TB is one of the most infectious and critical ailment that cause high mortality rate worldwide. Diabetes patients with active TB infection are more susceptible to death than those who are not infected with TB. The morbidity and mortality rate due to the dual epidemic of diabetes and TB is massive and create considerable healthcare burdens in both families and society. In the present scenario, it is highly crucial to comprehend the mechanism and complications behind the diabetes mellitus (DM)-TB interaction to provide a rational basis for the development of preventive and treatment measures.

PATHOPHYSIOLOGY, RISK FACTORS AND COMPLICATIONS

The number of people infected with *Mycobacterium tuberculosis* is remarkably high in India. People infected with *Mycobacterium tuberculosis* bacteria have 10% risk of developing the active TB. However, persons with compromised immune systems, such as people living with HIV, diabetes or malnutrition, or people who use tobacco, have a higher chance of converting it into an active disease. Earlier studies, conducted in diabetic subjects to assess the prospect of developing an active TB, also reported that people with diabetes have a 3-fold elevated risk of contracting TB, as compared to those without diabetes. Furthermore, the evidences are also indicating that poor glycemic control forecasts the enhanced TB risk and insulin dependence can serve as a marker for the severity of disease. Patients with glycated hemoglobin (HbA1c) > 7 showed a three times higher risk of active TB compared with those with HbA1c < 7.[5] Factors like body mass index (BMI), central obesity, age, positive family history of diabetes, sedentary occupation, smoking and existence of pulmonary TB are found to trigger the complications among diabetic TB patients.[4]

The pathogenesis of the association between DM and TB is relatively complex. Diabetes weakens the immune system making the subjects more susceptible to the microbial infections.[6,7] Diabetes impairs both innate and adaptive immune responses to Mycobacterium tuberculosis. The cytokines associated with the innate and adaptive immune response were reported to be up-regulated in diabetic TB patients, especially in those with poor metabolic control.[6,8] Insights from animal models suggest that the T-cell response in patients having both diabetes and TB would be quantitatively larger than that happening in the nondiabetic TB subjects. A study using diabetic mice exhibited a critical delay in adaptive immune priming attributable to defective sentinel function of resident alveolar macrophages.[8-10] There is also evidence that DM enhances the risk of development of respiratory infection.[11]

The relationship between diabetes and TB is bidirectional i.e. diabetes exerts a negative effect on the clinical course of TB with elevated risk of treatment failure, relapse and death;[12] while TB depreciates the glycemic control in diabetes subjects.[13] One of the major concerns among the complications of diabetic TB patients is stress-induced hyperglycemia. A number of studies indicated that TB patients with diabetes expressed higher bacillary load in sputum, delayed myobacterial clearance and higher incidence of multi-drug resistance (MDR).[14] Another important clinical challenge in treating the diabetic TB patients is the drug-drug interaction between anti-TB agents and some of the sulphonylurea group of oral hypoglycemic agents, which may lead to severe adverse effects. Rifampicin, a potent hepatic enzyme-inducer, used in anti-TB treatment accelerates the metabolism of oral antidiabetic drugs and lowers their plasma levels causing hyperglycemia.[15] TB adversely affects the glycemic control of diabetic patients which ultimately lead to other critical complications of diabetes, including chronic kidney diseases and ischemic heart disease. Studies also reported that TB patients with DM require more time to cure than the subjects without DM. Patients with co-epidemic of TB and DM are estimated to have four to five times higher risk of mortality than that of nondiabetic TB patients.

SCREENING, DIAGNOSIS AND TREATMENT

Active screening measures for DM are recommended in patients with TB that could improve the diagnosis and early management of DM and its complications. All the TB patients should be thoroughly screened for diabetes. Patients with DM, particularly those with suboptimal control, should be screened for active TB in areas of high TB prevalence. Early detection can assist progressive care and treatment outcomes of both diseases.[13] Fasting plasma glucose (FPG) and glucose tolerance test (GTT) are the two common methods used to diagnose diabetes in India. Diagnostic tools that measure only plasma glucose concentration cannot differentiate diabetes from the stress hyperglycemia associated with TB. Studies comparing the performance of both the diagnostic tools i.e. HbA1c and FPG, in the patients affected with both the diseases, reported the better efficiency of HbA1c.[16] Previous studies proposed that in patients with TB, it is more reliable to screen for DM later in the course of anti-treatment rather than at the start.[12] If investigations are performed too early, TB being a chronic infectious disease may elevate blood glucose levels, because of cytokine stimulation, resulting in false positive DM diagnoses. However, delayed screening will miss the opportunity for subsequent modification of treatment in the case of positive DM patients.[17,18] More analytical research has to be conducted to establish the optimal time and best methods for diagnosing DM in patients with TB.

Active TB and reactivation of latent infection have long been known to be a risk of DM. TB infection deteriorates the glycemic control and diminishes the effectiveness of DM management. The patients of pulmonary TB with DM experienced poor rate of sputum conversion along with higher rates of treatment failure and deaths at the end of treatment as compared to patients without diabetes.[19] For the effective management of diabetes and TB, key strategies are required to ensure the availability of optimal treatment to the people affected with both the diseases. Early detection of TB in people with diabetes and vice versa is very important. The anti-TB therapy includes a long-time, wide spectrum of drugs, which can predispose patients to develop adverse drug reactions. The use of anti-DM medication may lead to interactions with anti-tubercular drugs. A subjective assessment is therefore essential to elucidate the factors associated with anti-TB medication adverse reaction, which may determine adherence and therefore, therapy success.

AWARENESS PROGRAMS

Even though India has instituted various national TB control programs and follows an excellent 'DOTS' model for TB control, there is a quite large number of people getting affected with the disease day by day and absolute eradication of the ailment still is a herculean task. There is an imperative requirement to sensitize the TB health care providers on this dual burden. Screening persons with DM for TB could be one of the strategies for early and increased TB case detection. World Health Organization and the International Union against Tuberculosis and Lung Diseases (IUATLD) have constituted a collaborative framework for care and control of TB and diabetes in order to ensure the availability of trained health care providers as well as basic diagnostic and therapeutic facility to screen and manage the complications of both TB and DM.[20] The training programs of this kind were found to be highly successful in recuperating the knowledge as well as the skills of primary care physicians in South India.[21]

Prof M Viswanathan Diabetes Research Centre which is a World Health Organization collaborating center for research, education and training in diabetes in India, has initiated a DM-TB project in 2010, in the state of Tamil Nadu, to train and help the healthcare personals in the warfare against this dual burden. The major goals of the project were to construct a team of 1,000 trained doctors for the diagnosis, prevention and management of DM and TB and also to advance the knowledge and expertise of 300 paramedical staffs and 350 health workers in the screening and detection of DM-TB. Programs were also intended to generate awareness about the complications of DM-TB and necessity of optimal care among 2,510 TB patients in the primary healthcare setting in three districts of Tamil Nadu, India.

CONCLUSION

With the startling augment in the co-existence of TB and DM, India has to combat an immense burden of eradicating two potentially complicated diseases. As the link between TB and DM has been well established, implementation of screening and research programs to prevent, monitor as well as eradicate the dual burden is becoming a prime necessity. Early detection of TB in people with diabetes and vice versa is extremely important to guarantee best possible treatment for persons affected with both the diseases. Integration of national-level awareness and screening programs for DM and TB among people, especially who lives in rural and low socio economic set ups will serve as an immediate solution to tackle the situation in the developing countries like India.

REFERENCES

1. World Health Organization. Gobal Tuberculosis Report 2015 WHO Press, Geneva 2015.
2. Stevenson CR, Forouhi NG, Roglic G, et al. Diabetes and tuberculosis: the impact of the diabetes epidemic on tuberculosis incidence. BMC Public Health. 2007;7:234.
3. Jeon CY, Murray MB. Diabetes Mellitus increases the risk of active tuberculosis: a systematic review of 13 observational studies. PloS Medicine. 2008;5:e152.
4. Viswanathan V, Kumpatla S, Aravindalochanan V, et al. Prevalence of diabetes and pre-diabetes and associated risk factors among tuberculosis patients in India. PLoS One. 2012;7(7):e41367.
5. Leung CC, Lam TH, Chan WM, et al. Diabetic control and risk of tuberculosis: a cohort study. Am J Epidemiol. 2008;167:1486-94.
6. Martinez N, Kornfeld H. Diabetes and immunity to tuberculosis. Eur J Immunol. 2014;44:617-626.
7. Restrepo BI, Fisher-Hoch SP, Pino PA, et al. Tuberculosis in poorly controlled type 2 diabetes: altered cytokine expression in peripheral white blood cells. Clin Infect Dis. 2008;47:634–641.
8. Vallerskog T, Martens G, Kornfeld H. Diabetic mice display adaptive immune response to *Mycobacterium tuberculosis*. J Immunol. 2010;184: 6275-6282.
9. Martens GW, Arikan MC, Lee J, et al. Tuberculosis susceptibility of diabetic mice. Am J Respir Cell Mol Biol. 2007;37(5):518-524.
10. Martinez N, Ketheesan N, West K, et al. Impaired recognition of Mycobacterium tuberculosis by alveolar macrophages from diabetic mice. J Infect Dis. 2016;214:1629-1637.
11. Leegaard A, Riis A, Kornum JB, et al. Diabetes, glycemic control, and risk of tuberculosis. A population-based case-control study. Diabetes Care. 2011;34:2530-2535.
12. Dooley KE, Chaisson RE. Tuberculosis and diabetes mellitus: convergence of two epidemics. The Lancet Infectious Diseases. 2009;9:737-46.
13. Jeon CY, Harries AD, Baker MA, et al. Bi-directional screening for tuberculosis and diabetes: a systematic review. Tropical Medicine & International Health. 2010;15:1300-14.
14. Fisher-Hoch SP, Whitney E, McCormick JB, et al. Type 2 diabetes and multidrug-resistant tuberculosis. Scand J Infect Dis. 2008;40(11-12):888-893.
15. Heysell SK, Moore JL, Keller SJ, et al. Therapeutic drug monitoring for slow response to tuberculosis treatment in a state control program, Virginia, USA. Emerging Infectious Diseases. 2010;16:1546-53.
16. Kumpatla S, Aravindalochanan V, Rajan R, et al. Evaluation of performance of A1c and FPG tests for screening newly diagnosed diabetes defined by an OGTT among tuberculosis patients – a study from India. Diab Res Clin Pract. 2013;102:60-64.
17. Edginton ME. Tuberculosis patient care decentralised to district clinics with community-based directly observed treatment in a rural district of South Africa. Int J Tuberc Lung Dis. 1990;3:445-450.
18. Drabo KM, Dauby C, Cost T, et al. Decentralising tuberculosis case management in two districts of Burkina Faso. The International Journal of Tuberculosis and Lung Disease. 2006;10:93-98.
19. Wang CS, Yang CJ, Chen HC, et al. Impact of type 2 diabetes on manifestations and treatment outcome of pulmonary tuberculosis, Epidemiology and Infection. 2009;137(2):203-210.
20. Maurice J. WHO framework targets tuberculosis–diabetes link. The Lancet. 2011; 378 (9798):209-1210.
21. Tharkar S, Kathiresan K, Abraham P, et al. Development and evaluation of a training programme on primary prevention of diabetes for primary care physicians. International Journal of Health Research. 2009;2:307-314.

Chapter 87

Peculiar Infections in Diabetes

Jayanta Kumar Panda, Manoranjan Behera

INTRODUCTION

Diabetes mellitus (DM) is considered as a secondary immune deficiency disorder by World Health Organization (WHO) as the disease is characterized by frequent, severe, prolonged and recurrent infections due to alteration of at least one of the immune response mechanisms and elimination of underlying cause leads to resolution.[1] This immunocompromised state predisposes the patient to increased risk of infection and sepsis which are contributing factors for increasing rate of morbidity and mortality in diabetic subjects. Several factors contribute to increased propensity for infection in patients of diabetes which includes, importantly, an altered immunity. The innate immunity is predominantly affected manifesting as dysfunction of polymorphonuclear cells (PMN) which includes dysfunction in adhesion, impaired migration, altered chemotaxis, reduced phagocytosis, oxidative burst and capacity of microbial killing.[2] Abnormalities in monocyte/macrophage chemotaxis and phagocytic function have also been found. Diabetes has direct inhibitory effect on the adaptive immune system as well. Certain infections associated with increased incidence in DM are genitourinary tract infections, respiratory tract infections, skin and soft tissue infections and gastrointestinal infections. Some peculiar infections are exclusively associated with DM are rhino-orbital-cerebral-mucormycosis (ROCM), invasive malignant otitis externa, emphysematous cholecystitis (EC), emphysematous pyelonephritis (EPN), emphysematous cystitis (ECy), necrotizing fasciitis (NF) and fournier's gangrene (FG) as shown in Box 1.

Box 1: Peculiar infections associated with diabetes.

- Emphysematous pyelonephritis
- Emphysematous cystitis
- Emphysematous cholecystitis
- Necrotizing fasciitis
- Fournier's gangrene
- Malignant otitis externa
- Rhinocerebral mucormycosis

These infections are peculiar in the sense they occur most commonly or exclusively in uncontrolled diabetic patients, uncommon or rare in ouccurrence, rapidly progressive, potentially fatal, needs high index of suspicion for early diagnosis and aggressive multimodality treatment which includes urgent hemodynamic stabilisation, glycemic control, broad spectrum antibiotics and surgical interventions as and when necessary. Despite best of treatment the morbidity and mortality is alarming.

Emphysematous Pyelonephritis

Emphysematous pyelonephritis is an acute severe necrotizing infection of the renal parenchyma and its surrounding tissues resulting in accumulation of gas in the renal parenchyma, collecting system or perinephric tissue.[3] Uncontrolled DM is the single most common underlying associated factor found in up to 95% of patients with EPN.[4] Most commonly found in women, female to male ratio 6:1 in small studies possibly due to increased susceptibility to urinary tract infections. *E. coli* is the most common causative organism, isolated from urine or pus cultures in about 70% of the reported cases. Other organisms reported are *Proteus, Klebsiella,* Enterobacteriaceae spc, Group D *streptococcus* and coagulase negative *staphylococcus*. Bacteremia is found in more than half of the patients and the organisms are the same as those in pus or urine culture.[5]

Various postulated factors responsible for pathogenesis of EPN in diabetes are high level of glucose within the renal tissues, presence of gas-forming microorganisms, impaired blood supply due to microvascular angiopathy and deranged host immunity.[5] A high level of tissue glucose along with vasculopathy associated ischemia of the kidneys facilitates the process of anaerobic metabolism. Gram-negative organisms like *E. coli* behave as facultative anaerobes (in absence of oxygen) and produce gas via the fermentation of glucose and lactates, resulting in accumulation of high levels of carbon dioxide and hydrogen at the site of inflammation. The air is a combination of various gases like carbon dioxide, hydrogen, nitrogen, oxygen and traces of ammonia. Gas may extend from site of inflammation to the sub capsular, perirenal and pararenal spaces.[5]

The presenting clinical features are like those of acute pyelonephritis such as fever with chills/rigors, dysuria, hematuria, nausea, vomiting and flank pain or pneumaturia. Other clinical manifestations may be acute renal dysfunction, altered sensorium and rapid progression to septic shock. Among the physical signs loin tenderness is the most common finding elicited and in some cases crepitus around the renal area and the scrotum may be found. Laboratory investigations may show neutrophilic leukocytosis in 70–80% cases, thrombocytopenia in 15–20% cases, hyperglycemia, acute renal failure, microscopic/macroscopic hematuria and severe proteinuria.[5]

The EPN is a radiological diagnosis as most of the clinical and laboratory investigations will indicate sepsis of renal origin. A plain X-ray of abdomen shows an abnormal gas shadow in the renal area raising suspicion, where as an ultrasonography (USG) or computerized tomography (CT) of abdomen will confirm the presence of intrarenal gases (Fig. 1). CT scan is the diagnostic procedure of choice as it is more sensitive and shows the extent of EPN.[5]

Patients of DM with acute pyelonephritis and fail to respond to standard medical therapy should always be subjected to CT scan to exclude the possibility of emphysematous complications of genitourinary tract.

The EPN is a life threatening condition and requires urgent attention. Most of the mortality from EPN is attributable to septic complications. The bad prognostic factors are systolic blood pressure (SBP) <90 mm of Hg, altered sensorium, increased serum creatinine, thrombocytopenia and bilateral EPN. Medical management (MM) with antibiotics alone is associated with higher mortality when compared with additional interventions like percutaneous drainage (PCD) of the gas/abscess or nephrectomy.[4]

Management includes basic resuscitation, judicious antibiotic and glycemic control. It is necessary to maintain SBP >100 mm of Hg. As gram-negative bacteria is the most common pathogen, the empirical antibiotics like aminoglycosides, β-lactamase inhibitors, cephalosporins and quinolones can be used and should be guided by local

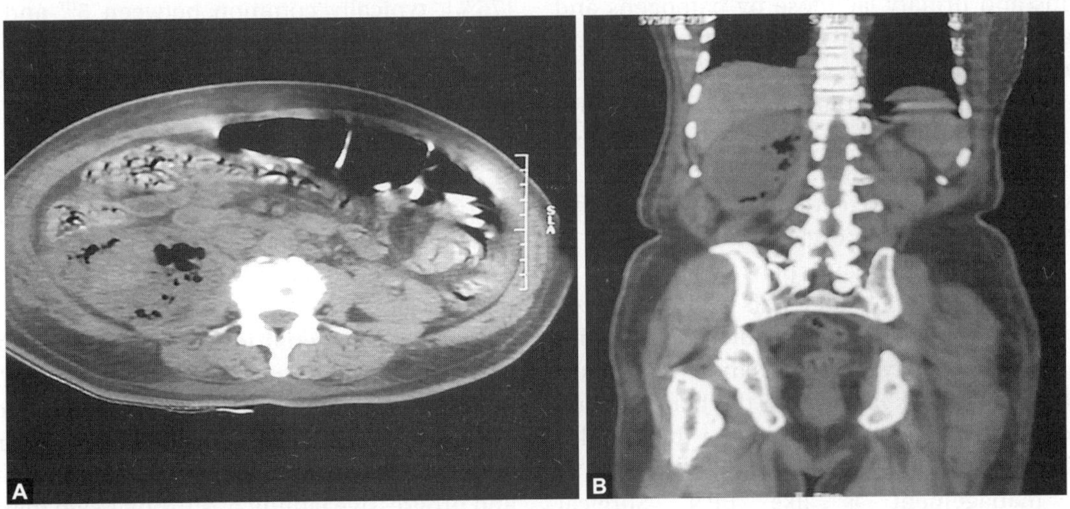

Figure 1 CT Scan of abdomen showing emphysematous pyelonephritis of right kidney.

hospital policy. Aminoglycoside can be combined with any of the above three groups till culture and sensitivity report is available. Antibiotics are usually required for 6–8 weeks. The mortality from EPN is 70–80% with MM alone.[6] Over the last few years, there is a nephron saving approach with PCD, with or without elective nephrectomy at a later stage has reduced the mortality significantly to 21%.[6]

PCD is the procedure of choice in patients who have localized collection of gas and having functional renal tissue.[5] Recent treatment strategies include MM alone, MM plus PCD, MM plus emergency nephrectomy and MM plus PCD plus emergency nephrectomy.[(6)] Recent evidences suggests that most successful strategy was MM with PCD (30–100%) and was associated with lowest mortality rate i.e. 13.5%.[6]

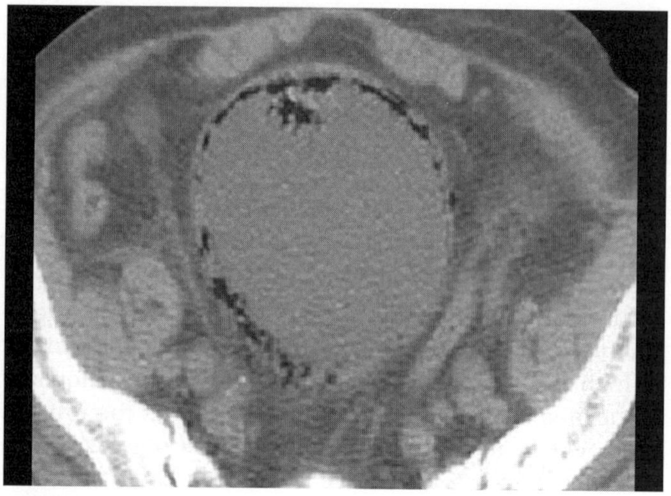

Figure 2 CT Scan of pelvis showing emphysematous cystitis.

Emphysematous Cystitis

Emphysematous cystitis (ECy) is a relatively rare, potentially fatal infection characterized by presence of gas in urinary bladder wall and/or lumen.[7] DM is the major risk factor for ECy. The exact incidence and prevalence of ECy are unknown but according to one series the mean age was 62.7 years, most were women (63.4%), DM was present in 66.7% cases and overall death rate was 6.6 %.[8]

The clinical presentation is like uncomplicated cystitis and is characterized by fever, dysuria, hematuria, urgency and frequency, abdominal pain except the presence of an unique finding of pneumaturia. The presentation may range from asymptomatic accidental detection to subcutaneous emphysema and/or severe sepsis. Though the exact mechanism of pneumaturia is poorly understood it is postulated to be due to fermentation of glucose, tissue proteins and urinary lactulose by pathogens and impaired gas transport due to local inflammation. It is highly suggestive but rarely reported by patients. It should always be suspected in diabetic subjects with UTI not responding to medical therapy or having unusual presentations.

About two-third of ECy are caused by *E. coli* and rest one-third are caused by similar organisms as EPN.

Plain X-ray of abdomen and pelvis may reveal a radiolucency outlining the bladder wall with or without luminal gas. USG may reveal abnormal thickened bladder wall but has a low sensitivity. CT scan is the investigation of choice which can show gas around the bladder wall, diffuse thickening of bladder wall or gas in the bladder lumen (Fig. 2).[7]

Medical management is like EPN. Surgical interventions like debridement or partial cystectomy may be needed for patients poorly responding to MM or have necrotizing tissue. The potential complications due to delay in diagnosis and appropriate treatment are septicemia, rupture of bladder, peritonitis and death. Mortality rate is around 10% in failure to diagnose early.[7]

Emphysematous Cholecystitis

Emphysematous cholecystitis is a rare but potentially fatal form of acute cholecystitis characterized by ischemia of gall bladder wall and collection of air in lumen and wall of gall bladder (GB).[9] It occurs in 1% to 4% cases of acute cholecystitis (AC).[9] Patients with uncontrolled DM are at higher risk of developing EC. Around 50% of EC patients have a history of DM. It affects males more commonly (75%), typically common between 5th and 7th decades of life. Gallstones are found less commonly (~40%) than AC but gangrene of GB is 5–10 times (~75% of cases) and perforation of GB is 30 times (~20% of cases) more common than AC.[10]

Most common microorganisms attributed to EC are *C. perfringens* and *E. coli* but other organisms like *P. vulgaris, A. aerogenes, staphylococcus, streptococcus, Klebsiella* and *B. fragilis* are reported.[10] Diabetes related microangiopathy leads to ischemia and necrosis of GB followed by bacterial invasion and anaerobic glycolysis and gas formation. Diabetic neuropathy facilitating multiple entry of micro-organisms and altered immunity are also responsible for growth of micro-organisms.[11]

Clinical features are that of AC with marked toxicity and progressive jaundice. Murphy's sign may be absent.[10] Crepitus on abdominal palpation is the ominous sign.

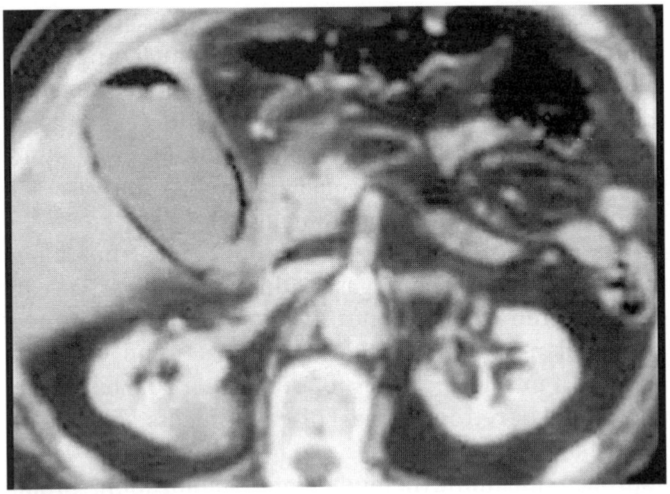

Figure 3 CT Scan of abdomen showing emphysematous cholecystitis.

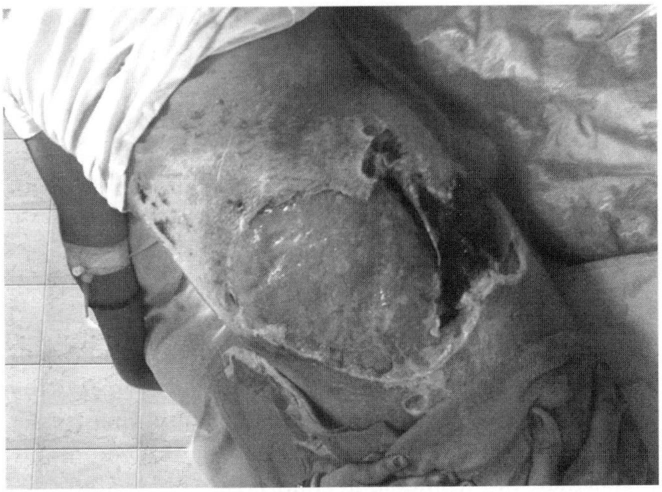

Figure 4 Necrotizing fasciitis of abdomen and chest wall. ***(For color version, see Plate 8)***

The common complications apart from gangrene and perforation are sepsis, pericholecystic abscess and generalized/biliary peritonitis.

Abdominal radiography and USG have sensitivity up to 95% for diagnosis of EC. Sonographically, EC is diagnosed by demonstration of air in the GB lumen (stage 1), air in the GB wall (stage 2) or air in the pericholecystic fluid (stage 3).[12] CT scan of abdomen have 100% sensitivity as it is able to detect the exact location of gas in GB wall/lumen/biliary tree and various complications of EC (Fig. 3).[10] Air if found in hypochondrium, suggests perforation. Magnetic resonance imaging (MRI) is also accurate in diagnosis of EC.

Treatment strategies for EC include conservative MM, laparoscopic/open cholecystectomy, percutaneous cholecystostomy or hyperbaric oxygen therapy.[10] Conservative therapy includes proper glycemic control, intravenous fluids, broad spectrum antibiotics (covering gram-negative, gram-positive and anaerobic organisms) and analgesics and this can be successful in managing mild form of EC. Hemodynamically stable moderate to severe cases of EC and patients unresponsive to MM in 72-96 hours, cholecystectomy is ideal. In critically ill, unstable or very old patient's cholecystostomy can be attempted. The overall mortality is 15–20%.

Necrotizing Fasciitis

Necrotizing fasciitis is a rapidly progressive necrotizing infection of the soft tissues spreading along fascial planes with or without overlying cellulitis.[13] About 75% of patients with NF have DM.[14] It has no sex predilection. It usually follows trauma, insect bites, abrasions or lacerations of skin. It can occur in any part of the body but most common sites involved are extremities, abdomen followed by groin. It usually begins as a tender, erythematous, hot and swollen area of cellulitis which doesn't respond to the standard regimen of antibiotics, heat application or elevation of the affected part. This follows extensive fascial necrosis and wide spread undermining of the skin with sparing of muscles and tendons initially, which standout almost as an anatomic dissection (Fig. 4). The reason for muscle sparing is not known but muscle and bone can be affected if the original injury exposes these structures or if the fascial envelope surrounding a muscle is entirly involved by the disease process. The patients are usually febrile and toxic. During early part of the necrotic process, lymphatic obstruction occurs and lymphatic channels are rapidly destroyed, so lymphadenitis and lymphangitis are rare.

The NF is usually polymicrobial being caused by both aerobic and anaerobic gram-positive cocci and gram-negative bacilli and categorized as two clinically undifferentiable but bacteriologically distinct group by Giuliano.[15] Type 1- This is most common type, isolating anaerobic bacteria including Bacteroides with facultative anaerobic bacteria, enterobacteriaceae and non-group *A. streptococcus*. Anaerobes were never cultured exclusively. Type 2 - This is less common and isolate Group A *streptococcus* alone or in combination with bacteria other than anaerobes or enterobacteriaceae.

It needs early diagnosis, aggressive surgical debridement along with broad spectrum antibiotics. Despite appropriate therapy mortality range from 9–64%. Death is usually due to sepsis, respiratory failure, renal failure or multi-organ failure.

Fournier's Gangrene

Fournier's gangrene is a rare, life threatening form of NF of the perineal, genital and perianal region.[16] NF of scrotum rapidly causes dermal gangrene due to lack of subcutaneous tissue and usually the first sign of necrotizing infection arising from the perineal area. An estimated 20–70% of patients with FG are associated with DM.[17] The most common sources of infection include the lower gastrointestinal tract (30–50%), genitourinary tract (20–40%) and cutaneous injuries (20%).[17] This commonly affects male but women and children are not spared.

It is usually polymicrobial caused by aerobes and anaerobes which include Coliforms, *Klebsiella, Streptococci, Staphylococci, Bacteroides, Clostridia* and *Corynebacterium.* Most of these are commensals in perineum and genitalia area. At least three organisms are cultured from each patient on an average.[17] The impaired host defense mechanism along with synergistic effect of aerobes and anaerobes leading to production of various exotoxins and enzymes facilitates tissue destruction and ultimately expedite spread of infection. The aerobes cause platelet aggregation and complement fixation and anaerobes produce heparinase and collagenase lead to microvascular thrombosis and dermal necrosis.[17]

The clinical presentation varies from insidious onset and slow progression to rapid onset and fulminant course. This starts as a cellulitis adjacent to the portal of entry with profound pain, swelling and severe systemic signs disproportionate to the local extent of the disease. As the subcutaneous inflammation progresses necrotic patches appear over the underlying skin which progresses to extensive necrosis if untreated (Fig. 5).[17] Crepitus over the affected part is usually found. Infection can spread to involve penis, scrotum, anterior abdominal wall up to clavicle.[17] The testes are usually spared as the vascular supply originates intra-abdominally.

The diagnosis of FG is primarily clinical but plain radiograph may show gas within tissues, USG can delineate intrascrotal abnormality as well as thickened and swollen scrotal wall with gas within. CT and MRI scan are useful in selected cases to establish or rule out intra-abdominal or retroperitoneal disease process.[17]

Treatment comprises aggressive multimodal approach including hemodynamic stabilization, broad spectrum antibiotics, glycemic control and early surgical debridement.[17] Despite best of treatment the mortality is still high (20–30%) and the causes of mortality are sepsis and multi organ failure.[17]

Malignant Otitis Externa

Malignant otitis externa is an invasive infection of the external auditory canal and skull base, which typically occurs in elderly patients with DM. Majority of the cases are caused by *Pseudomonas,* sometimes secondary to colonization by *Aspergillus* of the external auditory canal, rarely by S. *aureus, Proteus mirabilis* and *Klebsiella oxytoca.*

Patients present with severe otalgia, otorrhea and headache. Erythema with oedema of ear canal is common but tympanic membrane is usually normal (Fig. 6). The important predisposing factors are increased

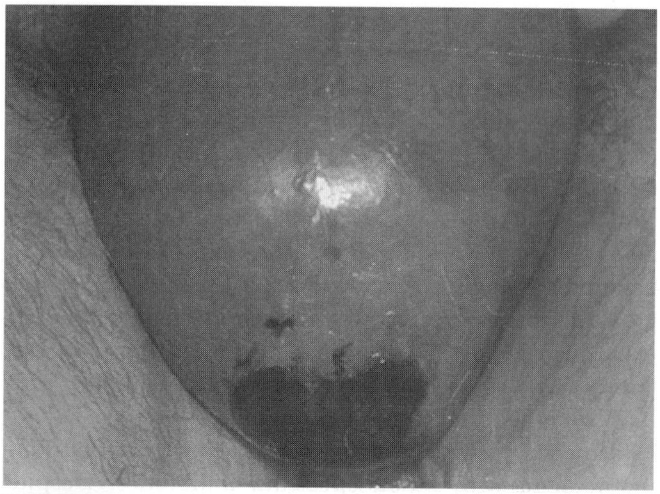

Figure 5 Fournier's gangrene. ***(For color version, see Plate 8)***

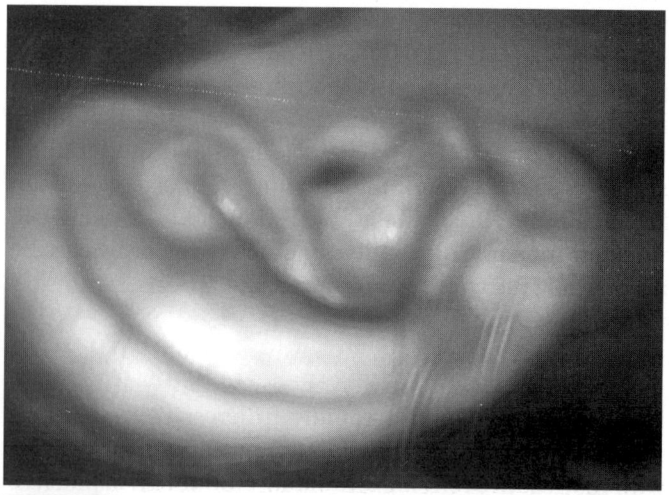

Figure 6 Malignant otitis externa. ***(For color version, see Plate 8)***

pH in diabetic cerumen, microangiopathy of ear canal, poor glycemic control, use of hearing aids, swimming in contaminated swimming pools and use of non-sterile water for ear irrigation. Spread of infection leads to cranial osteomyelitis, facial nerve palsy, lower canial nerve palsies and involvement of sigmoid sinus and the meninges.[18]

Early diagnosis depends on demonstration of pseudomonas by gram stain and culture. Tissue biospy is mandatory to exclude non-invasive otitis. MRI and radionuclide scans are useful as further diagnostic investigations.[19]

Management includes surgical debridement of necrotic tissue and appropriate antipseudomonal therapy. Ciprofloxacin is the treatment of choice (750 mg twice daily orally or intrevenous ciprofloxacin for initial few days). Total duration of the therapy is 6–8 weeks to prevent relapse. In suspected osteomyelitis ceftazidime or cefepime intravenously can be used. There is no role of topical antimicrobials.

Rhino-orbital-cerebral-mucormycosis

Rhino-Orbital-Cerebral-Mucormycosis is a rare, rapidly progressive and often fatal opportunistic fungal infection, almost always associated with DM and especially diabetic ketoacidosis (DKA) in up to 70% of the cases.[20] It is caused by a fungi of the order mucorales. *Mucor* is ferrophilic, acidophilic and angioinvasive fungus. Qualitative and quantitative abnormalities of neutrophils, monocytes and macrophages along with altered iron metabolism are critical factors in the pathogenesis of mucormycosis in patients with DM.[20] In patients with uncontrolled DM the inhaled sporangiospores germinate to form hyphae leading to angioinvasion with thrombosis and tissue necrosis which is a key pathophysiological feature. The ethmoid sinus is a critical site from which sinus mucormycosis may extend through lamina papyracea into the orbit, extraocular muscles, eye and the optic nerve. The brain may be seeded by invasion of ethmoidal and orbital veins, which drain into cavernous sinus.[20] The presenting features are nasal congestion, dark blood tinged rhinorrhea or epistaxis, sinus tenderness, retro orbital headache, fever and malaise. Rapid extension into cranial cavity leads to neurological deficits like proptosis, ophthalmoplegia, visual loss and cranial nerve palsies (Fig. 7). Cerebral involvement is suspected where there is abnormal mentation, seizures, focal neurological deficit and cranial nerve deficits. Biopsy with histopathological examination of tissue collected

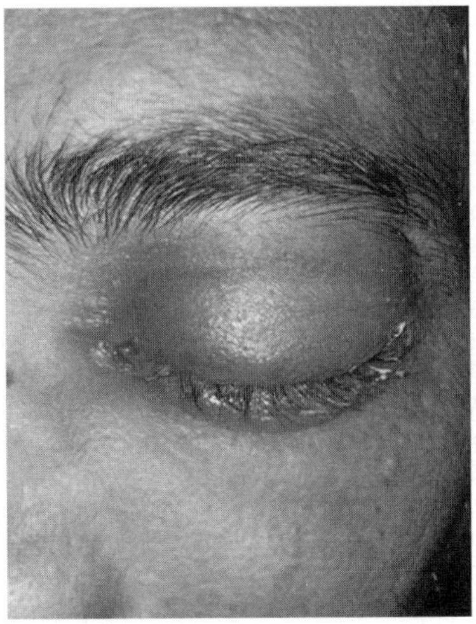

Figure 7 Rhino-orbital-cerebral-mucormycosis showing proptosis and drooping of left eyelid. ***(For color version, see Plate 8)***

from sinuses demonstrating wide, thick walled, ribbon like aseptate hyphae branching at right angles establishes the diagnosis. CT and MRI scan of sinuses and brain can further aid in delineating the extension of lesion. Early diagnosis, rapid correction of glycemic status, medical therapy with lyophilised Amphotericin-B and surgical debridement of sinuses are the cornerstone of management.[20] If untreated, the disease is universally fatal.

CONCLUSION

Many specific and some exclusive peculiar infections are seen in patients with diabetes contributing to high morbidity and mortality. These peculiar infections are uncommon and usually found in subjects with uncontrolled glycemic status. They are rapidly progressive and potentially lethal. They need early recognition, hemodynamic stabilisation good glycemic control, broad spectrum antibiotics, and surgical intervention as and when necessary. Despite best of management mortality rate is alarming.

REFERENCES

1. WHO. Immunodeficiency: Report of a scientific group. Technical Report Series 630. Geneva: World Health Organization, 1978.
2. Delamaire M, Maugendre D, Moreno M, et al. Impaired leucocyte functions in diabetic patients. Diabet Med. 1997;14:29-34.
3. Pantine AR, Barnes RD, Joffe J, et al. Emphysematous pyelonephritis in diabetic patients. Br J Urol.1995;75:71-4

4. Falagas ME, Alexiou VG, Giannopoulou KP, et al. Risk factors for mortality in patients with emphysematous pyelonephritis: A meta-analysis. J Urol. 2007;178:880-5
5. Ubee SS, McGlynn L, Fordham M. Emphysematous pyelonephritis: BJU international 2010;107:1474-8.
6. Somani BK, Nabi G, Thorpe P, et al. Is percutanous drainage the new gold standard in the management of emphysematous pyelonephritis? Evidence form a systemic review. J Urol 2008;179:1844-9.
7. Thomas AA, Lane BR, Thomas AZ, et al. Emphysematous cystitis: a review of 135 cases, BJU International 2007;100:17-20.
8. Toyota N, Ohawa D, Ishii K, et al. Emphysematous Cystictis in a patient with Type 2 diabetes Mellitus. Acta med oayama. 2011:65:129-33.
9. Safioleas. M, Stamatakus M. Kanakis M, et al. Soft tissue gas gangrene: a severe complication of emphysematous cholecystitis. Tohoku J Exp Med. 2007;213:323-28.
10. Safwan M, Penny SM. Emphysemetous cholecystitis: A deadly twist to a common disease. Journal of Diagnostic Medical Sonography. 2016;32(3):131-7.
11. Delgado-plasencia L, Gonzalez-Garcia I, Rodriguez - Gonzalez D, Torres-Monzon AE. Pneumomediastinum as a complication of emphysematous cholecystitis: case report. BMC Gastroenterol. 2010;10:99.
12. Sunnapwar A, Rout AA, Nagar AM, Katre R. Emphysematous cholecystitis: Imaging findings in nine patients. Indian J Radiol Imaging. 2011;21(2): 142-46.
13. Ahrenholz DH. Necrotising Soft-tissue infections Surg clin North Am. 1988;68:199-214
14. Wheat LJ. Infection and diabetes mellitus. Diabetes care. 1980;3: 187-97.
15. Giuliano A, Lewis F Jr, Hadley K, et al. Bacteriology of nectotising fasciitis Am J Surg 1977;134:52-7.
16. Smith GL, Bunker CB, Dineeen MD. Fornier's gangrene. Br J Urol. 1988;81:347-555.
17. Thwaini A, Khan A, Malik A, et al. Fourniers gargrene and its emergency management postgrad. Med J. 2006;82:516-19.
18. Sapico F, Bessman A. Infections in the diabetic patient. Infect Dis Clin Pract. 1995;1:339.
19. Carfrae MJ, Kesser BW. Malignant otitis externa. Otolaryngol Clin North Am. 2008;41:537-49.
20. Gamaletsou MN, Sipsas NV, Roilides E, et al. Rhino-orbital–cerebral mucormycosis. Curr infect Dis Rep. 2012;14:423-34.